Companion Animal Care and Welfare

The Universities Federation for Animal Welfare

UFAW, founded in 1926, is an internationally recognised, independent, scientific and educational animal welfare charity that promotes high standards of welfare for farm, companion, laboratory and captive wild animals, and for those animals with which we interact in the wild. It works to improve animals' lives by:

- Funding and publishing developments in the science and technology that underpin advances in animal welfare;
- Promoting education in animal care and welfare;
- Providing information, organising meetings and publishing books, videos, articles, technical reports and the journal Animal Welfare;
- Providing expert advice to government departments and other bodies and helping to draft and amend laws and guidelines;
- Enlisting the energies of animal keepers, scientists, veterinarians, lawyers and others who care about animals.

Improvements in the care of animals are not now likely to come of their own accord, merely by wishing them: there must be research...and it is in sponsoring research of this kind, and making its results widely known, that UFAW performs one of its most valuable services.

Sir Peter Medawar CBE FRS, 8 May 1957

Nobel Laureate (1960), Chairman of the UFAW Scientific Advisory Committee (1951–1962)

UFAW relies on the generosity of the public through legacies and donations to carry out its work, improving the welfare of animals now and in the future. For further information about UFAW and how you can help promote and support its work, please contact us at the following address:

Universities Federation for Animal Welfare
The Old School, Brewhouse Hill, Wheathampstead, Herts AL4 8AN, UK
Tel: 01582 831818 Fax: 01582 831414 Website: www.ufaw.org.uk
Email: ufaw@ufaw.org.uk

UFAW's aim regarding the UFAW/Wiley-Blackwell Animal Welfare book series is to promote interest and debate in the subject and to disseminate information relevant to improving the welfare of kept animals and of those harmed in the wild through human agency. The books in this series are the works of their authors, and the views they express do not necessarily reflect the views of UFAW.

Companion Animal Care and Welfare

The UFAW Companion Animal Handbook

Edited by
James Yeates, MRCVS
Cats Protection, Chelwood Gate
Sussex, UK

WILEY Blackwell

Registered Office(s)
John Wiley & Sons, Inc., 111 River Street, Hoboken, NJ 07030, USA
John Wiley & Sons Ltd, The Atrium, Southern Gate, Chichester, West Sussex, PO19 8SQ, UK

Editorial Office
9600 Garsington Road, Oxford, OX4 2DQ, UK

For details of our global editorial offices, customer services, and more information about Wiley products visit us at www.wiley.com.

Wiley also publishes its books in a variety of electronic formats and by print-on-demand. Some content that appears in standard print versions of this book may not be available in other formats.

Library of Congress Cataloging-in-Publication Data

Names: Yeates, James, 1980– editor. | Universities Federation for Animal Welfare.
Title: Companion animal care and welfare : the UFAW companion animal handbook / edited by James Yeates.
Description: Hoboken, NJ : Wiley-Blackwell, 2019. | Includes bibliographical references and index. |
Identifiers: LCCN 2018024349 (print) | LCCN 2018025479 (ebook) |
  ISBN 9781118688762 (Adobe PDF) | ISBN 9781118688786 (ePub) |
  ISBN 9781118688793 (pbk.)
Subjects: LCSH: Pets. | Animal welfare. | MESH: Pets | Animal Welfare | Animal Diseases
Classification: LCC SF411.5 (ebook) | LCC SF411.5 .C644 2019 (print) | NLM SF 411.5 |
  DDC 636.08/3–dc23
LC record available at https://lccn.loc.gov/2018024349

Cover Design: Wiley
Cover Image: Courtesy of Marit Emilie Buseth;
Courtesy of Dr. James Yeates; Courtesy of Dr. Peter Burgess;
© jgareri / iStock / Getty Images

Set in 9.5/12pt Sabon by SPi Global, Pondicherry, India

10 9 8 7 6 5 4 3 2 1

Contents

Contributor List

Sophie Adwick
Independent, Horsham, UK

Vera Baumans
Laboratory Animal Science Specialist, Department of Animals, Science and Society, Division Laboratory Animal Science, Utrecht University, Utrecht, the Netherlands

Culum Brown
Department Biological Sciences, Macquarie University, Sydney, Australia

Oliver Burman
School of Life Sciences, University of Lincoln, Lincoln, UK

John Chitty
Anton Vets, Unit 11, Andover, UK

Victoria Cussen
Department of Animal Science, University of California, Davis, CA, USA

Kevin Eatwell
Hospital for Small Animals, Royal (Dick) School of Veterinary Studies, Midlothian, UK

Joanna Hedley
Beaumont Sainsbury Animal Hospital, The Royal Veterinary College, London, UK

Andrew C. Highfield
Casa Karma, Almeria, Spain

Bryan Howard
The University of Sheffield, Sheffield, UK

Robert Johnson
Zoologica Consulting, Mosman, Australia

Kirk Klasing
Department of Animal Science, University of California, Davis, CA, USA

Graham Law
College of Medical, Veterinary & Life Sciences, University of Glasgow, Glasgow, UK

Anne McBride
School of Psychology, University of Southampton, Southampton, UK

Paul McGreevy
The University of Sydney, Sydney, Australia

Joy Mench
Department of Animal Science, University of California, Davis, CA, USA

Anna Meredith
Hospital for Small Animals, Royal (Dick) School of Veterinary Studies, University of Edinburgh, Midlothian, UK

Siobhan Mullan
Department Clinical Veterinary Science, University of Bristol, Bristol, UK

Rudolf Nager
Institute of Biodiversity, Animal Health and Comparative Medicine, University of Glasgow, Glasgow, UK

Joanne Paul-Murphy
School of Veterinary Medicine, University of California, Davis, CA, USA

Irene Rochlitz
Department of Veterinary Medicine, Centre for Animal Welfare and Anthrozoology, University of Cambridge, Cambridge, UK

Nicola Rooney
Department of Clinical Veterinary Science, University of Bristol, Bristol, UK

Richard Saunders
Bristol Zoological Society Ltd., Clifton, Bristol, UK

Elke Scheibler
School of Applied Sciences, Faculty of Computing, Engineering and Science, University of South Wales, Pontypridd, UK

Nico J. Schoemaker
Division of Zoological Medicine
Department of Clinical Sciences of Companion Animals
Faculty of Veterinary Medicine, Utrecht University, Utrecht, The Netherlands

Lynne Sneddon
Institute of Integrative Biology, University of Liverpool, Liverpool, UK

Kevin Stafford
Institute of Veterinary Animal and Biomedical Sciences, Massey University, Palmerston North, New Zealand

Claudia Vinke
Department of Animals in Science & Society, Faculty of Veterinary Medicine, Utrecht, The Netherlands

Eva Waiblinger
Independent, Ebmatingen, Switzerland

Michael Wilkinson
Biological Services Division, Veterinary Research Facility, Glasgow, UK

David Wolfenden
Blue Planet Aquarium, Longlooms Road, Cheshire Oaks, UK

James Yeates
Cats Protection, Chelwood Gate, Sussex, UK

Yvonne R. A. van Zeeland
Division of Zoological Medicine, Department of Clinical Sciences of Companion Animals, Faculty of Veterinary Medicine, Utrecht University, Utrecht, The Netherlands

Foreword

Humans have kept animals as pets for at least 12 000 years, but possibly for much longer. During this time, most animals were kept for practical reasons as farmed animals for food or as working animals, but we know that pet keeping was widespread in recent hunter-gatherer societies, suggesting it may well have also occurred in Palaeolithic societies. In other words, many people just seem to like having an animal around. Keeping, feeding, and caring for animals can be a substantial cost, and until recently, it tended to be the better off who kept companion animals. Today, however, the practice is becoming much more widespread, and the number of companion animals throughout the world is increasing dramatically.

The vast majority of those people who keep companion animals do so because they have a love of animals. Most wish to keep them healthy and happy, and indeed, many treat their pet as a member of the family. However, it is all too easy to misunderstand animals' needs and to make mistakes that result in poor welfare or suffering. Although companion animals may be treated as one of the family, animals are not humans, and their needs are often quite different to those of humans. The fact is, that keeping and caring for animals properly requires knowledge gained through experience, research, or education, and it is not just owners who need this information. Others such as veterinarians, shelter and quarantine staff, and those responsible for setting or enforcing standards all need to understand how to meet companion animals' needs.

The Universities Federation for Animal Welfare (UFAW) was founded with the intention of using science to inform our understanding of how to care for and meet the needs of animals and, for many years, UFAW has produced handbooks on the care and management of animals used in research (first edition 1947) and farm animals (first edition 1971). In these 'handbooks', which have developed into quite heavy tomes, experts in the field sift and synthesise the available specialist and scientific knowledge to provide authoritative and accessible advice for those at the sharp end who have to make practical decisions on the care of these animals. We were therefore delighted when James Yeates approached us and offered to add to the series by producing a handbook using the same approach for companion animals. Yeates has already written a book for the UFAW/Wiley animal welfare series on Animal Welfare in Veterinary Practice and is eminently qualified to carry out this task, with a well-established academic interest in ethics and animal welfare.

Yeates has brought together experts from around the world to contribute chapters on a wide range of species and species groups, providing information on their natural history, husbandry and health, and signs of poor welfare. He also addresses the practicalities of euthanasia – a difficult and painful subject for many pet owners and veterinarians – but essential to avoid unnecessary suffering. The chapters also include suggestions for improving the welfare of the species or groups of species, providing some useful ideas for long-term strategies to improve the welfare of companion species through, for example, education, changes to legislation, or development of better products.

We are extraordinarily grateful to James Yeates and to the chapter authors who have put so much hard work and their expertise into a volume that, we hope, will improve the welfare of millions of animals around the world.

Robert Hubrecht
UFAW

April 2018

Prologue

This book aims to be a comprehensive and practical reference for everyone who cares about how we should care for our companion animals. Since 1926, Universities Federation for Animal Welfare (UFAW) has improved animal welfare through its publications, which are both robustly informed and engagingly readable. To date, UFAW publications have predominantly focused on farm and laboratory contexts, and the UFAW Farm Animal and Laboratory Animal Handbooks are now illustrious, popular, mainstream references and essential reading for all involved in animal welfare science, policymaking, and practice.

People are now beginning to give more attention to the welfare of companion animals because the animals are an increasingly important part of modern society. Pet keeping appears to be growing in popularity, acceptability, stature, and economic impact in many countries, with an estimated 202 million cats and 171 million dogs worldwide. In many Asian and African countries, pet keeping is only recently growing in popularity, but with limited 'folk wisdom' about pets' needs. In many American and European countries, the popularity of pets has generated multibillion-dollar industries based on traditional misinformation and pseudo-scientific fads, and it is only now being realised that owners' love does not make pets' lives a utopian ideal and that many welfare compromises are mainstream. Indeed, ignorance may be less dangerous than its progeny, misinformation. In many countries worldwide, there is an increasing awareness that pets (like spouses and children) are not things whose treatment can be considered merely a 'private' concern. And in many of the same countries, animal welfare is growing as a societal concern in general. These changes make it essential to critically examine pet keeping and to determine how pet breeding, care, and trade can deliver the best animal welfare outcomes.

Consequently, companion animal welfare is an area of increasing scientific investigation because researchers have begun to reflect and satisfy that need. There is growing international literature on companion animal welfare within veterinary, ethology, and clinical animal behaviour texts, as well as more 'popular' guides. At the same time, our most august institutions are turning to companion animal welfare – for example, the relatively new Companion Animals Department in the RSPCA. Therefore, there is a *demand* for accessible scientific information about companion animal welfare and a *supply* of such information, but not yet in a form that is scientific and accessible for owners and policymakers. It is that gap that this book aims to bridge.

This created some challenges for the book. It is a book based on science, not mere opinion. So as editor, I've tried to keep to the rule that readers are given only facts for which there is convincing supporting evidence (albeit always with the risk of new information challenging those facts) or where doing scientific studies would be inappropriate (either because of the harm to animals or the waste of resources). But guidance on what *should* be done cannot be solely scientific because guidance relies on expertise. I've prevented authors from quoting others' guidance (i.e. most references are to scientific studies or similar, rather than merely referring to others' opinions), especially because I've chosen some of the most informed and expert scientists on the planet to write for this book. Other good sources of expertise are given in the references section, which can be taken as 'further reading'. Such scientific information needed to be presented without oversimplification or technical terminology (I have never understood the need for experts to replace everyday words with technical phrases – especially as the latter often just use either the ancient Latin or Greek everyday word or use another English everyday word in an esoteric way). One deliberate exception to the latter is that each chapter uses both the everyday and scientific names of animals and their groups, to serve as a reminder that pets are still animals that evolved most of their biology long before we existed (although, of course, we are animals, too, who share much of that biology). At the same time, the book needed to avoid overly focusing on basic biology or veterinary health issues to cover all welfare issues.

Writing the overarching chapters on biological groups ('Birds', 'Reptiles', etc.) was a particularly difficult task of providing valuable overviews as a starting point, while recognising the wide variety within each biological group. Readers should note the strong caveat that there can be substantial differences even between closely related species; more specific chapters, then, focus on particular companion animal species (hence, the somewhat esoteric examples used where readers' own minds will be screaming better examples for more common pets). More generally, readers may be well advised to dip into particular chapters, albeit always with reference to the overarching chapters both overall (Chapters 1 and 22) and for those animals.

The choice of which species to give their own chapters was particularly tricky. Essentially, this book focuses on companion animals that are (i) commonly kept, (ii) not clearly unsuitable for keeping, and (iii) where there is sufficient scientific information to make an informative science-based book. These three factors inter-relate insofar as there is more information on popular pets and more information can lead to greater suitability, and popularity may have enhanced domestication. I thought about limiting the book to animals that are domesticated 'enough' to provide genuine mutual companionship, but I did not want to exclude popular species who can suffer considerably. My final rule of thumb was to include animals whose knowledge of their pet care will increase and exclude (or at least not explicitly include) rare and unsuitable animals of which I personally hope our knowledge about them as pets will be replaced only by knowledge of them as wild animals, such as amphibians, invertebrates, marsupials, pigs, primates, and pygmy hedgehogs. Perhaps specialist individuals may continue to keep these animals, but that is different to their being 'pets' kept by 'normal' members of the public. Indeed, one argument to limiting the species allowed to be kept is to focus on generating and disseminating knowledge on those animals, and I suggest that the animals in this book provide a basis for such a 'positive list' as well as kick-starting that knowledge generation and dissemination. This is not to say that the animals in this book are 'easy' or cannot suffer considerably, but simply that they are ones that debatably can be kept in captivity by (and only *by*) people who are sufficiently knowledgeable, committed, and resourced.

My enormous thanks to all the authors for their time – especially with my less-than-subtle timekeeping pressures. All these authors are busy people (part of being so illustrious) and have prioritised this work because of the immense potential influence it can have on improving animals' lives. In particular, my thanks for the information they gave for the overarching chapters. Specific thanks to the authors, both for their chapters and for their contributions for the overarching chapters (all the interesting bits are from them; all the errors my own). Thanks to the anonymous reviewers and the identifiable ones who assisted various authors: Vera Baumans; Emily Blackwell; John Bradshaw; Rachel Casey; Samantha Gaines; Maggie Jennings; Maeve Moorcroft; Christopher Newman; Anna Olsson; Russell Parker; Clifford Warwick; John Webster; Katie Wonham, and particularly Jane Tyson and Nicola White.

As John Webster said in the foreword for the Farm Handbook: 'caring *about* animals is not enough. Caring *for* them is what matters. This requires compassion, understanding and a great deal of skill.' With the different (sometimes) human-animal relationships for companion versus farm animals, this book uses the term *care* more than *management*, but both ideas apply equally to each context. This book seeks to promote the best possible care of our companion animals. It provides the most comprehensive, accessible, and up-to-date guide available, covering, chapter by chapter, the husbandry and care of all major companion animal species from hamsters to horses to fish to amphibians. The book identifies what their needs are, how we know what their needs are, and gives clear advice how those needs can be met. Overarching chapters also provide fresh understanding of animal welfare science, ethics, and the role of society in ensuring the best possible care of companion animals. Owners also need compassion, temperance, self-awareness, resources, and knowledge. This book can help with the last.

James Yeates

Introduction: The Care and Animal Welfare of All Species

James Yeates

1.1 Introduction: Concepts in Companion Animal Welfare

Owners have a duty of care to their companion animals. This is an ethical obligation, a vital part of good owner-pet relationships, and a legal duty in many countries. The broad aim of this book is to provide an introduction to the welfare of companion animals. This chapter covers the key concepts in animal welfare, general principles of care, and signs of welfare that can, and should, be applied to our pets. Given the wide range of animals kept as pets and the limited amount of scientific data on some animals, this book focuses on certain groups of animals. For other animals, owners can use Chapters 2, 6, 12, 14, 18, and 22 or cautiously apply data from similar species. However, this chapter provides general guidelines that can apply to all species.

1.1.1 Natural Histories

Pets are *animals* and so are members of species with wild or feral relatives that may share many characteristics with their captive counterparts. We can therefore use information about animals' natural biology and motivations to predict what pets need (in practice, this may sometimes be difficult when wild populations are rare or extinct). Where this information exists, it needs to be used intelligently, and there are several

Companion Animal Care and Welfare: The UFAW Companion Animal Handbook,
First Edition. Edited by James Yeates.
© 2019 Universities Federation for Animal Welfare. Published 2019 by John Wiley & Sons Ltd.

caveats to consider. First, animals may suffer welfare compromises while in the wild that owners should *not* replicate (e.g. predation and disease). Second, animals' motivations and needs may depend on their personal experiences and learning (e.g. natural early life experiences) and the captive environment in which they are kept (e.g. animals may need extra ultraviolet [UV]-B or vitamin D supplementation to compensate for insufficient sunlight). Third, many animals have been altered significantly from their wild ancestors, and animals kept as pets may have needs that differ from those of their wild ancestors (e.g. an altered tolerance of human company or a need for medical care to treat breed-related diseases).

1.1.2 Domestic Histories

Pets are also *companions*. Humans have kept pets for at least 12 000 years (Serpell 1986), and some species are popular and widespread (Table 1.1). Some companion animals have been adapted to human company or captivity by 'domestication' through selective breeding and 'taming' through exposure and training. Knowing about this history may also help to determine what care these companions should receive. However, this information also needs to be used intelligently, and there are other caveats to consider before trying to domesticate or tame animals. First, animals may suffer welfare compromises during those processes (e.g. as a result of dystocia, fear of humans, starvation, or separation from their mother). Second, changes from artificial selection are not necessarily associated with improved welfare (e.g. breeding animals for different colours may be irrelevant to their welfare, and some breeding may create breed-related diseases). Third, selective breeding may mean animals have particular needs that are harder to meet (e.g. stronger motivations for company).

1.1.3 Sentience and Welfare

The expression *animal welfare* has two distinct uses. The first is a factual description of what animals experience. The second is an ethical prescription of what animals *should* experience. These two concepts overlap because we are concerned with understanding how our actions can harm or benefit animals. There are several different concepts of animal welfare. A classic division is among 'feelings', 'function', and 'naturalness' (Fraser et al. 1997; Fraser 2008). *Function* refers to the efficiency and effectiveness of biological processes, with particular regard to deviations from normality, disease, and injury. *Naturalness* refers to how animals live unaffected by human control. *Feelings* are subjective experiences of sentient animals.

Sentience may be defined as the ability to experience 'feelings that matter' (Webster 2005). These include affective feelings (e.g. pain and pleasure), motivations (e.g. wanting something), or moods (e.g. depression or happiness). Such feelings might matter more if they are more intense, long-lasting, or frequent. Ultimately, companion animal welfare is about whether pets suffer or are happy, although scientific papers often avoid those terms.

Animals' feelings depend on the interaction between each animal and their environment. The external environment acts on various senses (usually mediated by chemicals, movement, or electromagnetism) and animals' bodies stimulate other senses (e.g. gastric stretching and proprioception). These external and internal inputs prompt various responses that may be pathological (e.g. diarrhoea), physiological (e.g. stress hormone

Table 1.1 Estimated pet populations worldwide.

Group	Australia	Brazil	China	Europe[b]	Japan	New Zealand	South Africa	UK	USA
									Approximate Estimated Numbers (in Millions) of Owned Pets (2011–2016)
Carnivorans[a]	8	45	80	185	21–25	2	9	17	145–179
Glires[a]	—	—	—	27		2		2	18
Ungulates[a]	—					3		0.4	8
Birds	5			55		5		2	21
Reptiles[a]	—		6	7		—		1	12
Amphibians	—		—			—		0.2	—
Fish	11		—	17		9		40–45	159
Humans	24	200	1382	508	126	5	55	65	324

Source: American Health Alliance (Australia) (AHA 2014), American Pets Product Association (APPA 2014), Caixong (2015), Dray (2016), European Union (EU 2016), European Pet Food Industry Federation (FEDIAF 2017), Goldman Sachs (2014), New Zealand Companion Animal Council (NZCAC 2011), Pet Food Institute (PFI 2014), Pet Food Manufacturers Association (PFMA 2014), Zenoaq (2008).
[a] Carnivoran figures based on reports on cats and dogs numbers; Glires figures for New Zealand are specifically for rabbits; Ungulates figures generally exclude 'farm' or 'working' animals (i.e. often relate to horse numbers); Reptile figures for China are specifically for tortoises. All figures to nearest whole million (except where less then 1)
[b] Historic figures for Europe include the UK (accepting the discrepancy regarding fish).

levels), or behavioural (e.g. aggression). These responses may then alter the animal's environment (e.g. scaring off a competitor) and internal states (e.g. filling their stomach). These changes may, in turn, further affect the animal's future interactions with their environment. Such perceptions and responses may be associated with pleasant or unpleasant feelings.

Exactly what feelings each animal experiences, and how they respond, may depend on their particular needs, senses, and cognitive processes – and these may depend on their species, breed, age, sex, reproductive status, personality, abilities, learning, and personal preferences. This means animals cannot be treated as all the same. It also means there is debate about what forms of suffering different animals may experience and when. In fact, the ability to experience suffering need not actually require a high level of conscious cognitive reasoning, and there is increasing scientific evidence of subjective feelings such as pain in reptiles (e.g. Liang and Terashima 1993; Bennett 1998), amphibians (Machin 1999), and fish (e.g. Sneddon 2011, 2013). The evidence for invertebrates is less clear, but all pets should be given the benefit of the doubt (Figure 1.1).

The fact that all species differ in how they interact with their environment may also limit our ability to understand how other animals may be feeling. Our experiences of the world are probably different to our pets'. Animals' senses may have greater sensitivity (e.g. the ability to detect low concentrations of chemicals or quieter noises), extend outside humans' ranges (e.g. the ability to detect UV, infrared, ultrasound, and infrasound) or be senses that humans lack completely (e.g. the ability to detect particular chemicals or magnetic fields). Animals' responses may also differ, depending on their mental processes and their natural motivations. This makes it important to observe animals carefully, to avoid oversimplistic or uncritical anthropomorphism, and to have our views constantly challenged by ongoing scientific findings.

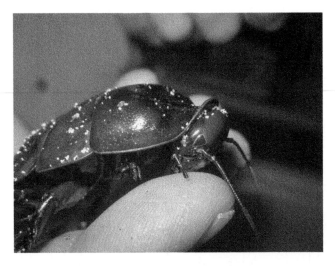

Figure 1.1   Pet invertebrates such as Giant burrowing cockroaches (*Macropanesthia rhinoceros*) should be treated as if they may suffer (*Source:* courtesy of Robert Johnson).

1.1.4 Stress and Suffering

Animals may be subjected to challenges, such as infections or the presence of potential predators. Within animal welfare, the term *stress* is used in a strict physiological sense, but in everyday language it is also used to refer to an unpleasant feeling. A stress response is related to a particular challenge and may not be associated with poor welfare as defined by feelings. Animals may attempt to adapt to challenges in their neurological (e.g. activation of the sympathetic nervous system), hormonal (e.g. secretion of glucocorticoids), immune (e.g. production of antibodies), or behavioural (e.g. elicitation of aggression) processes – all of which may or may not be associated with subjective experiences. Some responses return the animals to a set normal point (e.g. blood oxygen levels), but some lead the animal to a change (e.g. to survive periods of decreased food availability or low temperatures). When the animal's body is unable to re-establish acceptable levels, the animal's welfare may be seriously compromised.

Of particular significance to animal welfare are general physiological responses, including the release of hormones (e.g. cortisol, corticosterone, and noradrenaline), altered (e.g. heart rate), and associated changes behavioural changes (e.g. readiness for flight). These responses may occur in a wide range of situations and may also have a wide range of short- and long-term biological effects. However, the exact responses an animal makes may depend on the nature of the challenge (e.g. Maier and Watkins 2005; Lucas et al. 2014) and the animal (e.g. NRC 2008). For example, an animal's immunity may depend on the type of infection, animal (e.g. mammal versus reptiles), the animal's previous exposure (e.g. after vaccinations), and the presence of other challenges (e.g. malnutrition or pregnancy). This makes it impossible to find a single measure that universally and definitively indicates the absence or presence of stress in the everyday sense of poor welfare.

Responses may allow the animal to adapt to the challenge (e.g. by flight) or to reduce its effects (e.g. by forming an abscess around an infection). Over time, animals may get better at meeting repeated challenges, through learning or adapting their physiology (e.g. their bone density, hormonal sensitivity, or immune system) or behaviour (e.g. through learning). Some unpleasant challenges may therefore help animals to cope with future stresses in the long term. Concern for companion animal welfare therefore does not mean that pets should never be challenged, but that the challenges should be the right ones, with which the animal can cope.

However, companion animals may be unable to cope with challenges if they are too severe, multiple, unpredictable, or uncontrollable; if the animal lacks particular capacities (e.g. juveniles may be immunologically or psychologically naïve); or if owners prevent them from responding (e.g. by confinement or limited resources). Others may face chronic or cumulative stress, which may lead to harmful changes such as muscle break down, gastric ulceration, and skin problems or to animals learning *not to* respond because previous attempts have proved useless.

In everyday language, *suffering* is a general term (like 'enjoyment') that includes a wide range of different unpleasant feelings. More specifically, pain is an unpleasant sensory and emotional experience usually associated with actual or potential tissue damage. Fear is an unpleasant psychological emotion, usually associated with an actual or potential threat to the individual (although some fear occurs without real threat, e.g. in some hyper-anxiety syndromes). Malaise is the feeling associated with illness (in addition to any more specific feelings such as pain, nausea, etc.). Frustration is the feeling from unsatisfied motivations. Boredom is the feeling directly associated with a lack of challenge, interest, or stimulation.

The amount of suffering might be considered in terms of intensity, duration, number of animals affected, and frequency, while recognising that it is ultimately a subjective experience. Nevertheless, it is possible that animals may suffer while attempting to cope with challenges and may suffer more if they cannot cope or if challenges are sustained. Some processes may make animals more sensitive to suffering, for example when animals' injuries make animals more sensitised to pain or induce depression-like or anxiety-like moods. Conversely, drugs may also alter animals' propensity to suffer; for example, medical painkillers may reduce pain and tranquillisers may reduce anxiety.

1.1.5 Achievement and Enjoyment

Keeping pets is not all about avoiding them suffering. Owners want their pets not merely to cope but to flourish and to experience pleasant feelings. Animals may have positive motivations to achieve an outcome such as obtaining palatable food. They may experience short-term feelings of pleasure or enjoyment or longer-term moods that make them tend towards perceiving stimuli as positive (e.g. optimism). Such positive welfare may be associated with everyday sensational pleasures: engaging with their environment, their conspecifics, and their handlers and realising their own goals (Yeates and Main 2008). Many animals appear to play, including reptiles (Burghardt 2013) and fish (Burghardt 2014a, 2014b; Burghardt, Dinets, and Murphy 2014), and this may be associated with enjoyment.

Animals' capacity for pleasant experiences may relate to their genetics (Yeates 2010), although all species in this book can probably have enjoyable experiences. Capacity for pleasant experiences may also depend on animals' individual histories. Some processes may make animals more or less sensitive to pleasant experiences (e.g. optimistic cognitive biases) or to particular motivations (e.g. a pet may learn to associate human company with food). Perhaps most importantly, animals' enjoyment may depend on their opportunities to engage with rewarding stimuli. Animals need resources to be provided and not to be too inexperienced, scared, or ill to interact with them.

Often, pleasant experiences occur in the absence of suffering (Fraser and Duncan 1998; Spinka et al. 2001). Conversely, some positive experiences may reduce suffering, by improving animals' biological functioning and ability to cope with challenge and stress (Pressman and Cohen 2005; Kikusui, Winslow, and Mori 2006). Sometimes minor challenges may lead to pleasant experiences, for example in relief or the enjoyment of learning, and some stressors may be beneficial (e.g. Selye 1975). In other cases, achieving pleasant experiences may lead to later suffering; for example, the short-term enjoyment of high-energy foods may cause later obesity, and these competing issues need to be balanced.

1.2 Principles of Companion Animal Care

Humans determine most aspects of our pets' lives: often including their parentage, diet, environment, transportation, company, reproduction, health care, and death. Animals are given certain resources while being prevented from obtaining others.

This control makes it important for keepers to get it right by adequately meeting animals' needs while they are in the keepers' care.

Animals' needs may be considered using a framework such as the Five Freedoms. These were produced for assessing farm animal welfare but are also useful for companion animals if used alongside considerations of positive welfare and human company (Table 1.2). For each principle, there are a number of potential 'hazards' (good or bad) that risk suffering or enjoyment (Table 1.3). These are the bases for the principles around which this book's chapters are laid out. However, each principle cannot be considered in isolation because animals' needs may interact in complex ways. For example, how animals use environmental resources may depend on other animals, particularly if there is competition (e.g. in overstocked aquaria) or if animals are motivated to use facilities together (e.g. in communal nesting). There may also be conflicts between short- and long-term effects (e.g. eating versus obesity or surgery versus illness) or different principles (e.g. long-distance transportation versus being left at home alone). Mammals, birds, reptiles, amphibians, and fish are complex organisms with complex needs, which may depend on their species, personal history, and individual characteristics.

So how can keepers decide what is needed to meet animals' dietary, environmental, health, psychological, and other needs? There are three main approaches:

1) The first is to decide on specific provisions (e.g. providing hay to all rabbits).
2) The second is to let animals choose from a range of options (e.g. giving reptiles a thermal gradient).
3) The third is to assess the outcomes from the care given (e.g. monitoring body condition and behaviour).

Table 1.2 Five Freedoms and five opportunities.

Five Freedoms and Provisions	Five Opportunities and Provisions
Freedom from hunger and thirst – by ready access to fresh water and a diet to maintain full health and vigour	*Opportunity for dietary preferences* – by provision of a varied diet from which to choose
Freedom from discomfort – by providing an appropriate environment and a comfortable resting area	*Opportunity for control* – by allowing the achievement of motivations that alter the animal's environment
Freedom from pain, injury, and disease – by prevention or rapid diagnosis and treatment	*Opportunity for pleasure, development, and vitality* – by providing enjoyable and beneficial interactions
Freedom and Opportunity to express normal behaviour – by providing sufficient space, proper facilities, and the company of the animal's own kind	
Freedom from fear and distress – by ensuring conditions and treatment which avoid mental suffering	*Opportunity for interest and confidence* – by providing conditions and human interactions that allow mental enjoyment

Source: Adapted from Farm Animal Welfare Council (1993); Parker and Yeates (2012).

Table 1.3 Risks and hazards (good and bad) to companion animal welfare under each principle.

Principle	Hazard	Risk	Examples
Diet	Undernutrition	Hunger	Starvation in hibernating tortoises
	Overnutrition	Obesity-related disease	Type II diabetes in cats
	Specific malnutrition	Ill health	Calcium disorders in lizards
	Lack of enrichment	Boredom, frustration	Oral stereotypies in horses
Environment	Insufficient substrate	Frustration, fear	Inability to dig in gerbils
	Glass vivaria walls	Injury and pain	Rostral injuries in dragons
	Lack of security	Fear	Lack of hides for hamsters
	Extreme confinement	Frustration	Zebra finches in small cages
	Unpredictability	Anxiety	Variable light schedules in mice
	Barren environment	Boredom	Unenriched rat cages
	Toys	Play	Dogs playing with ball
Animal Company	Lack of company	Loneliness, fear	Isolation of rabbits
	Bullying	Fear, hunger	Bearded dragons of mismatched size
Human Company	Poor handling	Fear	Rough handling of parrots
	Pleasant handling	Tactile enjoyment	Stroking dogs and cats
Health	Poor hygiene	Infectious disease	Pigeon parasite infections
	Lack of foot care	Pain	Lameness in horses
	No vaccination	Infectious disease	Parvovirus in puppies
Euthanasia	Overhandling	Fear	Overhandling stray cats
	Stressful method	Pain, distress	Drowning kittens or freezing dragons

Which is the best approach depends on how much we can trust our judgement compared to that of the animals'. The first approach may be best when there is reliable scientific information about the necessary resources. The second may be best when the animals have evolved or learned adaptive behaviour. The third may be best when our information needs to be more tailored to the animal. We may also use the third approach to work out what resources to provide in the first two approaches.

This also means we can continuously improve how we care for animals, starting with options we think will be appropriate and then learning more accurately what resources are chosen by animals and are beneficial. We learn more about types of animals through animal welfare science and more about individual animals through interacting with them. Keepers should combine information both from experience and scientific research in determining exactly what their animals need. Keepers may initially give animals a limited range of safe options, then refine them using knowledge of the individual and outcome-assessments. At the same time, we can work out what outcomes to assess by seeing how they change when different resources are provided.

However, given the range of species kept, there is limited information known or available about many animals to make reliably accurate guesses about how to care for them. This is a good reason to keep more common pets. But if rarer pets are kept, what information should owners use? Sometimes it is valid to use information about other animals (e.g. related species or how animals are cared for in zoological and laboratory conditions). Whatever one thinks about animal research, zoos, or nature, pets' welfare should be no worse than that of animals kept for other purposes. Alternatively, it may be best to replicate how those animals' relatives live naturally (Figure 1.2), while also minimising the risks to which wild animals are exposed (e.g. starvation or predation). However, owners' homes usually cannot perfectly recreate animals' natural environments. Owners' homes are set up for humans. They may lack animals' natural climates, ecosystem, and space. It is probably impossible for homes, kennels, or pet shops to meet animals' needs and motivations completely while containing them, especially within cages or tanks (Figure 1.3) – unless their enclosures are made so big and complex that they do not constitute containment. Keepers should therefore minimise any compromises.

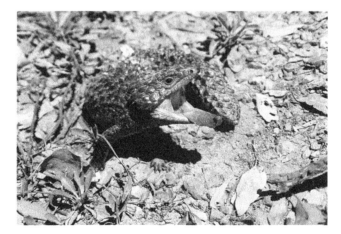

Figure 1.2   Shingleback (*Tiliqua rugosa*) in a naturalistic outdoor enclosure (*Source:* courtesy of Robert Johnson).

(a)   (b)

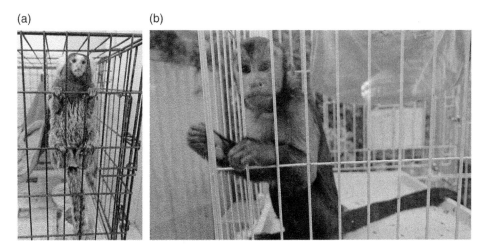

Figure 1.3 (a) Marmoset and (b) tufted capuchin in a pet shop in Hong Kong (*Source:* courtesy of Phillip Wilson).

1.2.1 Diet

All animals need a diet that ensures 'full health and vigour' and satisfies their motivations (Table 1.4). Pet animals may be carnivorous, omnivorous, or herbivorous, with the dietary proportion of meat comprising anywhere from 0% (excepting invertebrates in plants) to 100% (excepting vegetative matter in prey intestines). In general, each animal should take in a balanced supply of nutrients that is:

- Sufficient for the animal to maintain its body and meet any additional demands (e.g. reproduction and exercise),
- Ensures efficient, healthy digestion,
- Avoids excessive hunger and thirst,
- Adequately satisfies the animal's motivations to obtain and manipulate food, and
- Does no harm.

All animals require sufficient vitamins, minerals, amino acids (Table 1.5), and energy to meet their basal metabolic rate (for mammals and birds) or standard metabolic rate (for reptiles and amphibians) to avoid starvation and malnutrition. For example, many species need a particular amount of calcium, often linked to the amount of dietary phosphorus (i.e. the calcium-to-phosphorus ratio), the amount of vitamin D (from the diet or sunlight), and the calcium requirements (e.g. for growth and milk or egg production) to avoid metabolic syndromes that can affect bones and neurological functions (Figure 1.4). Many animals need adequate nutrients, particularly sufficient water and fibre, to allow their intestines to function properly. Animals also need to avoid excesses, both of particular nutrients (e.g. some vitamins, minerals, and carbohydrates) and of energy overall, which may lead to obesity, 'fatty liver', or insulin-resistance syndromes. Obesity often restricts animals' behaviour, particularly reducing exercise, thereby creating a 'vicious circle' of insufficient exercise and increased bodyweight.

Individual chapters have tables of nutritional requirements, where there is sufficient scientific evidence. When owners feed home-mixed diets, it is especially important to ensure

Table 1.4 Aims of suitable diets.

General aim	Specific aim	Example risks of failure
Ensuring health	Adequate nutrients	Starvation Vitamin deficiencies
	Avoids excessive nutrients	Obesity Vitamin excesses
	Is digestible	Gut blockages Poor absorption syndromes
	Matches biological process	Dental malocclusion Gut stasis
	Is safe	Toxicity Intestinal blockages
	Is delivered safely	Injuries from competing animals Food 'poisoning', e.g. salmonellosis
Allowing motivated behaviour	Sufficient quantity and type to satisfy hunger	Severe or chronic hunger Frustration
	Allow behaviours involved in obtaining and consuming food	Lack of appetite Oral stereotypies
	Sufficient 'pleasure' and interest	Inappetance Boredom

Source: Adapted from Webster 2011b.

a balance of nutrients. Alternatively, commercial diets may be available for many species, although they may not state the exact nutritional composition (beyond caloric value and raw protein, fibre, and ash contents). The availability of nutrients from the food also depends upon the nature of the ingredients, the presentation of the food (e.g. pelleting), and the conditions and duration of storage. For those species where nutritional requirements are not well known, the best option might be to offer a wide variety of foodstuffs from which animals can choose. Such a variety may allow animals to select nutritious foods (Manteca et al. 2008). However, animals may also selectively choose an unbalanced diet or food containing toxins, bacteria, or that may cause intestinal blockages in that species.

The principles also relate to how the food is provided, in particular in terms of frequency and method of provision. Although it may be impossible to avoid any feelings of hunger, these should be minimised by providing adequate fibre and feeding frequently often. The methods of provision also need to be suitable for the animal, for example whether they drink water, take it from foliage, or absorb it through the skin (Figure 1.5). Satisfying motivations requires a diet that allows feeding behaviours such as foraging, hunting, obtaining, grazing, manipulating, chewing, and storing food, especially because these motivations may be so strong that animals may choose to perform these behaviours rather than take freely available food. These behavioural needs may be met by activities that encourage physical activity (e.g. playing with toys or foraging) or mental activity (e.g. puzzle feeders and training), and for carnivorous pets, toys should be used instead of feeding sentient live prey.

Table 1.5 Key nutrients for many species.

Nutrient/requirement	Key functions
Energy	Fuel for biological processes, including active physiological processes and behaviour
Protein	Principal structural component of body organs, tissues (e.g. muscle), enzymes, signalling (e.g. hormones), and antibodies Energy production
Essential amino acids	Protein subunits that need to come from the diet
Carbohydrate	Short- and mid-term energy storage Source of glucose for energy and as building block of other nutrients
Fibre	Gut motility and water reabsorption; fermentation to short chain fatty acids and to help provide a feeling of stomach satiation
Fat/Lipid	Essential constituent of cell membranes, long-term energy storage, neuron and body insulation; production of steroid hormones; to allow absorption of fat-soluble vitamins
Calcium	Cellular signalling; ion gradients; body stability (bone and teeth); muscle contraction; blood clotting
Phosphorus	Production of DNA (for cell division), NADPH (for some body-building processes), and ATP (i.e. energy production); acid–base balance; body stability (bone, tooth enamel); muscle and reproductive functions
Magnesium	Skeletal and teeth structure, DNA and RNA metabolism, protein synthesis
Sodium	Acid–base balance, extracellular volume regulation; neuron/synapse functioning
Potassium	Acid–base balance; ion gradients for nerve transmission
Iron	Production of haemoglobin: Enzyme cofactor in O_2 transport and redox reactions
Copper	Production of enzymes (e.g. for respiration); iron metabolism and red blood cell production
Iodine	Production of thyroid hormones
Zinc	Enzyme component, cell replication, skin function, wound healing
Selenium	Antioxidant
Fat- and Water-soluble vitamins	Various enzymatic and transport functions
Water	Main solvent of life processes

ATP, adenosine triphosphate; NADPH, nicotinamide adenine dinucleotide phosphate.

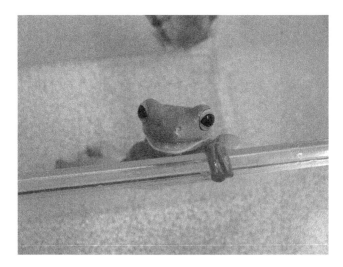

Figure 1.4 Green tree frog (*Litoria caerulaea*) with metabolic bone disease causing a deformed mandible (*Source:* courtesy of Robert Johnson).

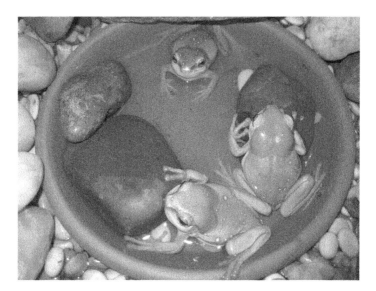

Figure 1.5 Magnificent tree frog (*Litoria splendida*) absorbing fluid through ventral drink patch (*Source:* courtesy of Robert Johnson).

Both nutritional needs and motivations may differ, depending on the animal's age, lifestyle, exercise, pregnancy, lactation, and diseases, whereas predation and competition may affect how much food each animal gets. So owners need to feed the right food in the right way. For rarer pets, a useful rule of thumb is to mimic natural diets as closely as possible. For more popular pets, owners can now buy commercial diets for many animals to reduce the risks of major errors or 'food poisoning' (e.g. salmonella or botulism), although these animals still need to be fed correctly to prevent boredom, dental problems, and obesity. Owners should also monitor each animal's intake, body condition, and body weight and compare these to ideal values, expected growth rates, the animal's normal (seasonal) weight, or generic body-condition scoring systems. They should also look for behaviour and health measures that might suggest malnutrition, disease, or other problems, such as not eating, oral stereotypies, and eating nonfood items.

1.2.2 Environment

Owners should have four key aims regarding their pets' environment:

- To ensure safety: Avoiding threats both real and perceived;
- To maintain hygiene: Minimising the risks of infection and feelings associated with being ungroomed;
- To provide comfort: Facilitating animals' use of their senses, movements, and resting;
- To provide stimulation: Allow (nonharmful) motivated behaviour.

Each should be considered from the owner's and the animal's point of view; animals need both to *be* and to *feel*: safe, clean, comfortable, and stimulated and to minimise disease, stress, and frustration. Better environments may also make animals respond better, physiologically and behaviourally, and thereby cope with other challenges. Various provisions help to meet these needs (Table 1.6).

A general environmental requirement is sufficient three-dimensional space. All animals need sufficient space to stretch to their full length in all dimensions and for enough movement and exercise. For many animals, this includes swimming and climbing. The space also needs to be large enough to allow other needs to be met, such as hiding, digging, burrowing, foraging, scatter-feeding, and company. For example, animals need to be able to maintain adequate distances from one another when they choose, and resources need to be spaced out and positioned to minimise competition. Some animals may not use all the available space frequently; for example, some animals may choose to sleep in contact with one another or to hide within smaller units, but this is not a reason to prevent access to enough space to perform other, less common needs. Indeed, animals should be given smaller shelters in which to hide and feel safely enclosed *within* larger spaces. Many animals may divide their space into different areas (e.g. for eating, sleeping, and toileting).

Within this space, there are certain physical requirements, such as temperature, humidity, ventilation, and lighting. These often interact, for example temperature, humidity, and ventilation interact, and owners need to ensure all three are correct. Physical requirements sound simple, but they can actually be complicated. For example, the right lighting depends on many factors. In many cases, animals should not be given a single ambient climate, but be allowed to choose between different environments. Environments also need to be appropriate in terms of the animals' senses, allowing them to use their senses, avoiding excessive stimulation (e.g. overly loud noises or unpleasant smells), and maintaining some familiar smells. Cleaning therefore needs to ensure adequate hygiene without impoverishing or oversanitising the space.

Table 1.6 Example effects of provisions on animals' environmental needs (including company).

Principle / Provision	Safety	Hygiene	Comfort	Stimulation
3-D Space	Opportunities for vigilance behaviours Width to turn around Ability to avoid and escape from others Ability to avoid perceived threats Ability to avoid unpleasant stimuli (e.g. bright lights or excessive noise) Cover and barriers Height for climbing Depth for diving or wallowing	Distances between toileting, bed, food, and water Dilution of pathogens Distancing between individuals Ability to groom	Ability to extend to full dimensions in all directions Ability to rest comfortably in any chosen posture Ability to groom Ability to maintain comfortable stocking density Opportunities to perform basic locomotion Thermal and humidity ranges for thermoregulation and hydroregulation	Environmental complexity Opportunities for exploration Opportunities to exercise and perform basic locomotion Opportunities to play alone Opportunities to interact with other animals Opportunities to interact with humans
Environmental Complexity	Vantage points and views for vigilance Barriers for escape Barriers and cover for hiding	Physical separation of areas for toileting, bed, food, and water Bathing areas Scratching areas	Thermal and humidity ranges	Opportunities to explore Toys for object play Barriers for social play Opportunities for locomotory play
Space to allow sufficient company	Reassurance of other animals' presence Shared vigilance Shared defence Minimised competition Minimised bullying	Mutual insect control Social learning about toileting Pathogens and parasites kept at low densities and away from feeding areas	Shared body-warmth Sufficient resources for each animal to use simultaneously	Social locomotory play Social toy play Social learning about how to interact with their environment Confidence in exploration, exercise, and interactions

Environments also need to be sufficiently complex to stimulate the animal. An impoverished environment may be cleanest, but it will not allow many behaviours to be met. In particular, environments should allow pets to play and interact with their environments. Many animals also benefit from opportunities to explore, for example by providing new areas or toys, to provide mental stimulation. This complexity needs to balanced with minimising stress resulting from unfamiliar objects. Animals should always be allowed to choose whether to interact with such enrichments, and owners should carefully observe their animals to ensure they strike the right balance. The correct environment often depends on the species and individual; for example, a captive-bred, precocious. and fast-learning juvenile carnivore may enjoy more excitement than a wild-caught, neophobic, and older prey animal.

1.2.3 Animal Company

The third key principle of companion animal welfare is to ensure social animals get the right company of other animals and that all animals avoid inappropriate company. Depending on their natural motivations, species are often described as 'social' or 'solitary'. Such descriptions may be oversimplification, especially when ascribed to whole groups such as 'reptiles' or where individual animals' experiences affect their responses to other animals. Nevertheless, these labels may be useful rules of thumb for pet owners to ensure they provide appropriate company for the former and not for the latter.

For social animals, company may be valuable both in itself and because of its impact on other sources of stress. Animal company may be pleasant and may also provide a necessary buffer against other challenges and increase resilience. Such company may provide mutual protection, improved predator vigilance, play, affiliation, thermoregulation, fly-swatting, mutual grooming, cooperative activities, learning, and (if allowed) mating and the care of offspring. However, animal company may also be unpleasant and may also exacerbate other challenges and increase vulnerability (Table 1.6). Such company may create competition for resources, social stress from overcrowding or social defeat, disease risks, cannibalisation, or aggression. More specifically, breeding also brings risks during intercourse (e.g. sexually transmitted infections), pregnancy (e.g. nutritional imbalances), birth (e.g. dystocia), and raising offspring (e.g. cannibalisation).

The value of company may depend on each individual, the relationships between them, group stability, the resources provided, and any external threats (Table 1.7). Even animals of 'social species' may become unsociable as a result of pain, previous unpleasant experiences, or mismanaged introductions, and any animals' relationships may be strained by insufficient space and resources. When keeping animals together, owners should therefore:

- Ensure that animals are healthy, vaccinated, socialised, and minimally stressed;
- Match animals carefully for size and gender, neutering before puberty when safe;
- Manage introductions carefully (Table 1.8) and maintain stable groups (excepting deaths);
- Give opportunities for animals to avoid, escape, and communicate with each other;
- Provide sufficient resources for all animals to use at the same time;
- Maintain appropriate (and not excessive) hygiene; and
- Closely observe the animals and have contingency plans in place.

Table 1.7 Factors that affect the value of animal company.

Factor	Description and examples
The Animals	
Species	Animals of species that have evolved to be social may suffer from isolation.
	Animals of species that have evolved to be more solitary may suffer from company.
	Most pet species are rarely naturally sociable with other pet species.
	Some pet species are potential predators or competitors of others.
	Some species may transfer infections between species.
Age, gender, and reproductive status	In some species, males or females or adults or juveniles may be more or less social.
	Some may show aggression during reproductive periods.
	Neutering may alter some levels of aggression or other interactions.
Patho-physiological conditions	Infectious diseases present risks of infection.
	Birthing, disease, or pain may decrease sociability.
	Breeding of animals with extreme shapes may lead to problems giving birth.
Personal histories	Learning that other animals may be safe or dangerous
	Learning how to determine which animals are safe or threatening
	Learning how to communicate with other animals
Matching	Discrepancies in size may lead to bullying.
	Some personalities may be incompatible.
	Animals of mixed genders (if unneutered) may mate (even if related).
Personal relationships	Siblings and offspring may be more compatible.
	Some animals may fear particular species, breeds, or genders.
	Some individuals may form particular pleasant or unpleasant relationships.
Animals' responses	Each animal may signal to others about their state or preferences.
	Each animal may read others' signals.
Context	
Space	Space may affect how well animals can observe one another.
	Space may affect how well animals can avoid or carefully approach one another.

(*Continued*)

Table 1.7 (Continued)

Factor	Description and examples
Environmental design	Light, vantage points, and shelters affect animals' abilities to see each other and hide. Barriers and high perches can prevent or permit escape or chasing.
Resources	Insufficient resources can lead to bullying or competition. Poorly located resources can allow individual to prevent others' access to resources.
Cleanliness	Lack of hygiene can lead to disease spread. Excessive cleaning can remove familiar, reassuring smells. Cleaning can remove or transfer smells of other animals.
Owners	Owners can worsen problems through inappropriate interventions.

Table 1.8 General principles for introducing unfamiliar animals humanely.

Factor to consider	Good general principles
Area	Neutral to both animals, i.e. not either's territory Familiar to each animal Quiet and calm No specific sources of stress No dangers during flight (e.g. sharp edges or clear barriers) No dead ends Plenty of escape routes and visual barriers Introduction of sensory stimuli (e.g. mixing smells first)
Resources	Sufficient basic resources (e.g. space) No highly valued resources that might cause competition Plenty and well spaced-out resources as distractions
Humans	Experienced and knowledgeable Relaxed Carefully observing Unseen by the animals but close to intervene Contingency plans in place
Animals	Well fed Relaxed and otherwise not fearful anxious or stressed Healthy Matched (e.g. similar size) Good temperament Not in heat (and, for some animals, neutered)

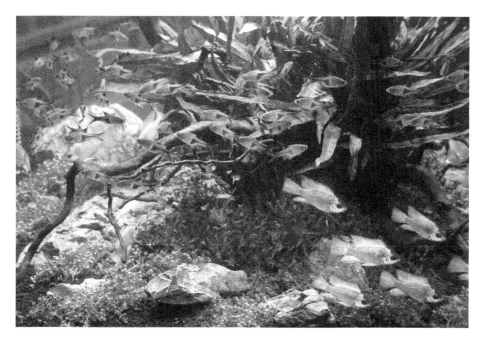

Figure 1.6 Mixed species freshwater tropical aquarium (*Source:* courtesy of Peter Burgess).

Owners may be poor judges of how their animals respond to company and may fail to notice signs of isolation or of incompatibility. However, some more obvious signals may be useful. For example, owners may notice positive signs (e.g. animals voluntarily spending more time together, playing and engaging in mutual grooming) or signs of incompatibility (e.g. avoiding one another). Fighting may indicate an incompatibility or a lack of resources. However, animals usually fight only when other strategies such as avoidance or threats have failed, so a lack of fighting is not evidence of compatibility.

Some animals may enjoy or tolerate the company of other species, for example, in 'community tanks' of fish (Figure 1.6), but mixing species may cause problems for one or both animals. Some infectious diseases may spread between species. Predator species may enjoy hunting potential prey animals (if permitted), but the prey animals may be caused fear (especially if unable to escape). There is some suggestion that deliberately inducing mild fear of predators may improve welfare overall (e.g. tamarins, Chamove and Moodie 1990), although this is controversial (Roush et al. 1992). Predator animals may also experience frustration through being unable to reach their prey. The safest rule is to keep predators and prey – and their smells and sounds – completely separate.

1.2.4 Human Interactions

The third key principle is to ensure human interactions are suitable. As 'companions' to humans, pets often interact with humans more than with other animals. Some animals appear motivated to interact with humans or find particular interactions rewarding, such as stroking, tickling, and praise. Others may associate humans with other rewards (e.g. food). Some social animals may also find human company directly rewarding, although not necessarily in ways similar to that of their own species (so human company is not an appropriate substitute for company of their own kind). However, human company may also be stressful for many animals. Humans may be unfamiliar or natural predators for some species and may also be noisy, unpredictable, and interfering.

Some animals do not want to be handled at particular times, such as reptiles during shedding or during the daytime for nocturnal animals (unless owners reverse the daily lighting schedules). Some animals simply do not enjoy human presence or contact. In such cases, owners should minimise stressful interactions, perhaps allowing animals to feel hidden while still being visible by using hidden video cameras, camouflage netting, one-way glass, peep holes, mirrors, by red lighting and handling these animals only when necessary. Owners' desires to interact with their animals should not compromise the animals' welfare by failing to allow them to perform their natural motivations.

All handling should be gentle, calm, and predictable. Handlers should also avoid anything that might be stressful for the particular species, such as lifting animals to fear-inducing heights, acting like that species' natural predator (e.g. not coming from above) or like an aggressive competitor (e.g. approaching from the front for some species). Handlers should also ensure they do not hold animals in a way that causes pain or discomfort (e.g. lifting animals only by their limbs, tail, or head) or that risks injury (e.g. from escape attempts). Owners should also not use methods that rely on stress, such as prey showing immobility as a response to predators. In some cases, stress may be minimised by tranquillisers that reduce animals' anxiety and the length of handling.

Breeders and owners should ensure their animals are used to all types of humans with whom they are likely to come into contact (e.g. male, female, adults, and children), in ways that do not cause additional stress. Positive 'socialisation', especially early in life, may mean some animals find human company rewarding. Other animals may be 'tamed', so they may at least tolerate human interactions. In either case, this process should minimise stress, so that animals do not simply learn that it is useless to respond. Unpleasant interactions may actually increase animals' fear of humans and lead to problematic behaviours such as fear-related aggression if animals use that as a last resort after escalating efforts to escape or deter humans or learn that it is the only successful tactic to avoid stressful handling.

Handling may also be improved by training animals to perform certain behaviours such as walking onto their owner's hand, walking on a lead, or to enter animal carriers voluntarily. Owners may also want to train animals to perform certain behaviours. Active punishment or attempts to 'dominate' animals may cause pain or fear (and be ineffective or counterproductive), and animals may then associate that pain or fear with humans or their owners. Instead, owners should reward the desired behaviours, while not rewarding any unwanted behaviours (even with attention when animals find that rewarding). Owners should expect gradual improvements and not expect animals to perfectly mind-read what their owners want them to do. Instead, owners should respect animals' own preferences as much as possible, by training animals to perform behaviours that are as close as possible to their natural behaviour and own motivations.

1.2.5 Health

The fifth key principle of companion animal welfare is to keep the animal as healthy as possible. All animals may suffer from infections or infestations such as viruses, bacteria, fungi, protozoa, worms, flukes, insects, or arthropods (Table 1.9). In many cases, some parasites may carry other diseases. Sometimes multiple species may be susceptible to different microorganisms, although different species may be affected in different ways. Some infections may spread to humans, particularly to owners who live in close contact with their pets and elderly, young, or immunocompromised people. Important zoonotic diseases include rabies, plague, salmonellosis, pasteurellosis, chlamydiosis, toxoplasmosis, and mycobacteriosis.

Owners should source healthy animals, screening and quarantining animals to reduce the spread of infections. They should also provide adequate hygiene and preventative

Table 1.9 Selected health issues in companion animals.

Condition	Causes	Generic examples
Infectious/ Parasitic	Viruses (V)[a]	Influenza Retroviruses Parvoviruses
	Bacteria[a]	Coliforms Rickettsial Clostridial
	Fungi[a]	Aspergillus Yeasts
	Protozoa[a]	Intestinal protozoa
	Internal Parasites[a]	Worms Flukes
	External Parasites[a]	Fleas Ticks Mites Lice
Noninfectious diseases	Hormonal disorders	Hyperadrenocrticoidism Diabetes mellitus
	Neoplastic	Benign tumours Malignant tumours
	Inherited	Genetic disorders Extreme shapes
	Degenerative/Geriatric conditions	Dental disease Osteoarthritis
	Toxic	Heavy metals Drug overdoses
	Traumatic	Road accidents Being dropped

(V) denotes vaccines are available in some countries for some strains.
[a]Denotes the potential for spread to humans.

care, such as vaccinations, anti-parasitics, and neutering, as appropriate. Owners should also ensure animals are otherwise well cared for generally because stress may also increase animals' susceptibility to infectious diseases, or mean animals' may lack the resources to fight off infections. When problems are identified, they should be rapidly diagnosed, isolated, if appropriate, and treated. The risks of zoonotic diseases may be reduced by simple precautions such as avoiding contact with wild animals, regular veterinary examinations, and good hygiene while handling any animals (especially dead or sick animals) and while preparing food and thorough cooking of food. Where appropriate and possible, owners should try to use specialist veterinary practitioners (Table 1.10).

Because pets often live longer than many wild or farm animals, they also experience a number of age-related or degenerative conditions (although sometimes such conditions may occur in earlier life). Many animals experience dental disease (except those without teeth), particularly if they are not fed adequate material to chew. Dental disease may be painful, may cause damage to the oral cavity, and may reduce animals' ability to eat food. Some carnivores may cope without teeth, but herbivores often need to be able to chew their food for adequate digestion. Many animals may also suffer from arthritis, which may cause pain and reduced mobility, although this may be mistaken as animals simply slowing down in old age. Animals may also experience cancers, such as skin, fatty tissue, mammary glands, or womb tumours.

Breeders should avoid breeding animals who have an increased likelihood of experiencing health problems, that is, from animals with genes for heritable conditions. These conditions might be intrinsically associated with the animal's physical characteristics that breeders want to achieve, such as exaggerated body shapes. Alternatively, they might be conditions that are coincidentally associated with the breed's ideal because the genes for both are closely linked or because the animals that have these conditions are seen as the best show animals. Animals should not be bred if they are too genetically similar because this may increase the risk of their offspring having recessive genes that encode physical abnormalities and mean that breeds are less biodiverse. Owners should therefore avoid breeding from animals who are closely related, part of a small, closed breed, or overly bred (e.g. males being mated to many females) and should match mates who have the lowest risks of heritable health problems (UFAW 2016).

Companion animals may be subjected to various surgeries not aimed at treating a particular condition (Table 1.11). Some owners may want their animals to be altered aesthetically by cosmetic 'mutilations' that may cause pain and prevent locomotory or communicative behaviours. Although some surgery may be clinically necessary for the health of the animal (e.g. neutering may bring health benefits for many animals), other surgery may instead be aimed at the benefit of the human (e.g. removing vocal cords, claws, teeth, or horns to reduce noise, damage to property, or injuries to humans). Other elective, nontherapeutic surgeries are aimed at making animals fit a management system, for example, pinioning birds' wings so they cannot fly away. Each chapter has a table of such interventions (unless there are no justifiable surgeries for those species). In all cases, other methods should be used instead of surgery, except where these would lead to greater welfare compromises.

Table 1.10 Examples of veterinary specialisations.

Recognising organisation	Example veterinary specialties
American Veterinary Medical Association	American Board of Veterinary Practitioners in Avian Practice
	American Board of Veterinary Practitioners in Canine and Feline Practice
	American Board of Veterinary Practitioners in Equine Practice
	American Board of Veterinary Practitioners in Exotic Companion Mammal Practice
	American Board of Veterinary Practitioners in Reptile and Amphibian Practice
	American College of Animal Welfare
	American College of Veterinary Behaviourists
	American College of Veterinary Nutrition
	American College of Zoological Medicine
European Board of Veterinary Specialisation	European College of Aquatic Animal Health
	European College of Zoological Medicine
	European College of Animal Welfare and Behavioural Medicine
	European College of Veterinary and Comparative Nutrition
	European College of Animal Welfare and Behavioural Medicine
Australian and New Zealand College of Veterinary Scientists	Australian and New Zealand College of Veterinary Scientists: Avian Health Chapter
	Australian and New Zealand College of Veterinary Scientists: Animal Welfare Chapter
	Australian and New Zealand College of Veterinary Scientists: Veterinary Behaviour Chapter
	Australian and New Zealand College of Veterinary Scientists: Zoo and Wildlife Medicine Chapter
	Australian and New Zealand College of Veterinary Scientists: Unusual Pets Chapter
United Kingdom (RCVS)	Diploma in Animal welfare science, ethics, and law
	Diploma in Zoological Medicine
	RCVS Recognised Specialists in Animal welfare science, ethics, and law
	RCVS Recognised Specialists in Exotic animal medicine
	RCVS Recognised Specialists in Zoo and wildlife medicine

RCVS, Royal College of Veterinary Surgeons.

Table 1.11 Examples of elective nontherapeutic surgery in companion animals.

Rationale	Examples	Possible alternatives	Key chapters
Reduction of reproductive behaviour/breeding	Spaying Castration	Chemical suppression Isolation	2, 6, 12 2, 6
Reduction of noise or scent production	Removal of vocal chords Removal of scent glands	Training	4 6
Reduction of damage to human property	Removal of claws Nose-ringing to reduce rooting	Provision of specific enrichments to allow behaviour	3 12
Making animals easier or safer to handle	Removal of antlers or horns Nose-ringing to attach rope	Training Halters etc.	12 12
Improvement of performance	Surgery on upper respiratory tract	Medical treatment Retirement	13
Prevention of escape	Pinioning or clipping of wings to prevent flight	Training to return Housing design to allow safe, contained flight	14
For identification	Ear-notching	Microchipping	12
Cosmetic	Tattooing Tail-docking and ear-cropping	Microchipping	4, 22 4

1.2.6 Euthanasia

Animals should receive timely and humane euthanasia when in their welfare interests. Owners are often responsible for when and how pets die (but not whether they do) and should try to provide a humane death when their animal would otherwise suffer severely (and then still die eventually). Shelters also need to provide euthanasia when death is better than other realistic options available, given any limitations in resources or potential adopters. In such cases, euthanasia is better than continued suffering. In some countries, companion animals are also culled in an (often unsuccessful) attempt to control populations or slaughtered to eat.

The best euthanasia method is one that minimises the duration and the intensity of any suffering involved and risks of error or ineffectiveness. The ideal procedure is one that causes immediate death or at least immediate unconsciousness followed by death before consciousness is recovered. Where unconsciousness is not immediate, methods should be minimally irritant, painful, malodorous, or otherwise aversive. All methods of pet euthanasia should be performed by a competent veterinary surgeon, except where delay or transportation would cause increased suffering, to minimise the risks of error. Those performing euthanasia should also ensure they minimise risks to human safety, for example as a result of free gases, needle injuries, or ricocheting bullets. With any method, death should be ensured by using an irreversible method and by checking for the absence of life signs. For example, 'pithing' involves using a needle or rod to macerate the brain tissue (in the correct location), thereby ensuring death.

The best method is also one that minimises any suffering during handling, transportation, and restraint before euthanasia. Some animals may benefit from their owners staying until they lose consciousness, so long as this is safe, and the owners' presence does not add to the distress. Injecting local anaesthetics at injection sites or catheters placed before the injection can refine the procedure. Tranquillisers and sedatives can reduce anxiety and make handling easier and speed up drug effects. They may sometimes be given at higher doses than would normally be considered safe, so that animals' last moments are more comfortable. Some animals can be fully anaesthetised beforehand – in which case, some other permanent methods may become acceptable if they reliably prevent animals regaining consciousness before experiencing any adverse effects. Any efforts to reduce suffering should be evaluated to ensure they do not actually increase distress compared to euthanasia alone.

Finally, the best method depends on the species (e.g. some burrowing species find hypoxic gas mixtures more aversive), age (e.g. the tolerance of high carbon dioxide [CO_2] levels by neonates), individual animal (e.g. their level of fear during handling), person (e.g. competence for different methods), circumstances (e.g. the degree of animal suffering during any delay), and any postmortem requirements (e.g. to ensure intact brain material or avoid anaesthetic chemicals precipitating within tissues or if the animal is going to be eaten). Some methods may be generally suitable for many pets (Table 1.12). Other methods may cause levels of suffering that are unsuitable for any pets (Table 1.13) except when they are the only available method to prevent greater suffering or where the animal is already unconscious. For example, CO_2 inhalation can cause pain (as a result of acidic reactions on eye and respiratory tissues), fear (by directly stimulating brain ion channels), feelings of breathlessness (by stimulating respiration while impairing gas exchange), signs of stress (particularly corticosteroid and catecholamine increases), and avoidance behaviours (in some cases) and should not be used for companion species.

1.3 Signs of Companion Animal Welfare

Good care requires owners to assess each pet's welfare carefully, primarily by recognising and interpreting signs of their pathology, physiology, and behaviour. Such signs may also help to determine what changes in the animal's care actually make a difference. Owners' familiarity with their pets may help them assess their welfare but may still allow owners to miss signs that are subtle, gradual, or shown only in their absence (e.g. separation-related behaviours). All assessors need to have adequate knowledge and understanding of the species and the individual, in particular to avoid ignoring signs that are normal in a breed or misinterpreting signs as if the animals were human.

Table 1.12 Methods of euthanasia suitable for (some) conscious companion animals.

Method	Restraint required	Welfare benefits	Welfare risks
Anaesthetic overdose injected into a vein	Tight handling for vein access Sedation advised	Fast	Minor pain of injection Pain from chemical in tissues if vein missed
Anaesthetic overdose injected into the liver, abdomen, or coelom	Handling Sedation or anaesthesia advised	Less tight restraint	Moderate to severe pain of injection (depending on chemical used and whether pH buffered or local anaesthetic added) Slow if accidentally placed into intestines, bladder, or air sacs
Overdose of volatile anaesthetic inhaled	Containment in chamber	Reduced handling	Odour may be unpleasant (depending on chemical, concentration, and species) Relatively slow (depending on chemical, concentration, and species) May induce breath-holding, further slowing loss of consciousness
Immersion (for aquatic or amphibian species) in anaesthetic overdose	Containment in tank	No handling Animal may be left in familiar environment	Relatively slow Irritation (depending on chemical, concentration, and species) Risk of ineffectiveness because of underdosage
Head or brain trauma	Restraint of head and body to ensure accuracy (where possible)	Instantaneous prevention of any experiences	Severe pain if inaccurate
Neck dislocation	Tight handling	Very fast	Severe pain if ineffective

1.3.1 Pathophysiological Signs

An animal's pathology and physiology may indicate various welfare compromises (Table 1.14). Additionally, insofar as other welfare compromises may increase diseases risks, pathophysiological signs may also suggest other, noninfectious welfare compromises. For example, stress may predispose some pets to particular pathophysiological signs such as hair loss, gastric ulcers, or urinary tract disease.

Because different animals respond differently, animals (like us) may suffer without any observable physical signs. Conversely, some pathophysiological changes may not

Table 1.13 Methods of euthanasia not (usually) suitable for conscious companion animals.

Method	Restraint required	Welfare risks
Carbon dioxide (CO_2) inhalation	Containment	Slow respiratory distress and pain as a result of acidic reactions in mucous membranes
Drowning	Handling or containment within vessel	Slow Severe distress
Hanging	Noose restriction	Slow when death as a result of asphyxiation Distress, pain, and respiratory distress
Neuromuscular blocking agents[a]	Handling for injections	Slow Distress and confusion Respiratory distress
Decapitation	Handling or restraint to allow incision	Pain and distress May be especially long duration in animals able to tolerate hypoxia
Exsanguination	Handling or restraint to allow incision	Slow (depending on method and species anatomy) Pain and distress
Electrocution[a]	Restraint to allow application	Pain Inaccuracy may allow continued or regained consciousness Inappropriate parameters may lead to ineffectiveness
Freezing in commercial freezer	Containment in freezer	Slow Thermal discomfort Pain resulting from ice-crystal formation within tissues
Poisoning	None (if oral)	Depending on chemical, species, and dosage

[a] NB Some methods may be acceptable if performed under anaesthetic or in conjunction with or after another method to ensure death.

correspond to suffering (e.g. normal hibernation or season changes in reproduction) or even correspond to pleasant feelings (e.g. stress hormones may rise during play). Owners therefore need to interpret pathophysiological signs in relation to the context, the individual in which they occur, and other signs, in particular their pet's behaviour.

The choice of pathophysiological signs should depend on the context and the decisions being made. Some measures may themselves stress the animal (e.g. handling or restraint for blood sampling), making it harder to interpret the cause of their results. Other measures may be more remote (e.g. breathing rate or faecal cortisol, Palme 2012) but may provide limited information. Many of the pathophysiological signs used by scientists are hard to measure in the home without expensive scientific equipment or training or be hard to interpret where we lack reliable baseline (i.e. normal

Table 1.14 Potential welfare signs in companion animals.

Type of measure	Examples
Pathophysiological signs	
Hormone levels	Plasma glucocorticoids (+ metabolites)
	Faecal, salivary, and urinary glucocorticoids (+ metabolites)
Blood chemical levels	Lactate dehydrogenase
	Glucose
	Creatine kinase
	Plasma osmolarity
	Albumin concentrations
	Globulin concentrations
	Measures of particular antibodies
Blood cell levels	White blood cell counts
	Packed cell volume
Physiological responses	Heart rate
	Heart rate variability
	Respiratory rate
	Urination rate
Immune responses	Signs of inflammation
	Body temperature
	Specific clinical signs
Biological performance	Body weight
	Size
	Body condition
	Fertility
	Lactation
	Exercise tolerance
	Gastric ulceration
	Hair or plumage condition
	Shedding and skin condition
	Longevity or mortality
Behavioural signs	
Activity levels	Sleeping
	Exercise
Levels of maintenance behaviours	Eating
	Drinking
	Grooming
	Seeking high temperatures
Repetitive behaviours	Stereotypies
	Obsessive compulsive disorders

Table 1.14 (Continued)

Type of measure	Examples
Interactions with pleasant stimuli	Social interactions
	Play
	Engagement
	Appetite
Interactions with unpleasant stimuli	Vigilance
	Hiding and voluntary isolation
	Flight
	Marking
	Aggression
Sickness behaviours and signs of injury	Vomiting
	Diarrhoea
	Limping
Species-specific signs of stress	Particular postures (for the species)
	Types of mouth licking (dogs)

reference ranges for the species). Owners should therefore record normal measures for their own animals (e.g. body weight) to assess trends over time, such as growth rates or weight loss.

1.3.2 Behavioural Signs

Animals use behaviour to respond to their environment. At its simplest, an animal's behaviour may represent an animal's choices (e.g. approach or avoidance). Behaviour may indicate an animal's particular neuromuscular or other health issues (Table 1.15).

Some behaviours may suggest particular welfare states. Indeed, some are characterised as 'sickness behaviour' or 'pain-related' or 'fear-related' behaviour in a particular species. Stereotypies or other repetitive behaviours may be caused by strong, unmet motivations, excitement or anticipation, attempts to cope with previous welfare compromises, and neurological conditions. Aggression may indicate pain, fear, or neurological disorders. Owners should get to know what is normal for the species and the individual. For example, animals may stop or reduce the time spent eating, grooming, or playing when they are ill. Owners should also try to assess their animal's overall behaviour or demeanour.

The absence of behavioural signs of problems – or at least the absence of owners' noticing them – does not mean that an animal has perfect welfare. Solitary or prey animals may be less likely to show behavioural signs of poor welfare, including in the presence of humans they perceive as potential predators. For example, immobility may be a stress response rather than an indication that the animal tolerates human contact. Owners may also make some animals less able to show certain behaviours (e.g. as a result of breeding or surgical mutilations). A particular behaviour may also suggest several possible underlying feelings. Animals may jump and move around when frustrated, in anticipation, during play, or when trying to escape. Owners need to interpret behaviours in relation to the individual (e.g. species, previous experiences), the context (e.g. time of day and what prompted the behaviour), and other current or previous behaviour and physiological responses.

Table 1.15 Key behavioural signs of possible welfare compromises in companion animals.

Aspect of behaviour	Specific responses
Altered activity or responsiveness	Increased vigilance or activity
	Attention to particular threats
	Startling
	Reaction on palpation or withdrawal of body part from contact
	Lethargy, immobility, or decreased mobility (e.g. less movement or play)
	Playing dead
	Slow or absent reflexes (e.g. righting reflex)
	Altered performance
Avoidance	Avoiding particular areas
	Hiding
	Immobility or 'freezing'
	Preparation for flight
	Escape attempts during handling
	Flight
Altered posture or expression	Altered head, neck, body, tail, or ear position
	Altered hair, colour, or feathers
	Altered eye opening (e.g. wide or closed eyes)
	Looking 'smaller' or 'bigger'
	Tongue or tail movements
	Open-mouthed threats
	Particular repetitive movements (e.g. head bobbing)
Altered metabolic processes and maintenance or other common behaviour	Increased respiratory rate
	Altered appetite
	Increased swallowing
	Increased drinking
	Urination or defaecation
	Altered toileting
	Altered grooming or bathing
	Altered time spent resting or sleeping
	Reduced time spent playing or hunting
Altered interactions with the environment or other animals	Manipulating environmental objects
	Altered social interactions
Vocalisations	Social calls
	Alarm calls
	Pain-related sounds

Table 1.15   (Continued)

Aspect of behaviour	Specific responses
Attack or preattack behaviours (NB may often be employed defensively)	Preparation for attack
	'Fake' or 'symbolic' attack behaviours
	Actual attack behaviours
	Spraying urine, scent, or faeces
Abnormal or repetitive movements	Circling or pacing
	Pecking at particular spots
	Spinning or flipping
	Self-mutilation
	Regurgitation
Specific local signs of local pain	Hunched or tucked up abdomen
	Rigid posture or area
	Biting or scratching a specific area
	Lameness

All behavioural responses may also indicate other welfare issues than those listed, and the absence of any particular sign in any individual does not mean they are not experiencing that welfare compromise.

1.4 Action Plans

1.4.1 Ethics and Values in Companion Animal Welfare

Concern for animal welfare is a moral principle. Most humans are moral 'agents' who have moral responsibilities and who *can* and *should* act morally. People may obtain animals altruistically, particularly when adopting animals needing homes but may also obtain animals for other reasons (Table 1.16). Whatever the reason, owners and those who have responsibility for animals have a duty of care for the animals in their charge.

1.4.2 Setting Priorities

The most common and severe welfare compromises vary depending on species and country. Most animals can suffer from overfeeding, nutritional deficiencies, inappropriate temperature and lighting, insufficient space or places in which to take refuge or hide, inappropriate company or isolation, insufficient socialisation, mishandling, punishment, inherited disorders, insufficient preventive health care or health checks, and a failure to provide timely euthanasia.

Good breeding, capture, and raising is a priority for all species. Where animals are wild-caught, priorities include using humane catching methods, better transportation, or simply reducing the numbers of wild animals kept captive. For captive-bred animals, priorities include breeding animals with fewer inherited disorders and infectious

Table 1.16 Reasons other than 'companionship' for keeping 'companion animal species'.

Reason	Common examples
Hunting	Dogs
Pest control	Cats
Herding	Dogs
Transportation	Horses
Communication	Horses
	Pigeons
Assistance	Dogs
Guarding	Dogs
Weapons or threats	Dogs
	Horses
Owner appearing 'exotic'	Var. (rare species)
Owner appearing 'expert'	Var. (difficult species)
Symbols of owner's social class or club	Horses
membership	Var. (pedigree animals)
	Var. (expensive animals)
Owner decoration	Handbag dogs
Entertainment	Horses
	Parrots
Sport and show success	Dogs
	Horses
Home ornamentation	Fish
Zoological collections	Marine fish
Species conservation	Various
Scientific research	Rats or zebra fish
Meat	Dogs
	Rabbits
	Guinea pigs
	Horses
Profit	Var. (as above)
	Var. (breeding for above)

diseases, ensuring breeding animals get sufficient care, and that vulnerable young animals get their immediate needs met (e.g. for maternal care) and are prepared for their later lives as pets (e.g. taming or socialisation). For all animals, trade practices should avoid starvation, transportation, exposure or heat stress, isolation, social stress, handling, injury, and disease.

The numbers of animals abandoned, straying, or entering shelters needs to be reduced, and those who are abandoned or lost should be humanely helped by government or nongovernment organisations. Rehoming allows animals to have an additional life; this is expected to be of a good quality of life but may itself involve significant welfare compromises during kennelling, particularly in unfamiliar or overcrowded environments. Widespread culling should be avoided wherever possible, and if done, should use humane methods and be done alongside other efforts such as neutering to prevent populations increasing again. However, shelters that are under resourced or overcrowded might be worse for the animals than being left on the street or euthanised. Charities also have a responsibility to set good examples (e.g. in providing timely neutering and euthanasia) and to ensure they adopt only to good owners.

1.4.3 Methods of Achieving Welfare Improvements

Improving companion animal welfare needs to both promote good care by owners and keepers and to promote companion animal welfare in society at large. Situations may differ between species, owner sociodemographics, countries, and continents, but many themes are surprisingly consistent.

Education is important both to supply knowledge and to correct *mis*information or inappropriate attitudes, such as outdated behavioural theories, perceptions that certain species are easy, or assumptions that purebreds are better quality. Owners need to get the right information, taking care to ensure that self-appointed 'authorities' really do have the required expertise. This should help owners ensure they have the resources and commitment needed for animals' whole lives *before* getting them (and ideally before the emotional event of meeting them). In particular, owners should choose suitable animals in terms of species, breed, and individual. Owners need to use resources such as UFAW's (2016) guidance on inherited disorders or the Swiss federal veterinary office's information for adults (www.meinheimtier.ch; www.animauxdecompagnie.ch; www.animalidacompagnia.ch) and children (www.neutierig.ch; www.passibete.ch; www.animalando.ch).

Those involved in the supply chain of pets should check and educate would-be owners before selling a pet, prevent impulse purchases, or animals being bought as gifts or prizes. Breeders and vendors should also ensure they only sell animals whose needs can be met by their future owners and avoid adding to problems of overproduction and oversupply or breeding 'fancy' animals with inherited disorders or extreme conformations. The pet 'industry' requires an adequate profit, but profit may be increased by marketing better-quality products (e.g. vaccinated and well-socialised animals or welfare-friendly products). Consumers could drive such changes in their consumer behaviour, particularly if there were reliable assurance schemes.

Societies at large should develop the infrastructure to assist breeders and owners, such as veterinary services, animal training, and behaviourist services. Veterinary professionals need to educate and advise on their patients' health, diet, environment, company, and interactions. Behaviourists need to use only welfare-friendly methods and avoid outdated or inaccurate theories about animals' 'natural' relationships. Some countries need more basic infrastructure (e.g. the first commercial veterinary practices in Malawi). Others need increased expertise in shelter medicine and in 'exotic' species of increasing popularity, with increasing development of specialists who owners should preferentially use (Table 1.10).

Finally, appropriate legislation is needed to protect animals' welfare. Specific legislation should aim to prevent cruelty (e.g. dog fighting), licence certain activities to competent individuals (e.g. veterinary services, breeding, transportation, and sale), and ensure animals are kept as companion animals only in ways that meet their needs.

Governments also need to ensure their commercial and public laws do not cause unnecessary welfare problems, for example, by preventing dogs interacting with other dogs off the lead. All such laws need to be properly interpreted and enforced, which requires adequate resources and training, and keep pace with scientific progress.

Bibliography

American Pet Products Association (APPA). (2014). Pet Industry Market Size & Ownership Statistics. Available at http://www.americanpetproducts.org/press_industrytrends.asp. Accessed 27 November 2014.

Animal Health Alliance (Australia) (AHA). (2014). Pet Ownership in Australia (2014). Available at https://petsinaustralia.com.au/wp-content/themes/_TBST-BusinessAccelerator-v3/library/Downloads/Pet-Ownership-in-Australia-2013.pdf. Accessed 27 November 2014.

AVMA (American Veterinary Medical Association). (2013). AVMA Guidelines for the Euthanasia of Animals: 2013 Edition. Available at https://www.avma.org/KB/Policies/Pages/Euthanasia-Guidelines.aspx. Accessed 7 October 2015.

Bateman, A., Singh, A., Krahl, T., and Solomon, S. (1989). The immune-hypothalamic-pituitary-adrenal axis. *Endocrine Reviews* 10: 92–112.

Beauchamp, T.L. and Childress, J.F. (1979). *Principles of Biomedical Ethics*. Oxford, UK: Oxford University Press.

Bennett, R.A. (1998) Pain and analgesia in reptiles and amphibians. In *Annual Conference of the American Association of Zoo Veterinarians* and American Association of Wildlife Veterinarians, Omaha, NE, 17-22 October 1998, pp. 461–465.

Bonnet, X., Shine, R., and Lourdais, O. (2002). Taxonomic chauvinism. *Trends in Ecology & Evolution* 17: 1–3.

Burghardt, G.M. (2013). Environmental enrichment and cognitive complexity in reptiles and amphibians: concepts, review, and implications for captive populations. *Applied Animal Behaviour Science* 147 (3): 286–298.

Burghardt, G.M. (2014a). Play in fishes, frogs and reptiles. *Current Biology* 25 (1): R10.

Burghardt, G.M. (2014b). A brief glimps at the long evolutionary history of play. *Animal Behaviour Cognition* 1: 90–98.

Burghardt, G.M., Dinets, V., and Murphy, J.B. (2014). Highly repetitive object play in a chichlid fish (*Tropheus duboisi*). *Ethology* 120: 1–7.

Caixong, Z. (2015). China's pet tally reaches 100 million, mostly cats and dogs. *China Daily*. Available at http://www.chinadaily.com.cn/china/2015-10/16/content_22203711.htm. Accessed 16 October 2015.

Cartner, S.C., Barlow, S.C., and Ness, T.J. (2007). Loss of cortical function in mice after decapitation, cervical dislocation, potassium chloride injection, and CO2 inhalation. *Comparative Medicine* 57 (6): 570–573.

CAWC (2006). *Companion Animal Welfare Council Report: Welfare Aspects of Modifications, through Selective Breeding or Biotechnological Methods, to the Form, Function, or Behaviour of Companion Animals*. Cambridge, UK: Companion Animal Welfare Council.

CCAC (2009). *CCAC Guidelines on: The Care and Use of Farm Animals in Research, Teaching and Testing*. Ottawa, Canada: Canadian Council on Animal Care.

CEC (2006). *Appendix A of the European Convention for the Protection of Vertebrate Animals Used for Experimental and Other Scientific Purposes*. Guidelines for Accommodation and Care of Animals. Strasbourg, France: Council of Europe.

Chamove, A. and Moodie, E. (1990). Are alarming events good for captive monkeys? *Applied Animal Behaviour Science* 276: 169–176.

Close, B., Bannister, K., Baumans, V. et al. (1996). Recommendations for euthanasia of experimental animals. Part 1. *Laboratory Animals* 30: 293–316.

Close, B., Bannister, K., Baumans, V. et al. Recommendations for euthanasia of experimental animals. Part 2. *Laboratory Animals* 31: 1–32.

Council of Europe. (2009). European Convention ETS 123 for the Protection of Animals Used for Experimental and other Scientific Purposes (revised 2007) Appendix A.

Dray, T. (2016). Number of Dogs and Cats in Households Worldwide. *The Nest.* Available at http://pets.thenest.com/number-dogs-cats-households-worldwide-8973.html. Accessed 22 August 2016.

Dudek, B.C., Adams, N., Boice, R., and Abbott, M.E. (1983). Genetic influence on digging behaviours in mice (*Mus muscularis*) in laboratory and seminatural settings. *Journal of Comparative Psychology* 3: 249–259.

Edgar, J.L., Nicol, C.J., and Clark, C.C.A. (2012). Paul ES 2012 measuring empathic responses in animals. *Applied Animal Behaviour Science* 138: 182–193.

Elgar, M.A. (1989). Predator vigilance and group size in mammals and birds: a critical review of the empirical evidence. *Biological Reviews* 64 (1): 13–33.

European Directive 2010/63/EU (86/609/EEC) for the Protection of Animals used for Experimental and other Scientific Purposes (revised 2010) Annex III.

European Pet Food Industry Federation (FEDIAF). (2017). Facts and Figures 2017. Available at http://www.fediaf.org/52-dcs-statistics. Accessed 26 June 2018.

European Union (EU). (2016). Living in the EU. Available at https://europa.eu/european-union/about-eu/figures/living_en. Accessed 22 August 2016.

Farm Animal Welfare Council. (1993). Five Freedoms. Available at http://webarchive.nationalarchives.gov.uk/20121010012427/http://www.fawc.org.uk/freedoms.htm. Accessed 4 May 2018.

FASS (1999). *Guide for the Care and Use of Agricultural Animals in Agricultural Research and Teaching*, 1st rev. ed. Savoy, USA: Federation of Animal Science Societies.

Fox, C., Merali, Z., and Harrison, C. (2006). Therapeutic and protective effect of environmental enrichment against psychogenic and neurogenic stress. *Behavioural Brain Research* 175 (1): 1–8.

Fraser, D. (2008). *Understanding Animal Welfare*. Oxford, UK: UFAW/Wiley Blackwell.

Fraser, D. and Duncan, I.J. (1998). 'Pleasures', 'pains' and animal welfare: Toward a natural history of affect. *Animal Welfare* 7 (4): 383–396.

Fraser, D., Weary, D.M., Pajor, E.A., and Milligan, B.N. (1997). A scientific concept of animal welfare that reflects ethical concerns. *Animal Welfare* 6: 187–205.

Galef, B.G. and Giraldeau, L.A. (2001). Social influences on foraging in vertebrates: causal mechanisms and adaptive functions. *Animal Behaviour* 61: 3–15.

Gentry, A., Clutton-Brock, J., and Groves, C. (2004). The naming of wild animal species and their domestic derivatives. *Journal of Archaeological Science* 31: 645–651.

Goldman Sachs. (2014). Womenomics 4.0: Time to Walk the Talk. Available at http://www.GoldmanSachs.com/our-thinking/pages/macroeconomic-insights-folder/womenomics4-folder/womenomics4-time-to-walk-the-talk.pdf. Accessed 11 May 2018.

Hawkins, P. (2002). Recognizing and assessing pain, suffering and distress in laboratory animals: a survey of current practice in the UK with recommendations. *Laboratory Animals* 36: 378–395.

Hopkins, W.A., Mendonça, M.T., and Congdon, J.D. (1999). Responsiveness of the hypothalamo-pituitary-interranel axis in an amphibian (*Bufo terrestris*) exposed to coal combustion wastes. *Comparative Biochemistry and Physiology – Part C* 122: 191–196.

Hosey, G., Melfi, V., and Pankhurst, S. (eds.) (2009). *Zoo Animals*. Oxford, UK: Oxford University Press.

Hubrecht, R. and Kirkwood, J. (eds.) *The UFAW Handbook on the Care and Management of Laboratory and Other Research Animals*. Oxford, UK: UFAW/Wiley.

International Association for the Study of Pain (IASP). (2015). IASP Taxonomy. Available at http://www.iasp-pain.org/Taxonomy#Pain. Accessed 2 December 2015.

International Union for the Conservation of Nature (IUCN). (2016). *The IUCN Red List of Threatened Species*. www.iucnredlist.org. Accessed 22 August 2016.

Kikusui, T., Winslow, J.T., and Mori, Y. (2006). Social buffering: relief from stress and anxiety. *Philosophical Transactions of the Royal Society B* 361: 2215–2228.

Kristensen, A.T. (2008). Companion animals. In: *Ethics of Animal Use* (ed. P. Sandøe and S.B. Christiansen), 119–136. Oxford, UK: Blackwell Publishing.

Leach, M.C., Bowell, V.A., Allan, T.F. et al. (2004). Measurement of aversion to determine humane methods of anaesthesia and euthanasia. *Animal Welfare* 13: S77–S86.

Leach, M., Raj, M., and Morton, D. (2005). Aversiveness of carbon dioxide. *Laboratory Animals* 39 (4): 452–453.

Liang, Y.F. and Terashima, S.I. (1993). Physiological properties and morphological characteristics of cutaneous and mucosal mechanical nociceptive neurons with A-δ peripheral axons in the trigeminal ganglia of crotaline snakes. *Journal of Comparative Neurology* 328 (1): 88–102.

Lucas, M., Ilin, Y., Anunu, R. et al. (2014). Long-term effects of controllability or the lack of it on coping abilities and sress resilience in the rat. *Stress* 17 (5): 423–430.

Machin, K.L. (1999). Amphibian Pain and analgesia. *Journal of Zoo and Wildlife Medicine* 30 (1): 2–10.

Maier, S.F. and Watkins, L.R. (2005). Stress controllability and learned helplessness: the roles of the dorsal raphe nucleus, serotonin and corticotrophin-releasing factor. *Neuroscience and Biobehavioral Reviews* 21: 699–703.

Manteca, X., Villalba, J.J., Atwood, S.B. et al. (2008). Is dietary choice important to animal welfare? *Journal of Veterinary Behavior-Clinical Applications and Research* 3: 229–239.

Mason, G., CLubb, R., Latham, N., and Vickery, S. (2007). Why and how should we use environmental enrichment to tackle stereotypic behaviour? *Applied Animal Behaviour Science* 102: 163–188.

Mason, G.J. (1991). Stereotypy: A critical review. *Animal Behaviour* 41: 1015–1038.

McKenna, M.C. and Bell, S.G. (1997). *Classification of Mammals above the Species Level*. Columbia, USA: Columbia University Press.

Meehan, C.L. and Mench, J.A. (2007). The challenge of challenge: can problem solving opportunities enhance animal welfare? *Applied Animal Behaviour Science* 102: 246–261.

Mellen, J.D. and MacPhee, M.S. (2001). Philosphy of environmental enrichment: past, present and future. *Zoo Biology* 20: 21–226.

Mellor, D., Patterson-Kane, E., and Stafford, K.J. (2009). *The Sciences of Animal Welfare*. Oxford, UK: UFAW/Wiley-Blackwell.

Mench, J.A. and Mason, G. (1997). Behaviour. In: *Animal Welfare* (ed. M.C. Appleby and B.O. Hughes), 127–141. Wallingford: CABI.

Mendl, M. (1999). Performing under pressure: stress and cognitive function. *Applied Animal Behaviour Science* 65: 221–244.

Mepham. B., Kaiser, M., Thorstensen, E. et al. (2006). *Ethical Matrix Manual* ECCR. Available at www.ethicaltools.info. Accessed 27 May 2018.

Mintline, E.M., Stewart, M., Rogers, A.R. et al. (2013). Play behavior as an indicator of animal welfare: disbudding in dairy calves. *Applied Animal Behaviour Science* 144: 22–30.

Moberg, G.P. (1999). When does stress become distress? *Laboratory Animals* 28 (4): 422–426.

Moberg, G.P. (2000). Biological response to stress: implications for animal welfare. In: *The Biology of Animal Stress* (ed. G.P. Moberg and J.A. Mench). Wallingford, UK: CAB International.

Mogil, J.S. (1999). The genetic mediation of individual differences in sensitivity to pain and its inhibition. *Proceedings of the National Academy of Sciences* 96: 7744–7751.

Mogil, J.S., Wilson, S.G., Bon, K. et al. (1999). Heritability of nociception I. Responses of eleven inbred mouse strains on twelve measures of nociception. *Pain* 80: 67–82.

Mohammed, A.H., Zhu, S.W., Darmopil, S. et al. (2002). Environmental enrichment and the brain. In: *Progress in Brain Research* (ed. M.A. Hoffman, G.J. Boer, A.J.G.D. Holtmaat, et al.), 109–133. Amsterdam, The Netherlands: Elsevier Science BV.

New Zealand Companion Animal Council (NZCAC). (2011). Companion Animals in New Zealand. Available at http://www.pijaccanada.com/en/commonDocs/Membership/IndustryStats/New%20Zealand%20Companion%20Animals%20in%20NZ%20Report%202011.pdf. Accessed 27 November 2014.

Newberry, R.C. (1995). Environmental enrichment: increasing the biological relevance of captive environments. *Applied Animal Behaviour Science* 44: 229–243.

NRC (National Research Council) (US) Committee on Recognition and Alleviation of Distress in Laboratory Animals (2008). *Recognition and Alleviation of Distress in Laboratory Animals*. Washington, D.C: National Academies Press.

NRC (National Research Council) (US) Committee on Recognition and Alleviation of Distress in Laboratory Animals (2011). *Guide for the Care and Use of Laboratory Animals*, 8e. Washington, DC: The National Academies Press.

Palme, R. (2012). Monitoring stress hormone metabolites as a useful, non-invasive tool for welfare assessment in farm animals. *Animal Welfare* 21: 331–337.

Panksepp, J. (2011). Cross-species affective neuroscience decoding of the primal affective experiences of humans and related animals. *PLoS One* 6 (8): e21236. doi: 10.1371/journal.pone.0021236.

Parker, R.A. and Yeates, J.W. (2012). Assessment of quality of life in equine patients. *Equine Veterinary Journal* 44 (2): 244–249.

Pet Food Institute (PFI). (2014). Cat and Dog Population. Available at http://www.petfoodinstitute.org/?page=PetPopulation. Accessed 27 November 2014.

Pet Food Manufacturers Association (PFMA). (2014). Pet Population Statistics. Available from www.pfma.org.uk/pet-population-2014. Accessed 27 November 2014.

Pressman, S. and Cohen, S. (2005). Does positive affect influence health? *Psychological Bulletin* 131: 925–971.

Roush, R.S., Burkhardt, R., Converse, L. et al. (1992). Comment on "Are alarming events food for captive monkeys?". *Applied Animal Behaviour Science* 33: 291–293.

RSPCA (2011). *Good Practice for Humane Killing: Supplementary Resources for Members of Local Ethical Review Processes*. Horsham, UK: RSPCA.

Sambrook, T.D. and Buchanan-Smith, H.M. (1997). Control and complexity in novel object enrichment. *Animal Welfare* 6: 207–216.

Sapolsky, R.M., Romero, L.M., and Munck, A.U. (2000). How do glucocorticoids influence stress responses? Integrating permissive, suppressive, stimulatory, and preparative actions. *Endocrine Reviews* 21 (1): 55–89.

Selye, H. (1975). Homeostasis and heterostasis. In: *Trauma* (ed. S.B. Day), 25–29. Boston: Springer.

Serpell, J.A. (1986). *In the Company of Animals*. Oxford, UK: Blackwell.

Seyfarth, R.M. (2003). Cheney DL. (2003). Signallers and receivers in animal communication. *Annual Review of Psychology* 54: 145–173.

Shape of Enrichment (2013). Available at www.enrichment.org. Accessed 27 November 2014.

Shi, Y. and Yokoyama, S. (2003). Molecular analysis of the evolutionary significance of ultraviolet vision in vertebrates. *Proceedings of the National Academy of Sciences of the United States of America* 100: 8308–8313.

Sneddon, L.U. (2011). Pain perception in fish: Evidence and implications for the use of fish. *Journal of Consciousness Studies* 18: 209–229.

Sneddon, L.U. (2013). Do painful sensations and fear exist in fish? In: *Animal Suffering: From Law to Science* (ed. T. Auffret Van Der Kemp and M. Lachance), 93–112. Toronto: Carswell.

Spinka, M., Newbury, R.C., and Bekoff, M. (2001). Mammalian play: Training for the unexpected. *Quarterly Review of Biology* 76: 141–168.

Stolba, A. and Woodgush, D.G.M. (1989). The behaviour of pigs in a semi-natural environment. *Animal Production* 48: 419–425.

Thornton, P.D. and Waterman-Pearson, A.E. (2002). Behavioural responses to castration in lambs. *Animal Welfare* 11 (2): 203–212.

UFAW. (2016). Genetic disease website. www.ufaw.org.uk/genetic-welfare-problems-intro/genetic-welfare-problems-of-companion-animals-intro. Accessed 1 August 2016.

Webster, J. (2005). *Animal Welfare: Limping Towards Eden*. Oxford, UK: UFAW/Wiley-Blackwell.

Webster, J. (2011a). *Management and Welfare of Farm Animals: The UFAW Farm Handbook*, 5e. Oxford, UK: UFAW/Wiley-Blackwell.

Webster, J. (2011b). Husbandry and animal welfare. In: *Management and Welfare of Farm Animals: The UFAW Farm Handbook* (ed. J. Wester), 1–30. Oxford, UK: UFAW/Wiley-Blackwell.

Wemelsfelder, F., Hunter, T.E.A., Mendl, M.T., and Lawrence, A.B. (2001). Assessing the 'whole animal': a free choice profiling approach. *Animal Behaviour* 62: 209–220.

Wildpro. (2015). *Wildpro – the electronic encyclopaedia and library for wildlife*. Available at http://wildpro.twycrosszoo.org/List_Vols/Wildpro_Gen_Cont.htm. Accessed 13 June 2015.

Wiepkema, P.R. and Koolhas, J.M. (1993). Stress and animal welfare. *Animal Welfare* 2: 195–218.

Wiltschko, W. and Wiltschko, R. (2005). Magnetic orientation and magnetoreception in birds and other animals. *Journal of Comparative Physiology A* 191: 675–693.

Yeates, J. (2010). Breeding for pleasure: the value of pleasure and pain in evolution and animal welfare. *Animal Welfare* 19 (Suppl): 29–38.

Yeates, J. and Main, D.C.J. (2008). Positive welfare: a review. *The Veterinary Journal* 175: 293–300.

Zenoaq. (2008). Recent Pet Stats for Japan. Available at http://www.zenoaq.jp/english-test/aij/0804.html. Accessed 11 July 2018.

Carnivorans (*Carnivora*)

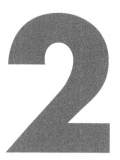

James Yeates

2.1 History and Context

2.1.1 Common Natural History

Carnivora is a mammalian order of about 300 carnivoran species (Table 2.1). They are divided into 'catlike' (*Feliformia*) and 'doglike' (*Caniformia*) suborders, differentiated by their ear anatomy. Carnivorans are found in a wide range of habitats, including deserts (e.g. fennecs [*Vulpes zerda*]), forests (e.g. kinkajou [*Potos flavus*]), savannah (e.g. meerkats [*Suricata suricatta*]), and polar tundra (e.g. arctic foxes [*Vulpes lagopus*]), plus several species have adapted to urban environments (e.g. racoons [*Procyon lotor*] and red foxes [*Vulpes vulpes*]). Several species have been introduced by humans into new areas, usually for sport or pest control or by accidental release, where they may predate on, compete with, or spread disease to native species.

Catlike carnivorans are usually obligate carnivores who stalk or ambush a variety of vertebrate and invertebrate prey. In contrast, several doglike carnivorans also obtain a considerable proportion of their food by opportunistic scavenging. Many doglike carnivorans are actually omnivorous (e.g. North American racoons [*P. lotor*]) or even

Companion Animal Care and Welfare: The UFAW Companion Animal Handbook,
First Edition. Edited by James Yeates.
© 2019 Universities Federation for Animal Welfare. Published 2019 by John Wiley & Sons Ltd.

Table 2.1 Examples of Carnivorans kept as companion animals.

Catlike carnivores (*Feliformia*)	Doglike carnivores (*Caniformia*)
Domestic cats (*Felis silvestris catus*; Chapter 3)	Domestic dogs (*Canis familiaris*; Chapter 4)
Bobcats (*Lynx rufus*)	Coatis (especially *Nasua* spp.)
Caracal (*Caracal caracal*)	Fennecs (*Vulpes zerda*)
Genets (*Viverrinae*)	Ferrets (*Mustela putorius furo*; Chapter 5)
Jungle cats (*Felis chaus*)	Grey wolves (*Canis lupus*)
Meerkats (*Suricata suricatta*)	Kinkajous (*Potos flavus*)
Ocelots (*Leopardus pardalis*)	North American Racoons (e.g. *Procyon lotor*)
Servals (*Leptailurus serval*)	Racoon dogs (*Nyctereutes procyonoides*)
	Ringtail cats (*Bassariscus astutus*)

herbivorous (e.g. kinkajous). Nevertheless, most carnivorans share anatomical adaptations for hunting and eating prey such as carnassial teeth, simple stomachs, claws (which are retractable for catlike carnivorans), binocular and good low-intensity 'night' vision, and partially fused forearm bones to improve power and speed. Many carnivorans range widely, and even those who burrow usually spend considerable time outside (e.g. fennecs). A few carnivorans hibernate (e.g. racoon dogs).

Some carnivorans are relatively solitary and secretive and avoid meeting other individuals even when their ranges overlap, except for mating. Other carnivorans live in pairs (e.g. racoon dogs) or larger groups (e.g. meerkats, Van Staaden 1994). These often collaborate in hunting, vigilance, defence, and care of juveniles and use highly developed vocal and behavioural repertoires and a variety of senses to communicate, including scent marking and vocalisations. Social structures are varied, often complicated and precisely adapted to the ecosystem and the food niche in which these species evolved (e.g. meerkats, Clutton-Brock et al. 2004). Carnivorans give birth to live young and provide various degrees of parental care, usually largely from the mother, although some canids may provide paternal care, sometimes with additional care from older offspring in the group.

2.1.2 Common Domestic History

Carnivoran species have different histories of captive management and domestication. Carnivorans have rarely been farmed for meat (except dogs), but they are farmed for fur (e.g. American mink [*Neovison vison*] and foxes [*V. vulpes*]) and musk gland chemicals for perfumes (e.g. civet). Others have been kept for hunting and pest control (e.g. smooth coated otters [*Lutrogale perspicillata*]).

Cats and dogs are now popular pets in many countries. This familiarity risks owners assuming they know all about the animals' care without needing any research and assuming that catlike or doglike species can be cared for similarly. Many carnivorans are kept in shelters and rehomed through animal-protection agencies.

Some pet species are nearly all caught from wild populations; others have been captive bred across many generations; and a few may even have initially interacted with human environments voluntarily (e.g. dogs, cats, and ringtail cats). Some species are bred commercially, the offspring may be hand-reared, and breeder registers have been established for several species (e.g. fennecs). In some populations, selective breeding has changed body shapes and behaviour (e.g. silver foxes) or colour varieties (e.g. mink), thereby creating a variety of 'types' or 'breeds'. There has also been some hybridisation, such as 'Bengals' (hybrids of domestic cats [*Felis sylvestris catus*] and Asian leopard cats [*Prionailurus bengalensis bengalensis*]), 'khonoriks' (hybrids of European mink [*Mustela lutreola*] with European polecats [*Mustela putorius*]), and 'coydogs' (hybrids of coyote [*Canis latrans*] and domestic dogs).

2.2 Principles of Carnivoran Care

2.2.1 Diets

Although not all carnivorans are carnivorous, many do require a source of meat-based protein. For those animals, raw whole cadavers may provide more naturalistic food, including organs, muscle, bones, and intestinal contents. However this method of feeding can risk parasite transfer, infections, and intestinal impactions, and owners may be unable to provide a balanced diet of this food. Commercial food preparations may reduce these risks, so long as they are appropriately formulated for the particular species. Foods formulated for dogs or cats (or humans) may lead to malnutrition when fed to other carnivorans. Some may be willing to eat unsuitable human scraps (e.g. racoons). Carnivorans can become obese from excessive energy, particularly when combined with unnaturally sedentary lifestyles, and some can develop high levels of cholesterol (e.g. meerkats, Allan et al. 2006). Most species do not have validated body condition scores, but owners can regularly weigh and monitor changes, noting that some wild carnivorans may have beneficial seasonal variations in body condition (e.g. American mink, Dunstone 1993).

Carnivorans obtain their food through active and complex behavioural sequences, including ranging, tracking, stalking, waiting, catching, immobilising, killing, and disembowelling. When carnivorans are not hunting for food (e.g. when kept inside homes), these experiences should be simulated through enrichments that allow the relevant behaviours (e.g. kinkajous: Blount and Taylor 2000; Johnson et al. 2005). These should include opportunities to find food and to play, ideally ending in the consumption of some food. Some animals are also motivated to chew bones or man-made chews, which may improve dental health.

Although carnivorans obtain some water from food, all animals should be provided ad libitum fresh water. Most can drink from still water (e.g. in bowls), although many prefer to drink running water (e.g. from fountains or directly from taps).

2.2.2 Environments

Carnivorans often need to be kept contained to prevent predation of native species or to comply with local legal constraints. However, domestic environments usually cannot replicate the spaces that carnivorans are motivated to utilise in ranging and exercise. Correlations between natural range sizes and display of stereotypies such as pacing suggest carnivorans of naturally wide-ranging species need particularly extensive space allowances (Clubb and Mason 2003, 2007). Owners should therefore try to provide as much

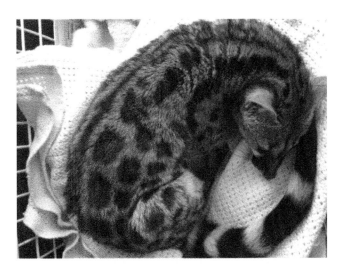

Figure 2.1 Rescued genet in transportation cage (*Source:* courtesy of RSPCA).

safe space as possible. This space should extend in three dimensions because many carnivorans climb (e.g. kinkajous, racoons, raccoon dogs, and stoats) or use vantage points
to monitor their environment (e.g. mongooses), and vigilance behaviour is important to
reduce fear of unseen threats (e.g. meerkats, Clutton-Brock et al. 1999; Manser 1999).
Some animals may also be highly motivated to create burrows, dig, hide food, or swim
(e.g. mink, Warburton and Mason 2003). Several may enjoy exercise for its own sake.

As warm-blooded, furred animals, most carnivorans can regulate their body temperature, so long as they are kept within an appropriate range. Some carnivorans are
more active at night or dawn and dusk and need appropriate light intensities and schedules. Carnivorans can be stressed by particular events (e.g. noises) or unpredictable
change (e.g. moving house or transportation; Figure 2.1). Predator species still need
places to hide when scared, with some (particularly naturally arboreal) animals preferring to hide up high. Their use of smell means they may find unfamiliar or overpower-
ing smells disruptive but familiar smells (e.g. of themselves) or species-specific
pheromones reassuring. Scent-based communication can also affect toileting behaviour
such as spraying, and further disrupting smells (e.g. with perfumed cleaners) can cause
further disturbances. Many carnivorans otherwise choose to, or can be trained to, toilet
in designated areas away from feeding and sleeping areas.

Carnivorans can have highly developed cognitive abilities and actively explore and
interact with their environment. In human homes, this risks them obtaining poisonous
products or human foods (including from closed cupboards or high shelves) or escaping
to become strays or feral animals, placing burdens on rehoming charities or harming
local wildlife. Many carnivorans play with toys but may become rapidly bored with
familiar toys, and so constantly need new toys or toys rotated regularly. Many
carnivorans are also motivated to play with objects that their owners might not consider
toys, for example destroying household objects (although such behaviour may have
many different possible causes).

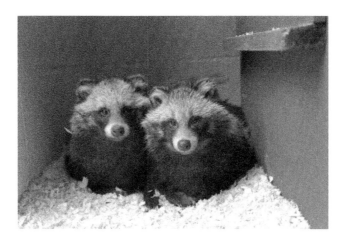

Figure 2.2   Pair of racoon dogs (*Nyctereutes procyonoides*) in captivity (*Source:* courtesy of RSPCA).

2.2.3 Animal Company

Many carnivorans are very sociable, particularly many larger canids (Bekoff et al. 1981), fennecs, and meerkats. Such carnivorans may engage in close physical contact, mutual grooming, and social play. Some may form pairs (Figure 2.2) or complex relationships, being highly aware of, and responding to, each other's behaviour, and many learn from one another (Galef and Giraldeau 2001; e.g. meerkats, Thornton 2008; Thornton and Brock 2011). Such species need adequate company, particularly in early life. Other carnivorans attack or avoid other animals of the same species (e.g. most mustelids), although owners may fail to notice their behaviour or stress. These differences are not simply matters of species; individual differences, particular relationships (e.g. siblings), and resources can affect each animal's motivations to avoid or obtain company.

In any groups, each animal should have plenty of opportunities to avoid and escape one another. Owners need to provide additional resources, suitably located to avoid competition and aggression (although some compatible animals may share food, which is a highly valued resource), and places to hide and escape. Owners also need to match and introduce animals carefully to ensure they are compatible. Introductions may sometimes familiarise animals with one another's smells before actual contact, but conversely, masking smells during introductions may decrease aggression in some animals (e.g. meerkats [*S. suricatta*]). Where an animal of a usually social species responds to other animals by aggression or avoidance, then expert veterinary and behavioural advice should be sought.

As mammals, carnivorans' relationships with their mothers are particularly important, for nutrition, immunity, and learning. Although carnivorans can learn later in life (i.e. this period is not always 'critical'), they may learn best during early 'sensitive periods'. Later learning also risks unpleasant experiences actually making them more sensitive to the presence of other animals. Carnivorans should therefore not be separated from their mother, except in some cases of illness, stress, or mis-mothering. Young animals should certainly not be removed from their mothers when there is not a problem,

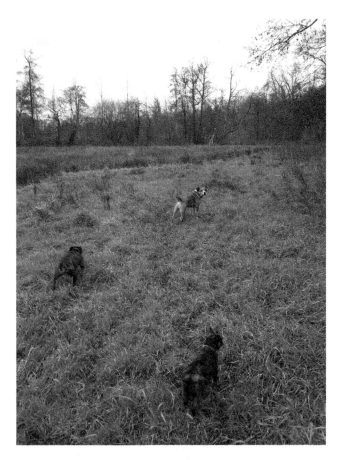

Figure 2.3 Domestic cat (*Felis catus*) accompanying domestic dogs (*Canis lupus*) on a walk (*Source:* courtesy of James Yeates).

purely to establish a bond with humans through hand-rearing (although human contact can be beneficial).

Carnivorans may occasionally form relationships with animals of other species (Figure 2.3). However, others may prey on (or be preyed on by) other species. Being in sight, smell, or hearing of those animals may not only be stressful for the potential prey but may also prove a source of frustration for the carnivorous predator. Some social carnivorans may interact with other species together, including in hunting (e.g. some larger canids) or 'mobbing' predators (e.g. meerkats, Graw and Manser 2007).

2.2.4 Human Interactions

Some carnivorans are motivated to obtain human company, depending on their personal experiences and the quality of that company. Some may also become distressed when they are isolated or separated from particular humans. However, others may find humans or particular individuals frightening. This fear may prompt aggression as a defensive strategy, particularly biting, scratching, and sometimes odour projection (e.g. striped skunks [*Mephitis mephitis*]). Any carnivorans *can* show aggression, depending on their upbringing and treatment, but some seem anecdotally particularly likely to show aggression to humans (e.g. racoons during mating).

Carnivorans' responses to humans partly depend on species; dogs, cats, and ferrets have been domesticated over many years, whereas others are effectively captive wild animals even if captive bred. They also often depend on previous interactions. Pleasant contact, especially while they are young, is important for 'taming' wild animals and 'socialising' domestic ones. If carnivorans are kept as pets, they need adequate interactions while young (without separating them from their mothers too early). Training carnivorans can also facilitate handling and other interactions, for example, training to walk on a lead can allow animals to be taken outside with a lower risk of escape. Training can also be rewarding in itself, so long as it is based on rewarding the desired behaviour. For all species, training should be done using reward-based methods (regardless of views as to how animals interact in the wild or in other captive populations). Owners should not assume their pets can understand them, even if they do seem particularly skilled at responding appropriately to human behaviour. Carnivorans should always be treated in ways appropriate to their species, even if they tolerate a degree of inappropriate anthropomorphic interaction (Figure 2.4).

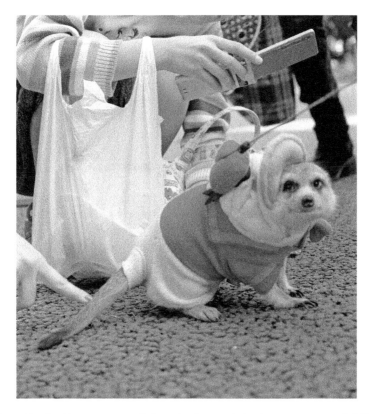

Figure 2.4 Meerkat (*Suricata suricatta*) dressed in human clothes (*Source*: courtesy of Phillip Wilson).

Table 2.2 Examples of veterinary specialisations specifically relevant to carnivorans kept as companion animals (see also Chapter 1).

Recognising organisation	Example veterinary specialties
American Veterinary Medical Association	American Board of Veterinary Practitioners in Canine and Feline Practice
	American Board of Veterinary Practitioners in Exotic Companion Mammal Practice
European Board of Veterinary Specialisation	European College of Zoological Medicine
Australian and New Zealand College of Veterinary Scientists	Australian and New Zealand College of Veterinary Scientists: Unusual Pets Chapter

Note: There are also many groups specialising in particular aspects of canine or feline medicine and surgery.

2.2.5 Health

Some diseases are common to several carnivorans species. Viral diseases include distemper, herpes, calici, parvo, and rabies virus infections; bacterial infections include zoonotic diseases such as tuberculosis, campylobacter, and salmonella; and parasites include gastrointestinal worms, fleas, mites, and lice. In many cases, prevention, and treatment used in common species may be used in others (e.g. some inactivated cat or dog vaccinations against distemper, rabies, panluecopaenia, herpes, or calicivirus). However, similar pathogens may cause different symptoms and need different treatment, and some dog or cat drugs may be harmful to some other species (e.g. some live or combination vaccines). All carnivorans should receive regular health checks from specialist veterinary surgeons where possible and appropriate (Table 2.2).

Carnivorans may also experience dental problems and should receive regular dental checks and preventive care as appropriate. Some carnivorans also need regular grooming and nail trimming, although nails should usually be kept at the right length by sufficient exercise and scratching opportunities. Many carnivorans should be routinely neutered when necessary to avoid unwanted pregnancies, straying, or the frustration of unmet sexual motivations, using either surgical or chemical methods. However, there are also risks from neutering such as surgical complications or reduced confidence through decreased testosterone. Neutering should not be used to stop a behaviour that is actually caused by inadequate care (e.g. to reduce aggression as a result of fear or incompatible animals). Similarly, no pet carnivorans should undergo surgery purely to improve the ease with which they can be kept as pets. Surgeries to remove vocal cords, claws, scent glands, or other body parts are acceptable only for specific medical reasons and in the animals' own interests.

2.2.6 Euthanasia

The best method of euthanasia of carnivorans is usually an overdose of pentobarbitone injected into a vein because most carnivorans have relatively accessible veins (Table 2.3). Where the animal would be stressed by close restraint, previous sedation may be

Table 2.3 Methods of euthanasia suitable for (some) Carnivorans kept as companion animals.

Method	Restraint required	Welfare benefits	Welfare risks
Anaesthetic overdose injected into a vein	Very high	Very fast loss of consciousness	Pain from chemical in tissues if vein missed
Head or brain trauma	None to Moderate	Instantaneous if accurate	Severe pain if inaccurate

necessary, and painkillers can also be beneficial where euthanasia solutions are irritating to tissues. Because of their large size, neck dislocation is usually impossible, but for larger carnivorans, trauma to the brain (e.g. accurate use of a firearm or captive bolt) may cause instantaneous brain death and can reduce handling. Carbon dioxide (CO_2) and hypoxic gas mixtures appear to cause aversion (e.g. mink, Cooper et al. 1998; Raj and Mason 1999) and should be avoided; similarly drowning is unacceptable even for large numbers of carnivorans.

2.3 Signs of Carnivoran Welfare

2.3.1 Pathophysiological Signs

As well as measures of health, heart rate and respiratory rate may also indicate short-term stress. Biochemical and haematological measures of stress include increased levels of catecholamines, corticosteroids, glucose, and 'stress leucograms'. However, there are only limited data available on normal ranges or clinical guidance on the use physiological measures for many species (except cats and dogs), so the use of such measures would be largely speculative.

2.3.2 Behavioural Signs

Social carnivorans may show clear behavioural signals to elicit beneficial responses from other animals. However, these signs still need to be interpreted correctly by human carers (Table 2.4). For example, particular vocalisations (e.g. growls), postural changes, raised hair, displayed teeth, or attacks may be associated with aggression, but there are a number of experiences that could underlie such behaviour, including pain and fear. Social withdrawal, aggression, or anorexia may indicate depression or illness. Similarly play may reduce if animals are ill or stressed (e.g. mongooses, Hinton and Dunn 1967). Social carnivorans may have specific alarm calls (e.g. meerkats, Manser et al. 2002; Hollén and Manser 2006). Carnivorans may also show 'abnormal' or excessive behaviours such as overgrooming; self-trauma; eating faeces, soil, or plants; excessive drinking; and inappropriate urination or marking, although these signs may be difficult to distinguish from normal, appropriate behaviours. Repetitive behaviours may also suggest a variety of welfare problems (e.g. for fennecs, Carlstead 1991).

Table 2.4 Key behavioural signs of possible welfare compromises in Carnivorans.

Aspect of behaviour	Specific responses	Example potential welfare issues
Altered activity or responsiveness	Increased vigilance or activity Attention to particular threats Startling Reaction on palpation or withdrawal of body part from contact Lethargy, immobility, or decreased mobility (e.g. less climbing or jumping)	Fear, agitation, pain, or illness
Avoidance	Hiding Immobility or 'freezing' Looking smaller Playing dead Preparation for flight (e.g. arched back) 'Wriggling' during handling Flight (jumping, running)	Fear or pain
Altered posture or expression	Pilo-erection Lowered body, head, or tail position Altered ear position (e.g. lowered) Displayed teeth Yawning Tense jaw Tail flicks (e.g. flicks of tail end or slow wags)	Fear, response to threats, or pain
Vocalisations	Barking, hissing, or growling Whining Alarm calls	Fear, response to threats, signalling, social separation, or excitement
Altered maintenance or other behaviours (short or long term)	Increased respiratory rate or panting Trembling Wide pupils Sweating paws Reduced appetite Increased salivation or swallowing Increased drinking or urination Altered toileting behaviour Increased or decreased grooming	Fear, distress, stress, heat, fatigue, illness, pain, itchiness, or excitement

Table 2.4 (Continued)

Aspect of behaviour	Specific responses	Example potential welfare issues
Attack or preattack behaviours	Altered time spent resting or sleeping Reduced time spent playing or hunting Raised paw to strike 'Symbolic' lunges Spraying urine, scent, or faeces Biting	Fear, pain, or aggression
Specific local signs of local pain	Hunched posture or tucked up abdomen Rigid posture Biting or scratching a specific area Lameness	Pain

All behavioural responses may also indicate other welfare issues than those listed; some behaviours in some contexts may not indicate a welfare issue and the absence of any particular sign in any individual does not mean they are not experiencing that welfare compromise.

2.4 Action Plan for Improving Carnivoran Welfare Worldwide

A key priority is to reduce the numbers of strays and relinquished animals needing rehoming (or euthanasia). Many rehoming charities focus on dogs and cats, suggesting that these are priority species, whereas rarer carnivorans may be difficult to rehome to appropriate owners, especially if they are species that are generally unsuitable to be kept as pets. All breeders need to ensure they do not breed too many animals and ensure future owners make good decisions and can meet the needs of carnivorans that may differ from those of animals with which they are familiar.

Society needs to ensure that animals deliberately bred are not from an overly restricted gene pool, whereas buyers and sellers of carnivorans need to tackle owners' biases that prevent them making rational decisions about what animals to keep. This latter is especially important for prospective owners who want particular popular species or breeds for reasons that ignore any associated welfare issues, who respond to emotive 'cute' appearances of many juvenile carnivorans, or who seek exoticism or novelty. Potential owners should question their own desire for a carnivoran pets, ensuring they obtain all the necessary information and explicitly evaluate the animals' compatibility with their lives *before* choosing any individual animals. More widely, the media and celebrities should also avoid promoting cultural prejudices towards exotic or cute species, where they are unsuitable as pets.

The seller or rehomer has an important role in helping to ensure good welfare. Breeders and vendors should check they are satisfied that the new owner has the right motivations, knowledge, and commitment *before* handing over an animal. Sellers should provide adequate information, particularly regarding dietary and social needs. Sellers of more 'exotic' animals should also make it clear to potential owners that although exotic carnivorans are 'doglike' or 'catlike', they have not been domesticated over millennia, that they may be very different to dogs or cats, and that there is much less information available about their care and professional services to assist owners. Governments or pet shops could also limit carnivoran ownership to carnivoran species that are suitable and safe as pets.

Bibliography

Allan, K.J., Waters, M., Ashton, D.G., and Patterson-Kane, J.C. (2006). Meningeal cholesterol granulomas in two meerkats (Suricata suricatta). *Veterinary Record* 158 (18): 636.

Allen, M.E., Oftedal, O.T., and Baer, D.J. (1996). The feeding and nutrition of carnivores. In: *Wild Mammals in Captivity: Principles and Techniques* (ed. D.G. Kleinman), 139–147. Chicago, USA: University of Chicago Press.

Bekoff, M., Diamond, J., and Mitton, J. (1981). Life-history patterns and sociality in canids: body size, reproduction, and behavior. *Oecologia* 50: 386–390.

Bekoff, M., Daniels, T.J., and Gittleman, J.L. (1984). Life history patterns and the comparative social ecology of carnivores. *Annual Review of Ecology and Systematics* 15: 191–232.

Blount, J.D. and Taylor, N.J. (2000). The relative effectiveness of manipulable feeders and olfactory enrichment for Kinkajous. *International Zoo Yearbook* 37 (1): 381–394.

Bush, M. and Gray, C.W. (1975). Dental prophylaxis in carnivores. *International Zoo Yearbook* 15: 223.

Carlstead, K. (1991). Husbandry of the Fennec fox: Fennecus zerda: environmental conditions influencing stereotypic behaviour. *International Zoo Yearbook* 30 (1): 202–207.

Clubb, R. and Mason, G. (2003). Captivity effects on wide-ranging carnivores. *Nature* 425: 473–474.

Clubb, R. and Mason, G.J. (2007). Natural behavioural biology as a risk factor in carnivore welfare: how analysing species differences could help zoos improve enclosures. *Applied Animal Behaviour Science* 102: 303–328.

Clutton-Brock, T.H., O'Riain, M.J., Brotherton, P.N.M. et al. (1999). Selfish sentinels in cooperative mammals. *Science* 284 (5420): 1640–1644.

Clutton-Brock, T.H., Russell, A.F., and Sharpe, L.L. (2004). Behavioural tactics of breeders in cooperative meerkats. *Animal Behaviour* 68: 1029–1040.

Cooper, J., Mason, G., and Raj, M. (1998). Determination of the aversion of farmed mink (*Mustela vison*) to carbon dioxide. *Veterinary Record* 143: 359–361.

Creel, S. and Macdonald, D. (1995). Sociality, group-size, and reproductive suppression among carnivores. *Advances in the Study of Behaviour* 4: 203–257.

Dempsey, J.L., Hanna, S.J., Asa, C.S., and Bauman, K.L. (2009). Nutrition and behavior of fennec foxes (*Vulpes zerda*). *Veterinary Clinics of North America: Exotic Animal Practice* 12 (2): 299–312.

Doolan, S.P. and MacDonald, D.W. (1996 Aug 1). Diet and foraging behaviour of group-living meerkats, Suricata suricatta, in the southern Kalahari. *Journal of Zoology* 239 (4): 697–716.

Dunstone, N. (1993). *The Mink*. London, UK: T and AD Poyser.

Galef, B.G. and Giraldeau, L.A. (2001). Social influences on foraging in vertebrates: causal mechanisms and adaptive functions. *Animal Behaviour*. 61: 3–15.

Graw, B. and Manser, M.B. (2007). The function of mobbing in cooperative meerkats. *Animal Behaviour* 74: 507–517.

Hinton, H.E. and Dunn, A.M.S. (1967). *Mongooses, Their Natural History and Behaviour*. Oliver and Boyd Ltd: London, UK.

Hollén, L.I. and Manser, M.B. (2006). Ontogeny of alarm call responses in meerkats, *Suricata suricatta*: the roles of age, sex and nearby conspecifics. *Animal Behaviour* 72: 1345–1353.

Johnson, S., Pullen, K., Robbins, A. and Nicklin, A. (2005). Kinkajou environmental enrichment and activity levels. In *Proceedings of the 7th Annual Symposium on Zoo Research, Twycross Zoo, Warwickshire, UK, 7-8th July 2005* (pp. 136–141). London: British and Irish Association of Zoos and Aquariums.

Manser, M.B. (1999). Response of foraging group members to sentinel calls in suricates, *Suricata suricatta*. *Proceedings of the Royal Society of London B* 266: 1013–1019.

Manser, M.B., Seyfarth, R.M., and Cheney, D.L. (2002). Suricate alarm calls signal predator class and urgency. *Trends in Cognitive Sciences* 6: 55–57.

Mason, G., Cooper, J., and Clarebrough, C. (2001). Frustrations of fur-farmed mink. *Nature* 410: 35–36.

O'Regan, H.J. and Kitchener, A.C. (2005). The effects of captivity on the morphology of captive, domesticated and feral mammals. *Mammal Review* 35: 215–230.

Raj, M. and Mason, G. (1999). Reaction of farmed mink (*Mustela vison*) to argon-induced hypoxia. *Veterinary Record* 145: 736–737.

Thornton, A. (2008). Social learning about novel foods in young meerkats. *Animal Behaviour* 76 (4): 1411–1421.

Thornton, A. and Clutton-Brock, T. (2011). Social learning and the development of individual and group behaviour in mammal societies. *Philosophical Transactions of the Royal Society B* 366 (1567): 978–987.

Van Staaden, M.J. (1994). Suricata suricatta. *Mammalian Species* 483: 1–8.

Warburton, H. and Mason, G. (2003). Is out of sight out of mind? The effects of resource cues on motivation in mink, Mustela vison. *Animal Behaviour* 65: 755–762.

Cats (*Felis silvestris catus*)

3

Irene Rochlitz and James Yeates

3.1 History and Context

3.1.1 Natural History

Domestic cats (*Felis silvestris catus*, sometimes classified as *F. catus*) are felid members of the class Mammalia, order Carnivora, and family Felidae. Domestic cats are descended from the 'North African' or 'Near Eastern' wildcat (*Felis silvestris libyca*). North African wildcats are relatively common across northern and western Africa (Driscoll et al. 2007). There are also many populations of feral *F. s. catus* in most continents. The domestic cat has not been included in the IUCN Red List, but *F. s. catus* is classified as of 'Least Concern'.

North African wildcats are most active at night, whereas feral domestic cats hunt by day and night. Both North African wildcats and feral cats prey upon small rodents, especially mice, birds, rabbits, and occasionally reptiles, depending on the geographical area. They spend a significant proportion of their time hunting to catch sufficient food to survive because not all attempts are successful. Feral cats usually spend most of their time in their territory: eating, sleeping, and playing in the core area and performing marking behaviours in the peripheral territory (Figure 3.1). They then travel

Companion Animal Care and Welfare: The UFAW Companion Animal Handbook,
First Edition. Edited by James Yeates.
© 2019 Universities Federation for Animal Welfare. Published 2019 by John Wiley & Sons Ltd.

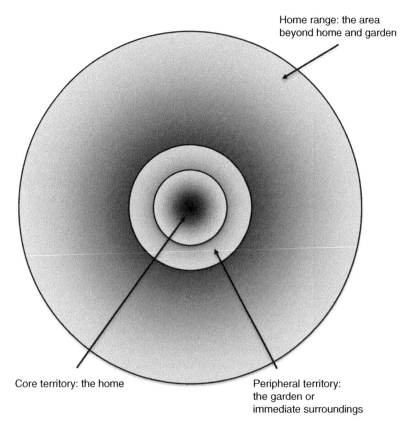

Home range: the area
beyond home and garden

Core territory: the home

Peripheral territory:
the garden or
immediate surroundings

Figure 3.1 Territory and home range. The area where a pet cat lives and travels divided into a territory (core and periphery) and a home range (positions and proportions not to scale – for illustration only).

throughout a wider range to find mates and food, usually bringing prey back to eat in the safety of the core territory. The size of this range can vary depending on factors such as local conditions (rural, suburban, or urban), cat population density, and gender. Consequently, different studies have found various average and maximum range sizes, although most find that feral cats range across multiple hectares.

North African wildcats are largely solitary-living animals. Feral cats also hunt alone but often form groups of mainly female relatives around food sources (Macdonald et al. 1987, 2000), and females may cooperate extensively in rearing kittens (Macdonald et al. 2000). Some individuals may form close relationships, especially if they are familiar and related (Figure 3.2), which they maintain through sleeping in close contact, licking one another's head and neck, touching noses, and rubbing foreheads, cheeks, flanks, or tails together (Bradshaw et al. 2012; Brown and Bradshaw 2014). Mating can be promiscuous, with queens occasionally gestating multiple litters simultaneously or having litters fathered by multiple males.

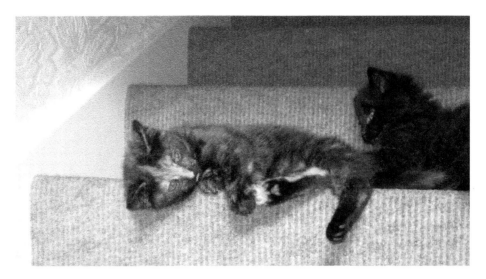

Figure 3.2 Related kittens playing. Familiar sibling cats who have formed a close relationship with one another (*Source:* courtesy of K. McLennan).

Vocalisation between cats is infrequent (Brown and Bradshaw 2014). Cats communicate remotely using long-lasting scent marking via urine spraying, urination, defaecation, scratching claws, and rubbing skin, although the information transmitted by these signals is largely unknown. Such scents appear to be in secretions from specialised glands found particularly on the chin, cheeks, forehead, and feet (e.g. rubbed or scratched onto inanimate objects) and ear and tail base (e.g. rubbed onto other cats). Because of this remote communication, feral cats are usually able to maintain an adequate distance between themselves and avoid physical conflicts.

3.1.2 Domestic History

The initial association between humans and cats probably started around 12 500 to 11 500 years ago at various locations in the 'Fertile Crescent' of Western Asia (O'Brien et al. 2008), when *F. s. libyca* were attracted to grain stores to prey on rodents, and some of them became tame (Cameron-Beaumont et al. 2002). As well as being used to control rodents, writings, paintings, and other records show them sharing human activities such as eating and hunting (Serpell 2014). From about 3500 years ago, cats had an important role in Egyptian religions (e.g. associated with the cat-goddess Bastet). Domesticated cats then spread along trade routes to virtually all parts of Asia and Europe. In the seventeenth century they were taken to North America and later to Australia to help settlers control rodent populations.

Cats are now common pets in many Western countries and increasingly popular in many Asian, African, and South American countries. In the United States in 2016, there were around 86 million pet cats in 35% of households (Human Society of the United States [HSUS] 2016). In Australia in 2013, there were approximately 3.3 million cats in 29% of households (Animal Health Alliance (Australia) [AHAA] 2016). In the United Kingdom in recent years, there were more than 8–10 million cats in 17–26% of households (Murray et al. 2010; Westgarth et al. 2010; Pet Food Manufacturers' Association [PFMA] 2015), and in 2014 there were an estimated 72.1 million pet cats in the European Union and 99.2 million in Europe as a whole, within 24% of households (European Pet Food Industry Federation [FEDIAF] 2014).

The terminology used to discuss domestic cats can be confusing and inconsistent. One approach is to divide the population into owned cats confined indoors, owned cats free to roam, and unowned 'community' cats (Sparkes et al. 2013; Rochlitz 2014; Figure 3.3). Community cats are often cared for by certain individuals within a community, who may be more likely to regard themselves as their guardians than owners. Community cats vary across a spectrum of sociability, from well-socialised strays to feral cats who do not tolerate human contact and are resistant to attempts to tame them. In between these two extremes is a range of cats tolerating varying degrees of human presence, contact, or interaction. It is thought that there are at least 1 million community cats in the United Kingdom and between 70 and 90 million in the United States (Levy 2011).

Partly because of community cats, there has been relatively little control over cats' reproduction (Bradshaw et al. 1999). Many of the female community cats are unneutered and mate with feral males (Horsfield 1998). Few owned cats are deliberately bred, with only 6–23% of pet cats being of pedigree breeds, depending on the country (Bradshaw et al. 2012). Cats are therefore unlikely to have undergone major changes

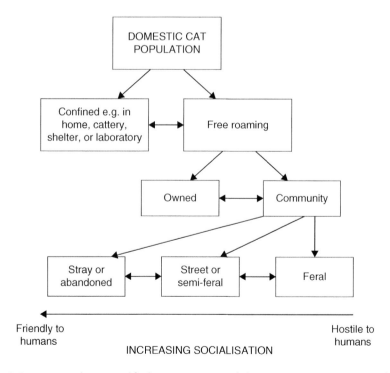

Figure 3.3 Cat population modified. Categorisation of domestic cats (cats may move between categories to another, e.g. with increasing socialisation) (*Source:* Adapted from Sparkes et al. 2013 and Rochlitz 2014).

through deliberate selection. Nevertheless, there may have been some selection pressure to increase cats' tolerance of humans and other cats. For example, one particular product of domestication may be miaowing to elicit human attention because pet cats produce shorter, higher-pitched miaows than feral cats (Yeon et al. 2011) and North African wildcats (Nicastro 2004). Similarly, purring is highly characteristic of domestic cats. The limited amount of pedigree breeding and showing has also produced various different breeds and various colour differences. Breeding has also created hybrids between *F. s. catus* and other species; for example Bengals are hybrids with Asian leopard cats, one of the least tameable of all the Felidae, but which achieves a popular aesthetic appearance of the offspring.

3.2 Determinants of Cat Welfare

3.2.1 Diet

Cats are obligate carnivores, and their nutritional requirements are largely provided by meat (Table 3.1). Cats have specific nutritional requirements for high protein levels, particular amino acids (e.g. taurine for retinal, heart, and reproductive functions and arginine within the urea cycle), fats (e.g. arachidonic acid), vitamins (e.g. vitamin A), and low levels of carbohydrates. Many commercial, especially dry, foods aim to include those necessary components but often also contain significant amounts of carbohydrates. Cats are also able to digest only low levels of lactose, and some are intolerant, so cats should not usually be given unmodified cows' milk. Cats are also unable to

Table 3.1 Nutritional requirements of normal adult cats.

Nutrient	Amount required
Energy density	4.0–5.0 kcal ME/g (16.7–20.9 kJ ME/g)
Protein	30–45% DMB
Taurine	>0.1% DMB
Arginine	1.04% DMB
Fat	10–30% DMB
Fibre	<5% DMB
Carbohydrate	No absolute dietary requirement
Calcium	0.5–1.0% DMB
Phosphorus	0.5–0.8% DMB
Calcium-to-phosphorus ratio	1:1 to 1.5:1 (depending on vitamin D levels and other factors)
Water daily requirement	1.2 × resting energy requirement (approx. 30 × BW kg + 70 mL day^{-1})

Source: Hand and Novotny (2002) and Sturgess and Hurley (2005).
DMB: dry matter basis.
All figures assume animals are of normal physiology, healthy, and non-breeding.

digest cellulose, although some cats deliberately eat grasses or other plants, and small amounts of vegetative matter may be found in prey intestines. Cats should therefore not be kept on vegetarian diets (Case et al. 2010).

In terms of the amount of food, obesity affects approximately 11–40% of pet cats in countries within Western Europe (Colliard et al. 2009; Courcier et al. 2010, 2012), the United States (Scarlett and Donoghue 1998; Lund et al. 2005), and Australia (Robertson 1999). Not all such studies have found the same causes, but risk factors generally include being male, neutered, middle age, fed ad-libitum, inactive, confined indoors, and non-pedigree. Obesity can lead to many welfare compromises such as osteoarthritis and diabetes mellitus (German 2006). Controlled intake and specific commercial diets may help prevent weight gain or promote weight loss, although it can be difficult to prevent a hungry outdoor cat hunting or entering other cats' homes and eating their food.

In terms of the presentation of food, cats are usually offered two or three meals a day, but their preferred pattern of feeding is often for frequent small meals throughout the day and night. Techniques have been devised to increase the time the cat spends in feeding behaviour (Figure 3.4), in particular in performing parts of the predatory sequences before consuming food. Examples include hiding kibble in the environment for the cat to find or putting it in containers with holes for the cat to extract individual pieces and playing with toys such as fishing rods and laser pointers. Such toys should be regularly replaced to maintain interest (Hall et al. 2001), and it seems sensible to ensure that play sometimes ends in a simulated catch and consumption. Allowing cats outside to prey provides excellent dietary enrichment but has significant welfare and ecological impacts upon the live prey (Kays and Dewan 2004), especially because cats may play with their prey before killing them. This may be avoided by keeping cats

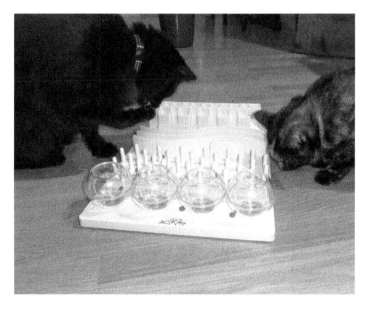

Figure 3.4 Cat feeding activity board. An 'activity board' feeding-enrichment device in which the cats have to make an effort to obtain dry food (*Source:* courtesy of K. McLennan).

indoors either permanently or at specific times when prey is most active (e.g. dawn and dusk). If cats are let out, their collars may be fitted with bells (which make noise as the cat moves), bibs (which interfere with pouncing), colourful collar covers (which alert prey with good colour vision such as birds), or devices that emit ultrasonic noise to alert prey (Nelson et al. 2005; Hall et al. 2015).

Domestic cats can live on the moisture from meat or moist commercial foods alone without drinking. Their kidneys are efficient and can excrete relatively small amounts of highly concentrated urine. Nevertheless, the risks of kidney, lower urinary tract, and metabolic diseases make adequate water intake essential, especially for cats fed dry foods or with particular water requirements as a result of disease, age, or lactation. All cats should therefore be provided with fresh water at all times. Some cats prefer to drink fresh or running water, for example, from running taps and water fountains.

3.2.2 Environment

At a bare minimum, space for cats to express their normal behaviours requires at least 2 m height and 1.5 m² of floor space (Council of Europe 2006). Additional space is provided by shelves. Kessler and Turner (1999b) recommend at least 1.7 m² floor space per cat for group-housed cats in shelters, while ensuring that each cat can maintain sufficient distance from others. The addition of stand-alone shelving can increase the space available for cats' use and may reduce agonistic interactions in groups of cats (Desforges et al. 2016).

Many cats are unrestricted within their owner's whole house and outside. Others are kept permanently indoors, sometimes within just a few rooms, or permanently outdoors, sometimes without any specific shelter provided. The popularity of each option differs considerably between countries. For example, only 8–9% of cats are kept permanently indoors in the United Kingdom (Rochlitz 2005a) compared to 50–60% in the United States (Patronek et al. 1997). Each option has both risks and benefits, which makes it difficult to categorically recommend one or the other (Table 3.2). Cats given outdoor access may generally show less spraying inside the home (Rochlitz 2009), which might be taken as indicating less stress, but this might simply represent that these behaviours are instead performed in the outdoor peripheral territory.

The welfare effects of allowing cats outdoors can depend on the environment (e.g. climate and road traffic), the individual (e.g. experiences and motivation to hunt), the presence of other cats (e.g. in the house or neighbourhood), and whether the cat is neutered (which may reduce the risks of roaming, fighting, some infectious diseases, and pregnancies). Furthermore, when owners are unwilling to keep a cat that performs an undesirable behaviour such as scratching or which urinates indoors, outdoor access may be preferable to declawing or euthanasia. In general, cats should not be confined indoors unless they are used to it, are kept singly or with demonstrably compatible cats, and show no frustration from being contained. Cats should not be allowed outdoors unless they are neutered and microchipped, but ultimately the choice should be tailored to each individual cat and situation. In either case, owners need to ensure the cat's welfare needs are met (Table 3.3).

Cats tolerate a wide range of temperatures, with kittens usually able to thermoregulate by around 4 weeks of age (Bradshaw et al. 2012). An ambient temperature of 18–24 °C is recommended. This is easily met within the home and assessed by owners

Table 3.2 Benefits of indoor versus outdoor housing.

Indoors	Outdoors
Decreased risk of road accidents, infectious diseases (e.g. FeLV and FIV), straying from home, and theft	Reduced incidence of idiopathic cystitis and some infectious diseases (e.g. flu viruses if in multicat household)
Decreased fighting with or social stress from neighbourhood cats	Reduced social stress from other cats within the house
Increased welfare of wild animals	Increased performance of natural hunting behaviours
Easier to observe	More exercise opportunities
Easier to limit diet	Access to grasses and other plants
Shelter from the elements	Access to sunlight, a range of environmental stimuli
Easier to avoid unwanted pregnancies	

Source: Buffington (2002), Rochlitz (2009), and Seawright et al. (2009).
FeLV = feline leukaemia virus, FIV = feline immunodeficiency virus.

Table 3.3 Additional requirements for cats kept permanently indoors or permanently outdoors.

Indoors	Outdoors
Adequate environmental complexity	Access to shelter
Microchip identification (in case of escape or theft)	Microchip identification
Stimulating play to simulate hunting	Protection from road traffic accident
Cat grass	Neutering
Visual access to outside	Escape routes to safety in case of challenge from other cats
Access to a fenced outdoor area	Daily surveillance by and contact with humans
Single cat or very compatible cats in household	

Note: These provisions are especially important in each case, but all may be beneficial in both cases or for cats allowed both indoors and outdoors.

in terms of their own comfort. Shelters, boarding establishments, and veterinary hospitals should measure maximum and minimum temperatures. Young, geriatric, sick, or thin cats may require higher ambient temperatures. Ventilation should aim for a rate of air exchange of 15 times per minute, and owners should avoid high levels of humidity because they may promote mould growth and contagion (Gilman 2004). Lighting should provide naturalistic 24-hour light–dark cycles, with night-time lighting of 5–10 lx so cats can see at night.

Cats spend large periods of time sleeping, dozing, or resting, preferring to do so high up and within hides. They therefore need resting places that provide comfort, conceal-ment, and for many cats, height. These places should be free from loud and unpredict-able noises (e.g. dogs barking), although some background noise may be reassuring (Newberry 1995). More sites should be provided than there are cats in the house, both to minimise competition and to satisfy cats' motivations to regularly change resting places and to hide when threatened. However, outdoor views may cause anxiety for some cats, so owners should monitor the effect of providing such vantage points on other signs of anxiety.

Cats are highly motivated to rub and scratch (Figure 3.5), probably both for visual and scent marking and to sharpen and maintain claws (Casey 2009). In the core terri-tory, cats may use surfaces such as furniture legs or stair carpets if owners do not pro-vide them with adequate secure scratching posts. Cats need locations to urinate and defaecate that are safe, clean, hidden, away from the core area, not shared with other cats, and that have sufficient substrate to bury faeces. Inability to access a suitable toilet area may lead to toileting in other places. Owners should avoid excessively cleaning areas used for rubbing or toileting, which can disrupt familiar and reassuring smells, especially if using scented cleaning products. Owners can also maintain familiar smells in the cat's resting area by providing two pieces of bedding and washing one at a time.

Maintaining familiar smells is especially important when moving cats from one loca-tion to another. Cats can find changing their environment extremely stressful, for exam-ple. in moving house or being taken to a shelter. Most cats are rarely transported and often only to unpleasant places. Consequently, they usually find transport frightening, and this stress can be fatal. Transport stress may be reduced by minimising disturbances and using familiar smells, pheromones, food supplements, enjoyable distractions, and

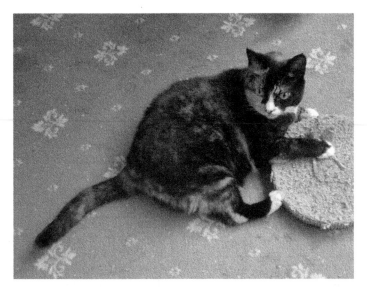

Figure 3.5 Cat scratch post. Cardboard disc provided as a surface for scratching within a cat's core territory (*Source:* courtesy of I. Rochlitz).

cat baskets or carriers to prevent excessive movement and make cats feel hidden. Kittens can be habituated to carriers and car journeys, ideally making the experiences pleasant through food or toys.

3.2.3 Animal Company

The social motivations of many domestic cats are not necessarily the same as those of *F. s. libyca*. Pet cats' social systems can be variable and flexible, with a complex range of behaviours that allow some cats to live in groups of varying size or alone. Differences between individuals' responses to company may be as a result of differences in population density and resource availability, incompatibility or unfamiliarity, and temporary factors such as each individual's background level of contentment or stress (Gourkow and Fraser 2006; Stella et al. 2014). For example, entire males from farms may come into conflict with other cats when moved into higher population densities such as suburban neighbourhoods. Whatever the reasons, considering cats as all 'social' or as all 'solitary' are often both oversimplifications.

Some cats may seek out, sleep alongside, groom, and play with other cats whom they appear to perceive as being within their social group (Curtis et al. 2003; Casey 2009). This compatibility is most likely amongst mother-offspring relationships or between juvenile related cats (Crowell-Davis et al. 2004). However, many cats tend to prefer not to closely interact with one another, and the presence or scent of incompatible or unfamiliar cats can cause stress. Moreover, there is no evidence that isolation from other cats often causes problems for cats, apart from any disruption to established relationships, suggesting cats do not always need social contact. Indoor neutered cat pairs tend to keep one to three metres apart (Barry and Crowell-Davis 1999), many cats prefer playing and sleeping alone (Podberscek et al. 1991), and the scent of socially incompatible cats can precipitate signs of anxiety and marking behaviour (Pryor et al. 2001). Signs of social stress may be subtle, such as going out less, or they may cause problems for the owners, such as spraying in the house. Contact and close proximity can also spread infectious diseases, particularly upper respiratory tract viruses and feline parvovirus.

Cats are generally relatively poor at giving obvious signals of appeasement to avoid or diffuse conflicts or to reconcile relationships afterwards (van den Bos 1998). They therefore rely largely on avoidance and aggression. Some cats may actively patrol their territory. Others may reduce their territory or range to the minimum necessary to find food and toilet, which can be small when provided with food and toilet areas. Some pet cats' core territories are therefore limited to the house or, for multicat households, particular rooms (Bernstein 2005). Similarly, some cats' ranges are limited to 0.4 ha (Schmidt et al. 2007); some cats barely leave their territory. However, sometimes cats may overlap their ranges (Crowell-Davis et al. 1997; Bernstein 2005) and may 'time-share' parts of the environment such as paths along high fences, facilitating both avoidance and ranging. New arrivals or departures within a house or neighbourhood can disrupt these 'arrangements'.

Boarding catteries and shelters should house cats individually or in their original groups and avoid creating groups with unfamiliar cats (Rochlitz 2014). Individual housing appears preferable for unsocialised cats (Kessler and Turner 1999a), and creating new groups involves mixing large numbers of unfamiliar and potentially infectious cats. Catteries should therefore err on the side of caution. However, once cats have adapted to a new environment, it may be possible to try moving them into communal housing, provided they appear sociable, the group is healthy and small, and the cats have plenty of space and resources (Dantas-Divers et al. 2011; Rochlitz 2014). If so, the cats should be carefully monitored, any incompatible animals separated, and the group kept otherwise stable.

In homes, the safest option for owners is usually to keep a single cat, except where groups are already established. If necessary, other local cats should be kept away from the home or certain rooms by the use of magnetic collars and cat flaps, thereby allowing the resident cat to leave the room or house while preventing intrusion of their core territory. If owners do keep multiple cats, they should be neutered, ideally related (Crowell-Davis et al. 2004), and introduced as juveniles (because even adult cats may tolerate kittens better than adults). Owners should manage introductions carefully and pay close attention to how the cats interact and respond (Rochlitz 2009). Once established, owners should keep groups stable.

For both owners and catteries, it can be difficult to assess cats' compatibility, especially when cats are forced close together for food or sleeping, thereby making proximity an unreliable method. Nevertheless, some signs can be taken as indicative of compatibility for practical purposes; for example, cats who rub against or groom each other or who deliberately choose to sleep together may be considered compatible (Heath 2005; Ellis et al. 2013), whereas fighting injuries and avoidance can be usually taken to represent incompatibility. Shelters can also try to assess cats' responses to unfamiliar socialised cats (Kessler and Turner 1999a) to evaluate sociability for rehoming purposes.

When cats are kept together, they should be given enough space to keep an adequate distance from one another, escape routes (e.g. letting them go outside the house), and vantage points to see one another (DeLuca and Kranda 1992; Rochlitz 2005a). They should also have enough litter trays, food and water bowls, beds, and hides so that all cats are able to access resources at the same time and without one cat having to get too close to another. Where cats appear stressed by one another's presence, the environment can also be segregated into home territories, using physical barriers or magnetic cat flaps. Cats can be given bells on their collars so they can hear each other's approach. Owners should also remember that altering one room may affect the cat whose territory it is and disrupt social patterns throughout the house.

Unwanted breeding should be prevented in cats kept together, either by using neutered animals or by single-sex groups. Differences between mature entire males and females include a pair of easily visible external testicles beneath the anus in the male and a vulval opening in the female. Adult males also tend to be larger and have well-developed jowls, compared with females.

Many households keep other species as pets as well as cats. The impact of dogs can depend on the behaviour of the dog (e.g. displaying chasing behaviour), the socialisation experience of each species to the other, and the familiarity of individuals. It has also been suggested that having the cat present in a household before the dog's arrival may increase the chance of a good relationship (Feuerstein and Terkel 2008). Many other small pets may be seen as potential prey animals. Allowing a cat to see them while preventing them from hunting them may cause frustration.

3.2.4 Human Interactions

Cats can show a variety of responses to human company, ranging from aversion to enjoyment. Some variation may be as a result of differences between cats' personalities, previous experiences, early socialisation and current stress levels (Casey and Bradshaw 2008; Stella et al. 2014). Some may be because of breeding. For example, Bengals are unsurprisingly described as showing low levels of affection and high levels of aggression towards humans and other cats (Hart et al. 2014). Breeding and hybridisation may also focus on aesthetics rather than on their temperament and suitability for living with humans. Some variation may also be a result of differences between humans, in particular regarding their skill, sensitivity, manner of handling, and mood (Rieger and Turner 1999). Many cats establish particular relationships with individual familiar people.

Fearful cats may try to avoid humans through flight, climbing, hiding, and using defensive aggression (Heath 2009). Aggression can include both biting and scratching, often preceded by hissing and postural changes. Some cats may also treat handlers' hands like prey, by grabbing them and performing disembowelling actions when their stomachs are stroked, although the underlying feelings are unclear. There is no established standard for assessing cats' relationships with humans (Slater et al. 2013a), although there are many suggestions on how to assess particular reactions (e.g. Siegford et al. 2003; Slater et al. 2010, 2013a, 2013c; American Society for the Prevention of Cruelty to Animals [ASPCA] 2014).

When cats require handling, stress may be minimised by handlers ensuring they are calm, quiet, and deliberate, approaching from the side and avoiding direct and unblinking eye contact. It is unclear whether covering the cat's head, swaddling, or scruffing reduces or increases fear. Cats do grasp the scruff of the neck of other cats, but only in limited circumstances such as mothers carrying kittens and during sexual intercourse, and it is not naturally used as a method of discipline (Rodan et al. 2011). Nevertheless, in some cases, such methods may protect owners and perhaps lead to shorter handling. Pinching the cat's skin may also inhibit reactions, but this may be by causing pain, so this method should not be used until more is known about its effects (Tarttelin 1991; Pozza et al. 2008; Nuti et al. 2016). Cats can be trained to interact through positive reward, for example, using clicker training, and this is preferable for repeated handling.

Young kittens should be provided with a range of positive human interactions from a variety of people, especially from 2 to 7 weeks of age, their sensitive period for socialisation. Feral kittens socialised from a very young age may be tameable, although there is considerable debate about how early that contact needs to begin. Once cats are older, humans should adapt to the established preferences of each cat, allowing cats to choose and direct the interactions wherever possible. As a general approach, it is best to start by allowing the cats to approach an unfamiliar human. If they do so, then caregivers can progress to more intimate contact (e.g. stroking) or active interaction (e.g. playing). Cats should never be forced into contact. In particular, truly feral adults typically remain too frightened of humans and should not be placed into home environments.

Without forcing their cat, owners should offer them opportunities for company, and if welcome, for stroking, grooming, resting together, and playing with interactive toys. These may be enjoyable, and may reduce anxiety, frustration, susceptibility to respiratory disease, and problem behaviours (Heidenberger 1997; Gourkow et al. 2014b), although these findings may be partly because of interactions causing owners to have a more positive perception of the cat or greater motivation to provide good husbandry. Individual cats may like or dislike particular interactions; for example, different cats may prefer being stroked on the head than on their back end (Soennichsen and Chamove 2002); prefer noncontact play to physical contact (Rochlitz 2005a); or dislike being picked up at all (Ellis et al. 2013).

3.2.5 Health

Cats can suffer from many diseases including 'flu', fleas, and worms (Table 3.4). Many viral infections can be fatal, including feline leukaemia, feline infectious peritonitis, and rabies. Some infections and infestations are interlinked (e.g. life cycles of the flea [*Ctenocephalides felis*] and the tapeworm [*Dipylidium caninum*] and some parasites can transmit other disease), and some viruses can alter or reduce cats' immunity to other diseases. Relatively uncommon zoonotic diseases include rabies, toxoplasmosis, worms, ringworm (*Microsporum canis*), cat scratch disease (*Bartonella henselae*), and mycobacterial infections.

Inherited disorders include Persian cats' flat faces and shortened heads, which make them prone to problems such as respiratory difficulties, chronic nasal discharge, chronic ocular discharge, and skin disease (UFAW 2011). In severe cases, displacement and rotation of facial bones and teeth affect the efficacy of the tear-duct drainage system, leading to persistent discharge from the eyes and skin irritation (Schlueter et al. 2009). Breeds' head shapes may also be associated with problems giving birth (Gunn-Moore and Thrusfield 1995). Selection and inbreeding has also led inadvertently to a number of inherited diseases, such as retinal degeneration in several breeds (Menotti-Raymond et al. 2010) and polycystic kidney disease in the Persian and exotic shorthairs, which affects an estimated 30–38% of Persians worldwide (Barrs et al. 2001; Cannon et al. 2001; Barthez et al. 2003). For the latter disease, a DNA test can detect affected cats who should not be used for breeding.

Geriatric conditions are common because of the age many cats reach. Reduced kidney function has multiple (and somewhat unclear) causes and is largely incurable, although supportive care can improve cats' quality of life. Increased thyroid function, diabetes, and altered cognition (Gunn-Moore et al. 2007) may also be common in older cats. Dental disease and joint conditions can be common in cats of different ages and can cause chronic pain. However, dental disease is often missed by owners, who do not examine their cats' mouths sufficiently often or miss signs of oral pain. Some dental conditions can be reduced by dental care or treated medically or surgically. Many cats cope better with few or no teeth than with a severely painful mouth.

All cats should receive routine preventive veterinary care, including dental checks, parasite control, and core vaccinations (Day et al. 2010; Mathews et al. 2014). Some vaccines only need to be administered every 3 years, but adult cats should be checked annually, and older and younger cats biannually, for early signs of disease or other problems (Hoyumpa Vogt et al. 2010). Kittens should also be presented soon after weaning for neutering, health checks, and parasite control. However, some owners do not take their cat to the veterinarian because of the difficulty in getting the cat into its carrier and transporting it to the surgery and because of the signs of stress the cat shows during the visit (Volk et al. 2011).

Table 3.4 Selected health problems in domestic cats.

Condition			Welfare effects
Infectious or Parasitic	Viral	Feline infectious enteritis/ panleucopaenia	Diarrhoea; malaise; reduced appetite Cerebellar hypoplasia in kittens
		Feline herpesvirus Feline calicivirus	Usually mild upper respiratory symptoms but can be severe in kittens Lifelong carriers can be minimally affected, with flare ups occasionally, especially during stress
		Feline leukaemia virus	Anaemia; reduced immune function (and secondary infections); tumours
		Feline immunodeficiency virus	Reduced immune function (and secondary infections)
		Feline infectious peritonitis	Various problems
		Rabies[a]	Various neurological symptoms
	Fungal	Ringworm[a] (Microsporum spp.)	Sometimes itchiness
	Internal Parasites	Toxoplasma[a] gondii Toxocara cati[a]	May be asymptomatic
	External Parasites	Ctenocephalides felis[a] (cat flea)	Itchiness; self-trauma; anaemia; may spread worms
Hormonal disorders		Hyperthyroidism	Increased thirst; weight loss; further problems
		Diabetes mellitus	Altered appetite; increased thirst; lethargy; collapse
Neoplastic		Lymphoma; squamous cell carcinoma; mammary adenocarcinoma; soft-tissue sarcoma	Pain; discomfort; malaise
Inherited		Polycystic kidney disease	Decreased appetite; weight loss; increased thirst; lethargy; malaise; secondary problems

(Continued)

Table 3.4 (Continued)

Condition		Welfare effects
Degenerative or Geriatric conditions	Osteoarthritis	Reduced mobility and activity; changes in temperament and in grooming behaviour
	Chronic renal disease or renal insufficiency	Increased thirst; weight loss; malaise
	Dental disease	Pain; altered appetite
Toxic	Permethrins (in some flea products)	Increased sensitivity; increased salivation; fever; muscle twitching; disorientation; loss of balance; convulsions; blindness
	Lilies	Vomiting; depression; dehydration; reduced appetite
Traumatic	Road accidents	Pain; tissue damage

Source: Rochlitz (2003), Sturgess (2005), Sturgess and Hurley (2005), Blackwood (2013), Gerhold and Jessup (2013), and American Association of Feline Practitioners (AAFP 2015).
[a] zoonosis

Table 3.5 Nontherapeutic elective surgical procedures performed on cats.

Mutilation	Benefits for animals	Benefits for humans	Perioperative welfare risks	Behaviour prevented	Acceptability
Castration	May facilitate social housing; reduced sexual frustration	Reduced spraying; reduced roaming	Minor to moderate pain; anaesthetic complications	Loss of breeding and related behaviours	Yes
Spaying	Prevention of breeding and related risks	Reduced disruptive behaviour while in season	as above	as above	Yes

Neutering is commonly performed on males and females to reduce unwanted pregnancies, behaviours such as spraying, fighting and roaming, road accidents, some infections, and some tumours (Table 3.5). Cats can be neutered safely from 6 weeks of age, and this should be done before puberty, which can occur from around 16 weeks (Joyce and Yates 2011; Porters et al. 2014). Immunocontraception also has the potential to be a practical and cost-effective method to control breeding of community cats (Levy 2011), but such products are not yet widely commercially available.

Table 3.6 Methods of euthanasia for cats kept as companion animals.

Method	Restraint required	Welfare benefits	Welfare risks
Intravenous injection of barbiturate	Secure and precise handling by trained person Sedation advised	Rapid loss of consciousness	Possible pain at injection site Reversible at low dosages Needs restraint

Source: American Veterinary Medical Association (AVMA 2013) and Human Society of the United States (HSUS 2013).

Cats are sometimes declawed (either surgically or using a laser) or undergo a tendonectomy (cutting the deep digital flexor of each digit) to reduce damage to the owner's property. Some argue that such procedures may indirectly help some cats, where the alternative is poor management, relinquishment, or euthanasia. However, declawing can cause both short- and long-term pain (possibly including phantom pains) and complications as a result of bandaging, infection, bleeding, tissue necrosis, and lameness. Declawing can also make cats unable to mark their territory visually, protect themselves from aggressors, climb, or hold objects, thereby frustrating the cats' unaffected motivations. The procedure is banned in more than 25 countries, including the United Kingdom, but it is legal in the United States (Sandøe et al. 2016).

3.2.6 Euthanasia

Acceptable methods of euthanasia of cats are listed in Table 3.6. The best method is usually sedation if needed, followed by the injection of an overdose of pentobarbitone into the cephalic vein. Injections into the heart, liver, or kidney are usually appropriate only in unconscious cats. Cats that cannot be humanely restrained may need to be restrained in a crush cage or similar holding device for sedation or given oral sedation initially.

3.3 Indicators of Welfare Problems

3.3.1 Pathophysiological Signs

Physiological assessments can use measures such as heart rate and respiratory rate (Table 3.7), with some highly stressed cats exhibiting dyspnoea. Potential biochemical measures include glucose (Yeates 2013) and urinary cortisol-to-creatinine ratios (Carlstead et al. 1993; Rochlitz et al. 1998), although such measures may not be perfectly reliable (Gourkow et al. 2014a). Pain may be indicated by increases in respiratory and heart rates and raised blood pressure (Hellyer et al. 2007).

Body-condition score (BCS) is a semi-quantitative assessment of body condition and is assessed by physical examination, visual observation, and palpation (Freeman et al. 2011; Aiello and Moses 2016). On a 9-point scale BCS ranges from cachectic (1/9) to severely obese (9/9) (see http://www.wsava.org/nutrition-toolkit; Freeman et al. 2011). Many geriatric conditions have somewhat similar effects such as weight loss or loss of

Table 3.7 Basic measures and clinical standards of cats (*Felis catus*).

Parameter	Normal measures	
Life expectancy	Up to 20 years or more, mean 12–14 years (great variation)	
Mean weight	Males: varies with breed; are usually larger than females	Females: varies with breed; are usually smaller than males
Body-condition score (BCS)	4–5 out of 9 is optimal	4–5 out of 9 is optimal
Body temperature	38.0–39.2 °C	
Respiratory frequency	16–40 per min (may be lower in home environment)	
Heart rate	120–240 per min (may be lower in home environment)	
Pubescence	Males: 4–9 months	Females: 4–9 months
Blood volume	6.5% of body weight, approximately 66 mL kg^{-1}	
Haematocrit	30–45	

Source: Freeman et al. (2011), Rudd (2013), Scherk (2013), and Aiello and Moses (2016).

body condition and increased drinking and may occur simultaneously. Such signs may therefore be considered generic signs of a problem that requires further investigation. Several feline diseases may also indicate underlying stress, including infectious respiratory diseases and lower urinary tract conditions such as cystitis (Buffington 2002; Buffington et al. 2006; Westropp et al. 2006; Seawright et al. 2008; Stella et al. 2011; Tanaka et al. 2012).

3.3.2 Behavioural Signs

Cats often seem to express few or subtle signs of welfare problems. This may partly be because of the lack of explicit signalling by cats and partly as a result of our inability to identify their behavioural expressions, especially because many of the signs involve cats *not* doing something (e.g. reduced activity or lack of interaction). However, there are also several more active signs that owners can notice quite easily; indeed, some behavioural indicators are noticed as behavioural problems for the owners.

Cats produce a range of vocalisations including yowls, snarls, hisses, and shrieks. Miaows often include other elements, such as clicks and growls, which enable different calls to be distinguished, for example 'trills' as social greetings (Nicastro 2004). Purring can be heard in kitten-cat, cat-cat, and cat-human interactions and seems to be associated with soliciting care (Brown and Bradshaw 2014), although purrs can also be combined with other noises to change their meaning (McComb et al. 2009). Cats may purr when being groomed but also when fearful, in severe pain, and even when moribund. Purring is therefore not a reliable sign of contentment.

Signs of pain may be subtle and difficult to recognise, and the severity of the pain difficult to judge (Lascelles and Robertson 2010; Robertson and Lascelles 2010). Various behaviours can indicate pain, although there is no single sign that present in

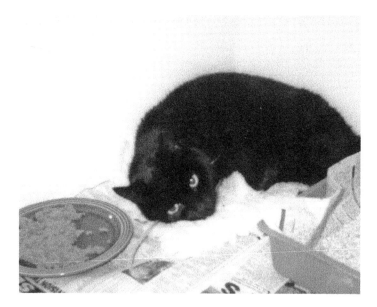

Figure 3.6 Cat in pain. This cat is in pain and has become withdrawn and timid (*Source:* courtesy of I. Rochlitz).

every case (Merola and Mills 2016). Cats in acute pain may vocalise (growling, hissing, spitting, yowling, or purring) or be silent. They are often withdrawn, immobile. and tense, with a reduced appetite and changes in demeanour such as aggression or extreme timidity (Figure 3.6). A crouched sternal posture with a stiff, ventro-flexed neck, or other abnormal postures may be seen (Waran et al. 2007), and cats may resent palpation of the painful area. Signs of chronic pain include changes in behaviour and lifestyle, alongside response to painkillers (Table 3.8). Methods for pain identification, scoring, and management have been developed for cats (e.g. Hellyer et al. 2007; Robertson 2008; Brondani et al. 2011, 2013; Calvo et al. 2014; Epstein et al. 2015; Merola and Mills 2016).

Stress, fear, and anxiety can be assessed by a range of similar behaviours or alterations in the performance of maintenance, avoidance, and affiliative behaviours (Carlstead et al. 1993; Stella et al. 2014). Some activities may be reduced, such as eating, exploration, and interactions. Some may increase, such as resting, hiding, or vomiting. Others may increase or decrease, such as grooming and sleeping, which may represent that fact that different cats cope with challenges in different ways, both actively and passively (Iki et al. 2011). Acute fear may also be indicated by postural changes (largely that make cats appear smaller or their fur stand on end), preparation for flight, and aggression. Owners may draw on structured methods to assess stress and fear, such as the Cat Stress Score (Kessler and Turner 1997). This has reasonable reliability between assessors, although its complexity, training requirements; and length may make it impractical for some owners; its effectiveness, too, has been questioned (McMillan 2012).

Urination can change with several welfare problems, such as marking in intercat communication, stress-related spraying, urinary tract disease caused or exacerbated by

Table 3.8 Common signs of chronic pain in domestic cats.

Lifestyle, behaviour, and temperament	Direction of change	Examples
Mobility	Decreased	Difficulty jumping onto surfaces, less graceful jumping, difficulty climbing up or down stairs
Activity	Decreased	Increased time spent resting or sleeping, reduced time spent playing or hunting, increased time spent hiding
Grooming behaviour	Increased or decreased	Change in time spent grooming, poor coat, increased time spent grooming the painful areas (can lead to alopecia)
Appetite	Decreased	Weight loss, anorexia, difficulty accessing feed bowl
Elimination	Change in habits	Difficulty or reluctance to use litter tray, urination, or defaecation in inappropriate places
Scratching with claws and other marking behaviour	Decreased	Difficulty accessing or using scratch posts, overgrown claws
Temperament	Change in demeanour	Less friendly, irritability, aggression, less willing to interact positively with other cats or with owner, withdrawal

stress, insufficient toileting resources, or bullying and conditions such as obesity, kidney disease, hyperthyroidism, or urinary crystals. The volume, frequency, and location of urination may help to determine the cause; for example, spraying around entrances may suggest threats outside the house (e.g. neighbourhood cats) or room (e.g. household cats), spraying on objects in the house may suggest anxiety or other emotional disturbance, and urination near toileting areas may suggest inappropriate litter facilities or urinary disease (Bowen and Heath 2005; Levine 2008).

3.4 Action Plan for Improving Cat Welfare

Many of the major actions needed can be considered as elements of tackling overpopulation. Although it is difficult to determine actual and optimal cat numbers, this can be assessed by the excessive numbers of community cats and cats in shelters. For example, it has been estimated that in 2009 more than 130 000 cats, and in 2010 more than 150 000 cats, entered UK animal welfare organisations (Clark et al. 2012). A range of strategies can be adopted to tackle overpopulation; each one must be adapted to fit the local conditions and available resources. All of them require cooperation between animal welfare organisations and veterinary organisations to educate existing and potential owners, discourage breeding, support owners who are considering relinquishment, promote adoption, and manage cats in the community.

An important area for improvement is to raise shelter standards. Cats in shelters experience confinement, noise, isolation, and exposure to diseases. Some cats may adapt to the shelter environment within 4 days, and others may take 5 weeks or more (Kessler and Turner 1997; Rochlitz et al. 1998). In general, the longer cats are kept in a shelter, the more likely they are to suffer diseases and undergo behavioural changes that indicate deteriorations in their quality of life. Shelters should therefore aim to keep the 'time to adoption' to the minimum needed for treatment and rehabilitation before rehoming and not keep cats permanently caged. Shelters should also ensure they are not overcrowded, which is difficult when so many cats need help. More responsible shelters may respond by prioritising intake or, as a last resort, increasing euthanasia rates – which are both better than causing widespread and long-term suffering.

The role of the veterinary profession in the rescue, rehabilitation, and rehoming of cats needs to be increased by the growth of shelter medicine as a specialist discipline in its own right and by altruistic collaboration between the veterinary profession and animal welfare organisations. At the same time, formal inspection and licensing schemes should be put in place to prevent shelters having inadequate standards of care, and in particular, to prevent the number of cats exceeding the capacity of the shelter to provide adequate care. Shelters are regulated in some U.S. states and European countries such as Austria and Germany, but not in many other countries. However, shelters are not a panacea for the cat overpopulation problem. It is better to prevent overpopulation, which is a societal problem and requires societal changes such as reducing breeding, microchipping, and public education. For some charities, investing funds in these activities may be more beneficial than maintaining a shelter.

Despite major recent efforts by the veterinary profession, animal charities, and other organisations preventing the birth of unwanted litters is proving difficult to achieve, and litters of kittens are commonly presented to shelters. In many developed countries, more than 80% of cats may be neutered (Chu et al. 2009, Murray et al. 2009, Toribio et al. 2009), but many cats are allowed to breed beforehand (Welsh et al. 2014). Prepubertal neutering (i.e. by 12 weeks old) should be practiced and promoted by all shelters, welfare charities, veterinary clinicians, and veterinary bodies. Future research should aim to unravel the complex reasons for owner resistance to neutering and how to overcome this resistance in different groups of owners. For example, surveys of cat owners, both in the United States (New et al. 2000) and the United Kingdom (Welsh et al. 2014) show that misconceptions regarding cat reproduction are common. Owners may believe that a female cat should have a litter before being neutered or that related cats would not mate with each other. Other owners may simply delay making a decision, in which time their queen has become pregnant. These beliefs need to be overcome through education or limiting ownership.

Efforts should also be made to promote and facilitate identification. A large proportion of cats entering shelters are strays who have become accidentally separated from their owners or deliberately abandoned. These cats are unlikely to be reunited because of a lack of identification (Lord et al. 2007b). As a striking example, only 2–5% of cats in U.S. shelters are reunited with their owners (Lord et al. 2007a). Cats should be identifiable by microchips, registered with up-to-date details, and tags on well-fitting and quick-release collars, so they can be rapidly reunited with their owners, and shelter resources redirected to help unowned cats (Figure 3.7). Governments should consider

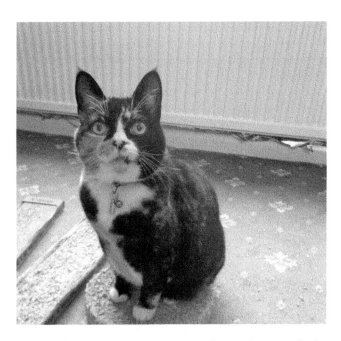

Figure 3.7 Cat identification. A cat wearing a collar and tag (and also microchipped) (*Source:* courtesy of I. Rochlitz).

making microchipping and registration mandatory. At the same time, rather than hastily taking them to a shelter, healthy stray cats in a safe environment should be left to make their way home. Charities or members of the public trying to help apparently stray cats can often determine if they are roaming owned cats or genuinely lost or feral cats by placing a paper collar on them with contact details for an owner to call if the cat is theirs, and only removing the cats if such contact is not made.

Community cat populations need to be humanely managed to improve the welfare of these cats, reduce the negative effects of such populations on the welfare of owned cats, maintain public health, and limit the effects of predation on wildlife. Widespread culling is likely to be ineffective and inhumane (an exception might be killing all cats on an island to protect other animals if there is no alternative). Moving community cats into shelters may result in unsocialised cats being unable to adapt to the shelter or rehomed environment, and so either suffering or being euthanised. Ideally, such cats should be caught and neutered (and treated as necessary) and then either released back into their colony or relocated as a colony to another site. Where possible, designated guardians should be identified to monitor for health problems and ensure basic needs are met. This challenge of managing community cats humanely and effectively must be tackled constructively by all interested groups, including those involved in wildlife conservation. For any effort, the effects on the overall population should be closely monitored to avoid wasting resources and having adverse welfare impacts.

Another strategy in the action plan is to address inadequate standards of cat ownership, which can lead to abandonments and relinquishments, neglect, and overbreeding. Some problems may be obvious, but owners may nevertheless fail to notice or act upon them, for example, in tackling obesity or incompatible multicat households. Some problems may only be seen when it too late to do anything, such as fear and other signs of poor adaptation experienced by cats in later life who have been raised indoors in impoverished environments. Others may not be recognised at all, such as chronic pain, which may be ignored or attributed to inevitable and untreatable ageing. All owners should obtain proactive education on reasonable responsibilities and expectations of cat ownership, either at point of sale, rehoming, or within licensing schemes. Important topics include expected veterinary costs; neutering; what constitutes normal cat behaviour and how their lives may be affected by it; signs of poor cat welfare such as house soiling and fighting; and how to address problematic behaviour.

Bibliography

American Association of Feline Practitioners (AAFP). (2015). Feline Disease and Medical Conditions. Available at https://catfriendly.com/feline-diseases/. Accessed 24 August 2018.

American Society for the Prevention of Cruelty to Animals (ASPCA). (2014). Meet Your Match Feline-ality™ Assessment. Available at http://aspcapro.org/feline-ality. Accessed 22 November 2016.

Animal Health Alliance (Australia) Ltd (AHAA). (2016). Pet Ownership in Australia (2013) Available at http://www.cabi.org/animalscience/news/23457. Accessed 22 November 2016.

AVMA (American Veterinary Medical Association). (2013). AVMA Guidelines for the Euthanasia of Animals: 2013 Edition. Available at https://www.avma.org/KB/Policies/Pages/Euthanasia-Guidelines.aspx. Accessed 7 October 2015.

Barrs, V.R., Gunew, M., Foster, S.F. et al. (2001). Prevalence of autosomal dominant polycystic kidney disease in Persian cats and related-breeds in Sydney and Brisbane. *Australian Veterinary Journal* 79: 257–259.

Barry, K.J. and Crowell-Davis, S.L. (1999). Gender differences in the social behavior of the neutered indoor-only domestic cat. *Applied Animal Behaviour Science* 64: 193–211.

Barthez, P.Y., Rivier, P., and Begon, D. (2003). Prevalence of polycystic kidney disease in Persian and Persian related cats in France. *Journal of Feline Medicine and Surgery* 5: 345–347.

Bernstein, P.L. (2005). The human-cat relationship. In: *The Welfare of Cats* (ed. I. Rochlitz), 47–89. Dordrecht, The Netherlands: Springer.

Blackwood, L. (2013). Cats with Cancer: where to start. *Journal of Feline Medicine and Surgery* 15: 366–377. doi: 10.1177/1098612X13483235.

van den Bos, R. (1998). Post-conflict stress-response in confined group-living cats (Felis silvestris catus). *Applied Animal Behaviour Science* 59: 323–330.

Bradshaw, J., Horsfield, G., Allen, J., and Robinson, I. (1999). Feral cats: their role in the population dynamics of *Felis catus*. *Applied Animal Behaviour Science* 65: 273–283.

Bradshaw, J.W.S., Casey, R.A., and Brown, S.L. (2012). *The Behaviour of the Domestic Cat*, 2e. Wallingford, UK: CAB International.

Brondani, J.T., Luna, S.P., and Padovani, C.R. (2011). Refinement and initial validation of a multidimensional composite scale for use in assessing acute postoperative pain in cats. *American Journal of Veterinary Research* 72: 174–183.

Brondani, J.T., Mama, K.R., Luna, S.P. et al. (2013). Validation of the English version of the UNESP-Botucatu multidimensional composite pain scale for assessing postoperative pain in cats. *BMC Veterinary Research* 9: 143.

Brown, S. and Bradshaw, J.W.S. (2014). Communication in the domestic cat: within- and between- species. In: *The Domestic Cat: The Biology of Its Behaviour*, 3e (ed. D.C. Turner and P. Bateson), 37–59. Cambridge, UK: Cambridge University Press.

Buffington, C.A. (2002). External and internal influences on disease risk in cats. *Journal of the American Veterinary Medical Association* 220: 994–1002.

Buffington, C.A., Westropp, J.L., Chew, D.J., and Bolus, R.R. (2006). Clinical evaluation of multimodal environmental modification (MEMO) in the management of cats with idiopathic cystitis. *Journal of Feline Medicine and Surgery* 8: 261–268.

Calvo, G., Holden, E., Reid, J. et al. (2014). Development of a behaviour-based measurement tool with defined intervention level for assessing acute pain in cats. *Journal of Small Animal Practice* 55: 622–629.

Cameron-Beaumont, C., Lowe, S.E., and Bradshaw, J.W.S. (2002). Evidence suggesting pre-adaptation to domestication throughout the small Felidae. *Biological Journal of the Linnean Society* 75: 361–366.

Cannon, M.J., MacKay, A.D., Barr, F.J. et al. (2001). Prevalence of polycystic kidney disease in Persian cats in the United Kingdom. *Veterinary Record* 149: 409–411.

Carlstead, K., Brown, J.L., and Strawn, W. (1993). Behavioral and physiological correlates of stress in laboratory cats. *Applied Animal Behaviour Science* 38: 143–158.

Case, L.P., Daristotle, L., Hayek, M.G., and Raasch, M.F. (2010). *Canine and Feline Nutrition: A Resource for Companion Animal Professionals*, 3e. Missouri, USA: Mosby Elsevier.

Casey, R.A. and Bradshaw, J.W.S. (2008). Owner compliance and clinical outcome measures for domestic cats undergoing clinical behaviour therapy. *Journal of Veterinary Behavior: Clinical Applications and Research* 3: 114–124.

Casey, R.A., Vandenbussche, S., Bradshaw, J.W.S., and Roberts, M.A. (2009). Reasons for relinquishment and return of domestic cats (*Felis Silvestris catus*) to rescue shelters in the UK. *Anthrozoös* 22: 347–358.

Chu, K., Anderson, W.M., and Rieser, M.Y. (2009). Population characteristics and neuter status of cats living in households in the United States. *Journal of the American Veterinary Medical Association* 234: 1023–1030.

Clark, C.C.A., Gruffydd-Jones, T.J., and Murray, J.K. (2012). Number of cats and dogs in UK welfare organisations. *Veterinary Record* 17: 493–496.

Colliard, L., Paragon, B.-M., Lemuet, B. et al. (2009). Prevalence and risk factors of obesity in an urban population of healthy cats. *Journal of Feline Medicine and Surgery* 11: 135–140.

Council of Europe. (2006). Appendix A of the European Convention for the Protection of Vertebrate Animals Used for Experimental and Other Scientific Purposes (ETS No. 123): Guidelines for Accommodation and Care of Animals (Article 5 of the Convention) Approved by the Multilateral Consultation. Council of Europe: Strasbourg, France. Available at http://conventions.coe.int/Treaty/EN/Treaties/PDF/123-Arev.pdf. Accessed 6 April 2016.

Courcier, E., O'Higgins, R., Mellor, D.J., and Yam, P.S. (2010). Prevalence and risk factors for feline obesity in a first opinion practice in Glasgow, Scotland. *Journal of Feline Medicine and Surgery* 12: 746–753.

Courcier, E., Mellor, D.J., Pendlebury, E. et al. (2012). An investigation into the epidemiology of feline obesity in Great Britain: results of a cross-sectional study of 47 companion practises. *Veterinary Record* 171: 560. doi: 10.1136/vr.10095.

Crowell-Davis, S.L., Barry, K., and Wolfe, R. (1997). Social behavior and aggressive problems of cats. *Veterinary Clinics of North America: Small Animal Practice* 27: 549–568.

Crowell-Davis, S.L., Curtis, T.M., and Knowles, R.J. (2004). Social organization in the cat: a modern understanding. *Journal of Feline Medicine and Surgery* 6: 19–28.

Curtis, T.M., Knowles, R.J., and Crowell-Davis, S.L. (2003). Influence of familiarity and relatedness on proximity and allogrooming in domestic cats (*Felis catus*). *American Journal of Veterinary Research* 64: 1151–1154.

Dantas-Divers, L.M., Crowell-Davis, S.L., Alford, K. et al. (2011). Agonistic behavior and environmental enrichment of cats communally housed in a shelter. *Journal of the American Veterinary Medical Association* 239: 796–802.

Day, M.J., Horzinek, M.C., and Schultz, R.D. (2010). WSAVA guidelines for the vaccination of dogs and cats. *Journal of Small Animal Practice* 51: 338–356.

DeLuca, A.M. and Kranda, K.C. (1992). Environmental enrichment in a large animal facility. *Laboratory Animals* 21: 38–44.

Desforges, E.J., Moesta, A., and Farnworth, M.J. (2016). Effect of a shelf-furnished screen on space utilisation and social behaviour of indoor group-housed cats (*Felis silvestris catus*). *Applied Animal Behaviour Science* 178: 60–68.

Driscoll, C.A., Menotti-Raymond, M., Roca, A.L. et al. (2007). The Near Eastern origin of cat domestication. *Science* 317: 519–523.

Ellis, S. (2009). Environmental enrichment: practical strategies for improving feline welfare. *Journal of Feline Medicine and Surgery* 11: 901–912.

Ellis, S.L.H., Rodan, I., Carney, H.C. et al. (2013). AAFP and ISFM feline environmental needs guidelines. *Journal of Feline Medicine and Surgery* 15: 219–230.

Epstein, M.E., Rodan, I., Griffenhagen, G. et al. (2015). The American Animal Hospital Association and the American Association of Feline Practitioners (AAHA/AAFP) pain management guidelines for dogs and cats. *Journal of Feline Medicine and Surgery* 17: 251–272.

European Pet Food Industry Federation (FEDIAF). (2014). [Online] Available: http://www.fediaf.org. Accessed 6 April 2016.

Farnworth, M., Dye, N., and Keown, N. (2010). The legal status of cats in New Zealand: a perspective on the welfare of companion, stray, and feral domestic cats (*Felis catus*). *Journal of Applied Animal Welfare Science* 13: 180–188.

Feuerstein, N. and Terkel, J. (2008). Interrelationships of dogs (*Canis familiaris*) and cats (*Felis catus L.*) living under the same roof. *Journal of Applied Animal Behaviour Science* 113: 150–165.

Freeman, L., Becvarova, I., Cave, N. et al. (2011). WSAVA nutritional assessment guidelines. *Journal of Small Animal Practice* 52 (7): 385–396.

Gerhold, R.W. and Jessup, D.A. (2013). Zoonotic diseases associated with free-roaming cats. *Zoonoses and Public Health* 60: 189–195. doi: 10.1111/j.1863-2378.2012.01522.x.

German, A.J. (2006). The growing problem of obesity in dogs and cats. *Journal of Nutrition* 136: 1940S–1946S.

Gilman, N. (2004). Sanitation in the animal shelter. In: *Shelter Medicine for Veterinarians and Staff*, 2e (ed. L. Miller and S. Zawistowski), 67–78. Oxford, UK: Blackwell Publishing.

Gourkow, N. and Fraser, D. (2006). The effect of housing and handling practices on the welfare, behaviour and selection of domestic cats (*Felis sylvestris catus*) by adopters in an animal shelter. *Animal Welfare* 15: 371–377.

Gourkow, N., LaVoy, A., Dean, G.A., and Phillips, C.J.C. (2014a). Associations of behaviour with secretory immunoglobulin A and cortisol in domestic cats during their first week in an animal shelter. *Applied Animal Behaviour Science* 150: 55–64.

Gourkow, N., Hamon, S.C., and Phillips, C.J.C. (2014b). Effect of gentle stroking and vocalization on behaviour, mucosal immunity and upper respiratory disease in anxious shelter cats. *Preventive Veterinary Medicine* 117: 266–275.

Gunn-Moore, D.A. and Thrusfield, M.V. (1995). Feline dystocia: prevalence and association with cranial conformation and breed. *Veterinary Record* 136: 350–353.

Gunn-Moore, D.A., Moffat, K., Christie, L.A., and Head, E. (2007). Cognitive dysfunction and the neurobiology of ageing in cats. *Journal of Small Animal Practice* 48: 546–553.

Hall, S.L., Bradshaw, J.W.S., and Robinson, I.H. (2001). Object play in adult domestic cats: the roles of habituation and disinhibition. *Applied Animal Behaviour Science* 79: 263–271.

Hall, C.M., Fontaine, J.B., Bryant, K.A., and Calver, M.C. (2015). Assessing the effectiveness of the Birdsbesafe® anti-predation collar cover in reducing predation by pet cats on wildlife in Western Australia. *Applied Animal Behaviour Science* 173: 40–51.

Hand, M.S. and Novotny, B.J. (2002). *Pocket Companion to Small Animal Clinical Nutrition*, 4e. Kansas, USA: Mark Morris Institute.

Hart, B.L., Hart, L.A., and Lyons, L.A. (2014). Breed and gender behaviour differences: relation to the ancient history and origin of the domestic cat. In: *The Domestic Cat: The Biology of its Behaviour*, 3e (ed. D.C. Turner and P. Bateson), 155–165. Cambridge, UK: Cambridge University Press.

Heath, S.E. (2005). Behaviour problems and welfare. In: *The Welfare of Cats* (ed. I. Rochlitz), 91–118. Dordrecht, The Netherlands: Springer.

Heath, S. (2009). Aggression in cats. In: *BSAVA Manual of Behavioural Medicine*, 2e (ed. D. Horwitz and D.F. Mills), 223–235. Quedgeley Gloucester, UK: BSAVA.

Heidenberger, E. (1997). Housing conditions and behavioural problems of indoor cats as assessed by their owners. *Applied Animal Behaviour Science* 52: 345–364.

Hellyer, P., Rodan, I., Brunt, J. et al. (2007). The AAHA/AAFP pain management guidelines for dogs and cats. *Journal of Feline Medicine and Surgery* 9: 466–480.

Horsfield, G.F. (1998). Behavioural Aspects of the Population Genetics of the Domestic Cat. PhD thesis, University of Southampton, UK.

Hoyumpa Vogt, A., Rodan, I., Brown, M. et al. (2010). AAFP/AAHA: feline life stage guidelines. *Journal of Feline Medicine and Surgery* 12: 43–54. Available at http://www.catvets.com/guidelines/practice-guidelines/life-stage-guidelines. Accessed 6 April 2016.

Humane Society of the United States (HSUS). (2013). *Euthanasia Reference Manual*, 2e. The Humane Society of the United States. Available at https://www.animalsheltering.org/sites/default/files/content/euthanasia-reference-manual.pdf. Accessed 2 July 2018.

Humane Society of the United States (HSUS). (2016). *APPA National Pet Owners Survey 2015–2016*. Available at http://www.humanesociety.org/issues/pet_overpopulation/facts/pet_ownership_statistics.html. Accessed 13 April 2016.

Iki, T., Ahrens, F., Pasche, K. et al. (2011). Relationships between scores of the feline temperament profile and behavioural and adrenocortical responses to a mild stressor in cats. *Applied Animal Behaviour Science* 132: 71–80.

Joyce, A. and Yates, D. (2011). Help stop teenage pregnancy! Early-age neutering in cats. *Journal of Feline Medicine and Surgery* 13: 3–10.

Kays, R.W. and Dewan, A. (2004). Ecological impact of inside/outside house cats around a suburban nature preserve. *Animal Conservation* 7: 273–283.

Kessler, M.R. and Turner, D.C. (1997). Stress and adaptation of cats (Felis silvestris catus) housed singly, in pairs and in groups in boarding catteries. *Animal Welfare* 6: 243–254.

Kessler, M.R. and Turner, D.C. (1999a). Socialization and stress in cats (Felis silvestris catus) housed singly and in groups in animal shelters. *Animal Welfare* 8: 15–26.

Kessler, M.R. and Turner, D.C. (1999b). Effects of density and cage size on stress in domestic cats (Felis silvestris catus) housed in animal shelters and boarding catteries. *Animal Welfare* 8: 259–267.

Lascelles, D. and Robertson, S. (2010). DJD-associated pain in cats – what can we do to promote patient comfort? *Journal of Feline Medicine and Surgery* 12: 200–212.

Levine, E.D. (2008). Feline fear and anxiety. *Veterinary Clinics of North America: Small Animal Practice* 38: 1065–1079.

Levy, J.K. (2011). Contraceptive vaccines for the humane control of community cat populations. *American Journal of Reproduction and Immunology* 66: 63–70.

Lord, L.K., Wittum, T.E., Ferketich, A.K. et al. (2007a). Search and identification methods that owners use to find a lost dog. *Journal of the American Veterinary Medical Association* 230: 211–216.

Lord, L.K., Wittum, T.E., Ferketich, A.K. et al. (2007b). Search and identification methods that owners use to find a lost cat. *Journal of the American Veterinary Medical Association* 230: 217–220.

Lund, E.M., Armstrong, P.J., Kirk, C.A., and Klausner, J.S. (2005). Prevalence and risk factors for obesity in adult cats from private US veterinary practices. *International Journal of Applied Research in Veterinary Medicine* 3: 88–95.

Macdonald, D.W., Apps, P.J., Carr, G.M., and Kirby, G. (1987). Social dynamics, nursing coalitions and infanticide among farm cats. *Ethology* 28 (Supplement Adv Ethology): 1–66.

Macdonald, D.W., Yamguchi, N., and Kerby, G. (2000). Group living in the domestic cat: its socio-biology and epidemiology. In: *The Domestic Cat: The Biology of Its Behaviour*, 2e (ed. D.C. Turner and P. Bateson), 95–115. Cambridge, UK: Cambridge University Press.

Mathews, K., Kronen, P.W., Lascelles, D. et al. (2014). WSAVA guidelines for recognition, assessment and treatment of pain. *Journal of Small Animal Practice* 55: E10–E68.

McComb, K., Taylor, A.M., Wilson, C., and Charlton, B.D. (2009). The cry embedded within the purr. *Current Biology* 19: R507–R508.

McMillan, F.D. (2012). Stress versus fear in cats. *Journal of the American Veterinary Medical Association* 240: 936.

Menotti-Raymond, M., David, V.A., Pflueger, S. et al. (2010). Widespread retinal degenerative disease mutation (rdAc) discovered among a large number of popular cat breeds. *Veterinary Journal* 186: 32–38.

Aiello, S.E. and Moses, M.A. (eds.) (2016). *Merck Veterinary Manual*, 11e. Kenilworth, NJ: Merck & Co.

Merola, I. and Mills, D.S. (2016). Behavioural signs of pain in cats: an expert consensus. *PLoS One* 11: 1–15.

Murray, J.K., Roberts, M.A., Whitmarsh, A., and Gruffydd-Jones, T.J. (2009). Survey of the characteristics of cats owned by households in the UK and factors affecting their neutered status. *Veterinary Record* 164: 137–141.

Murray, J.K., Browne, W.J., Roberts, M.A. et al. (2010). Number and ownership profiles of cats and dogs in the UK. *Veterinary Record* 166: 163–168.

Nelson, S.H., Evans, A.D., and Bradbury, R.B. (2005). The efficacy of collar-mounted devices in reducing the rate of predation of wildlife by domestic cats. *Applied Animal Behaviour Science* 94: 273–285.

New, J.C. Jr., Salman, M.D., King, M. et al. (2000). Characteristics of shelter-relinquished animals and their owners compared with animals and their owners in U.S. pet-owning households. *Journal of Applied Animal Welfare Science* 3: 179–202.

Newberry, R.C. (1995). Environmental enrichment: increasing the biological relevance of captive environments. *Applied Animal Behaviour Science* 44: 229–243.

Nicastro, N. (2004). Perceptual and acoustic evidence for species-level differences in meow vocalizations by domestic cats (*Felis catus*) and African wild cats (*Felis sylvestris libyca*). *Journal of Comparative Psychology* 118: 287–296.

Nuti, V., Cantile, C., Gazzano, A. et al. (2016). Pinch-induced behavioural inhibition (clip-thesia) as a restraint method for cats during veterinary examinations: preliminary results on cat susceptibility and welfare. *Animal Welfare* 25: 115–123.

O'Brien, S.J., Johnson, W., Driscoll, C. et al. (2008). The state of cat genomics. *Trends in Genetics* 24: 268–279.

Patronek, G.J., Beck, A.M., and Glickman, L.T. (1997). Dynamics of dog and cat populations in the community. *Journal of the American Veterinary Medical Association* 210: 637–642.

Pet Food Manufacturers' Association (PFMA) 2015 Pet Population 2015. Available: www.pfma.org.uk/pet-population-2015 Accessed 6 April 2016.

Pittari, J., Rodan, I., Beekman, G. et al. (2009). American Association of Feline Practitioners' senior care guidelines. *Journal of Feline Medicine and Surgery* 11: 763–778.

Podberscek, A.L., Blackshaw, J.K., and Beattie, A.W. (1991). The behaviour of laboratory colony cats and their reactions to a familiar and unfamiliar person. *Applied Animal Behaviour Science* 31: 119–130.

Porters, N., Polis, I., Moons, C. et al. (2014). Prepubertal gonadectomy in cats: different surgical techniques and comparison with gonadectomy at traditional age. *Veterinary Record* 175: 223.

Pozza, M.E., Stella, J.L., Chappuis-Gagnon, A.C. et al. (2008). Pinch-induced behavioral inhibition ('clipnosis') in domestic cats. *Journal of Feline Medicine and Surgery* 10: 82–87.

Pryor, P.A., Hart, B.L., Bain, M.J., and Cliff, K.D. (2001). Causes of urine marking in cats and effects of environmental management on frequency of marking. *Journal of the American Veterinary Medical Association* 219: 1709–1713.

Rieger, G. and Turner, D.C. (1999). How depressive moods affect the behavior of singly living persons towards their cats. *Anthrozoös* 12: 224–233.

Robertson, I.D. (1999). The influence of diet and other factors on owner-perceived obesity in privately owned cats from metropolitan Perth, Western Australia. *Preventive Veterinary Medicine* 40: 75–85.

Robertson, S.A. (2008). Managing pain in feline patients. *The Veterinary Clinics of North America. Small Animal Practice* 38: 1267–1290.

Robertson, S.A. and Lascelles, D. (2010). Long-term pain in cats – how much do we know about this important welfare issue? *Journal of Feline Medicine and Surgery* 12: 188–199.

Rochlitz, I. (2003). Study of factors that may predispose domestic cats to road traffic accidents: part 1. *Veterinary Record* 153: 549–553. doi: 10.1136/vr.153.18.549.

Rochlitz, I. (2005a). Housing and welfare. In: *The Welfare of Cats* (ed. I. Rochlitz), 141–176. Dordrecht, The Netherlands: Springer.

Rochlitz, I. (2005b). *The Welfare of Cats*. Dordrecht, The Netherlands: Springer.

Rochlitz, I. (2009). Basic requirements for good behavioural health and welfare in cats. In: *BSAVA Manual of Behavioural Medicine*, 2e (ed. D. Horwitz and D.F. Mills), 35–48. Quedgeley Gloucester, UK: BSAVA.

Rochlitz, I. (2014). Feline welfare issues. In: *The Domestic Cat: The Biology of Its Behaviour*, 3e (ed. D.C. Turner and P. Bateson), 131–153. Cambridge, UK: Cambridge University Press.

Rochlitz, I., Podberscek, A., and Broom, D.M. (1998). The welfare of cats in a quarantine cattery. *Veterinary Record* 142: 35–39.

Rodan, I., Sundahl, E., Carney, H. et al. (2011). AAFP and ISFM feline-friendly handling guidelines. *Journal of Feline Medicine and Surgery* 13: 364–375.

Rudd, S. (2013). QRG 20.2 blood transfusion. In: *BSAVA Manual of Feline Practice – A Foundation Manual* (ed. A. Harvey and S. Tasker), 456–460. Quedgeley, Gloucester, UK: BSAVA.

Sandøe, P., Corr, S., and Palmer, C. (2016). *Companion Animal Ethics*. Oxford, UK: UFAW/Wiley.

Scarlett, J.M. and Donoghue, S. (1998). Associations between body condition and disease in cats. *Journal of the American Veterinary Medical Association* 212: 1725–1731.

Scherk, M. (2013). Chapter 1: the cat friendly practice. In: *BSAVA Manual of Feline Practice – A Foundation Manual* (ed. A. Harvey and S. Tasker), 1–31. Quedgeley, Gloucester, UK: BSAVA.

Schlueter, C., Budras, K.D., Ludewig, E. et al. (2009). Brachycephalic feline noses: CT and anatomical study of the relationship between head conformation and the nasolacrimal drainage system. *Journal of Feline Medicine and Surgery* 11: 891–900.

Schmidt, P.M., Lopez, R.R., and Collier, B.A. (2007). Survival, fecundity and movements of free-roaming cats. *Journal of Wildlife Management* 71: 915–919.

Seawright, A., Casey, R., Kiddie, J. et al. (2008). A case of recurrent feline idiopathic cystitis: the control of clinical signs with behavior therapy. *Journal of Veterinary Behavior* 3: 32–38.

Serpell, J.A. (2014). Domestication and history of the cat. In: *The Domestic Cat: The Biology of Its Behaviour*, 3e (ed. D.C. Turner and P. Bateson), 83–100. Cambridge, UK: Cambridge University Press.

Siegford, J.M., Walshaw, S.O., Brunner, P., and Zanella, A.J. (2003). Validation of a temperament test for domestic cats. *Anthrozoös* 16: 332–335.

Slater, M.R., Miller, K.A., Weiss, E. et al. (2010). A survey of the methods used in shelter and rescue programs to identify feral and frightened pet cats. *Journal of Feline Medicine and Surgery* 12: 592–600.

Slater, M.R., Garrison, L., Miller, K.A. et al. (2013a). Practical physical and behavioral measures to assess the socialization spectrum of cats in a shelter-sike setting during a three day period. *Animals* 3: 1162–1193.

Slater, M.R., Garrison, L., Miller, K.A. et al. (2013c). Physical and behavioral measures that predict cats' socialization in an animal shelter environment during a three day period. *Animals* 3: 1215–1228.

Soennichsen, S. and Chamove, A.S. (2002). Responses of cats to petting by humans. *Anthrozoös* 15: 258–265.

Sparkes, A., Bessant, C., Cope, K. et al. (2013). ISFM guidelines on population management and welfare of unowned domestic cats (Felis catus). *Journal of Feline Medicine and Surgery* 15: 811–817.

Stella, J.L., Lord, L.K., and Buffington, C.A. (2011). Sickness behaviors in response to unusual external events in healthy cats and cats with feline interstitial cystitis. *Journal of the American Veterinary Medical Association* 238: 67–73.

Stella, J., Croney, C., and Buffington, C. (2014). Environmental factors that affect the behavior and welfare of domestic cats (Felis silvestris catus) housed in cages. *Applied Animal Behaviour Science* 160: 94–105.

Sturgess, K. (2005). Disease and welfare. In: *The Welfare of Cats* (ed. I. Rochlitz), 205–225. Dordrecht, The Netherlands: Springer.

Sturgess, K. and Hurley, K.J. (2005). Nutrition and welfare. In: *The Welfare of Cats* (ed. I. Rochlitz), 227–257. Dordrecht, The Netherlands: Springer.

Tanaka, A., Wagner, D.C., Kass, P.H., and Hurley, K.F. (2012). Associations among weight loss, stress, and upper respiratory tract infection in shelter cats. *Journal of the American Veterinary Medical Association* 240: 570–576.

Tarttelin, M. (1991). Restraint in the cat induced by skin clips. *Journal of Neuroscience* 57: 288.

Toribio, J.A., Norris, J.M., White, J.D. et al. (2009). Demographics and husbandry of pet cats living in Sydney, Australia: results of cross-sectional survey of pet ownership. *Journal of Feline Medicine and Surgery* 11: 449–461.

Turner, D.C. and Bateson, P. (2014). *The Domestic Cat: The Biology of Its Behaviour*, 3e. Cambridge, UK: Cambridge University Press.

UFAW. (2011). Genetic Welfare Problems of Companion Animals: Persian – Brachycephaly. Available at www.ufaw.org.uk/cats/persian-brachycephaly. Accessed 8 November 2016.

Volk, J.O., Felsted, K.E., Thomas, J.G., and Siren, C.W. (2011). Executive summary of the Bayer veterinary care usage study. *Journal of the American Veterinary Medical Association* 238: 1275–1282.

Waran, N., Best, L., Williams, V. et al. (2007). A preliminary study of behaviour-based indicators of pain in cats. *Animal Welfare* 16 (Suppt.1): 105–108.

Welsh, C.P., Gruffydd-Jones, T.J., Roberts, M.A., and Murray, J.K. (2014). Poor owner knowledge of feline reproduction contributes to the high proportion of accidental litters born to UK pet cats. *Preventive Veterinary Medicine* 174: 118–123. doi: 10.1136/vr.101909.

Westgarth, C., Pinchbeck, G.L., Bradshaw, J.W.S. et al. (2010). Factors associated with cat ownership in a community in the UK. *Veterinary Record* 166: 354–357.

Westropp, J.L., Kass, P.H., and Buffington, C.A. (2006). Evaluation of the effects of stress in cats with idiopathic cystitis. *American Journal of Veterinary Research* 67: 731–736.

Yeates, J. (2013). *Animal Welfare in Veterinary Practice*. Oxford, UK: UFAW/Wiley.

Yeon, S.C., Kim, Y.K., Park, S.J. et al. (2011). Differences between vocalization evoked by social stimuli in feral cats and house cats. *Behavioral Processes* 87: 183–189.

Dogs (*Canis familiaris*)

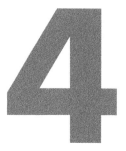

Nicola Rooney and Kevin Stafford

4.1.1 Natural History

Domestic dogs (*Canis lupus familiaris* or *Canis familiaris*) are members of the class Mammalia, order Carnivora, and family Canidae. The domestic dog is a social canid that descended from the grey wolf (*Canis lupus*) at least 15 000 years ago (Thalmann et al. 2013) and now lives in close association to human societies throughout the world. Wolves are found in parts of Asia, North America, and Europe and are classified as 'Of Least Concern', whilst the domestic dog is not included in the IUCN Red List (International Union for Conservation of Nature and Natural Resources 2016).

In the wild, wolves are highly social, wide-ranging animals, with a large, flexible behavioural repertoire, advanced communication, and signalling abilities. They naturally live in cohesive family-based groups, with less confrontational social organisation than had previously been assumed from studies of captive wolves (e.g. Mech 1999). Extrapolations from wolf populations to domestic dogs are common in the literature.

Companion Animal Care and Welfare: The UFAW Companion Animal Handbook,
First Edition. Edited by James Yeates.
© 2019 Universities Federation for Animal Welfare. Published 2019 by John Wiley & Sons Ltd.

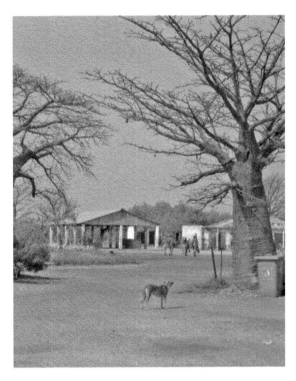

Figure 4.1 Free roaming dog in West Africa (*Source:* courtesy Nicola Rooney).

Dog behaviour has traditionally been interpreted in terms of 'alpha pairs' and hierarchical dominance structures (e.g. The Monks of New Skete 1978, 1991). However, recent scientific studies suggest that such interpretations about wolves and domestic dogs are flawed (Bradshaw et al. 2009; Bradshaw 2011). More meaningful comparisons can be yielded by considering the behaviour of feral and domestic dogs (Rooney and Bradshaw 2016).

Free-roaming dogs are found in many countries (Figure 4.1) including free-ranging dingoes in Australia and Southeast Asia. These dogs are highly social; for example, one population in West Bengal was recorded as forming groups of 5 to 10 adult dogs plus dependent offspring, sharing a territory that they defended against neighbouring groups (Pal et al. 1999; Pal 2011). Free-roaming dogs generally have large home ranges and spend much of their day active (Boitani et al. 1995), feeding, and exploring their surroundings (Prescott et al. 2004). All adult females within a population may come into oestrus every year and attempt to select males for mating, although there may also be forced matings (Pal et al. 1999). Amongst a wide variety of mating strategies, seasonal monogamy is common, with males guarding their litters for the first 6 to 8 weeks of life (Pal 2005). Free-living dogs do not appear to breed cooperatively, nor do they commonly hunt cooperatively, although some packs of dingoes have been recorded successfully hunting together (Thomson et al. 1992).

As hunters and social animals, dogs use postural signalling in communication. Thus, vision is important to dogs, and they are particularly sensitive to movement. However, smell is often described as the primary sense for dogs. Dogs' sense of smell is considerably more sensitive than that of humans (Prescott et al. 2004), and they use smell in preference to other senses in learning tasks (Williams and Johnston 2002). Dogs also use vocalisations in communication, and they have sensitive hearing, with the peak sensitivity in the range 4–8 KHz. Although their low frequency limit is similar to humans, they have considerably higher upper limits – 41–47 KHz, compared to 15–20 KHz in humans – and are able to hear 'ultrasonic' frequencies (Heffner 1983, 1998).

4.1.2 Domestic History

There are various theories as to how wolves were domesticated. It is commonly suggested that individual wolves who were less fearful of humans scavenged food close to human settlements. Natural selection favoured the individuals which were least afraid of people, until some wolves were sufficiently tame to live within human settlements, being fed and used as alarms and later as hunting companions (Clutton-Brock 1995). During the next phase of domestication, humans selected individual wolves to breed from, thereby producing the first domestic dogs. Subsequent selection led to additional behavioural changes, such as altered social cognitive abilities (Hare et al. 2002; Miklosi 2007; Rooney and Bradshaw 2014) and increased responsiveness to humans (Kaminski and Nitzschner 2013). As examples, domestic dogs are highly responsive to human gestures and play more than wolves (Virányi and Range 2014; Bradshaw et al. 2015).

With time, different sorts of dogs were required for different roles, and various 'types' were selected specifically for guarding, hunting, herding, and traction. In the 1850s, the hobby of dog showing emerged, and physical appearance became an important selection criterion (Sampson and Binns 2006). In dog shows, judges evaluate individuals against a 'breed standard' based predominantly on appearance. Breeding rules also decree that stud books are closed, and breeds of dog can only be bred within that breed's gene pool. This artificial selection has resulted in hundreds of dog breeds, which vary more in their anatomy, and particularly in their size, than those of any other species. This differentiation of breeds has led to extreme body shapes. Countries such as Brazil and China have recently embraced the sport of dog showing, which appears to be becoming a global phenomenon.

The physical differences between breeds can affect both the dogs' ability to communicate (Goodwin et al. 1997; Rooney 2009) and the way in which their emotional states are shown behaviourally. This makes it difficult to generalise or extrapolate needs across different breeds. For example, the environmental and behavioural needs of a Chihuahua might be very different to those of a Great Dane, 25 times its size (Bateson 2010), as might the needs of a Collie selected for its herding instinct to those of a Bull Terrier originally bred to fight.

Dogs now live in a wide range of environments and have many different relationships with humans. Some are considered family members and live in small apartments, whereas others are 'street dogs' living loosely connected with humans. Many free-roaming dogs are owned by humans (Hiby 2013), and there are perhaps very few, if any, dogs worldwide whose lives are unaffected by human influence.

4.2 Principles of Dog Care

4.2.1 Suitable Diet

Although within the order Carnivora, dogs have evolved to eat an omnivorous diet. Their nutritional requirements include specific amino acids, glucose precursors, fatty acids, and dietary fibre are important dietary elements (Bosch et al. 2009; Deka 2009). Dogs also need a range of vitamins and minerals, although they are able to synthesise their own vitamin C (Innes 1931 cited in Committee on Animal Nutrition 1985). Precise dietary requirements vary with each dog's age, lifestyle, health, and activity level (Arnold and Elvehjem 1939; Donoghue and Kronfield 1994; Fahey et al. 2008; Hill et al. 2009). Pregnant and lactating bitches need extra food to meet foetal and lactation requirements. From 3 weeks old, puppies should be offered small amounts of moist food in addition to their dam's milk. Puppies should be gradually weaned onto an appropriate, complete, high-protein diet from 6 to 8 weeks of age (Committee of Animal Nutrition 2006). Large breed puppies also need precise levels of calcium in their diet (Hazewinkel et al. 1991). Puppies should be weighed at least weekly to ensure that their weight gain is as predicted for their breed type.

A failure to provide the correct amount of food or the correct balance of nutrients can lead to malnutrition (Kienzle and Hall 1994; Stafford 2007) and increased susceptibility to disease (Slater et al. 1992; Medeiros and Angela 2008). Dogs may survive well on vegetarian diets (Brown 2009). However, there is doubt whether they can remain healthy on a vegan diet (Remillard et al. 2000), but this is still debated (Knight 2015). Home-made diets can provide adequate nutrition, but incomplete or unbalanced home-prepared diets can lead to malnutrition (Taylor et al. 2009). Some human foods can also be poisonous, for example, onions (Gault et al. 1995) and chocolate (Alsop and Albertson 2008). A myriad of commercial foods have been developed for dogs' general or particular needs. As specific examples, a dental prescription diet can result in less dental plaque and inflammation than a regular food (Logan et al. 2001).

The quantity of food required depends on the type of food, in particular, its energy content, the dog's health, and activity level (Hill et al. 2009). Because there is such a diversity of dogs' sizes, lifestyles, and body composition (Jeusette et al. 2010), it is impossible to have universal recommendations for quantities required for all breeds and ages. The quantity of food should be aimed at maintaining the dog at an optimal weight and body condition, whilst avoiding feelings of excessive hunger. As well as body weight, body condition should be monitored visually and by feeling areas that may accumulate fat (Burkholder and Bauer 1998; McGreevy et al. 2005), ideally using a validated scoring system (e.g. Laflamme 1997; Thatcher et al. 2010).

Free-roaming dogs often suffer from hunger, emaciation, and low body condition. However, overnutrition is now a problem for dogs in many postindustrial countries (Houpt et al. 2007; Stafford 2007). Estimates in various countries suggest 30–60% of dogs are overweight (Houpt et al. 2007; Holmes et al. 2007; Rohlf et al. 2010), and 15–20% are clinically obese (Mason 1970; Houpt et al. 2007; Courcier et al. 2010). Obesity limits a dog's ability to exercise, play, and groom. It can also increase the risk, and exacerbate the effects of, conditions such as diabetes, arthritis, hip dysplasia, respiratory disease, and neoplasia (German et al. 2010). Specifically, letting dogs become overweight in their first 2 years can increase the risk of hip dysplasia (Smith et al. 2006). Overall, lean dogs live an average of 1 to 2 years longer than overweight dogs (Kealy et al. 2002).

Risk factors for obesity include being older, female, neutered, and purebred (Colliard et al. 2006; Courcier et al. 2010; O'Neill et al. 2014), with some breeds being particularly susceptible (McGreevy et al. 2005). Owners are also more likely to own an obese dog if they feed them snacks, feed them only once a day, or provide infrequent or low-intensity forms of exercise (Crane 1991; Sloth 1992; Kienzle et al. 1998; Robertson 2003; Courcier et al. 2010). Ultimately most obesity can be prevented by careful monitoring of body condition and by appropriate feeding and exercise regimes (Burkholder and Toll 2000). Weight can be reduced by decreasing food intake (e.g. to around 60% of maintenance diet) and by giving appropriate exercise (German et al. 2010). Such programmes can lead to increased or constant hunger and frustration, which may additionally increase dogs' sensitivity to environmental stressors (Bosch et al. 2009). Weight-control diets must therefore be carefully planned to ensure dogs feel satiety and do not suffer excessive hunger (German et al. 2012). A high-protein, high-fibre diet may improve satiety and reduce hunger (German et al. 2010).

The method of presenting a dog's food is also important, and many commercial foods may not provide an adequate feeding experience (Stafford 2007). Owners should consider giving dogs interactive feeding devices (Rooney et al. 2009a), which are often included as part of the prevention of separation-related behaviour (RSPCA 2015). For example, food-filled Kongs™ can stimulate appetitive activity (Schipper et al. 2008), become anticipated, and be beneficial to dogs (Hiby 2005; Gaines 2008, Gaines et al. 2008; Rooney et al. 2009a).

All dogs should be given continuous access to clean drinking water (Prescott et al. 2004). Dogs have a limited capacity to store water and water deprivation can cause death considerably quicker than food deprivation (Maskell and Johnson 1993). When transporting dogs, journeys should incorporate breaks at least every 3 hours for dogs to be offered water and should recommence only after 30 minutes to allow absorption (Prescott et al. 2004). Some anti-bark muzzles put pressure on the jaw, which may prevent dogs drinking and panting (Juarbe-Diaz and Houpt 1996; Cronin et al. 2003) and should not be used.

4.2.2 Suitable Environment

There is currently little experimental evidence on which to base recommendations regarding the space required by dogs in their living environment or during confinement. A more useful approach is to consider the behaviours which a dog needs to perform (e.g. resting, running, and playing) and ensure that the environment is both of adequate size and complexity to permit these. In addition, most dogs generally show high levels of exploratory behaviour (Siwak et al. 2001) and therefore need a secure, safe, risk-free environment.

Worldwide, many dogs are allowed to roam freely (Hsu et al. 2003; Stafford 2007), although this is now rare in developed countries; for example, in the United Kingdom, only 1% of dogs are reported to roam freely (Westgarth et al. 2008). Free-roaming dogs can suffer from increased risks of disease and injury (Hsu et al. 2003), and straying may be responsible for a significant proportion of the dog deaths in road traffic accidents

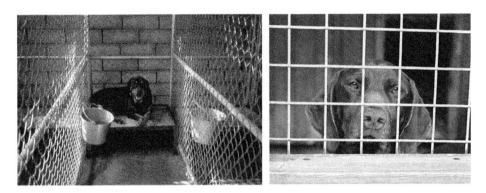

Figure 4.2 Kennel environments can provide safe resting places but can be stressful (*Source: courtesy Elly Hiby*).

(Johnston 1990). In comparison, many dogs are confined to kennels in owners' homes or gardens or in boarding establishments and rehoming establishments. Such confinement can improve safety but restricts behavioural freedom.

Confinement in kennels can be stressful for some dogs who are not accustomed to the experience (Hiby et al. 2006; Rooney et al. 2007). Dogs can show considerable distress (physiological and behavioural), especially during the initial period of kennelling (Hiby et al. 2006; Rooney et al. 2007; Figure 4.2). A large proportion of kennelled dogs exhibit repetitive behaviours, including pacing, circling, bouncing, spinning, tail-chasing, and wall bouncing (Hubrecht et al. 1992; Rooney et al. 2009a, 2000b; Denham et al. 2014) which suggests that kennels are often suboptimal (Burghardt 2003). Repetitive behaviour, however, may have multiple causes and present differently in different contexts and needs to be interpreted cautiously (Denham et al. 2014). In general, kennels may be appropriate as a resting area, for example, for dogs who have met many of their behavioural and psychological needs whilst outside the kennel (e.g. in work). However, kennels are largely inappropriate as a permanent home.

Crates and cages are used to confine dogs within homes, transport vehicles, veterinary surgeries, and markets. These can significantly restrict movement and prevent various species-typical behaviours (Prescott et al. 2004). Dogs confined in crates or cages should always have room to turn around, stand upright, and lie fully stretched out without touching another animal or the sides of the accommodation. Using crates for short periods of time will allow opportunities outside the crate for other elements of the dog's daily behavioural repertoire. Nevertheless, even short-term confinement in a cage can cause physiological stress, for example, in dogs hospitalised in veterinary surgeries (Siracusa et al. 2008) and dogs held in dark kennels while their enclosure is being cleaned (Gaines 2008). Hence, if kennels or cages are used, even for short periods, stress levels should be reduced by getting animals used to them gradually by rewarding calm behaviour and pairing the environment with positive experiences (e.g. food and play; Rooney et al. 2007).

Dogs are adaptable to a wide range of temperatures (Prescott et al. 2004) especially if allowed time to acclimatise. However, periods of inclement weather (Beerda et al. 1999) and low temperatures (Hiby 2005) can lead to physiological distress. Similarly, high temperatures, especially when accompanied by high humidity can result in heat stroke (Bruchim et al. 2006). Dogs should therefore always have rest areas which are dry, draught-free, away from climatic extremes, and at a temperature where dogs show no signs of distress (e.g. within 10–26 °C; CIEH 1995). Where movement is limited, for example in crates, then these must be positioned so as to avoid high and low temperatures. In particular, dogs should not be left in cars where rapidly rising temperatures and humidity can be distressing and even fatal. Provision of additional bedding, coats, or heating to avoid cold temperatures (Rooney et al. 2009a) and mechanical ventilation to ameliorate heat may also be necessary.

During resting periods, dogs have brief (e.g. each lasting for less than 10 minutes) and frequent (e.g. 4 per hour) sleep–wake cycles (Adams and Johnson 1994, 1995). However, provision of uninterrupted rest periods is still important. Most dogs prefer to rest on soft materials (Adams and Johnson 1995) and will generally use beds when available. These materials should be on a comfortable solid surface, which should not be wire mesh or slats. In multidog environments, there should be at least as many resting places as there are dogs.

Owners should pay attention to the visual features of a dog's environment but also consider their other senses, especially smell and hearing. Strong odours such as cleaning fluids may be aversive and even painful to dogs (Kore and Kieschenesselrodt 1990). Consistency of smells is commonly believed to be valuable to puppies newly separated from their mothers (Milan 2010) and possibly to newly kennelled dogs (Gaines 2008). Its value within the domestic environment is yet to be fully researched, but smells such as camomile have been shown to promote calm restful behaviours in kennelled dogs (Prescott et al. 2004; Graham et al. 2005a). Similarly, Dog Appeasing Pheromone (DAP®) may be beneficial, but this remains a source of debate (Cracknell and Mills 2008; Gaultier et al. 2009; Broach and Dunham 2016).

Noise levels in many kennel establishments can reach 100 db (Hubrecht et al. 1997; Sales et al. 1997; Coppola et al. 2006), and such high levels are likely to disrupt dog-resting patterns (Gaines 2008). In addition, up to half of all dogs show behaviours indicative of fear of loud noises such as fireworks or thunderstorms (Blackwell et al. 2006, 2013). Dogs should be gradually habituated to the range of sounds found within their environment (Blackwell et al. 2006). The use of classical music may have a calming effect on dogs (Wells et al. 2002; Kogan et al. 2012), although it remains unclear whether this acts directly on the dogs or indirectly by calming the caregivers. Aversive noises should also be avoided, including those undetectable by humans, such as sounds emitted by metal gates, audiovisual equipment, or ultrasonic flea collars (Roe and Sales 1992). If there is a lot of external ambient noise, then accommodation should be sound insulated, and all environments should provide dogs with access to a quiet space in which to hide away from excessive noise.

A dog's environment can be restrictive, uncontrollable, and understimulating (Beerda et al. 1997; Kobelt et al. 2003; Prescott et al. 2004). The provision of enrichment devices and toys, which dogs can chew and play with, can add interest to their environment and have some value to some singly and group-housed dogs (Hubrecht 1993; Wells 2004a, 2004b). Play is an important part of the dog's behavioural repertoire and should be promoted (Figure 4.3). However, the extent to which dogs utilise toys is variable (Hiby 2005) and differs according to toy type (Pullen et al. 2010). Toys are generally used

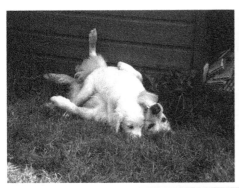
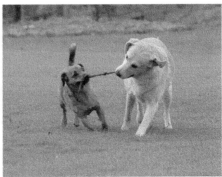
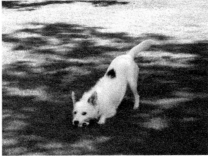

Figure 4.3   Dogs showing a motivation to play (*Source:* courtesy Nicola Rooney and Sam Gaines).

more if they are destructible and chewable, with bones and chew toys being most favoured (Hiby 2005; Gaines et al. 2008). The potential welfare benefits therefore depend on appropriate enrichment devices that are valued by the individual dog. Dogs should also be walked at least daily because walking can not only provide exercise and improve fitness, but also allows opportunities to investigate, explore, and interact with other dogs and people.

The predictability of daily routines has been shown to be important to dogs in kennels (Hennessy et al. 1997, 1998), but this is also likely to be the case for dogs kept in homes. Changes in walking schedules can result in considerable frustration (Meers et al. 2004). Similarly, dogs formerly receiving enrichment via feeding devices showed behaviours indicative of frustration and increased physiological stress levels when deprived of them (Hiby 2005; Gaines 2008). Routines and provision of enrichment and events that dogs find rewarding should be predictable whenever possible, and interruptions or cessation of routine activities should be avoided.

Routine is particularly relevant for toileting behaviour. Most dogs are unwilling to urinate or defecate in their resting place (Houpt 2005). Training often produces strongly conditioned responses not to urinate or defecate indoors or even on specific surface types. Therefore, dogs are likely to suffer if not given regular opportunities to toilet in suitable places, causing psychological distress and ultimately pain and discomfort. This highlights the importance of a predictable routine and ensuring dogs are regularly removed from any cage or let loose from a tether to allow toileting and never be restricted so long that they become distressed. Routines need to be tailored to the individual's needs because urination frequencies are likely to vary with age (Wirant and McGuire 2004).

Transportation can be a source of fear, anxiety, and stress (Mills and Mills 2003; Wohr and Erhard 2004). Individual responses will depend on the dog's previous experiences, temperament, and the conditions during transportation. Hence it is important to gradually introduce dogs to transport in a positive way. As a general rule, dogs should not be transported within 2 hours of feeding and should be exercised immediately before they are loaded to stimulate elimination. If dogs become fearful during transportation, remedial action should be taken to overcome those fears using behavioural modification techniques (Crowell-Davis et al. 2003; Cracknell and Mills 2008; Levine and Mills 2008). In specific cases, drugs may be required, and the use of DAP has been demonstrated to help overcome some established fears of transport (Estelles and Mills 2006).

4.2.3 Animal Company

Dogs are generally social animals. Most well-socialised dogs are strongly motivated to establish contact and interact with other dogs, for example on a walk (Westgarth et al. 2010). Even when unable to interact physically in a kennelled environment, dogs often take the opportunity to gain visual contact with conspecifics (Wells and Hepper 1998). Group and pair-housing has been shown to enhance the welfare of kennelled dogs (Hetts 1991; Hubrecht 2002; Wells 2004a; Taylor and Mills 2007) and having a second dog in the house may help some dogs to cope with fears such as during thunderstorms (Dreschel and Granger 2005).

Solitary kennelled dogs show more repetitive behaviours than dogs in groups (Hubrecht et al. 1992; Mertens and Unshelm 1996), and when removed from a group, dogs show behaviours indicative of distress including autogrooming, paw lifting, vocalisation, coprophagy (eating faeces), and repetitive behaviours (Beerda et al. 1999). Dogs should therefore be kept in amicable pairs or social groups whenever possible. When multidog housing is not possible, dogs should be allowed to interact with other dogs at least daily. Pet dogs walked on leads are limited in the quality of interaction in which they can engage (Westgarth et al. 2010) and are less likely to be able to play with other dogs (Allen 2010). This may frustrate those dogs with a strong motivation to play (Rooney et al. 2001), so interaction with other dogs should be off the lead when safe (Figure 4.4).

Individual dogs differ in their motivation and ability to interact amicably with other dogs. Some individuals can be incompatible (Marston et al. 2005), or fearful, which can manifest as aggression. Therefore, new dogs need to be carefully integrated into established groups of dogs (Sonderegger and Turner 1996). It is also important that dogs are able to choose to interact or withdraw from one another. They should always be provided with adequate resources to avoid competition for, and monopolisation of, hiding places, beds, toys, feeding, and resting places. Dogs should always have the opportunity to avoid and to rest out of sight of other animals (Graham et al. 2005a, 2005b). The relative value of social housing will depend on the caregivers' ability to achieve good standards of husbandry and monitoring (Hubrecht and Buckwell 2004). When an individual dog shows persistent fear or aggression towards other dogs, owners should seek

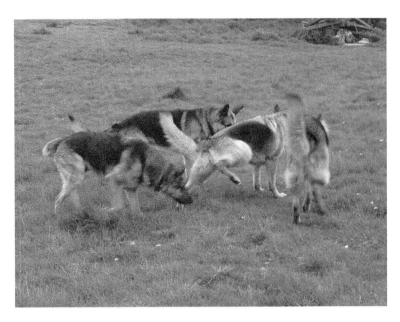

Figure 4.4 Dog-dog interactions between dogs off lead (*Source:* courtesy Sam Gaines).

specialist advice from a clinical animal behaviourist (ASAB 2016) for treatment, which may permit their dog to later benefit from social interaction.

Dogs' motivation and ability to interact may be influenced by past experiences, in particular, their experience during sensitive phases of their development (Overall 1997). Puppy socialisation classes, during which puppies are gradually introduced to a range of stimuli and conspecifics in a controlled manner, are widely regarded as being very good at improving the dog's later social behaviour. For example, dogs who have attended puppy socialisation classes are less likely to show undesirable reactions such as aggression to dogs from outside the household or to unfamiliar people (Blackwell et al. 2008; Casey et al. 2014). Dogs' sociability may also be affected by their ability to give appropriate signals, which depends partly on social learning and partly on their anatomy, including tail length (Leaver and Reimchen 2008) and snout length (Kerswell et al. 2010).

It is general practice for puppies to be weaned and removed from the litter and dam between the ages of 6 and 8 weeks. Opinions vary as to the optimum weaning age. On the one hand, in an optimal maternal environment where puppies are well cared for, introduced to a range of new environments, and the dam has a favourable temperament, later weaning can allow puppies to benefit from longer maternal influence (Goddard and Beilharz 1986) and to learn social behaviours from their littermates (O'Farrell 1992). Consequently, puppies weaned at 12 weeks as compared to 6 weeks show better weight gain and health (Slabbert and Rasa 1993). On the other hand, in an imperfect early-rearing environment, as occurs in some establishments (Bateson 2010; McMillan et al. 2011, 2013), puppies may lack stimulation, complexity, and opportunities for socialisation. Consequently, puppies may develop better outside that environment. As a general

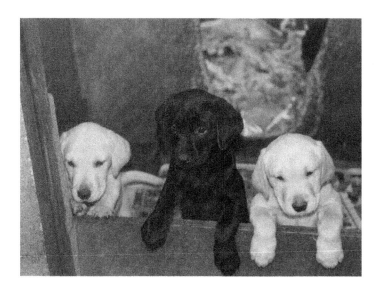

Figure 4.5 Puppies in their early-rearing environment (*Source:* courtesy Nicola Rooney).

rule, puppies should not be permanently removed from their litter before 8 weeks of age, but the best time for weaning will depend on the relative quality of breeder and the environment with the new owner (Figure 4.5).

Most dogs live in an environment in which they will encounter multiple species. Interactions with other species can be enriching, but only if neither individual shows any signs of fear or aggression. Dogs should not be housed in close proximity to any animals of whom they may be afraid or have frustrated motivations to chase. Young dogs should be gradually introduced in a positive manner to all species which they will encounter later. This has been shown to help dogs and cats learn each other's body language and establish amicable relationships (Feuerstein and Terkel 2008).

4.2.4 Human Interactions

Human contact has beneficial effects for many dogs. Positive interactions such as stroking, scratching, talking, and playing may result in increased beta-endorphin, oxytocin, prolactin, beta-phenylethylamine, and dopamine (Odendaal and Meintjes 2003) and reduced cortisol levels during stressful periods such as arriving in rehoming kennels or blood sampling (Hennessy et al. 1998, 2006; Coppola et al. 2006; Shiverdecker et al. 2013). Indeed, providing human contact to dogs which arrive in a rehoming centre can also reduce stress when those dogs are subsequently presented with a novel environment or person (Hennessy et al. 2002; Bergamasco et al. 2010). Military dogs whose handlers provide additional contact showed increased confidence and less howling, destructive behaviour, and biting than dogs left in centralised kennels (Lefebvre et al. 2007; Haverbeke et al. 2010).

Importantly, a dog's need for, and reaction to, human company is affected by its temperament and early experiences (Scott and Fuller 1965). For example, puppies which receive gentle handling between the ages of 3 and 21 days are generally calmer at

8 weeks of age (Gazzano et al. 2008). Puppies obtained from pet stores, and probably bred in commercial establishments, are more likely to be reported as fearful or aggressive to family members, unfamiliar people, and other dogs (McMillan et al. 2013). This is likely to be a result, at least in part, of insufficient or inappropriate 'socialisation', particularly during the sensitive period of development from approximately 3–14 weeks of age. In this period, dogs show enhanced learning through interaction with people and other dogs (Howell and Bennett 2011) and have an increased propensity to later develop fear responses to stimuli, including types of people, that they have not encountered at this time (McCune et al. 1995).

For many dogs, human contact may be more valuable for well-being than contact with other dogs (Wells 2004a; Valsecchi et al. 2007), and contact with familiar people produces greater inhibition of stress in novel environments than does contact with familiar dogs (Tuber et al. 1996). However, dogs do not respond to humans and other dogs in the same way (Rooney et al. 2000, 2001). Their interaction with each species is likely to be separately motivated, not simply part of an overall need for social contact. Therefore, human company should not be viewed as a substitute for canine company nor vice versa.

Humans and dogs can form such close relationships that many dogs suffer in their owner's absence. Dogs may vocalise, eliminate, or destroy things when their owners are away and can become distressed or even aggressive shortly before they leave. Past surveys have recorded 24% of dogs in the United Kingdom currently or previously exhibiting separation-related behaviours (Bradshaw et al. 2002a), whilst in a longitudinal study almost 50% of Collies and Labradors showed separation-related behaviour by 18 months of age (Bradshaw et al. 2002b). Similarly, 56% of dogs living in urban Rio de Janeiro were seen to show clinical signs of separation anxiety (Soares et al. 2010). Dogs who exhibit separation-related behaviours may be more likely to experience negative emotions at other times, not just when they are actually performing these behaviours (Mendl et al. 2010). Furthermore, many dogs which show no apparent behavioural signs of distress have urinary cortisol levels which suggest that they too may be suffering (Channel Four 2014).

Pet dogs often live in households where all humans are absent for at least part of the day; for example, in Sweden, 73% are routinely left for periods in excess of 4 hours a day (Norling and Keeling 2010). Many owners do not appreciate that their dog becomes anxious when left alone and then punish them for 'misbehaviour' when they return on the mistaken assumption that dogs have the cognitive capacity to connect events that have occurred several hours apart. As a general principle, dogs should gradually be introduced to being left alone and should never be left for so long as to cause them distress. A useful guide is that dogs should not be left alone for more than 4 hours in daytime, depending on the individual's behaviour. Where dogs start to show separation-related behaviour, behavioural advice should be sought from a trained clinical animal behaviourist to reduce their anxiety (e.g. see ASAB 2016).

The quality of interaction between dog and owner is important. In particular, owners should ensure they interact with their dogs positively and consistently. Inconsistent owner behaviour such as rewarding or punishing responses to the same behaviour by the dog on different occasions is associated with increased reported behaviour problems, disobedience, fear, and anxiety (Casey et al. 2007; Arhant et al. 2010). Owners should also avoid training methods that cause physical pain and distress, such as punishment using electric shock collars, prong or choke collars, or methods that restrict a dog's air supply using chains or pinning it to the ground, as well as verbal chastisement. In fact, such methods may cause more fear and anxiety (Blackwell et al. 2008; O'Sullivan et al. 2008; Tami et al. 2008; Herron et al. 2009; Arhant et al. 2010; Hsu and Sun 2010; Casey et al. 2013), reduce subsequent learning ability (Rooney and Cowan 2011) and obedience, and increase the chances of behaviour problems such, as aggression, developing (Hiby et al. 2004; Casey et al. 2014). In particular, using remotely activated electric shock collars may cause chronic fear to a greater degree than other types of positive punishment (Schilder and van der Borg 2004; Schalke et al. 2007). In comparison, reward-based training can be beneficial (Haverbeke et al. 2010) and may be a way to improve pet dogs' quality of life (Hiby et al. 2004).

Owners may respond to problem behaviours inappropriately, especially because those behaviours often result from negative emotional states such as fear and anxiety. For example, some owners may isolate or not walk dogs who are poorly trained, pull on the lead, or who show fear-related aggression (Marston et al. 2005). Dogs with toileting problems can be left outside, and hyperactive dogs ignored, shouted at, or confined. Dogs that bark may be fitted with anti-bark muzzles that prevent them panting and drinking. Other owners punish their dogs for 'disobedience', for example, by using collars that spray citronella, which are aversive. The use of punishment is often advocated by owners misinterpreting dogs' behaviour as a result of excessive anthropomorphism, outdated views of 'wolf society' and 'dominance theory', or assuming behaviour is motivated by higher cognitive processes such as guilt (Horowitz 2009) and by owners erroneously trying to replicate dog-dog interactions. Other owners respond by relinquishing or euthanasing their dog (and, in some countries, selling them into the meat trade), and this is particularly likely for human-directed aggression and separation-related behaviours (Bailey 1992; Mondelli et al. 2004; Diesel et al. 2007; Kim et al. 2009; O'Neill et al. 2013).

Problem behaviours should be improved by tackling the underlying causes. For example, there are validated protocols to treat separation-related behaviours, producing improvements in 81% of dogs (Blackwell et al. 2006). More widespread use of such techniques, and associated clinical behavioural advice from skilled professionals, has the capacity to improve quality of life for many dogs and reduce relinquishment rates. Protocols for prevention (e.g. Blackwell et al. 2016) are even better, with dogs gradually introduced to periods of being alone, being rewarded for calm behaviours, and never punished for separation-related behaviours. Such habituation programmes have been effective at training dogs to be left in crates or kennels (Rooney et al. 2007) and homes (Blackwell et al. 2016).

4.2.5 Health

Dogs can suffer from many diseases, including several infectious agents that are found worldwide, (Table 4.1; Figure 4.6). External parasites cause itchiness and anaemia (Totton et al. 2011; Yoak et al. 2014) and act as vectors for other diseases such as tick paralysis (Eppleston et al. 2013). Rabies is an important disease internationally, affecting millions of dogs yearly (Wandeler et al. 2013), and extrapolating from human experiences, may cause respiratory distress and pain prior to death (Jackson 2011). Studies

Table 4.1 Selected health problems in domestic dogs.

Condition				Welfare effects
Infectious and parasitic diseases	Viral		Rabies[a] (V)	Pain, distress
			Distemper (V)	Malaise
			Parvo disease (V)	Diarrhoea
			Hepatitis (V)	Malaise
			Kennel cough (V)	Cough, malaise
	Bacterial		Leptospirosis (V)	Jaundice, malaise
	Internal parasites		*Toxocara canis*	Discomfort, diarrhoea
			Hookworms	Anaemia
			Dirofilaria immitis	Exercise intolerance
	External parasites		Ticks	Irritation, paralysis
			Fleas	Irritation
			Demodex and Sarcoptes mites	Itchiness, irritation
Nutritional			Obesity	Exercise intolerance, exacerbates other conditions
			Emaciation	Susceptible to disease
Inherited			Upper airway disfunction	Exercise intolerance, stress, sleep problems
			Hip dysplasia	Pain, exercise intolerance
			Retinal atrophy	Poor sight, blindness
Degenerative or geriatric			Arthritis	Pain, behavioural restriction
			Periodontitis	Pain, restricted chewing activity
Allergic			Atopic dermatitis	Irritation
Trauma			Brutality, road traffic accidents (RTA), fighting	Pain, blood loss, fear

Source: Jackson (2011); Bugg et al. (1999); Morgan (2008); Bowman and Atkins (2009); Totton et al. (2011); and Yoak et al. (2014).
[a] Zoonotic disease.
V = vaccination available.
Note: Kennel cough is theoretically zoonotic but appears to be of limited risk.

vary, possibly partly because of the wide variety of movement and social patterns of dogs, but some suggest canine rabies can be prevented by restricting dog movement and vaccinating approximately 60–70%, or more, of dogs (Hampson et al. 2009).

Dogs should be inspected by a veterinarian at least once yearly, and in the interim, parasite infestations can be prevented by regular treatment. All dogs should be routinely vaccinated against conditions such as distemper, infectious canine hepatitis, parvovirus, leptospirosis, and rabies, although the availability and cost of vaccines often limits their use. Kennel cough is associated with exposure and stress, and dogs at

(a)   (b)

(c)   (d)

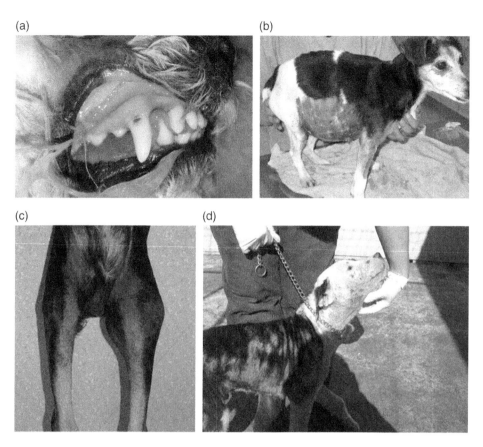

Figure 4.6 Physical signs of ill health: (a) Jaundice; (b) abdominal swellings; (c) ostreosarcoma; (d) demodectic mange (*Source:* courtesy Ian Scott and Keith Thompson).

risk should be vaccinated against it, for example before entering boarding kennels, and efforts made to ameliorate stressful conditions.

Dental problems and gum disease are common in dogs. Teeth and gums should be checked regularly and kept healthy using appropriate diets, brushing (Ingham and Gorrel 2001), or dental chews, although the value of such regimes is still open to some debate (Rawlings 1996; Roudebush et al. 2005). Ears may be affected by infections, parasitic infestation, or foreign bodies such as grass seeds, which may cause inflammation of the ear canals with resultant pruritus, pain, and swelling or haematomas (Cote 2011). Gastrointestinal disease can be caused by, amongst others, infectious agents, parasites, foreign body ingestion, dietary problems, and poisoning. Urinary diseases include urolithiasis (Osborne et al. 1999), which may result in painful urethral blockage (Collins et al. 1998) and urinary incontinence (leaking), which is not thought to be painful but may cause distress for dogs previously taught not to soil indoors.

Geriatric problems such as osteoarthritis and cancer can be common in dogs. For example, osteoarthritis affects about 20% of adult pet dogs (Lascelles and Main 2002; Walton et al. 2013) and cancer may be found in about 50% of dogs older than 10 years of age in some countries (de Lorimier and Fan 2005; Fan et al. 2007). Dogs with such conditions may experience both pain (Lascelles and Main 2002) and frustration because of a reduction in normal behaviours (e.g. running or climbing stairs; Morgan 2008). Dogs with arthritis should be given adequate pain relief, controlled exercise, and put on a weight loss programme if necessary. The welfare implications of any proposed treatment, needs to be considered. For example, treatment for cancer may cause pain, malaise, and nausea, although chemotherapeutic side effect may be less unpleasant than in humans because lower doses are used. Other treatments, such as providing paraplegic dogs with wheels to replace their back legs, may prevent some behaviours. In some such cases, treatment may be inappropriate and the welfare of the dog may be better served by euthanasia.

Inherited health problems are especially common in pedigree and purebred dogs. There are more than 500 identified genetic diseases in dogs (Sargan 2004), with all the 50 most popular UK dog breeds having at least one conformation-related disorder (Asher et al. 2009) and at least one inherited disorder (Summers et al. 2010). More diseases are usually identified for the most common breeds, although this is likely simply a result of increased surveillance (Rooney and Sargan 2009). One underlying problem is breed standards that have promoted exaggerated physical characteristics such as extremely short faces and compressed skulls (Figure 4.7). These can cause pain and suffering (Asher et al. 2009; Rooney and Sargan 2009) and hamper the ability of dogs to communicate and carry out various behaviours (Rooney 2016). Another cause is that dog breeds were generally produced from a few ancestors and then inbred to 'fix'

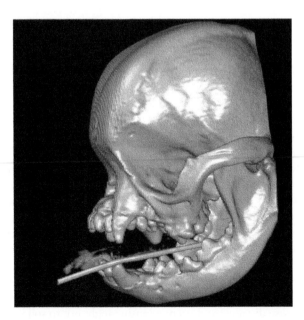

Figure 4.7 A brachycephalic shaped skull – an extreme physical feature common in several breeds and associated with a number of health problems including breathing difficulties (*Source: courtesy Andrew Worth*).

characteristics. Furthermore, these characteristics are related mainly to appearance, hence selection for them presents a corresponding lack of attention to health, temperament, and welfare. The tendency to use show champion males extensively for breeding further reduces genetic variety. In general, crossbred dogs live longer than purebred dogs of an equivalent size (Rooney and Sargan 2009; O'Neill et al. 2013).

Breeders should avoid mating dogs with heritable conditions and should try to reverse existing exaggerations where these affect welfare (advice on various heritable conditions is available at www.ufaw.org.uk/genetics). Some diseases may be avoided by not breeding animals who have the condition or the gene responsible. For example, the Irish Setters breeders in the United Kingdom are believed to have substantially reduced canine leucocyte adhesion deficiency through screening, selective breeding, and conditional registration. Other diseases are more difficult to eliminate, in particular if breeders also select for appearance (Mäki et al. 2005). For example, efforts to reduce hip dysplasia (Figure 4.8) have been disappointing, although combining pedigree records, hip scores, and genotyping may help reduce its incidence in the future (Zhu et al. 2009). Increasing genetic diversity, whilst actively selecting against heritable disorders and phenotypic extremes is critical as is selection for dogs of a temperament well-suited to life as a pet.

Neutering is the most common surgery carried out on pet dogs (Adin 2011). It prevents mating and can also have significant health and behaviour benefits in both sexes. Castrated dogs are uninterested in mating, may not be as inclined to roam or fight as intact animals (Maarschalkerweerd et al. 1997), and cannot get testicular cancers. Spayed bitches avoid oestrus, pregnancy, and parturition and are less likely to get mammary cancer, uterine, or ovarian diseases (Cote 2011). Neutering should be carried out

(a)   (b)

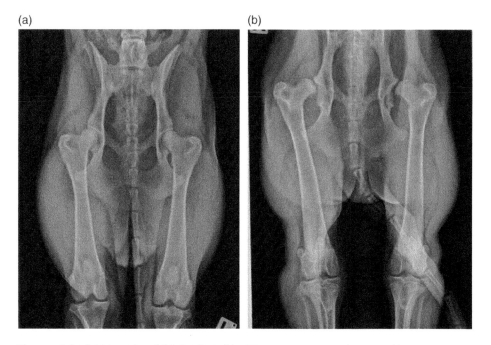

Figure 4.8 (a) Normal and (b) dysplastic hips (*Source:* courtesy Andrew Worth).

under general anaesthesia with preoperative analgesia (Weber et al. 2012). In some scenarios, surgical complications have been found in 20% of cases (Burrow et al. 2005). There is ongoing discussion about the consequences of neutering at different ages, but there is little evidence that earlier neutering of females results in urinary incontinence (Beauvais et al. 2012). In situations where it is otherwise impossible to prevent unwanted mating, owners should usually neuter their puppy before puberty.

Surgeries such as tail docking and ear cropping are commonly performed on puppies in some countries, often either for cosmetic purposes or to prevent injuries during blood sports or fieldwork (Table 4.2). However, it is unlikely that tail docking will significantly reduce tail injuries (Darke et al. 1985) and an estimated 500 dogs would need to be docked to prevent a single injury (Diesel et al. 2010). Tail docking can cause intense shrieking during the procedure (Noonan et al. 1996) and can lead later to urinary incontinence (Holt and Thrusfield 1993; de Bleser et al. 2011), neuromas (Gross and Carr 1990), adhesions (Carr 1979), and self-trauma, often resulting in the need for further tail shortening (Scott et al. 1995). This makes tail docking an unnecessary and harmful mutilation.

4.2.6 Euthanasia
Acceptable methods of euthanasia of dogs are listed in Table 4.3. A good method is sedation followed by the injection of an overdose of pentobarbitone into the cephalic vein (AVMA 2013). Street dogs who are not habituated to humans may be more humanely euthanased by accurate cranial shooting with a shotgun, free bullet, or captive bolt.

4.3 Signs of Dog Welfare

4.3.1 Pathophysiological Signs
The normal weight and body-condition score varies greatly between breeds and with age of the dog (Table 4.4). Extremely low body weight and severe emaciation usually reflects undernutrition or systemic disease, although some dogs with low bodyweight or poor body condition may actually be very fit animals; for example, racing greyhounds are often heavily muscled but have light fat cover over their ribs and flanks when in ideal body condition. Dehydration may be indicated by decreased skin elasticity ('skin tenting'), sunken eyes, and dry oral mucous membranes (Nelson and Couto 1998). Increased salivation and drooling saliva can be indicative of rabies, hunger, objects lodged in the mouth, oral lesions such as gum disease or distress (Beerda et al. 1997; Cote 2011; Fisher 2011), or be normal for some breeds with loose facial skin folds. Loose faeces and vomiting can indicate pathological states or occur following stressful or exciting situations (Gaines 2008). Skin lesions and conditions such as mange may also provide a general indication of the physical welfare of dogs in a population (Garde et al. 2016; Sankey et al. 2012; Steinberger 2012).

Rapid shallow 'panting' is normal in excited dogs, whereas laboured breathing may indicate pneumonia or anaemia. Increases in respiration rate (above 35 breaths/min), heart rate (above 140 beats/min), or rectal temperature (above 39 °C) can

Table 4.2 Nontherapeutic elective surgical procedures performed on dogs.

Procedure	Benefits to animals	Benefits to the humans	Perioperative health risks	Behaviour prevented	Acceptability
Castration	Reduced roaming, RTAs; escaping; fighting; and intermale aggression	Dog can be easier to manage and contain	Pain (which can be easily alleviated); infection; bleeding; wound breakdown	Mating, natural courtship, and sexual behaviour	Acceptable
Spaying	Prevention of pregnancy, uterine, and ovarian disease Reduced risk of mammary cancers	No concerns around mating and whelping	Involves general anaesthetic risks		Acceptable
Tail docking	None. Tail injury protective effect disproven	Aesthetic for some owners	Pain (which can be alleviated).	Ability to signal emotional state and intent and hence initiate safe social interaction Balance and swimming ability	Unacceptable
Ear cropping	None		Pain (which can be alleviated). Haemorrhage.	Ability to signal emotional states and intent using ear position	Unacceptable
Dew claw removal	May reduce the incidence of damage to claw	Show ring requirement	Minor pain or infection		Acceptable under anaesthetic
Vocal cord removal	Cannot bark as loudly or correctly	Can reduce inappropriate barking but may be replaced by other noise	General anaesthetic effects; haemorrhage, coughing; gagging; aspiration Infection of larynx or trachea may result in permanent narrowing of the air passages Scarring of the vocal cord tissue with regrowth may lead to difficulty breathing	May make it difficult for the animal to communicate inter- and intra-specifically And may reduce ability to interact socially and to deter predators or competitors	Unacceptable
Teeth removal	Cannot bite effectively	Dog not so dangerous	General anaesthetic effects.	Reduced ability to chew and perform natural oral behaviours	Unacceptable (except for clinical need)

RTAs = road traffic accidents.

Table 4.3 Methods of euthanasia of dogs kept as companion animals.

Method	Restraint required	Welfare benefits	Welfare risks
Intravenous injection of barbiturate	Sedation recommended	Quick and pain free	Poor injection procedure slows effect Pain of injection May be excessive resistance to restraint if not sedated
Free bullet (0.22 calibre) or shotgun (410 gauge or larger)	Needs secure and short leashing	Immediate death if done correctly	If inaccurate shooting, serious injury Danger of bullet ricochet
Captive bolt	Needs secure and short leashing	Immediate concussion	Need ensanguination after shooting

Source: AVMA (2013).

Table 4.4 Basic measures and clinical standards of dogs (*Canis familiaris*).

Parameter	Normal measures	
Life expectancy (median)	Great Dane 6 years	Mini Poodle 14 years
	Bulldog: avg. 8 years	Crossbred 13 years
Common weight range	Chihuahua: 1.5–3 kg (2.7)	Great Dane: 55–80 kg
Resting respiratory frequency	18–34 min	
Heart rate	60–140 beats/min	
Haematocrit	35–57%	

Source: O'Neill et al. (2013); Fraser et al. (1991); Debraekeleer (2010).

indicate heat stroke, fever, disease, exercise, physiological stress, pain, fear, or excitement (Sjaastad et al. 2012). However, there is significant normal variation in different dogs' normal resting heart rates from around 80 to 140 beats per minute (Sjaastad et al. 2012). A slow capillary refill time of dogs' gums above 2 seconds may suggest dehydration or blood loss (Nelson and Couto 1998), whereas a quick refill time of less than 1 second suggests stress, fever, or pain (Cote 2011). Cortisol and its breakdown products can be detected and measured in urine, saliva, faeces, and blood plasma. Cortisol concentration can remain high in saliva for several minutes after a dog experiences a stressor, so this can be a useful measure of acute stress (Glenk et al. 2013). It increases in urine over several hours, so this can be a useful indicator of longer-term distress (Rooney et al. 2007; Figure 4.9). Increased cortisol can also indicate hyperadrenocorticism.

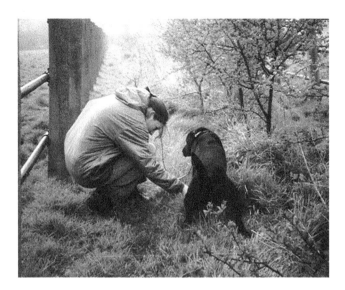

Figure 4.9   Researchers (a) collecting urine for analysis of cortisol levels (*Source:* courtesy Nicola Rooney).

4.3.2 Behavioural Signs

The behavioural responses of an individual dog are influenced by its breed, type, rearing, and current environment. Dogs also vary in their physical conformation and thereby the range of behaviours which they are able to show. Dogs have individual temperaments and varying coping styles, both proactive and passive (Blackwell et al. 2010). Animals also have different past experiences and have learned to exhibit different behaviour in particular situations. For example, one dog may have learned that hiding is an effective way to avoid stressful situations, whilst another has learned that barking results in their being removed from the source of distress by their owner. This makes it difficult to derive a single list of behavioural signs shown in all situations by all dogs. The most effective way of monitoring welfare is therefore to pay attention to changes in an individual dog's behaviour to detect causes for concern (Rooney et al. 2009a).

Nevertheless, some generic behavioural indicators are useful (Table 4.5). Play is rewarding and is generally seen at high levels when an animal's welfare needs are met, hence reduced levels or an absence of play, is potentially an important welfare indicator (Rooney and Bradshaw 2003). Behaviours that are most reliably linked to physiological indicators of acute stress (such as plasma cortisol concentrations) include paw lifting, yawning, snout or lip licking, lowered body positions, vocalising, panting and increased salivation, repetitive behaviours, increased activity, 'nosing' (not defined but possibly nudging a person or exploring the surroundings), increased urination, and decreased drinking (Beerda et al. 1997, 2000; Hiby et al. 2006). There are also additional behavioural signs which tend to be seen in aversive situations, although not for every dog (Table 4.5). Chronic stress can also result in an increased likelihood or a lowered threshold for showing such behaviours over time. The categorisation of acute versus

Table 4.5 Behavioural indicators of distress in dogs.

Behavioural sign	Definitions	Main response type(s)
Startling	Moving or jumping suddenly in response to an external stimulus	A, P
Lethargy or inactivity	Reduction in movement or activity or reluctance to move	C, P
Loss of appetite	Reduction in eating behaviour or motivation to obtain food	C
Reduced playing	Decrease in playful interaction with objects, other dogs or humans	C
Hunched or rigid posture	Assuming a crouched, bent, or cramped body position	P
Low body position	Cowering or crouching with head and tail tucked lower than torso	A
Low tail position	Tail held vertically or tucked between the legs	A
Yawning	Jaws opening wide without vocalisation	A
Ears held low	Ears held back or against side of head	A
Trembling or body shaking	Rapid body spasms (in absence of low ambient temperatures)	A
Vocalisations	Oral noises of barking, whining, whimpering, groaning, or crying	A, P
Licking lips (also referred to as tongue out, tongue flicking, or snout licking)	Tongue extrudes from mouth or runs over lips	A, C
Increased salivation	Rise in drooling in absence of food	A
Increased vigilance	Rise in alertness with eyes open and head turning in response to stimuli	C
Reduced responsiveness to humans or to previous rewarding stimuli	Decreased interactivity with people or objects which would formerly elicit responses	C
Increased self-grooming	Rise in behaviours directed to own body including licking, stretching, and scratching.	A, C
Paw lifting	Single foot raised and held above the ground	A
Withdrawal or hiding	Moving out from view	C
Destructive behaviour	Chewing, scratching, or biting housing or other inedible object	C
Change in elimination patterns or indoor soiling	Altered positioning, timing or frequency of defecation or urination, or starting to eliminate in housing	A, C
Panting	Mouth opens with tongue hanging out (not related to ambient temperature)	A, C

Table 4.5   (Continued)

Behavioural sign	Definitions	Main response type(s)
Aggression	Rise in tendency to growl, snap, or bite (humans or other dogs) in response to touch or other stimuli	A, C, P
Increased activity level	Rise in locomotory activity	C
Coprophagy	Consuming of own faeces	C
Self-mutilation	Scratching or biting part of own body (e.g. paws or tail)	C, P
Paying attention to wound	Looking at, licking, rubbing, or chewing site of injury	P
Repetitive behaviours	Exhibiting multiple identical behaviours with no apparent function e.g. pacing, circling, spinning, bouncing, tail-chasing, flank sucking, shadow staring, or chasing	C

Source: Adapted from Rooney et al. (2009a) and Casey et al. (2011).
A = acute response; C = chronic response; P = response to pain.
Examples of studies using each of indicator given in Rooney and Bradshaw (2014).

chronic stress needs therefore to be interpreted with caution, and a change in the rate or frequency of any of these behaviours is a cause for concern.

Dogs show a range of behavioural responses to pain, but there are wide individual differences again suggesting passive and active coping styles (Vaisanen et al. 2005). Dogs in pain may be inactive, and appear unresponsive or may vocalise. Palpation of a painful tissue can result in the dog moving away, lying still or protecting the area by growling, flinching, growling, guarding, or by snapping, or biting. Altered gait or a reluctance to move may indicate pain, although signs may be subtle, for example, in the early stages of arthritis. Unsurprisingly, owners struggle to assess pain in their dogs (Wiseman et al. 2001), and a number of different scoring systems have been developed (e.g. Holton et al. 2001; Reid et al. 2007, Murrell et al. 2008). Reliable behavioural indicators of pain include vocalisations (e.g. 'scream', 'groan', or 'cry'), attention to a wound or injury site (licking, rubbing, looking, or chewing), poor mobility (e.g. refusing, or slow or reluctance to move, lameness, or stiffness), response to touch, subjective assessments of demeanour (e.g. uninterested, depressed, aggressive, nervous, anxious, or fearful) and specific postures (rigid or hunched). Although some breeds are claimed to have greater pain tolerance (e.g. Pit Bull Terriers, Clifford et al. 1983), it is likely that selection has produced breeds whose behavioural expression of pain differs.

Many behaviours commonly described as 'problematic' are in fact indicative of an underlying welfare concern, whereby the dog finds itself in an environment or situation with which it cannot cope (Verga and Michelazzi 2009). Some 'problem behaviours' occur only, or at higher rates, in suboptimal conditions. Many other owner-perceived problems are natural species–specific behaviours for the dog, such as barking (Mills and Zulch 2010), scavenging, roaming, destructiveness, house-soiling (Patronek et al. 1996; Evans et al. 2007; Kim et al. 2009), scent marking (Prescott et al. 2004), chasing, and hyperactivity (Marston et al. 2005). Aggression is similarly often a dog's response to something frightening or an unpredictable environment. These behaviours may be useful welfare indicators if their frequency or character changes. For example, barking can become repetitive or 'stereotypical' in suboptimal conditions (Prescott et al. 2004).

Repetitive behaviours such as pacing, circling, bouncing, flank sucking, shadow staring or chasing, spinning, tail-chasing, and wall bouncing may indicate previous or current chronic stressful environments (Hetts et al. 1992; Hubrecht et al. 1992; Beerda et al. 1999, 2000; Rooney et al. 2009b). However, dogs vary in when they show these behaviours (Rooney et al. 2009b; Denham et al. 2014). Repetitive behaviours, performed during particular events, may suggest that those dogs have been previously rewarded for their performance. In comparison, those performed under minimal stimulation may be associated with stress (Denham et al. 2014). Any repetitive behaviours should prompt consideration of enhancing the conditions in which the affected dog is kept, such as by providing increased human interaction or other forms of enrichment (Hiby 2005; Gaines et al. 2008). Some repetitive behaviours may be a result of clinical conditions (e.g. pruritis) or previous living conditions and hence may not benefit from such efforts.

Changes in feeding (Delaney 2006), drinking (Hiby et al. 2006), and elimination behaviour may indicate disease or other problems. The reasons why dogs eat plants, faeces, and nonfood materials such as material or stones are yet to be understood. Coprophagy, for example, may be a natural behaviour in specific circumstances (Gaines 2008), but may be because dogs try to create novelty in otherwise understimulating environments, a nutritional imbalance, or previous harsh treatment used during toilet training that causes the dog to try to hide evidence of faeces for fear of being punished (Wells 2003; Rooney et al. 2009a).

Dogs' responses to rewards and training may also indicate their mood or overall welfare. Dogs with poorer welfare may be more 'pessimistic' and less trainable (e.g. those exhibiting separation-related behaviours). After training on simple tasks, some dogs are less motivated to approach food bowls of uncertain rewards (Mendl et al. 2010), whereas dogs in rehoming kennels (Udell et al. 2010) or those that have been frequently punished by their owners (Rooney and Cowan 2011) are less trainable. Dogs' reduced responses to previously effective rewards may also indicate changes in their overall mood. Humans are often poor at interpreting canine signs, even if they live or work with dogs (Kerswell et al. 2009; Mariti et al. 2012). Owners seem better at interpreting dogs' facial expressions (Bloom and Friedman 2013) but often fail to notice or misinterpret other signs (Correia et al. 2007; Tami and Gallagher 2009; Mariti et al. 2012).

4.4 Action Plan for Improving Dog Welfare Worldwide

There is no one set of priorities for improving dog welfare worldwide given the variety of dogs and their environments, and the lack of validated methods to prioritise the different issues. However, some priorities for particular countries have been identified by surveying scientists (Houpt et al. 2007) or veterinary surgeons (e.g. Yeates and Main 2011; Buckland et al. 2014) or by using quantitative methods (e.g. for greyhound racing; Rooney 2011). For many welfare issues, there is also insufficient scientific information from which to draw firm recommendations. Dogs are so varied and live under such diverse conditions that research into their welfare is often piecemeal and the results may or may not be relevant to all breeds or management conditions. There is limited funding of research by any canine industry (Stafford 2007; Rooney and Bradshaw 2014), and there is a need for systematic research to develop better techniques to assess dogs' feelings in different situations; combining behavioural and physiological indicators into a universal welfare index (Hewson et al. 2007). Nevertheless, some priorities can be identified.

In some countries, dogs suffer because of breed-specific legislation and breed stereotypes. Owners and policy makers need to understand that each dog is an individual, shaped by their rearing and opportunities to learn, as well as their genetic predispositions. Although dogs of different breeds may show tendencies to behave in different ways, they are also very likely to have been reared in different ways. It has been shown that there is more variation within individuals of a given breed than between breeds (Scott and Fuller 1965). In many countries, breed-specific legislation can mean dogs of specific breeds need lifetime muzzling and on-lead exercise, cannot be rehomed, or are euthanased, regardless of temperament. Better legislation requires education of the public, the media, and policymakers to avoid harmful blanket rules.

The myriad of genetic problems caused by breeding need to be addressed urgently, both to redress problems in countries where pedigree breeding and showing is established and to prevent them where pedigree breeding is growing. Changes in attitudes are therefore needed on the part of multiple stakeholders, and a variety of actions may help this be achieved (Table 4.6). Dog breeders, breed societies, and show judges need to have health and welfare as their priority, rather than a secondary concern after aesthetics, tradition, or financial interests. All dog breeders have a responsibility to produce puppies with minimal risk of disease and with optimal temperaments. However, many currently place considerably more importance on appearance than on health, behaviour, and welfare (van Hagen et al. 2004). Breed societies need to change this. Veterinary professionals, insurance companies, and individual owners should all exert market pressure on breeders to produce healthy dogs using educational resources (e.g. UFAW 2013) or formalised assurances (e.g. AWF/RSPCA 2012). The media and celebrities should also promote images of happy healthy dogs instead of celebrating those with exaggerated features. Legislation should ensure breeding establishments give sufficient care to puppies' health, rearing environment, and behaviour. A global approach is critical as mass breeding and global movement of puppies continues to expand.

In many countries, large numbers of unowned dogs on the street or relinquished to kennels often outstrip shelters' capacities. Even in countries with fewer free-roaming dogs such as the United States, 3 to 4 million dogs are still culled annually (HSUS 2014), albeit significantly fewer than the estimated 13 million dogs and cats euthanased in 1973 (Scarlett 2004). Supply of some breeds of dogs also greatly exceeds availability of homes, for example, ex-racing greyhound dogs. In some countries, euthanasia is resisted for cultural or political reasons. In some such places (e.g. India), dogs are managed on the streets, with varying success (e.g. Reece and Chawla 2006). But in other locations (e.g. Italy and Greece), many dogs are placed in shelters which are

Table 4.6 Fourteen priority recommendations deemed most likely to improve pedigree dog welfare from systematic expert interviews and survey in 2010 (derived in United Kingdom but universally applicable).

Rank	Action recommended
1	Systematic collection of morbidity and mortality data from all registered dogs
2	Revision of registration rules to prevent the registration of offspring of matings between first- and second-degree relatives
3	Open stud books to allow more frequent introduction of new genetic material into established breeds
4	Setting up systems to monitor the effectiveness of any interventions and changes (including those listed here), regularly reviewing, assessing, and evaluating the changes in morbidity and mortality in all breeds
5	Researching and reviewing the specific problems pertinent to each specific breed, considering to what extent these can be overcome with the current gene pool and the value of outcrossing
6	Development of detailed management plans for each breed, taking into consideration the specific issues (both exaggerated features and inherited disorders) most relevant to the breed; constructed by collaborations of geneticists, welfare scientists, and breeders all aiming to optimise breed health and welfare
7	Refinement of diagnostic tests and DNA markers for inherited disorders
8	Increase genetic diversity by encouraging importation and intercountry matings
9	Make registration of pedigree dogs conditional upon both parents undergoing compulsory screening tests
10	Introduction of codes of practice that encourage breeders to consider health, temperament, and welfare
11	Training and accreditation of judges to prioritise heath, welfare, and behaviour in the show ring
12	Creating and fostering the image of a happy and desirable dog being one that experiences high welfare
13	Formulation of an independent panel of experts from multiple disciplines to facilitate dialogue and result in positive action amongst stakeholders. This panel would help with the execution of many of the listed actions but remain independent of any organisation
14	Development of schemes for calculating Estimated Breeding Values for multifactorial disorders; the Estimated Breeding Value for an animal for any trait predicts the average 'performance' of its progeny for that trait

Source: Adapted from Rooney and Sargan (2010).

overcrowded and inadequate (Dalla Villa et al. 2010). Shelters need to be controlled to ensure they are not causing greater welfare problems than they are trying to solve.

To prevent a surplus of puppies, neutering should be promoted as part of responsible pet ownership, perhaps subsidised by charity or government initiatives. For free-roaming and breeding populations of dogs, this requires effective catch, neuter, and release protocols. These should be part of dog-control programmes, which should also include education, legislation, basic health care, rehoming, and possibly short-term humane culling in some populations, as appears to have had some success in the United States (Rowan and Williams 1987). Such programmes need adequate, sustained financial and logistical support; competent personnel; local community engagement; and ongoing monitoring (ICAM 2015). Locations differ in their dog population dynamics and in people's attitudes towards the dogs (e.g. how much they tolerate roaming dogs and euthanasia). They also vary in the availability and affordability of surgical neutering, so nonsurgical methods of bitch contraception are needed that are effective for years rather than months. One such method has been developed (e.g. *New York Times* 2013) but is not yet widely available (Massei and Miller 2013).

In all countries, there is also a need for campaigns to encourage rehoming of unwanted dogs in preference to procuring a deliberately bred puppy, at the same time as working to reduce the reasons why dogs are most commonly surrendered or abandoned. The latter requires encouraging responsible dog acquisition, with owners considering their own lifestyle, commitment, resources, and possible changes to their circumstances during their dogs' whole lifetime and having reasonable expectations. For example, owners may value well-behaved dogs but fail to devote time to training (King et al. 2009). Breeders and sellers should educate and screen future owners, and owners should check that breeders are keeping bitches, stud dogs, and puppies in conditions conducive to good welfare. This is made more challenging by increased internet sales, importation, and smuggling. Welfare charities, local authorities, and law enforcement should adopt a concerted effort to improve dog sales and purchases. The registration or licensing of dogs has the potential to increase responsibility of owners and reduce the number of dogs relinquished, as has been demonstrated in Calgary, Canada (ASPCA 2007), and could also include compulsory insurance, microchipping, and owner competency tests. The value of such schemes is yet to be fully quantified, but some implementing nations believe them to be successful. Legislation should also ensure those failing to meet their dog's needs are prevented from causing further dogs to suffer.

Owners need to be educated so they recognise behaviour problems and know that these are both preventable and treatable. For example, anxiety caused by separation or noises may be reduced by avoiding the causes and by employing gradual habituation protocols to avoid fear development, whilst established fears can be reduced by using validated treatment plans. Increased understanding of which behaviours are 'normal' and which are symptomatic of problems is vital. Owners and dogs may benefit from the development of resources to help people recognise signs of their dogs' feelings and be able to respond appropriately (e.g. Loftus et al. 2012). Owners should be encouraged to use appropriately skilled and qualified trainers (e.g. APDT 2015) and behavioural experts (e.g. ASAB 2016). This may also reduce relinquishment rates, especially in the case of human-directed aggression and separation-related behaviours, which are common causes of dog surrender (Bailey 1992; Mondelli et al. 2004; Diesel et al. 2007; Kim et al. 2009; O'Neill et al. 2013). Such behaviourists should use therapies and training methods based on positive reinforcement and not punishment or outdated views of 'wolf society' (e.g. 'dominance theory') or excessive anthropomorphism (e.g. assuming behaviour is motivated by higher cognitive processes such as guilt).

Owner education is also vital to improve recognition of pain, illness, and poor body condition. Undernutrition remains a priority in developing countries, requiring tailored dog population-management strategies. In contrast, obesity is one of the most important welfare issues in dogs today (Houpt et al. 2007) and a growing epidemic in the Western developed world. Tackling it is the responsibility of owners, caregivers, pet food companies, and veterinary professionals. Weight-loss programmes require the motivation of owners. However, owners often have false ideas about whether a dog is overweight or obese (Bland et al. 2009). Education from veterinarians and pet food manufacturers on appropriate body weight is required. Veterinary medicine for dogs has developed dramatically in the last half-century, health insurance policies are common in many countries such as Sweden (Bonnett et al. 1997), and owners may be motivated to keep their dogs alive. This creates risks of overtreatment that veterinarians need to manage. Veterinarians therefore need dialogue to determine what constitutes excessive treatment, incompatible with the individual animal's welfare. Veterinary professionals need to be informed on wider welfare issues so that they can educate owners, for example on the best ways to obtain a new dog, the optimal rearing of puppies, and methods to avoid behavioural problems developing. The pet care industry and popular media can also help shift social norms. For example, in the United Kingdom, recent televisions documentaries have raised awareness about the likely suffering of dogs with separation-related behaviours (Channel Four 2014) and those bred to pedigree standards (BBC 2009). However, education must translate into behavioural change amongst owners. Most critically, we need a worldwide change in attitude from seeing dogs as disposable commodities to understanding that owning a dog brings responsibilities and should only be undertaken by those whose lifestyle and circumstances make them able to provide for their dogs' welfare needs throughout its entire life.

Bibliography

Adams, G.J. and Johnson, K.G. (1994). Sleep, work and the effects of shirt work in drugs detector dogs Canis familiaris. Applied Animal Behaviour Science 41 (1): 115–126.

Adams, G.J. and Johnson, K.G. (1995). Guard dogs: sleep, work and the behavioural responses to people and other stimuli. Applied Animal Behaviour Science 46 (1): 103–115.

Adin, C.A. (2011). Complications of ovariohysterectomy and orchidectomy in companion animals. The Veterinary Clinics of North America. Small Animal Practice 41: 1023–1039.

Allen, L. (2010) The influence of the lead on dog behaviour. BSc Dissertation. University of Bristol.

Alsop, J.A. and Albertson, T.E. (2008). A case of canine ingestion of buzz-bites chocolate energy chews. Clinical Toxicology 46 (7): 625.

APDT (Association of Pet Dog Trainers). (2015). Choosing a Trainer. Available at www.apdt.co.uk/dog-owners/choosing-a-trainer. Accessed 12 February 2016.

Arhant, C., Bubna-Littitz, H., Bartels, A. et al. (2010). Behaviour of smaller and larger dogs: effects of training methods, inconsistency of owner behaviour and level of engagement in activities with the dog. Applied Animal Behaviour Science 123 (3–4): 131–142.

Arnold, A. and Elvehjem, C.A. (1939). Nutritional requirements of dogs. Journal of the American Veterinary Medicine Association 95: 187.

ASAB (Association for the Study of Animal Behaviour). (2016). Register of Certified Practitioners. Available at http://www.asab.org/ccab-register. Accessed 12 February 2016.

Asher, L., Diesel, G., Summers, J.F. et al. (2009). Inherited defects in pedigree dogs. Part 1: disorders related to breed standards. *Veterinary Journal* 182 (3): 402.

ASPCA (American Society for the Prevention of Cruelty to Animals) (2007) City of Calgary Animal Services: Dog Licensing Program. http://www.aspcapro.org/sites/pro/files/city-of-calgary-idprogram-profile-by-aspcapro_0.pdf. Accessed 29th February 2018

AVMA (American Veterinary Medical Association) (2013). AVMA Guidelines for the Euthanasia of Animals: 2013 Edition. Available at https://www.avma.org/KB/Policies/Pages/Euthanasia-Guidelines.aspx. Accessed 7 October 2015.

AWF/RSPCA (Animal Welfare Foundation/ Royal Society for the Prevention of Cruelty to Animals). (2012). Puppy Contract. Available at https://puppycontract.rspca.org.uk/home. Accessed 12 March 2016.

Bailey, G. (1992). *Parting with a Pet Survey*. Burford: The Blue Cross.

Bateson, P. (2010). *Independent Inquiry into Dog Breeding*. Published privately by Patrick Bateson in 2010 and printed by Micropress Ltd.

BBC (2009). *Pedigree Dogs Exposed*. Available at http://news.bbc.co.uk/1/hi/uk/7569064.stm. Accessed 12 March 2016.

Beauvais, W., Cardwell, J.M., and Brodbelt, D.C. (2012). The effect of neutering on the risk of urinary incontinence in bitches – a systematic review. *Journal of Small Animal Practice* 53: 198–204.

Beerda, B., Schilder, M.B.H., van Hooff, J.A.R.A.M., and de Vries, H.W. (1997). Manifestations of chronic and acute stress in dogs. *Applied Animal Behaviour Science* 52 (3–4): 307–319.

Beerda, B., Schilder, M.B.H., Van Hooff, J.A.R.A.M. et al. (1999). Chronic stress in dogs subjected to social and spatial restriction I: behavioural responses. *Physiology and Behaviour* 66: 233–242.

Beerda, B., Schilder, M.B., van Hooff, J.A.R. et al. (2000). Behavioural and hormonal indicators of enduring environmental stress in dogs. *Animal Welfare* 9: 49–62.

Bergamasco, L., Osella, M.C., Savarino, P. et al. (2010). Heart rate variability and saliva cortisol assessment in shelter dogs: human-animal interaction effects. *Applied Animal Behaviour Science* 125: 56–68.

Blackwell, E., Casey, R.A., and Bradshaw, J.W.S. (2006). Controlled trial of behavioural therapy for separation-related disorders in dogs. *Veterinary Record* 158 (16): 551–554.

Blackwell, E., Twells, C., Seawright, A., and Casey, R.A. (2008). The relationship between training methods and the occurrence of behavior problems, as reported by owners, in a population of domestic dogs. *Journal of Veterinary Behavior: Clinical Applications and Research* 3 (5): 207–217.

Blackwell, E.J., Bodnariu, A., Tyson, J. et al. (2010). Rapid shaping of behaviour associated with high urinary cortisol in domestic dogs. *Applied Animal Behaviour Science* 124 (3–4): 113–120.

Blackwell, E.J., Bradshaw, J.W.S., and Casey, R.A. (2013). Fear responses to noises in domestic dogs: prevalence, risk factors and co-occurrence with other fear related behaviour. *Applied Animal Behaviour Science* 145: 15–25.

Blackwell, E., Casey, R.A., and Bradshaw, J.W.S. (2016). Efficacy of written behavioral advice for separation-related behaviour problems in dogs newly adopted from a rehoming center. *Journal of Veterinary Behaviour: Clinical Applications and Research* 12: 13–19.

Bland, I.M., Guthrie-Jones, A., Taylor, R.D., and Hill, J. (2009). Dog obesity: owner attitudes and behaviour. *Preventive Veterinary Medicine* 92 (4): 333–340.

de Bleser, B., Brodbelt, D.C., Gregory, N.G., and Martinez, T.A. (2011). The association between acquired urinary sphincter mechanism incontinence in bitches and early spaying: a case –control study. *The Veterinary Journal* 187: 42–47.

Bloom, T. and Friedman, H. (2013). Classifying dogs' (*Canis familiaris*) facial expressions from photographs. *Behavioural Processes* 96: 1–10.

Boitani, L., Francisci, F., Ciucci, P., and Andreoli, G. (1995). Population biology and ecology of feral dogs in Central Italy. In: *The Domestic Dog: Its Evolution, Behaviour and Interactions with People* (ed. J.A. Serpell), 216–244. Cambridge University Press.

Bonnett, B.N., Egenvall, A., Olson, P., and Hedhammar, A. (1997). Mortality in insured Swedish dogs: rates and causes of death in various breeds. *Veterinary Record* 141 (2): 40–44.

Bosch, G., Beerda, B., van de Hoek, E. et al. (2009). Effect of dietary fibre type on physical activity and behaviour in kennelled dogs. *Applied Animal Behaviour Science* 121 (1): 32–41.

Bowman, D.D. and Atkins, C.E. (2009). Heartworm biology, treatment, and control. *The Veterinary Clinics of North America. Small Animal Practice* 39 (6): 1127.

Bradshaw, J.W.S. (2011). *Dog Sense: How the New Science of Dog Behavior Can Make You a Better Friend to Your Pet*. New York: Basic Books.

Bradshaw, J.W.S., Blackwell, E.J., Rooney, N.J. and Casey, R.A. (2002a). Prevalence of separation-related behaviour in dogs in southern England. *Proceedings of the 8th European Society of Veterinary Clinical Ethology Meeting on Veterinary Behavioural Medicine*. Granada, Spain, October 2, 2002. Eds J. Dehasse, E. Biosca Marce. Paris, Publibook. Pp. 189–193.

Bradshaw, J.W.S., McPherson, J.A., Casey, R.A., and Larter, I.S. (2002b). Aetiology of separation-related behaviour in the domestic dog. *Veterinary Record* 151: 43–46.

Bradshaw, J.W.S., Blackwell, E.J., and Casey, R.A. (2009). Dominance in domestic dogs-useful construct or bad habit? *Journal of Veterinary Behavior: Clinical Applications and Research* 4 (3): 135–144.

Bradshaw, J.W.S., Pullen, A.J., and Rooney, N.J. (2015). Why do adult dogs play? *Behavioural Processes* 110: 82–87.

Broach, D. and Dunham, A.E. (2016). Evaluation of a pheromone collar on canine behaviors during transition from foster homes to a training kennel in juvenile military working dogs. *Journal of Veterinary Behavior: Clinical Applications and Research* 14: 41–51.

Brown, W.Y. (2009). Nutritional and ethical issues regarding vegetarianism in the domestic dog. *Recent Advances in Animal Nutrition in Australia* 17: 137–143.

Bruchim, Y., Klement, E., Saragusty, J. et al. (2006). Heat stroke in dogs: a retrospective study of 54 cases (1999–2004) and analysis of risk factors for death. *Journal of Veterinary Internal Medicine* 20 (1): 38–46.

Buckland, E.L., Corr, S.A., Abeyesinghe, S., and Wathes, C.M. (2014). Prioritisation of companion dog welfare issues using expert. *Animal Welfare* 23 (1): 39–46.

Bugg, R.J., Robertson, I.D., Elliot, A.D., and Thompson, R.C. (1999). Gastrointestinal parasites of urban dogs in Perth, Western Australia. *Veterinary Journal* 157: 295–301.

Burghardt, W.F. (2003). Behavioral considerations in the management of working dogs. *The Veterinary Clinics of North America. Small Animal Practice* 33 (2): 417–446.

Burkholder, W.J. and Bauer, J.E. (1998). Foods and techniques for managing obesity in companion animals. *Journal of the American Veterinary Medicine Association* 212 (5): 658–662.

Burkholder, W.J. and Toll, P.W. (2000). Obesity. In: *Small Animal Clinical Nutrition*, 4e (ed. M.S. Hand, C.D. Thatcher, R.L. Reimillard, et al.), 401–430. Topeka, KS: Mark Morris Institute.

Burrow, R., Batchelor, D., and Cripps, P. (2005). Complications observed during and after ovariohysterectomy in 142 bitches at a veterinary teaching hospital. *Veterinary Record* 157: 829–833.

Carr, T. (1979). Caudal adhesions subsequent to tail docking. *Canine Practice* 6: 63–64.

Casey, R.A., Twells, C. and Blackwell, E.J. (2007). An investigation of the relationship between measures of consistency in owners and the occurrence of "behaviour problems" in the domestic dog, *Proceedings of the 6th International Veterinary Behaviour Meeting* 17–20th July, Riccione, Italy, Pp. 94–95.

Casey, R.A., Rooney, N.J. and Clark, C.C.A. (2011). How best to achieve a fearless working dog. Report to Defence Science Technology Laboratory.

Casey, R.A., Loftus, B., Bolster, C. et al. (2013). Inter-dog aggression in a UK owner survey: prevalence, co-occurrence in different contexts and risk factors. *Veterinary Record* 172: 127.

Casey, R.A., Loftus, B., Bolster, C. et al. (2014). Human directed aggression in domestic dogs (*Canis familiaris*): occurrence in different contexts and risk factors. *Applied Animal Behaviour Science* 152: 52–63.

Channel Four (2014). *Dogs their secret lives*. Available at http://www.channel4.com/programmes/dogs-their-secret-lives/on-demand/58820-002. Accessed 12 March 2016.

CIEH, Chartered Institute of Environmental Health (1995). *Model Licence Conditions and Guidance for Dog Boarding Establishments: Animal Boarding Establishments Act 1963*. London: The Chameleon Press.

Clifford, D.H., Boatfield, M.P., and Rubright, J. (1983). Observations on fighting dogs. *Journal of the American Veterinary Medicine Association* 83: 654–657.

Clutton-Brock, J. (1995). Origins of the dog: domestication and early history. In: *The Domestic Dog: Its Evolution, Behaviour and Interactions with People* (ed. J.A. Serpell), 7–20. Cambridge: Cambridge University Press.

Colliard, L., Ancel, J., Benet, J.J. et al. (2006). Risk factors for obesity in dogs in France. *Journal of Nutrition* 136 (7 Suppl): 1951S–1954S.

Collins, R.L., Birchard, S.J., Chew, D.J., and Heuter, K.J. (1998). Surgical treatment of urate calculi in Dalmatians: 38 cases (1980–1995). *Journal of the American Veternarry Medical Association* 213 (6): 833.

Committee of Animal Nutrition (2006). *Nutrient requirements of Dogs and Cats*. Washington DC: Subcommittee on Dog and Cat Nutrition, National Research Council National Academy Press.

Committee on Animal Nutrition (1985). *Nutrient Requirements of Dogs*. Washington DC: Subcommittee on Dog Nutrition, Committee on Animal Nutrition, Board of Agriculture, National Research Council. National Academy Press.

Coppola, C.L., Grandin, T., and Enns, R.M. (2006). Human interaction and cortisol: can human contact reduce stress for shelter dogs? *Physiology and Behavior* 87 (3): 537–541.

Correia C, Ruiz de la Torre JL, Manteca X and Fatjo J 2007 Accuracy of dog owners to describe and interpret the canine body language during aggressive episodes, 6th IVBM/ECVBM-CA Meeting Riccione.

Cote, E. (2011). *Clinical Veterinary Advisor*. USA: Mosby Elsevier.

Courcier, E.A., Thomson, R.M., Mellor, D.J., and Yam, P.S. (2010). An epidemiological study of environmental factors associated with canine obesity. *Journal of Small Animal Practice* 51: 362–367.

Cracknell, N.R. and Mills, D.S. (2008). A double-blind placebo-controlled study into the efficacy of a homeopathic remedy for fear of firework noises in the dog (*Canis familiaris*). *The Veterinary Journal* 177 (1): 80–88.

Crane, S.W. (1991). Occurrence and management of obesity in companion animals. *Journal of Small Animal Practice* 32: 275–282.

Cronin, G.M., Hemsworth, P.H., Barnett, J.L. et al. (2003). An anti-barking muzzle for dogs and its short-term effects on behaviour and saliva cortisol concentrations. *Applied Animal Behaviour Science* 83 (3): 215–226.

Crowell-Davis, S.L., Seibert, L.M., Sung, W. et al. (2003). Use of clomipramine, alprazolam and behavior modification for treatment of storm phobia in dogs. *Journal of the American Veterinary Medicine Association* 222: 744–748.

Dalla Villa, P., Kahn, S., Stuardo, L. et al. (2010). Free-roaming dog control among OIE-member countries. *Preventitive Veterinary Medicine* 97: 58–63.

Darke, P.G.G., Thrusfield, M.V., and Aitken, C.G.G. (1985). Association between tail injuries and docking in dogs. *Veterinary Record* 116: 409.

De Lorimier, L.-P. and Fan, T.M. (2005). Treating cancer pain in dogs and cats. *Veterinary Medicine* 100: 364–379.

Debraekeleer, J. (2010). Feeding reproducing dogs. In: *Small Animal Clinical Nutrition* (ed. M.S. Hand, D.T. Craig, R.L. Remillard, et al.), 281–294. Topeka, KS: Mark Morris Institute USA.

Deka, R.S. (2009). Crude fiber deficiency in a dog – a case report. *Veterinary Practitioner* 10: 183–184.

Delaney, S.J. (2006). Management of anorexia in dogs and cats. *The Veterinary Clinics of North America. Small Animal Practice* 36 (6): 1243.

Denham, H.D.C., Bradshaw, J.W.S., and Rooney, N.J. (2014). Repetitive behaviour in kennelled domestic dog: stereotypical or not? *Physiology and Behaviour* 128: 288–294.

Diesel, G., Smith, H., and Pfeiffer, D. (2007). Factors affecting time to adoption of dogs rehomed by a charity in the UK. *Animal Welfare* 16 (3): 353–360.

Diesel, G., Pfeiffer, D., Crispin, S., and Brodbelt, D. (2010). Risk factors for tail injuries in dogs in Great Britain. *Veterinary Record* 166: 812–817.

Donoghue, S. and Kronfield, D.S. (1994). Feeding hospitalised dogs and cats. In: *The Waltham Book of Clinical Nutrition of the Dog and Cat* (ed. J. Wills and K.W. Simpson). Oxford, UK: Pergamon.

Dreschel, N.A. and Granger, D.A. (2005). Physiological and behavioral reactivity to stress in thunderstorm phobic dogs and their caregivers. *Applied Animal Behaviour Science* 95: 153–168.

Eppleston, K.R., Kelman, M., and Ward, M.P. (2013). Distribution, seasonality and risk factors for tick paralysis in Australian dogs and cats. *Veterinary Parasitology* 196: 460–468.

Estelles, M.G. and Mills, D.S. (2006). Signs of travel-related problems in dogs and their response to treatment with dog-appeasing pheromone. *Veterinary Record* 159 (5): 143–148.

Evans, R.I., Herbold, J.R., Bradshaw, B.S., and Moore, G.E. (2007). Causes for discharge of military working dogs from service: 268 cases (2000–2004). *Journal of the American Veterinary Medical Association* 231 (8): 1215–1220.

Fahey, G.C. Jr., Barry, K.A., and Swanson, K.A. (2008). Age-related changes in nutrient utilization by companion animals. *Annual Review of Nutrition* 28: 425–445.

Fan, T.M., de Lorimier, L.P., O'Dell-Anderson, K. et al. (2007). Single-agent pamidronate for palliative therapy of canine appendicular osteosarcoma bone pain. *Journal of Veterinary Internal Medicine* 21: 431–439.

Feuerstein, N. and Terkel, J. (2008). Interrelationships of dogs (*Canis familiaris*) and cats (*Felis catus L.)* living under the same roof. *Applied Animal Behaviour Science* 113 (1–3): 150–165.

Fisher, J. (2011). *Why Does My Dog?* London: Souvenir Press.

Fraser, C.M., Bergeron, J.A., Mays, A., and Aiello, S.E. (1991). *The Merck Veterinary Manual*, 7e. Rahway, NJ: Merck & CO.

Gaines SA (2008). Kennelled dog welfare – effects of housing and husbandry. Unpublished PhD Thesis University of Bristol.

Gaines, S.A., Rooney, N.J., and Bradshaw, J.W.S. (2008). The effect of feeding enrichment upon reported working ability and behavior of kenneled working dogs. *Journal of Forensic Science* 53 (6): 1400–1404.

Garde, E., Pérez, G., Vanderstichel, R. et al. (2016). Effects of surgical and chemical sterilization on the behavior of free-roaming male dogs in Puerto Natales, Chile. *Preventative Veterinary Medicine* 123: 106–120. doi: 10.1016/j. prevetmed.2015.11.011.

Gault, G., Berny, P., and Lorgue, G.P. (1995). Plants which are toxic for pets. *Recueil de Medecine Veterinaire* 171 (2–3): 171–176.

Gaultier, E., Bonnafous, L., Viemet-Legue, D. et al. (2009). Efficacy of dog appeasing pheromone in reducing behaviours associated with fear of unfamiliar people and new surroundings in newly adopted puppies. *The Veterinary Record* 164: 708–714.

Gazzano, A., Mariti, C., Notari, L. et al. (2008). Effects of early gentling and early environment on emotional development of puppies. *Applied Animal Behaviour Science* 110 (3–4): 294–304.

German, A.J., Ryan, V.H., German, A.C. et al. (2010). Obesity, its associated disorders and the role of inflammatory adipokines in companion animals. *The Veterinary Journal* 185 (1): 4–9.

German, A.J., Holden, S.L., Wiseman-Orr, M.L. et al. (2012). Quality of life is reduced in obese dogs but improves after successful weight loss. *Veterinary Journal* 192 (3): 428–434.

Glenk, L.M., Kothgassner, O.D., Stetina, B.U. et al. (2013). Therapy dogs' salivary cortisol levels vary during animal-assisted interventions. *Animal Welfare* 22: 369–378.

Goddard, M.E. and Beilharz, R.G. (1986). Early prediction of adult behaviour in potential guide dogs. *Applied Animal Behaviour Science* 15: 247–260.

Goodwin, D., JWS, B., and Wickens, S.M. (1997). Paedomorphosis affects agonistic visual signals of domestic dogs. *Animal Behaviour* 53: 297–304.

Graham, L., Wells, D.L., and Hepper, P.G. (2005a). The influence of olfactory stimulation on the behaviour of dogs housed in a rescue shelter. *Applied Animal Behaviour Science* 91: 143–153.

Graham, L., Wells, D.L., and Hepper, P.G. (2005b). The influence of visual stimulation on the behaviour of dogs housed in a rescue shelter. *Animal Welfare* 14: 143–148.

Gross, T.L. and Carr, S.H. (1990). Amputation neuroma of docked tails in dogs. *Veterinary Pathology* 27: 61–62.

Hampson, K., Dushoff, J., Cleaveland, S. et al. (2009). Transmission dynamics and prospects for the elimination of canine rabies. *PLoS Biology* 7 (3): e1000053. doi: 10.1371/journal. pbio.1000053.

Hare, B., Brown, M., Williamson, C., and Tomasello, M. (2002). The domestication of social cognition in dogs. *Science* 298: 1634–1636.

Haverbeke, A., Messaoudi, F., Depiereux, C. et al. (2010). Efficiency of working dogs undergoing a new Human Familiarization and Training Program. *Journal of Veterinary Behavior: Clinical Applications and Research* 5 (2): 112–119.

Hazewinkel, H.A.W., van den Brom, W.E., van T Klooster, A.T. et al. (1991). Calcium metabolism in Great Dane dogs fed diets with various calcium and phosphorus levels. *Journal of Nutrition* 121: 99S–106S.

Heffner, H.E. (1983). Hearing in large and small dogs: absolute thresholds and size of the tympanic membrane. *Behavioural Neuroscience* 97: 310–318.

Heffner, H.E. (1998). Auditory awareness in animals. *Applied Animal Behaviour Science* 57: 259–268.

Hennessy, M.B., Davis, H.N., Williams, M.T. et al. (1997). Plasma cortisol levels of dogs in a county animal shelter. *Physiology and Behaviour* 62 (3): 485–490.

Hennessy, M.B., Williams, M.T., Miller, D.D. et al. (1998). Influence of male and female petters on plasma cortisol and behaviour: can human interaction reduce the stress of dogs in a public animal shelter? *Applied Animal Behaviour Science* 61: 63–77.

Hennessy, M.B., Voith, V.L., Hawke, J.L. et al. (2002). Effects of a program of human interaction and alterations in diet composition on activity of the hypothalamic-pituitary-adrenal axis in dogs housed in a public animal shelter. *Journal of the American Veterinary Medical Association* 221 (1): 65–71.

Hennessy, M.B., Morris, A., and Linden, F. (2006). Evaluation of the effects of a socialization program in a prison on behavior and pituitary-adrenal hormone levels of shelter dogs. *Applied Animal Behaviour Science* 99 (1–2): 157–171.

Herron, M.E., Shofer, F., and Reisner, I.R. (2009). Survey of the use and outcome of confrontational and non-confrontational training methods in client-owned dogs showing undesired behaviors. *Applied Animal Behaviour Science* 117: 47–54.

Hetts, S. (1991). Psychologic well-being: conceptual issues, behavioural measures and implications for dogs. *Veterinary Clinics of North America: Small Animal Practice* 21: 369–387.

Hetts, S., Clark, J.D., Calpin, J.P. et al. (1992). Influence of housing conditions on beagle behaviour. *Applied Animal Behaviour Science* 34: 137–155.

Hewson, C.J., Hiby, E.F., and Bradshaw, J.W.S. (2007). Assessing quality of life in companion and kennelled dogs: a critical review. *Animal Welfare* 16: 89–95.

Hiby EF (2005). The Welfare of Kennelled Domestic Dogs. PhD Thesis, University of Bristol.

Hiby, E.F. (2013). Dog population management. In: *Dogs, Zoonoses and Public Health*, 2e (ed. C.N.L. Macpherson, F.-X. Meslin and A.I. Wandeler), 177–204. Oxfordshire, UK: CABI International.

Hiby, E.F., Rooney, N.J., and Bradshaw, J.W.S. (2004). Dog training methods: their use, effectiveness and interaction with behaviour and welfare. *Animal Welfare* 13 (1): 63–69.

Hiby, E.F., Rooney, N.J., and Bradshaw, J.W.S. (2006). Behavioural and physiological responses of dogs entering re-homing kennels. *Physiology and Behavior* 89 (3): 385–391.

Hill, P.B., Hoare, J., Lau-Gillard, P. et al. (2009). Pilot study of the effect of individual homeopathy on the pruritus associated with atopic dermatitis in dogs. *Veterinary Record* 164: 364–337.

Holmes, K.L., Morris, P.J., Abdulla, Z. et al. (2007). Risk factors associated with excess body weight in dogs in the UK. *Journal of Animal Physiology and Animal Nutrition* 91: 166–167.

Holt, P.E. and Thrusfield, M.V. (1993). Association in bitches between breed, size, neutering and docking and acquired urinary incontinence due to incompetence of the urethral sphincter mechanism. *Veterinary Record* 133: 177–180.

Holton, L., Reid, J., Scott, E.M. et al. (2001). The development of a behavioural based pain scale to measure acute pain in dogs. *Veterinary Record* 148: 525–531.

Horowitz, A. (2009). Disambiguating the "guilty look": salient prompts to a familiar dog behaviour. *Behavioural Processes* 81: 447–452.

Houpt, K.A. (2005). *Domestic Animal Behavior*, 4e. Ames, IO: Blackwell Scientific.

Houpt, K.A., Goodwin, D., Uchida, Y. et al. (2007). Proceedings of a workshop to identify dog welfare issues in the US, Japan, Czech Republic, Spain and the UK. *Applied Animal Behaviour Science* 106 (4): 221–233.

Howell, T. and Bennett, P.C. (2011). Puppy power! Using social cognition research tasks to improve socialization practices for domestic dogs (*Canis familiaris*). *Journal of Veterinary Behavior: Clinical Applications and Research* 6 (3): 195–204.

Hsu, Y. and Sun, L. (2010). Factors associated with aggressive responses in pet dogs. *Applied Animal Behaviour Science* 123 (3–4): 108–123.

Hsu, Y., Severinghaus, L.L., and Serpell, J.A. (2003). Dog keeping in Taiwan: its contribution to the problem of free-roaming dogs. *Journal of Applied Animal Welfare Science* 6: 1–23.

HSUS (Humane Society of the United States) (2014). U.S. shelter and adoption estimates for 2012–13. Available at http://www.humanesociety.org/issues/pet_overpopulation/facts/pet_ownership_statistics.html. Accessed 12 March 2016.

Hubrecht, R.C. (1993). A comparison of social and environmental enrichment methods for laboratory housed dogs. *Applied Animal Behaviour Science* 37: 345–361.

Hubrecht, R.C. (2002). Comfortable quarters for dogs in research institutions. In: *Comfortable Quarters for Laboratory Animals*, 2e (ed. V. Reinhardt and A. Reinhardt), 56–64. Washington DC, USA: Animal Welfare Institute.

Hubrecht, R.C. and Buckwell, A. (2004). The welfare of laboratory dogs. In: *The Welfare of Laboratory Animal* (ed. E. Kaliste), 245–273. Dordrecht; London: Kluwer Academic.

Hubrecht, R.C., Serpell, J.A., and Poole, T.B. (1992). Correlates of pen size and housing conditions on the behaviour of kennelled dogs. *Applied Animal Behaviour Science* 34: 365–383.

Hubrecht, R., Sales, G., Peyvandi, A. et al. (1997). Noise in dog kennels, effects of design and husbandry. *Animal Alternatives, Welfare and Ethics* 27: 215–220.

ICAM (International Companion Animal Management Coalition). (2015). Are We Making a DifferenA Guide to Monitoring and Evaluating Dog Population Managemnet Interventions. Available at http://www.icam-coalition.org/downloads/ICAM_Guidance_Document.pdf. Accessed 12 June 2016.

Innes, J.R.M. (1931). *Vitamin C requirements of the dogs. Attempts to produce experimental scurvy. Second Report of the Director of Anial Pathology*, 143–150. Cambridge.

Ingham, K.E. and Gorrel, C. (2001). Effect of long-term intermittent periodical care on canine periodontal disease. *Journal of Small Animal Practice* 42: 67–70.

IUCN (International Union for Conservation of Nature and Natural Resources). (2016). The IUCN Red List of Threatenend Species. Available at http://www.iucnredlist.org/search. Accessed 22 August 2016.

Jackson, A.C. (2011). Update on rabies. *Research and Reports in Tropical Medicine* 2: 31–43.

Jeusette, I., Greco, D., Aquino, F. et al. (2010). Effect of breed on body composition and comparison between various methods to estimate body composition in dogs. *Research in Veterinary Science* 88 (2): 227–232.

Johnston, D.E. (1990). Care of accidental wounds. *The Veterinary Clinics of North America. Small Animal Practice* 20 (1): 27–46.

Juarbe-Diaz, S.V. and Houpt, K.A. (1996). Comparison of two antibarking collars for treatment of nuisance barking. *Journal of the American Animal Hospital Association* 32 (3): 231–235.

Kaminski, J. and Nitzschner, M. (2013). Do dogs get the point?: a review of dog–human communication ability. *Learning and Motivation* 44 (4): 294–302.

Kealy, R.D., Lawler, D., Ballam, J.M. et al. (2002). Effects of diet restriction on life span and age-related changes in dogs. *Journal of the American Veterinary Medical Association* 220: 1315–1320.

Kerswell, K.J., Bennett, P., Butler, K.L., and Hemsworth, P.H. (2009). Self-reported comprehension ratings of dog behavior by owners of adult dogs. *Anthrozoös* 26 (1): 5–11.

Kerswell, K.J., Bennett, P., Butler, K.L., and Hemsworth, P.H. (2010). The relationship of adult morphology and early social signalling of the domestic dog (Canis familiaris). *Behavioural Processes* 81 (3): 376–382.

Kienzle, E. and Hall, D.K. (1994). Inappropriate feeding: the importance of a balanced diet. In: *The Waltham Book of Clinical Nutrition of the Dog and Cat* (ed. J.M. Wills and K.W. Simpson). Oxford: Pergamon Press.

Kienzle, E., Bergler, R., and Mandernach, A. (1998). A comparison of the feeding behavior and the human-animal relationship in owners of normal and obese dogs. *The Journal of Nutrition* 128: 2779S–2782S.

Kim, Y.M., El-Aty, A.M.A., Hwang, S.H. et al. (2009). Risk factors of relinquishment regarding canine behavior problems in South Korea. *Berliner und Munchener Tierarztliche Wochenchrift* 122 (1–2): 1–7.

King, T., Marston, L.C., and Bennett, P.C. (2009). Describing the ideal Australian companion dog. *Applied Animal Behaviour Science* 120: 84–93.

Knight, A. (2015). *Vegan animal diets: facts and myths.* Available at https://www.vegansociety.com/whats-new/blog/vegan-animal-diets-facts-and-myths. Accessed 12 April 2016.

Kobelt, A.J., Hemsworth, P.H., Barnett, J.L., and Coleman, G.J. (2003). A survey of dog ownership in 2135 suburban Australia – conditions and behaviour problems. *Applied Animal Behaviour Science* 82: 137–148.

Kogan, L.R., SchoLenfeld-Tacher, R., and Simon, A.A. (2012). Behavioral effects of auditory stimulation on kenneled dogs. *Journal of Veterinary Behavior: Clinical Applications and Research* 7 (5): 268–275.

Kore, A.M. and Kieschenesselrodt, A. (1990). Toxicology of household cleaning products and disinfectants. *The Veterinary Clinics of North America. Small Animal Practice* 20 (2): 525–537.

Laflamme, D. (1997). Development and validation of a body condition score system for dogs. *Canine Practice* 22 (4): 10–15.

Lascelles, B.D.X. and Main, D.J.C. (2002). Surgical trauma and chronically painful conditions – within our comfort level but beyond theirs? *Journal of the American Veterinary Medical Association* 221: 215–222.

Leaver, S.D.A. and Reimchen, T.E. (2008). Behavioural responses of Canis familiaris to different tail lengths of a remotely-controlled life-size dog replica. *Behaviour* 145 (3): 377–390.

Lefebvre, D., Diederich, C., Delcourt, M., and Giffroy, J.-M. (2007). The quality of the relation between handler and military dogs: influences efficiency and welfare of dogs. *Applied Animal Behaviour Science* 104 (1–2): 49–60.

Levine, E.D. and Mills, D.S. (2008). Long term follow-up of the efficacy of a behavioural treatment programme for dogs with firework fears. *The Veterinary Record* 162: 657–659.

Loftus, B.A., Rooney, N.J. and Casey, R.A. (2012). *Recognising Fear and Anxiety in Dogs.* Available at http://www.bris.ac.uk/vetscience/services/behaviour-clinic/dogbehaviouralsigns. Accessed 12 February 2016.

Logan, E.I., Wiggs, R.B., Zetner, L., and Hefferren, J.J. (2001). Dental disease. In: *Small Animals Clinical Nutrition* (ed. M.S. Hand, C.D. Thatcher, R.L. Remillard and P. Rouydeebush), 475–504. Topeka, USA: Mark Morris Institute.

Maarschalkerweerd, R.J., Endenburg, N., Kirpensteijn, J., and Knol, B.W. (1997). Influence of orchidectomy on canine behaviour. *Veterinary Record* 140: 617–619.

Mäki, K., Liinamo, A.-E., Groen, A.F. et al. (2005). The effect of breeding schemes on the genetic response of canine hip dysplasia, elbow dysplasia, behaviour traits and appearance. *Animal Welfare* 14: 117–124.

Mariti, C., Gazzano, A., Moore, J.L. et al. (2012). Perception of dogs' stress by their owners. *Journal of Veterinary Behavior: Clinical Applications and Research* 7 (4): 213–219.

Marston, L.C., Bennett, P.C., and Coleman, G.J. (2005). Adopting shelter dogs: owner experiences of the first month post-adoption. *Anthrozoös* 18 (4): 358–378.

Maskell, I.E. and Johnson, J.V. (1993). Digestion and absorption. In: *The Waltham Book of Companion Animal Nutrition* (ed. I. Burger), 25–44. Oxford: Pergamon Press.

Mason, E. (1970). Obesity in pet dogs. *Veterinary Record* 86 (21): 612–616.

Massei, G. and Miller, L.A. (2013). Nonsurgical fertility control for managing free-roaming dog populations: A review of products and criteria for field applications. *Theriogenology* 80 (8): 829–838.

McCune, S., McPherson, J.A., and Bradshaw, J.W.S. (1995). Avoiding problems: the importance of socialisation. In: *The Waltham Book of Human-Animal Interaction: Benefits and responsibilities of Dog Ownership* (ed. I. Robinson), 71–86. Oxford: Pergamon.

McGreevy, P.D., Thomson, P.C., Pride, C. et al. (2005). Prevalence of obesity in dogs examined by Australian veterinary practices and the risk factors involved. *Veterinary Record* 156 (22): 695–701.

McMillan, F.D., Duffy, D.L., and Serpell, J.A. (2011). Mental health of dogs formerly used as 'breeding stock' in commercial breeding establishments. *Applied Animal Behaviour Science* 135: 86–94.

McMillan, F.D., Serpell, J.A., Duffy, D.L. et al. (2013). Differences in behavioval characteristics between dogs obtained as puppies from pet stores and those obtained from noncommercial breeders. *Journal of the American Veterinary Medical Association* 242: 1359–1363.

Mech, L.D. (1999). Alpha status, dominance, and division of labor in wolf packs. *Canadian Journal of Zoology* 77: 1196–1203.

Medeiros, V. and Angela, P. (2008). Susceptibility to diabetes mellitus in obese dogs. *Acta Scientiae* 36 (3): 312.

Meers L, Normando S, Odberg FO and Bono G 2004 Behavioural responses of adult beagles to interruption in a walking program. In: Heath SE (Ed) *Proceedings of the 2004 Companion Animal Behaviour Therapy Study*.

Mendl, M., Brooks, J., Basse, C. et al. (2010). Dogs showing separation-related behaviour exhibit a 'pessimistic' cognitive bias. *Current Biology* 20: R939–R940.

Mertens, P.A. and Unshelm, J. (1996). Effects of group and individual housing on the behavior of kenneled dogs in animal shelters. *Anthrozoös* 9: 40–51.

Miklosi, A. (2007). *Dog Behaviour, Evolution and Cognition*. Oxford: Oxford University Press.

Milan, C. (2010). *Caesar's Way*. Available at http://www.cesarsway.com/tips/puppytips/sleeping-arrangements-for-puppies. Accessed 17 August 2010.

Mills, D.S. and Mills, C.B. (2003). A survey of the behaviour of UK household dogs. *Proceedings of the 4th International Veterinary Behaviour Meeting*, Proceedings Number 352. Eds K. Seksel, G. Perry, D. Mills, D. Frank, E. Lindell, P. McGreevy, P. Pageat. Sydney, August 18–20, 2003. Pp. 93–98.

Mills, D.S. and Zulch, H. (2010). Veterinary medicine and animal behaviour: barking up the right tree! *Veterinary Journal* 183 (2): 119–120.

Mondelli, F., Previde, E.P., Verga, M. et al. (2004). The bond that never developed: adoption and relinquishment of dogs in a rescue shelter. *Journal of Applied Animal Welfare Science* 7 (4): 253–266.

Morgan, R.V. (2008). *Handbook of Small Animal Practice*. Missouri, USA: Saunders Elsevier.

Murrell, J.C., Psatha, E.P., Scott, E.M. et al. (2008). Application of a modified form of the Glasgow pain scale in a veterinary teaching centre in the Netherlands. *Veterinary Record* 162 (13): 405–410.

National Research Council (2006). *Nutrient Requirements of Dogs and Cats (Nutrient Requirements of Domestic Animals: A Series)*. Washington DC: National Academy Press.

Nelson, R.W. and Couto, C.G. (1998). *Small Animal Internal Medicine*, 2e. Missouri: Mosby.

New York Times. (2013). New Strides in Spaying and Netering. Available at http://well.blogs. nytimes.com/2013/12/02/new-strides-in-spaying-and-neutering. Accessed 12 April 2010.

Noonan, G.J., Rand, J.S., Blackshaw, J.K., and Priest, J. (1996). Behavioural observations of puppies undergoing tail docking. *Applied Animal Behaviour Science* 49: 335–342.

Norling, A.Y. and Keeling, L. (2010). Owning a dog and working: a telephone survey of dog owners and employers in Sweden. *Anthrozoös* 23 (2): 157–171.

Odendaal, J.S.J. and Meintjes, R.A. (2003). Neurophysiological correlates of affiliative behaviour between humans and dogs. *Veterinary Journal* 165 (3): 296–301.

O'Farrell, V. (1992). *Manual of Canine Behaviour*, 2e. Cheltenham, England: British Small Animal Veterinary Association.

O'Neill, D.G., Church, D.B., McGreevy, P.D. et al. (2013). Longevity and mortality of owned dogs in England. *Veterinary Journal* 198 (3): 638–643.

O'Neill, D.G., Church, D., PD, M.G. et al. (2014). Prevalence of disorders recorded in dogs attending primary-care veterinary practices in England. *PLoS One* 9 (3): 1–16.

Osborne, C.A., Sanderson, S.L., Lulich, J.P. et al. (1999). Canine cystine urolithiasis – cause, detection, treatment, and prevention. *The Veterinary Clinics of North America. Small Animal Practice* 29 (1): 193.

O'Sullivan, E.N., Jones, B.R., O'Sullivan, K., and Hanlon, A.J. (2008). Characteristics of 234 dog bite incidents in Ireland during 2004 and 2005. *Veterinary Record* 163 (2): 37–42.

Overall, K. (1997). *Clinical Behavioral Medicine for Small Animals*. Mosby-Year Book Inc.

Pal, S.K. (2005). Parental care in free-ranging dogs, *Canis familiaris*. *Applied Animal Behaviour Science* 90: 31–47.

Pal, S.K. (2011). Mating system of free-ranging dogs (*Canis familiaris*). *International Journal of Zoology* doi: 10.1155/2011/314216.

Pal, S.K., Ghosh, B., and Roy, S. (1999). Inter- and intra-sexual behaviour of free-ranging dogs (*Canis familiaris*). *Applied Animal Behaviour Science* 62: 267–278.

Patronek, G.J., Glickman, L.T., Beck, A.M., and McCabe, G.P. (1996). Risk factors for relinquishment of dogs to an animal shelter. *Journal of The Americn Veterinary Medical Association* 209 (3): 572–581.

Prescott, M.J., Morton, D.B., Anderson, D. et al. (2004). Refining dog husbandry and care. 8th Reportof the BVA/AWF/FRAME/RSPCA/UFAW Joint Working Group on refinement. *Laboratory Animals* 38 (Suppl 1): S1–S94.

Pullen, A.J., Merrill, R.J.N., and Bradshaw, J.W.S. (2010). Preferences for toy types and presentations in kennel housed dogs. *Applied Animal Behaviour Science* 125 (3–4): 151–156.

Rawlings, J.M. (1996). The role of tooth-brushing and diet in the maintenance of periodontal health in dogs. *Journal of Veterinary Dentistry* 13 (4): 139–143.

Reece, J.F. and Chawla, S.K. (2006). Control of rabies in Jaipur, India, by the sterilisation and vaccination of neighbourhood dogs. *Veterinary Record* 159: 379–383.

Reid, J., Nolan, A.M., Hughes, J.M.L. et al. (2007). Development of the short-form Glasgow Composite Measure Pain Scale (CMPS-SF) and derivation of an analgesic intervention score. *Animal Welfare* 16: S97–S104.

Remillard, R.L., Paragon, B.M., Crane, S.W. et al. (2000). Making pet food at home. In: *Small Animal Clinical Nutrition*, 5e (ed. M.S. Hand, C.D. Thatcher and R.L. Remillard), 163–181. Topeka, KS: Mark Morris Institute.

Robertson, I.D. (2003). The association of exercise, diet and other factors with owner-perceived obesity in privately owned dogs from metropolitan Perth, WA. *Preventative Veterinary Medicine* 58: 75–83.

Roe, D.J. and Sales, G.D. (1992). Welfare implications of ultrasonic flea collars. *Veterinary Journal* 130 (7): 142–143.

Rohlf, V.I., Toukhsati, S., Coleman, G.J., and Bennett, P.C. (2010). Dog obesity: can dog caregivers' (owners') feeding and exercise intentions and behaviors be predicted from attitudes? *Journal of Applied Animal Welfare Science* 13 (3): 213–236.

Rooney, N.J. (2009). The welfare of pedigree dogs: cause for concern. *Journal of Veterinary Behavior: Clinical Applications and Research* 4 (5): 180–186.

Rooney, N.J. (2011). Welfare of racing greyhounds - prioritisation of issues. UFAW International Animal Welfare Symposium Historic Dockyard, Portsmouth UK 28–29th June 2011.

Rooney, N.J. (2016). Deleterious effects of pedigree dog breeding on behaviour. *European Journal of Companion Animal Practice* 26 (4): 24–28.

Rooney, N.J. and Bradshaw, J.W.S. (2003). Links between play and dominance and attachment dimensions of dog-human relationships. *Journal of Applied Animal Welfare Science* 6 (2): 67–94.

Rooney, N.J. and Bradshaw, J.W.S. (2014). Canine welfare science: an antidote to sentiment and myth. In: *Domestic Dog Cognition and Behavior: The Scientific Study of Canis familiaris* (ed. A. Horowitz), 241–274. New Year: Springer.

Rooney, N.J. and Bradshaw, J.W.S. (2016). Dog social behaviour and communication. In: *The Domestic Dog: Its Evolution, Behaviour and Interactions with People*, 2e (ed. J. Serpell). New York: Cambridge University Press.

Rooney, N.J. and Cowan, S. (2011). Training methods and owner-dog interactions: links with dog behaviour and learning ability. *Applied Animal Behaviour Science* 132: 169–177.

Rooney, N.J. and Sargan, D. (2009). Pedigree Dog Breeding in the UK: a major welfare concern? An independent scientific report commissioned by the RSPCA. Available at https://www.rspca.org.uk/adviceandwelfare/pets/dogs/health/pedigreedogs/report. Accessed 12 January 2016.

Rooney, N.J. and Sargan, D.R. (2010). Welfare concerns associated with pedigree dog breeding in the UK. *Animal Welfare* 19: 133–140.

Rooney, N.J., Bradshaw, J.W.S., and Robinson, I.H. (2000). A comparison of dog-dog and dog-human play behaviour. *Applied Animal Behaviour Science* 6: 235–248.

Rooney, N.J., Bradshaw, J.W.S., and Robinson, I.H. (2001). Do dogs respond to play signals given by humans? *Animal Behaviour* 61 (4): 715–722.

Rooney, N.J., Gaines, S.A., and Bradshaw, J.W.S. (2007). Behavioural and glucocorticoid responses of dogs (*Canis familiaris*) to kennelling: investigating mitigation of stress by prior habituation. *Physiology and Behavior* 92: 847–854.

Rooney, N.J., Gaines, S.A., and Hiby, E.F. (2009a). Practitioner's guide to working dog welfare. *Journal of Veterinary Behavior* 4: 127–134.

Rooney, N.J., Gaines, S.A., Denham, H.D.C., and Bradshaw, J.W.S. (2009b). Response to a standardized psychogenic stressor as an indicator of welfare status. *Journal of Veterinary Behavior: Clinical Applications and Research* 4 (2): 77–78.

Roudebush, P., Logan, E., and Hale, F.A. (2005). Evidence-based veterinary dentistry: a systematic review of homecare for prevention of periodontal disease in dogs and cats. *Journal of Veterinary Dentistry* 22 (1): 6–15.

Rowan, A. and Williams, J. (1987). The success of companion animal management programs: a review. *Anthrozoös* 1 (2): 110–122.

RSPCA. (2015). *Learning to be left alone*. Available at https://www.rspca.org.uk/adviceandwelfare/pets/dogs/behaviour/separationrelatedbehaviour/prevention. Accesssed 12 April 2016.

Sales, G., Hubrecht, R., Peyvandi, A. et al. (1997). Noise in dog kennelling: Is barking a welfare problem for dogs? *Applied Animal Behaviour Science* 5 (3–4): 321–329.

Sampson, J. and Binns, M.M. (2006). The kennel club and the early history of dog shows and breed clubs. In: *The Dog and Its Genome* (ed. E.A. Ostrander, U. Giger and K. Lindblad-Toh), 19–30. USA: CSHL Press.

Sankey C, Häsler B and Hiby E 2012 Change in public perception of roaming dogs in Colombo City. In *1st DPM conference*. York, UK. September 4–8 2012.

Sargan, D. (2004). IDID: inherited diseases in dogs: web-based information for canine inherited disease genetics. *Mammlian Genome* 15: 503–506.

Scarlett, J.M. (2004). Pet population dynamics and animal shelter issues. In: *Shelter Medicine for Veterinarians and Staff* (ed. L. Miller and S. Zawistowski). Ames, Iowa: Blackwell Publishing.

Schalke, E., Stichnoth, J., Ott, S., and Jones-Baade, R. (2007). Clinical signs caused by the use of electric training collars on dogs in everyday life situations. *Applied Animal Behaviour Science* 105 (4): 369–380.

Schilder, M.B.H. and van der Borg, J.A.M. (2004). Training dogs with help of the shock collar: short and long term behavioural effects. *Applied Animal Behaviour Science* 85 (3–4): 319–334.

Schipper, L.L., Vinke, C.A., Schilder, M.B.H., and Spruijt, B.M. (2008). The effect of feeding enrichment toys on the behaviour of kennelled dogs (*Canis familiaris*). *Applied Animal Behaviour Science* 114 (1–2): 182–195.

Scott, J.P. and Fuller, J.L. (1965). *Genetics and the Social Behavior of the Dog*. Chicago: University of Chicago Press.

Scott, D., Miller, W., and Griffin, C. (1995). *Muller and Kirk's Small Animal Dermatology*, 5e. Philadelphia: WB Saunders Company.

Shiverdecker, M.D., Schiml, P.A., and Hennessy, M.B. (2013). Human interaction moderates plasma cortisol and behavioral responses of dogs to shelter housing. *Physiology and Behavior* 109: 75–79.

Siracusa, C., Manteca, X., Ceron, J. et al. (2008). Perioperative stress response in dogs undergoing elective surgery: variations in behavioural, neuroendocrine, immune and acute phase responses. *Animal Welfare* 17 (3): 259–273.

Siwak, C.T., Tapp, P., and Milgram, N.W. (2001). Effect of age and level of cognitive function on spontaneous and exploratory behaviors in the beagle dog. *Learning and Memory* 8: 317–325.

Sjaastad, O.V., Sand, O., and Hove, K. (2012). *Physiology of Domestic Animals*. Oslo, Norway: Scandanavian Veterinary Press.

Slabbert, J.M. and Rasa, O.A.E. (1993). The effect of early separation from the mother on pups in bonding to humans and pup health. *Journal of the South African Veterinary Association* 64: 4–8.

Slater, M.R., Scarlett, J.M., Donoghue, S. et al. (1992). Diet and exercise as potential risk-factors for osteochondritis-dissecans. *Journal of the American Veterinary Medical Association* 53 (11): 2119–2124.

Sloth, C. (1992). Practical management of obesity in dogs and cats. *Journal of Small Animal Practice* 33: 178–182.

Smith, G.K., Paster, E.R., Powers, M.Y. et al. (2006). Lifelong diet restriction and radiographic evidence of osteoarthritis of the hip joint in dogs. *Journal of the American Veterinary Medical Association* 229 (5): 690–693.

Soares, G.M., Pereira, J.T., and Paixao, R.L. (2010). Exploratory study of separation anxiety syndrome in apartment dogs. *Ciencia Rural* 40: 548–553.

Sonderegger, S.M. and Turner, D.C. (1996). Introducing dogs into kennels: prediction of social tendencies to facilitate integration. *Animal Welfare* 5: 391–404.

Stafford, K. (2007). *The Welfare of Dogs Springer*. Dordrecht: The Netherlands.

Steinberger, R. (2012). A roadmap to creating successful measurable outcomes through high volume spay/neuter in chronic poverty on a Lakota Reservation in the US. In: *1st DPM conference*. York, UK. September 4–8 2012.

Summers, J.F., Diesel, G., Asher, L. et al. (2010). Inherited defects in pedigree dogs. Part 2: disorders that are not related to breed standards. *The Veterinary Journal* 183: 39–45.

Tami, G. and Gallagher, A. (2009). Description of the behaviour of domestic dog (*Canis familiaris*) by experienced and inexperienced people. *Applied Animal Behaviour Science* 120 (3–4): 159–169.

Tami, G., Barone, A., and Diverio, S. (2008). Relationship between management factors and dog behavior in a sample of Argentine dogs in Italy. *Journal of Veterinary Behavior-Clinical Applications and Research* 3: 59–73.

Taylor, K.D. and Mills, D.S. (2007). The effect of the kennel environment on canine welfare: a critical review of experimental studies. *Animal Welfare* 16: 435–447.

Taylor, M.B., Geiger, D.A., Saker, K.E., and Larson, M.M. (2009). Diffuse osteopenia and myelopathy in a puppy fed a diet composed of an organic premix and raw ground beef breeders. *Journal of the American Veterinary Medical Association* 234: 1041–1048.

Thalmann, O., Shapiro, B., Cui, P. et al. (2013). Complete mithochondrial genomes of ancient canids suggest a European origin for domestic dogs. *Science* 341: 871–874.

Thatcher, C.D., Hand, M.S., and Remillard, R.L. (2010). Small animal clinical nutrition: an iterative process. In: *Small Animal Clinical Nutrition*, 5e (ed. M.S. Hand, C.D. Thatcher and R.L. Remillard), 3–21. Marceline, Missouri: Walsworth Publishing Co.

The Monks of New Skete (1978). *How to Be Your Dog's Best Friend: A Training Manual for Dog Owners*. Boston: Little, Brown & Co.

The Monks of New Skete (1991). *The Art of Raising a Puppy*. Boston: Little, Brown & Co.

Thomson, P.C., Rose, K., and Kok, N.E. (1992). The behavioural ecology of dingoes in North-Western Australia. Population dynamics and variation in the social system. *Wildlife Research* 19: 565–584.

Totton, S.C., Wandeler, A.I., Ribble, C.S. et al. (2011). Stray dog population health in Jodhpur, India in the wake of an animal birth control (ABC) program. *Preventive Veterinary Medicine* 98: 215–220.

Tuber, D., Hennessy, M.B., Sanders, S., and Miller, J.A. (1996). Behavioural and glucocorticoid responses of adult domestic dogs (*Canis familiaris*) to companionship and social separation. *Journal of Comparative Psychology* 11: 103–108.

Udell, M.A.R., Dorey, N.R., and Wynne, C.D.L. (2010). What did domestication do to dogs? A new account of dogs' sensitivity to human actions. *Biological Reviews* 85 (2): 327–345.

UFAW (Universities Federation for Animal Welfare) (2013). *Genetic Welfare Problems for Companion Animals*. Available at https://www.ufaw.org.uk/genetic-welfare-problems-intro/ genetic-welfare-problems-of-companion-animals-intro Last accessed on 12 April 2016.

Vaisanen, M.A.M., Valros, A.E., Hakaoja, E. et al. (2005). Pre-operative stress in dogs – a preliminary investigation of behavior and heart rate variability in healthy hospitalized dogs. *Veterinary Anaesthesia and Analgesia* 32 (3): 158–167.

Valsecchi, P., Pattacini, O., Beretta, V. et al. (2007). Effects of a human social enrichment program on behavior and welfare of sheltered dogs. *Journal of Veterinary Behavior: Clinical Applications and Research* 2 (3): 88–89.

Van Hagen, M.A., Van der Kolk, J., Barendse, M.A. et al. (2004). Analysis of the inheritance of white spotting and the evaluation of KIT and EDNRB as spotting loci in Dutch boxer dogs. *Journal of Hereditary* 95: 526–531.

Verga, M. and Michelazzi, M. (2009). Companion animal welfare and possible implications on the human-pet relationship. *Italian Journal of Animal Science* 8 (1): 231–240.

Virányi, Z. and Range, F. (2014). On the way to a better understanding of dog domestication: aggression and cooperativeness in dogs and wolves. In: *The Social Dog* (ed. J. Kaminski and S. Marshall-Pescini), 35–62. Amsterdam, Netherlands: Elsevier.

Walton, M.B., Cowderoy, E., Lascelles, D., and Innes, J.F. (2013). Evaluation of construct and criterion validity for the 'Liverpool osteoarthritis in dogs' (LOAD) clinical metrology instrument and comparison to two other instruments. *PLoS One* 8 (3): e58125. doi: 10.1371/journal.pone.0058125.

Wandeler, A.I., Bingham, J., and Meslin, F.-X. (2013). Dogs and rabies. In: *Dogs, Zoonoses and Public Health* (ed. M. CNL, F.-X. Meslin and A.I. Wandeler), 43–66. Oxfordshie, UK: CABI.

Weber, G.H., Morton, J.M., and Keates, H. (2012). Postoperative pain and perioperative analgesic administration in dogs: practices, attitudes and beliefs of Queensland veterinarians. *Australian Veterinary Journal* 90: 186–193.

Wells, D.L. (2003). Comparison of two treatments for preventing dogs eating their own faeces. *Veterinary Record* 153: 51–53.

Wells, D.L. (2004a). A review of environmental enrichment for kennelled dogs, *Canis familiaris*. *Applied Animal Behaviour Science* 85: 307–317.

Wells, D.L. (2004b). The influence of toys on the behaviour and welfare of kennelled dogs. *Animal Welfare* 13 (3): 367–373.

Wells, D.L. and Hepper, P.G. (1998). A note on the influence of visual conspecific contact on the behaviour of sheltered dogs. *Applied Animal Behaviour Science* 60 (1): 83–88.

Wells, D.L., Graham, L., and Hepper, P.G. (2002). The influence of auditory stimulation on the behaviour of dogs housed in a rescue shelter. *Animal Welfare* 11: 385–393.

Westgarth, C., Pinchbeck, G.L., Bradshaw, J.W.S. et al. (2008). Dog-human and dog-dog interactions of 260 dog-owning households in a community in Cheshire 2008. *Veterinary Record* 162 (14): 436–444.

Westgarth, C., Christley, R.M., Pinchbeck, G.L. et al. (2010). Dog behaviour on walks and the effect of use of the leash. *Applied Animal Behaviour Science* 125 (1–2): 38–46.

Williams, M. and Johnston, J.M. (2002). Training and maintaining the performance of dogs (*Canis familiaris*) on an increasing number of odor discriminations in a controlled setting. *Applied Animal Behaviour Science* 78: 55–65.

Wirant, S.C. and McGuire, B. (2004). Urinary behavior of female domestic dogs (*Canis familiaris*) influence of reproductive status, location, and age. *Applied Animal Behaviour Science* 85 (3–4): 335–348.

Wiseman, M.L., Nolan, A.M., Reid, J., and Scott, E.W.M. (2001). Preliminary study on owner-reported behaviour changes associated with chronic pain in dogs. *Veterinary Record* 149 (14): 423–424.

Wohr, A.C. and Erhard, M.H. (2004). Travel with dogs – aspects of animal welfare. *Tierarztliche Praxis Ausgabe Kleintiere Heimtiere* 32 (3): 148–157.

Yeates, J. and Main, D.C.J. (2011). Veterinary surgeons' opinions on dog welfare issues. *Journal of Small Animal Practice* 52 (9): 464–468.

Yoak, A., Reece, J.F., Gehrt, S.D., and Hamilton, I.M. (2014). Disease control through fertility control: secondary benefits of animal birth control in Indian street dogs. *Preventive Veterinary Medicine* 113 (1): 152–156.

Zhu, L., Zhang, Z., Friedenberg, S. et al. (2009). The long (and winding) road to gene discovery for canine hip dysplasia. *Veterinary Journal* 181: 97–110.

Ferrets (*Mustela putorius furo*)

5

Claudia Vinke, Nico J. Schoemaker, and Yvonne R. A. van Zeeland

5.1 History and Context

5.1.1 Natural History

Ferrets (*Mustela putorius fero*) are members of the class Mammalia, order Carnivora, and family Mustelidae, which also includes mink and polecats. The ferret (Figure 5.1) is the result of humans crossbreeding two species of polecat. This makes it difficult to refer to their natural history, beyond considering information about polecats, feral ferrets, and polecat-ferret hybrids. The most probable ancestors of the ferret are the European polecat (*Mustela putorius putorius*) and the Steppe polecat (*Mustela eversmanni*) (Ashton et al. 1965; Tetley 1965; Fisher 2006; MacKay 2006). These are distributed across much of Europe and Central Asia, and both are designated as Least Concern by the International Union for Conservation of Nature (IUCN). The ferret has not been included in the IUCN Red List.

Feral ferrets and polecats live in wooded and semi-wooded areas near water sources (Duda 2003). They live in dens such as rabbit burrows, but spend a large proportion of their active time travelling and foraging across home ranges of up to 102 ha (Norbury et al. 1998; Fisher 2006). Mean home ranges of 102 ± 58 ha are reported for males,

Companion Animal Care and Welfare: The UFAW Companion Animal Handbook,
First Edition. Edited by James Yeates.
© 2019 Universities Federation for Animal Welfare. Published 2019 by John Wiley & Sons Ltd.

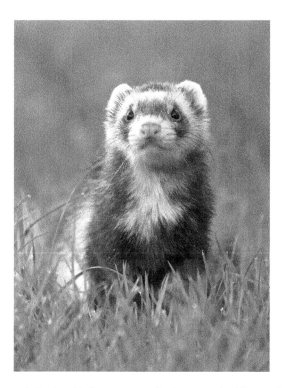

Figure 5.1   Ferret with the 'mask' characteristic of polecats and sable or wild-type coloured pet ferrets.

whereas mean home ranges of 76 ± 48 ha are reported for females (Norbury et al. 1998). Juvenile ferrets may disperse over distances up to 5 km (Caley and Morriss 2001). However, territoriality not only depends on gender and age, but also on environmental factors such as the abundance of prey in the area (Powell 1994). Polecats feed on a variety of vertebrate and invertebrate prey including rodents, small birds, reptiles, amphibians, spiders, beetles, slugs, snails, and earthworms (Bulloch and Tynes 2010).

(Feral) ferrets are solitary and territorial animals, except for breeding and before weaning. Their territories generally exclude other ferrets of the same sex (Powell 1979), whereas territories of opposite sexes may overlap extensively (Moors and Lavers 1981). Ferrets use anal gland secretions, faeces, and urine to obtain information on other individuals' identity, reproductive, and social status (Clapperton et al. 1988; Woodley and Baum 2003; Berzins and Helder 2008), and males use such olfactory cues to find mating partners (Baum 1976; Moors and Lavers 1981; Baum et al. 1983). The breeding season (in Europe) lasts from March to August, depending on daylight length (Fox et al. 2014). Ovulation is induced by the combination of vaginal stimulation and the hob gripping the jill's neck (Bibeau et al. 1991).

5.1.2 Domestic History
The ferret is a fully domestic species. Ferrets were first described before 1000 BCE in North Africa (Fisher 2006), and it is likely that ferret domestication started more than 2000 to 3000 years ago (Bulloch and Tynes 2010). Ferrets might have been kept initially to protect

Table 5.1 Number of ferrets kept as pets or for hunting in different countries.

Country	Number of ferrets	Reference
United States	≈ 800 000	(Jurek 1998)
United Kingdom	>100 000	(Vinke and Schoemaker 2012)
Germany	115 000	(Vinke and Schoemaker 2012)
Italy	105 000	(Vinke and Schoemaker 2012)
France	300 000	(Vinke and Schoemaker 2012)

human food from rodents (Price 2002); they were also commonly used for hunting – 'ferreting' – rabbits, mice, and rats (Thompson 1951; MacKay 1995). More recently, ferrets have also been used for research, especially as a model for the human influenza virus (Brown 2007), and a small number are bred for their fur (Anonymous 2001).

Contemporary estimates of pet ferret numbers are scarce, and most figures include both pets and ferrets used for hunting (Table 5.1). Ferret breeding varies from small-scale 'hobby-breeders' up to international commercial farming enterprises (United States, Fisher 2006). Domestic breeding has not created particular breeds of ferrets, but there is a variety of colours, including sable, white (onyx-eyed and albino), black, butterscotch, cinnamon, champagne, chocolate, and chocolate, with various additional markings (American Ferret Association [AFA] 2014).

5.2 Principles of Ferret Care

5.2.1 Diet

Ferrets are considered obligate carnivores, indicating that they need to be provided with food sources of animal origin to fulfil their nutrient requirements. The exact nutrient requirements for ferrets have not been well established, but some recommendations can been made (Table 5.2).

Insufficient protein or excessive carbohydrates may lead to health problems such as weight loss, poor coat condition, pancreatic endocrine disorders, insulinoma, and urinary calculi (Bell 1999). Conversely, feeding only muscle meat provides insufficient calcium and an overly low calcium-to-phosphorus ratio, leading to the 'All Meat Syndrome' (secondary nutritional hyperparathyroidism) in which loss of calcium in ferrets' bones increases the risk of bone fractures (Kronfeld 1985). Intestinal fermentation is limited by the ferrets' relatively simple intestinal flora and short colon (approximately 10 cm), so the digestion of fibre is minimal (Andrews and Ilman 1987; Brown 2004).

Excess energy can lead to obesity. It is therefore recommended to monitor the ferret's body weight and body condition monthly. Weights between males and females differ greatly, with males usually weighing between 1200 and 2100 g and females weighing between 700 and 1200 g (Fox et al. 2014). Ferrets' body weight may also vary 30–40% over the seasons because of increased deposition of fat during the autumn, which will decrease again the following spring (Moorman-Roest 1993). When food is ample and

Table 5.2 Nutritional requirements of normal adult ferrets.

Nutrient	Amount required, adult
Protein	30–40%
Carbohydrate	20–30%
Fibre	<3%
Lipid	15–20%
	(25–30% for lactating females)
Calcium-to-phosphorus ratio	1.5:1

Source: Wolf and Hebeler (2001), Brown (2004), Banks et al. (2010), Fox et al. (2014).
All figures assume animals are of normal physiology, healthy, non-breeding, and non-working.

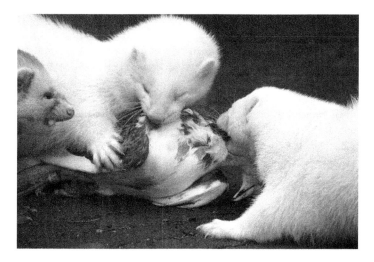

Figure 5.2 Ferrets sharing a frozen (and thawed) whole pigeon (*Source:* courtesy Birgit van der Laan).

freely available, ferrets typically eat 9–10 meals per day (Kaufman 1980). Ferrets have a tendency to hide excess food, which – if involving fresh food – may decay if not found in time by the owners.

Ferrets' nutritional requirements can be provided either by a commercial, balanced ferret kibble, soft food diet, or by whole prekilled prey animals. Whole prey addition-ally maintains dental health by cleaning the teeth without too much abrasion and pro-vides a source of enrichment by making ferrets work for and spend more time to obtain and consume their food, as well as create opportunities for chewing (Figure 5.2). It does, however, also pose an increased risk for bacterial infections, such as salmonellosis or campylobacteriosis. In addition, owners may find it easier and less gruesome to feed a complete commercial diet. All ferrets should also be given adequate and variable food enrichments, such as food placed in safe toys.

Wild polecat juveniles have a sensitive period between 60 and 90 days of age for the imprinting for the scent of their prey (Apfelbach 1986). If a ferret does not learn the smell of a prey species during this sensitive period, it is likely to refuse that food later in life. A similar process may explain why some individual ferrets have particular food preferences and why it may be difficult to convert to different types of food. Juveniles should therefore be offered a variety of foods during their first months of life to guarantee they will accept a broader range of foods later on in life (Fisher 2006).

Water intake is around 50 mL kg body weight per day (Kaufman 1980; Banks et al. 2010). Fresh water should be available at all times, especially when the ferret is fed dry kibble. This may be provided in either a bottle or a bowl, although ferrets often play with bowls and tip them over.

5.2.2 Environment

Guidelines for housing ferrets as animals used in research state that the minimum size is 4500 cm^2, although for hobs a space of at least 6000 cm^2 is required (EU Commission 2007). However, ferrets are inquisitive, active animals, and should therefore be kept in as extensive areas as possible, and if caged, given daily opportunities of supervised time outside of the cage (Figure 5.3). Ferrets need at least 50 cm height to stand on their hind legs and scan the surroundings (Schoemaker and van Zeeland 2013). Moreover, because ferrets are renowned escape artists, every effort should be made to ensure their enclosure is escape proof.

Ferrets can be housed indoors and outdoors, as long as protection against the elements is provided. Ferrets' preferred ambient temperature is 15–21 °C and should never exceed 29 °C because ferrets cannot transpire (Bulloch and Tynes 2010). It is therefore advisable to prevent ferrets from being kept in direct sunlight, without presence of

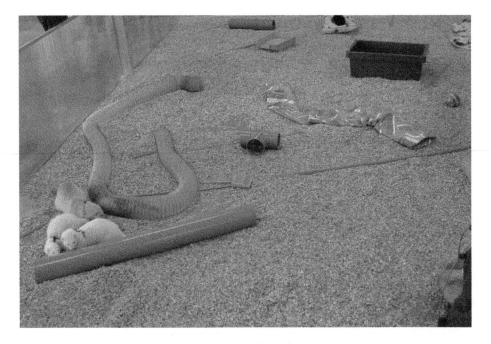

Figure 5.3 Ferrets exploring and using tubes and tunnels.

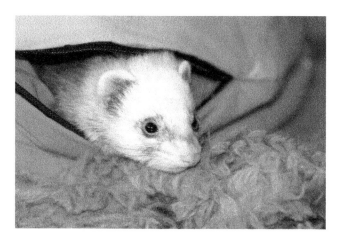

Figure 5.4 Ferret hiding in a sleeping tent.

sufficient shade or shelter (Schoemaker and van Zeeland 2013). Although mustelids are often more active in the twilight or night, most pet ferrets adapt to the activity cycle of their pet owners.

Because of the sensitivity of the ferrets' respiratory tract, ferrets need adequate ventilation, and aquaria are not adequate as housing systems for ferrets. This also means sawdust and straw are not advised as bedding materials (Jenkins and Brown 1993). Ferrets mostly eliminate in one or two favourite areas and can often be easily trained to eliminate in one location by creating an elimination point at a place that the ferret has already chosen (Schilling 2000; Bulloch and Tynes 2010). Healthy ferrets sleep between 18 and 20 hours a day (Fisher 2006) and need safe sleeping places, such as hammocks and sleeping tents. Tubes and pipes also allow pet ferrets to hide, rest, and sleep in constructions similar to their natural den choices (Figure 5.4).

Ferrets are active and inquisitive animals, which need varied and complex environments (Bays et al. 2006). This allows them to express various motivations and seems to improve alertness, emotional stability, and cognition. Digging opportunities are highly valued by ferrets and should be provided in addition to tubes and tunnels. Insufficient environmental enrichment may lead to behaviours such as destruction and plant digging (Bulloch and Tynes 2010). Enriched environments are particularly important for juvenile ferrets, which should come into contact with many novel objects and confronted with many different kinds of environments and situations during their early life because this is an important part of proper socialisation.

Tubes can also provide opportunities for play. Ferrets are playful animals and play may help ferrets to develop motor, mental, and social skills and to fulfil some behavioural needs. Play can also be used in a therapeutic way to help ferrets overcome stressful incidents or situations. Providing more enrichment may encourage more play (Talbot et al. 2014). Many ferret toys are now commercially available. Ferrets may habituate to familiar toys, so novel toys should be provided frequently, or toys rotated regularly. Ferrets are good destructors and often explore new objects with their mouths (Moorman-Roest 1993). Toys must therefore be chosen carefully to avoid ingestion and obstruction of the digestive tract. As many mustelids prefer the taste of rubber, soft rubber toys frequently lead to ingestion of rubber and gut obstruction and should be avoided. In general, hard, nondestructible toys should be chosen instead of toys with small parts (Bulloch and Tynes 2010).

5.2.3 Animal Company

Pet ferrets may react aggressively to each other, and this can be the most frequently reported behavioural problem (Staton and Crowell-Davis 2003). Inappropriate company can also cause chronic stress, which may lead to stress-induced elimination (personal communication Roest 2011) and increased vulnerability to diseases and infections such as *Helicobacter* infection (Fox and Marini 2001; Banks et al. 2010). Large groups may also increase the risk of problems such as *Helicobacter* infections. However, pet ferrets commonly sleep together, play, and groom each other, suggesting that these ferrets can appreciate certain forms of social interaction.

Ferrets can therefore best be kept in groups of up to four animals, although solitary housing or housing in larger groups may be possible, dependent on the preference of the individual ferret and the compatibility of the individuals. The success of matching highly depends on the animals' genetic predispositions, life history, familiarity, season, sexes, and neutering status (Staton and Crowell-Davis 2003). Ferrets may particularly reject new arrivals, so pairs or groups should be carefully introduced and kept stable. Groups should be given ample resources that are sufficiently spread out, so they are hard to monopolise.

Male and female ferrets are considerably different in their appearance, therefore making it easy to sex them. Hobs are usually bigger and broader than jills. Moreover, in jills, the vaginal opening and the anus are close together, whereas in hobs, a penile bone and testicles can easily be seen or felt. The genital opening and anus also lie further apart in the male, a feature which makes it easy to distinguish sexes even in juvenile ferrets (Figure 5.5) (MacKay 1995, 2006).

The bonding between mother and offspring is particularly important for the development of normal behaviour. Within the first weeks of life, their mother may help young ferrets learn many skills, elimination places, food preferences, and the limits of play and aggression. Similarly, young ferrets' socialisation phase is highly important for the development of normal social behaviour and interactions with other ferrets as well as acclimatisation to their future environment. Although the time of the socialisation period in ferrets has not been determined, it is assumed to be between 4 and 10 weeks, as suggested for polecats (Fisher 2006). Isolating pups during the first month of life may alter their later social interactions, sexual behaviour, learning abilities, drug tolerance, activity level, and body size (Einon 1996). Moreover, both socialisation deficiencies and early weaning may result in fear and fear-related aggression later in life. During their first months, ferrets should therefore be confronted with a variety of trustworthy ferrets and weaning should occur no earlier than around 8 weeks of age.

Ferrets may tolerate other species such as dogs or cats (Figure 5.6). Because of their motivation to hunt, they should not be kept with pet species that are their natural prey such as rabbits and rodents. If a juvenile ferret is to be expected to live in a household with other species, daily contact with these species should also be included in the socialisation programme.

(a)　　　　　　　　　　　　　　　　(b)

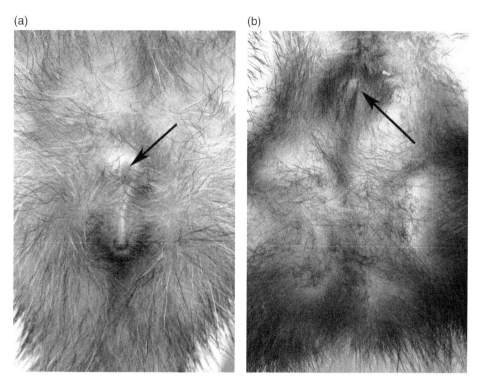

Figure 5.5 Determination of the gender in ferrets: (a) The urethral opening (arrow) in jills is located close to the anus. (b) In hobs, the penile opening (arrow) is much further located from the anus. In addition the penile bone and testicles, in intact hobs, can easily be palpated.

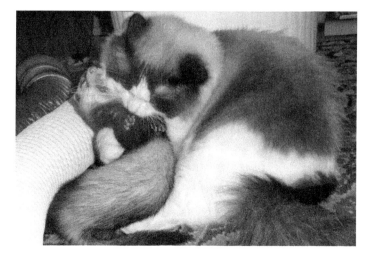

Figure 5.6 This ferret and cat (*Felis sylvestris catus*) live together in a household and enjoying rough play with each other.

5.2.4 Human Interaction

Ferrets may be fearful of humans, which can manifest as avoidance or aggression. Handling a fearful ferret can be difficult, poses a risk of injuries, and may result in owners relinquishing or even euthanizing their ferret. Inadequate exposure during the socialisation period is considered one of the main reasons for aggression towards humans (MacKay 1995; Fisher 2006). Aggression may also be learned, for example, when previous handling was unpleasant or when previous defensive behaviour had a positive outcome such as the removal of the threatening stimulus (i.e. the human or handling). Juvenile pet ferrets should be handled by familiar and unknown people daily from 28 days of age onwards (MacKay 2006), ensuring that this handling is positive and rewarding for the ferret.

A good way to pick up ferrets is by placing one hand around the thorax and supporting the hind legs with the other hand (Figure 5.7). If their hind legs are held too firmly, ferrets may struggle. Scruffing of the loose skin at the back of the neck may be necessary for restraining uncooperative ferrets (Schoemaker and van Zeeland 2013).

5.2.5 Health

Ferrets can suffer from several diseases, including many infectious agents (Table 5.3). Influenza is a common primary cause for respiratory disease in ferrets. Humans can infect ferrets and vice versa (Orcutt and Malakoff 2009). People with minor symptoms or risk of influenza should therefore not come close to ferrets or should wear a facemask. Many of the symptoms are similar to those of canine distemper but less severe. It is usually self-limiting and not fatal (Bell 1995), and the fever has usually gone down before the animal is presented to the veterinary surgeon. In comparison, canine distemper virus can be fatal.

Most ferrets carry *Helicobacter mustelae* bacteria within their gastrointestinal system. Previous studies have shown more than 80% of ferrets older than 1 year of

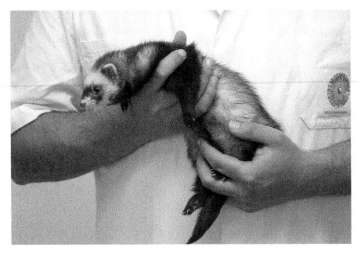

Figure 5.7 Ferret being picked up by the handler placing one hand around the thorax and supporting the hind legs with the other hand.

Table 5.3 Selected health problems in domestic ferret.

Condition			Possible welfare effects
Infectious or Parasitic diseases	Viral	Influenza[a]	Dyspnoea; fever; conjunctivitis; anorexia
		Rabies[a] (V)	Hypersensitivity; anorexia; behavioural changes; incoordination; paralysis; seizures
		Canine Distemper (paramyxo virus) (V)	Conjunctivitis; fever; severe dyspnoea; skin disease (hard pad); neurological signs
		Rotavirus	Severe diarrhoea; dehydration; emaciation
		Coronavirus	Systemic disease in rare cases (coronavirus)
		Aleutian disease (parvovirus)	Lethargy; anorexia; fever; hind leg weakness; emaciation; kidney failure
	Bacterial	*Helicobacter mustelae*	Stomach ulcers; nausea; anorexia; vomiting; lethargy; diarrhoea; melena; muscle wasting; abdominal pain
		Salmonella[a] or Campylobacter[a]	(Bloody) diarrhoea; vomiting; dehydration; emaciation
	Protozoal	Giardia	Intermittent diarrhoea; weight loss
		Coccidiosis Cryptosporidiosis	Diarrhoea at young age; dehydration; anal prolapse
	External parasites	Ear mites	Intense pruritus
		Fleas	Mild to intense pruritus
Metabolic or Hormonal problems	Persistent oestrus (jill)		Severe bone marrow suppression; immunosuppression; bleeding; anaemia
	Hyperadrenocorticism		Alopecia; pruritus; dysuria in hobs
	Insulinoma		Lethargy; hind leg weakness; nausea; coma
Cardiac disease	Dilated cardiomyopathy		Lethargy; exercise intolerance; anorexia; respiratory distress; liver failure; hind leg weakness
	Leaking heart valves		Often asymptomatic Coughing; difficulty breathing
Kidney disease	Chronic nephritis		Increased urination; dehydration; emaciation; nausea; vomiting; anaemia

(Continued)

Table 5.3 (Continued)

Condition		Possible welfare effects
Gastrointestinal disease	Dental disease or tartar	Pain; reduced food intake; hunger
	Foreign body ingestion or hair ball	Abdominal pain; vomiting; gut perforation; shock
	Immune-mediated inflammatory bowel disease	Abdominal pain; loss of appetite; nausea; vomiting; diarrhoea; emaciation
	Inflamed anal gland	Faecal straining; irritation; pain
Reproductive disease	Dystocia (especially in low litter size [<3 pups])	Abdominal pain; potential rupture of uterus
Neoplastic	Lymphoma	Loss of appetite; weight loss; organ failure
	Basal cell tumour	Benign skin tumour; ulceration
	Mast cell tumour	Benign skin tumour; itchiness
	Apocrine gland neoplasia	Locally invasive skin tumour; difficulty urinating
	Sebaceous epithelioma	Benign skin tumour
	Splenomegaly	Usually no welfare effects; lethargy
Traumatic	Bite wounds	Pain; irritation; infection; abscesses
Toxic	Incorrect vaccination	Delayed hypersensitivity reaction; high fever; anorexia; emaciation; muscle inflammation
	Rodenticide	Bleeding; blood loss
	Paracetamol or acetaminophen	Liver destruction

[a] zoonotic.
V = vaccine available to prevent the disease.

age to be carriers of the bacterium. Ferrets are thought to become infected at an early age and remain so until they are treated (Fox and Marini 2001; Morrisey 2004). *H. mustelae* has been associated with painful stomach ulcers, which frequently occur after stressful situations (Banks et al. 2010; Fox and Marini 2001). However, given the prevalence of carriers, confirmation of a causal relationship between ulcers and presence of *H. mustelae* infection is very difficult (Solnick and Schauer 2001).

Once ferrets get older, a variety of different diseases may be seen, including cardiac disease, renal disease, and neoplasia. Ferrets may get small tumours in the pancreas that produce an excess of insulin (so-called insulinomas), causing low blood glucose and resultant hind leg weakness. Checking the blood glucose on a regular basis may help in early recognition of the disease and allow for treatment (Schoemaker 2009). Other types of neoplasia that are common in ferrets include adrenal gland tumours, lymphoma, and skin neoplasia. Dental disease is relatively common and the oral cavity should be checked yearly.

Ferrets should be physically examined by a veterinary surgeon on at least an annual basis. Checking the teeth and blood glucose regularly may help in early recognition of diseases and allow for treatment (Schoemaker 2009). All ferrets should be vaccinated against distemper and against rabies in countries where it is prevalent. Veterinary surgeons should take care to use the correct vaccine because the administration of a vaccine cultured on a ferret cell line or containing wrong type of adjuvant can lead to a hypersensitivity reaction. Ferrets should also be treated regularly with antiparasitic drugs such as selamectin or fipronil. Ferrets may need regular grooming of their nails and hair, which can be done by their owners (Figure 5.8). Ferrets should preferably not be imported from other countries because this poses a risk of introducing new diseases. In addition, owners are recommended to take suitable safety measures when introducing a new animal into a group (e.g. keeping the new animal isolated from the others during a quarantine period of approximately 2 weeks) to prevent the spread of infectious diseases.

Jills need external stimulation to ovulate (Bibeau et al. 1991), otherwise oestrus persists for 6 months. During this period, elevated hormone concentrations can lead to lethally reduced levels of many blood cell types (Martin 1986). This may reduce immune function, bleeding, anaemia, and potentially death. Jills can also suffer from difficulty giving birth, especially for small litters of less than three pups. To prevent persistent oestrus and pregnancy, jills should be neutered before their first breeding season.

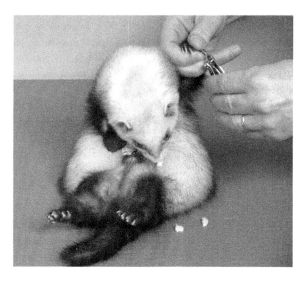

Figure 5.8 Nail-clipping a ferret while the ferret eats some of their favourite liquid or solid food placed on their belly by the owner.

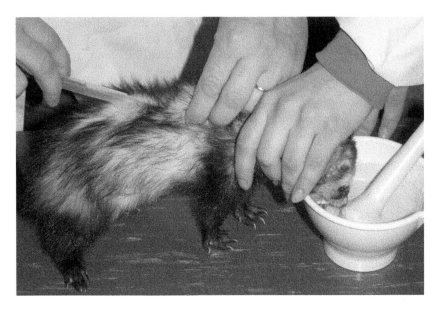

Figure 5.9 A jill being given a slow release implant containing deslorelin, while distracted with food.

Neutering may also reduce the incidence of repetitive behaviour in males and female (Talbot et al. 2014), perhaps by decreasing a frustrated motivation to roam. It furthermore reduces the distinct smell and fighting in males. However, in both sexes, neutering can be linked to the occurrence of hyperadrenocorticism, perhaps because of increased plasma concentrations of luteinizing hormone (Schoemaker et al. 2000, 2002), leading to severe alopecia, pruritus, and urinary blockage. For some people, this combination of risks has become a reason to consider ferrets as being unsuitable as pets. However, an alternative to neutering may be the use of a gonadrotropin-releasing hormone (deslorelin) implant to reduce plasma concentrations of luteinizing hormone (Prohaczik et al. 2010; Figure 5.9).

There is no need to remove ferrets' anal glands (Table 5.4). In fact, the typical odour in ferrets is caused by secretion of the sebaceous glands and *not* by the anal glands. It is therefore unnecessary as well as painful and can potentially impact on ferrets' social interactions or the smell of their home area. The removal of the anal glands should only be performed in case of a medical need.

5.2.6 Euthanasia
Before euthanasia, ferrets should be sedated, followed by the injection of an overdose of any of the available euthanasia solutions, such as those containing pentobarbitone or a mixture of embutramide, mebezonium iodide, and tetracaïne hydrochloride (e.g. T61) The solution can be administered into the cephalic vein, saphenous vein, cranial vena cava, or abdomen. The last route may be as effective and less stressful for the ferret but takes longer to take effect (Table 5.5).

Table 5.4 Nontherapeutic elective surgical procedures performed on ferrets.

Procedure	Reasons and benefits for the animal	Reasons and benefits for owners (or other humans)	Perioperative welfare risks	Welfare risks due to the behaviours prevented
Castration	Facilitates social housing; may reduce sexual frustration	Possible reduced odour; may increase sociability towards humans	Pain; Risk of hyperadrenocorticism	Precludes opportunity to mate and exhibit natural courtship and sexual behaviour
Spaying	Prevents persistent oestrus and associated pancytopenia; avoids pregnancy	May increase sociability towards humans		

Table 5.5 Methods of euthanasia for ferrets kept as companion animals.

Method	Restraint required	Welfare benefits	Welfare risks
Sedation or anaesthesia followed by intravenous, intracardiac, or intrathoracic injection of barbiturate or other euthanasia solution*	Restraint or handling for administration of sedation or anaesthesia	Sedation or anaesthesia prevents adverse reaction to euthanasia solution	Possible pain at injection site if sedation or anaesthesia is inadequate
Sedation or anaesthesia followed by intra-abdominal injection of barbiturate or other euthanasia solution*		May be less stressful	Generally takes longer time before death ensues Risk of pain on injection

Source: AVMA (2013).

* It is important to ensure that the animal is sedated or anaesthetised sufficiently by checking muscle tone and reflexes, including response to a painful stimulus (e.g. pinching of the toes), especially when administering the euthanasia solution via the intrathoracic, intracardiac, or intra-abdominal route. For these routes, a deep plane of anaesthesia, with loss of muscle tone and lack of response to a painful stimulus, is required.

5.3 Signs of Ferret Welfare

5.3.1 Pathophysiological Signs

Alongside basic measures (Table 5.6), signs of stomach ulcers such as nausea, vomiting, and dark faeces may indicate stress, for example associated with dietary changes, overcrowding, or the addition of a new animal in the group (Fox and Marini 2001; Banks et al. 2010). Alopecia (Figure 5.10) can be connected to several health problems including persistent oestrus, hyperadrenocorticism, allergic skin diseases, and parasites (Bowen and Heath 2005; Chitty 2009). Uncomfortable ferrets may also salivate, shiver, squint, and have more frequent, often shallow, respirations, and a pounding heartbeat. Weight loss may also indicate pain, starvation, dental disease, or other problems.

5.3.2 Behavioural Signs

Ferrets in pain are often lethargic, immobile, and anorexic, although some ferrets may become more anxious and restless (Fisher 2006). Other signs of discomfort or pain include trembling, collapse, crying, whimpering, not assuming their normal sleeping position or not grooming (Brown 2004; Johnson-Delaney 2009). Spasmodic teeth grinding may also indicate pain, with ferrets holding the head down and rhythmically moving the facial muscles back and forth and wriggling the ears (Fisher 2006). As abdominal pain is frequently associated with *H. mustelae* and stomach ulcers, signs of abdominal pain may be indicators of previous or continued stress. Abdominal pain may

Table 5.6 Basic measures and clinical standards of ferrets (*Mustela putorius*).

Parameter	Normal measures	
Life expectancy	up to 14 years, average 5–8 years	
Common weight range	Males: 1–2 kg	Females: 600–950 g
Body temperature	37.8–40.0 °C	
Respiratory frequency	33–36 breaths/min	
Heart rate	180–250 beats/min	
Pubescence	Males: 6–8 months	Females: 6–8 months
Blood volume	40 (female)–60 mL (5–7% of body mass)	
Haematocrit	36–55	

Source: Quesenberry and Orcutt (2012) and Fox et al. (2014).

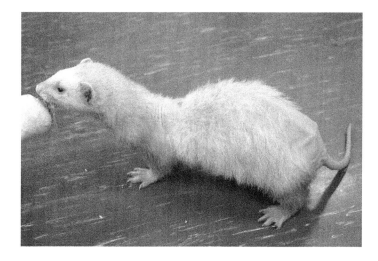

Figure 5.10 Alopecia, a potential sign of persistent oestrus or hyperadrenocorticism.

be indicated by a hunched posture, walking with an arched back or stilted gait. An arched back combined with raised hair on the tail ('bottle brush tail') may suggest fear or excitement (Fisher 2006). These postures are different from the normal posture which ferrets have during walking.

Signs of discomfort or pain also include crying and whimpering. Ferrets in fear, frustration, or pain may also squeal and scream (Fisher 2006). Continuous screaming can also be an indication of being alert to a serious danger, where the animal is excited or fearful and prepared to become aggressive. A barking-like sound can also be a sign of excitement or fear. Hissing can indicate fear, but it is sometimes difficult to interpret because it can also be heard during play patterns, particularly in situations of play escalation. A 'dook' or 'chuckling' noise may indicate excitement, for example, during play (Schilling 2000; Bulloch and Tynes 2010). Indeed, as ferrets are a very playful species, the observation of play patterns can be a useful indicator to assess a ferret's welfare status because play may not occur under severe stress. A normally playful ferret that suddenly stops to play might be unwell, in pain, or stressed. Ferrets in a good health and well-being, may dance, jerk, gallop, play fight with a partner, manipulate objects, and chase artificial prey (e.g. Poole 1978; Fisher 2006; Bulloch and Tynes 2010).

In mink, pacing along the side of the cage and scratching at the cage walls may be signs of stress (Heller 1991), frustration (Mason 1991), lack of enrichment (Hansen 1989; Mason et al. 2001; Poessel et al. 2011), or other problems (Hansen 1993; Mason 1993), and similar behaviour might indicate stress in ferrets (Talbot et al. 2014). Urinating outside the litter box, wiping the preputial sebaceous gland over surfaces, dragging the peri-anal sebaceous gland over surfaces, and defecating on objects (Fisher 2006) may all be considered as normal behaviours, quite probably related to ferrets' territorial natures (Fisher 2006). However, stress-induced elimination problems may be increased within instable social structures in multiferret households as a result of territoriality and social stress or individuals monopolising elimination places.

5.4 Worldwide Action Plan for Improving Ferret Welfare

Owners should be made more aware of ferrets' strong motivations for exploration, foraging, activity, play, and resting and of their natural social responses, especially those relating to aggression and territoriality. Owners need to know how to manage resources, carefully match company, avoid too many animals and respect some ferrets' preferences for solitary lives. Owners should be encouraged to fulfil ferrets' behavioural priorities by providing adequate and variable food enrichments, interesting toys, and comfortable hiding and resting places to prevent behaviours that are problematic for those owners. Encouraging more widespread feeding of whole prey animals should also be recommended to prevent dietary deficiencies and potentially decrease the occurrence of insulin-producing tumours. Owners should also be encouraged to present their ferrets for yearly veterinary check-ups, preventive health care, and vaccination against canine distemper. Knowledge of ferret medicine is increasing among veterinarians, thereby ensuring that ferrets may be provided with the best care possible.

Breeders and owners obtaining young ferrets should be encouraged to ensure they get adequate positive experiences in early life, particularly socialisation, to ensure they live with minimal stress as pets in human surroundings, who can easily be handled and can also live in good company with other ferrets. All breeders need to implement validated protocols inside and outside the ferrets' living environment with many stimuli and in many contexts, and these should be followed up by the new owner. Both breeders and owners have a responsibility to ensure that the latter are sufficiently knowledgeable and committed to look after each ferret forever. Information on the reasons for relinquishment is scarce, but a reasonable estimate is that 1–2% of the ferret population might be relinquished.

The historical need to neuter and the consequent risk of hyperadrenocorticism may be avoided with the development of hormone implants. Removing anal glands (for nomedical reasons) is illegal in many countries in Europe, but it is still common practice in the United States to remove the anal glands prior to selling a young ferret (Table 5.4). Finally, all ferrets should be microchipped and registered so they can be identified and returned to their owner if they escape.

Bibliography

American Ferret Association Inc (AFA). (2014). AFA Ferret Color and Pattern Standards. Available at http://www.ferret.org/events/colors/colorchart.html. Accessed 27 December 2014.

Andrews, P.L.R. and Illman, O. (1987). The ferret. In: *The UFAW Handbook on the Care and Management of Laboratory Animals*, 6e (ed. T.B. Poole and R. Robinson), 436–455. Harlow, England: Longman Scientific and Technical.

Anonymous 2001 EU report. *The welfare of animals kept for fur production*. Report of the scientific committee on animal health and animal welfare. Adopted on 12–13 December 2001, Brussels, Belgium.

Apfelbach, R. (1986). Imprinting on prey odours in ferrets (*Mustela putorius F. Furo* L.) and its neutral correlates. *Behavioural Processes* 12 (4): 363–381.

Applegate, J.A. and Walhout, M.F. (1998). Childhood risks from the ferret. *The Journal of Emergency Medicine* 16 (3): 425–427.

Ashton, E.H., Thomson, A.P.D., and Zuckerman, F.R.S. (1965). Some characters of the skulls and skins of the European polecat, the Asiatic polecat and the domestic ferret. *Proceedings of the Zoological Society of London* 125 (2): 317–333. (published online 20 Aug 2009).

AVMA (American Veterinary Medical Association). (2013). AVMA Guidelines for the Euthanasia of Animals: 2013 Edition. Available at https://www.avma.org/KB/Policies/Pages/Euthanasia-Guidelines.aspx. Accessed 7 October 2015.

Banks, R.E., Sharp, J.M., Doss, S.D., and Vanderford, D.A. (2010). *Exotic Small Mammal Care and Husbandry Ferrets*, 61–73. USA: Wiley-Blackwell.

Baum, J.M. (1976). Effects of testosterone propionate administered perinatally on sexual behavior of female ferrets. *Journal of Comparative and Physiological Psychology* 90: 399–410.

Baum, M.J., Canick, J.A., Erskine, M.S. et al. (1983). Normal differentiation of masculine sexual behaviour in male ferrets despite neonatal inhibition of brain aromatase or 5-alpha-reductase activity. *Neuroendocrinology* 36: 277–284.

Bays, T.B., Lightfoot, T., and Mayer, J. (2006). *Exotic Pet Behavior. Birds, Reptiles and Small Mammals*. St. Louis, Missouri, USA: Saunders Elsevier Inc.

Bell, J. (1995). Proven or potential zoonotic diseases of ferrets. *Journal of the American Veterinary Medical Association* 195: 990–994.

Bell, J.A. (1999). Ferret nutrition. *The Veterinary Clinics of North America. Exotic Animal Practice* 2: 169–192.

Berzins, R. and Helder, R. (2008). Olfactory communication and the importance of different odour sources in the ferret (*Mustela putorius f. furo*). *Mammalian Biology* 73 (5): 379–387.

Bibeau, C.E., Tobet, S.A., Anthony, E.L. et al. (1991). Vaginocervical stimulation of ferrets induces release of luteinizing hormone-releasing hormone. *Journal of Neuroendocrinology* 3 (1): 29–36.

Bowen, J. and Heath, S. (2005). *Behaviour Problems in Small Animals. Practical Advice for the Veterinary Team*. USA: Elsevier Saunders.

Brown, S.A. (2004). Basic anatomy, physiology and husbandry. In: *Ferrets, Rabbits and Rodents, Clinical Medicine and Surgery* (ed. E.V. Hillyer and K.E. Quesenberry), 3–14. UK: WB Saunders company.

Brown, S. (2007). History of the ferret. *The Small Animal health series*. Available at http://www.veterinarypartner.com/Content.plx?P=A&A=496. Accessed 24 August 2018..

Bulloch, M.J. and Tynes, V.V. (2010). Ferrets. In: *Behaviour of Exotic Pets* (ed. V.V. Tynes). USA: Wiley-Blackwell Publishing Ltd.

Caley, P. and Morriss, G. (2001). Summer/autumn movements, mortality rates and density of feral ferrets (*Mustela furo*) at a farmland site in North Canterbury, New Zealand. *New Zealand Journal of Ecology* 25 (1): 53–60.

Chitty, J. (2009). Ferrets: biology and husbandry. In: *BSAVA Manual of Rodents and Ferrets* (ed. E. Keeble and A. Meredith), 193–204. UK: BSAVA.

Clapperton, B.K., Minot, E.O., and Crump, D.R. (1988). An olfactory recognition system in the ferret *Mustela furo* L. (Carnivora: Mustelidae). *Animal Behaviour* 36 (2): 541–553.

Duda, J. (2003). Mustela putorius furo domestic ferret. *Animal Diversity Web*. Available at http://animaldiversity.org/accounts/Mustela_putorius_furo. Accessed 24 August 2018.

Einon, D. (1996). The effects of environmental enrichment in ferrets. In: *Environmental enrichment information resources for laboratory animals, 1965–1995: birds, cats, dogs, farm animals, ferrets, rabbits and rodents*, AWIC resource series, vol. 2, 113–126. Department of agriculture, Beltsville MD and Universities' federation for animal welfare (UFAW).

European Commission. (2007). Commission recommendation of 18 June 2007 on Guidelines for the accommodation and care of animals used for experimental and other scientific purposes. Annex II to European Council Directive 86/609, see 2007/526/EC. Available at https://eur-lex.europa.eu/LexUriServ/LexUriServ.do?uri=OJ:L:2007:197:0001:0089:EN:PDF. Accessed 13 May 2008.

Fisher, P.G. (2006). Ferret behavior. In: *Exotics Pet Behavior. Birds, Reptiles, and Small Mammals* (ed. T.B. Bays, T. Lightfoot and J. Mayer). Missouri, USA: Saunders, Elsevier Inc.

Fox, J.G. and Marini, R.P. (2001). Helicobacter mustelae infection in ferrets: pathogenesis, epizootiology, diagnosis and treatment. *Seminars in Avian and Exotic Pet Medicine* 10 (10): 36–44.

Fox, J.G., Bell, J.A., and Broome, R. (2014). Growth and reproduction. In: *Biology and Diseases of the Ferret*, 3e (ed. J.G. Fox and R.P. Marini), 187–210. Ames, Iowa: Wiley.

Hansen, C.P.B. (1993). Stereotypies in ranch mink: The effect of genes, litter size and neighbours. *Behavioural Processes* 29: 165–177.

Hansen SW. 1989. Activity in the daytime of lactating farm mink in cages with either water bath or net wire cylinder. In: Poster at the 21st International Ethological Congress, Utrecht, Netherlands, August 9–11.

Heller, K.E. (1991). Stress and stereotypies in farmed mink. *Applied Animal Behaviour Science* 30 (1–2): 179. (Abstract).

Jenkins, J.R. and Brown, S.A. (1993). *A practitioner's Guide to Rabbits and Ferrets*. USA: American Animal Hospital Association.

Johnson-Delaney, C.A. (2009). Ferrets: anaesthesia and analgesia. In: *BSAVA Manual of Rodents and Ferrets* (ed. E. Keeble and A. Meredith), 245–253. UK: BSAVA.

Jurek, R.M. (1998). A review of national and California population estimates of pet ferrets. In Calif. Dep. Fish and Game, Wild Manage. Div., Bird and Mammal Conservation Program 11p. Rep. 98–09. Sacramento, CA, USA.

Kaufman, L.W. (1980). Foraging cost and meal patterns in ferrets. *Physiology and Behavior* 25 (1): 139–141.

Kronfeld, D.S. (1985). Nutrition in orthopaedics. In: *Textbook of Small Animal Orthopaedics* (ed. C.D. Newton and D.M. Nunamaker). NY, USA: IVIS Ithaca.

MacKay, J. (1995). *Complete Guide to Ferrets*. Shrewsbury, UK: Swan Hill Press.

MacKay, J. (2006). *Ferret Breeding*. Shrewsbury, UK: Swan Hill Press, an imprint of Quiller Publishing Press.

Martin, D. (1986). Bone marrow depression associated with prolonged estrus in the European polecat or fitch ferret. *Veterinary Technician* 7 (7): 323–327.

Mason, G.J. (1991). Stereotypies and suffering. *Behavioural Processes* 25: 103–115.

Mason, G.J. (1993). Age and context affect the stereotypical behaviours of caged mink. *Behaviour* 127 (3–4): 191–229.

Mason, G.J., Cooper, J.J., and Clarebrough, C. (2001). Frustrations of fur-farmed mink. *Nature* 410: 35–36.

Moorman-Roest, J. (1993). De fret. In: *Diergeneeskundig memorandum*. Handleiding voor bijzondere dieren. Mycofarm/Janssen Pharmaceutica en Solvay Duphar: 82–88.

Moors, P.J. and Lavers, R.B. (1981). Movements and home range of ferrets (*Mustela furo*) at Puke puke lagoon. *New Zealand Journal of Zoology* 8 (1981): 413–423.

Morrisey, J.K. (2004). Ferrets: therapeutics. In: *BSAVA Manual of Rodents and Ferrets* (ed. E. Keeble and A. Meredith), 237–244. UK: BSAVA.

Norbury, G.L., Norbury, D.C., and Heyward, R.P. (1998). Space use and denning behaviour of wild ferrets (*Mustela furo*) and cats (*Felis catus*). *New Zealand Journal of Ecology* 22 (2): 149–159.

Orcutt, C. and Malakoff, R. (2009). Ferrets: cardiovascular and respiratory system disorders. In: *BSAVA Manual of Rodents and Ferrets* (ed. E. Keeble and A. Meredith), 282–290. UK: BSAVA.

Poessel, S., Biggins, D.E., Santymire, R.M. et al. (2011). Environmental enrichment affects adrenocortical stress responses in the endangered black-footed ferret. *General and Comparative Endocrinology* 172: 526–533.

Poole, T.B. (1978). An analysis of social play in polecats (Mustelidae) with comments on the form and evolutionary history of the open mouth play face. *Animal Behaviour* 26: 36–49.

Powell, R.A. (1979). Mustelid spacing patterns: variations on a theme by Mustela. *Zeitschift für Tierpsychologie* 90: 153–165.

Powell, R.A. (1994). Structure and spacing of Marten populations. In: *Biology and Conservation of Martens, Sables and Fishers* (ed. S.W. Buskirk, A. Harestad, M. Raphael and R. Powell), 101–121. NY, USA: Cornell University Press Ithaca.

Price, E.O. (2002). *Animal Domestication and Behaviour*. Wallington, Oxon, UK: CABI Publishing, CAB International.

Prohaczik, A., Kulcsár, N., Trigg, T. et al. (2010). Comparison of four treatments to suppress ovarian activity in ferrets (*Mustula putorius furo*). *Veterinary Record* 166: 74–78.

Quesenberry, K.E. and Carpenter, J.W. (2004). *Ferrets, Rabbits and Rodents: Clinical Medicine and Surgery*, 2e. Philadelphia, USA: WB Saunders Co.

Quesenberry, K.E. and Orcutt, C. (2012). Basic approach to veterinary care. In: *Ferrets, Rabbits and Rodents*, 3e (ed. K.E. Quesenberry and J.E. Carpenter), 13–26. Elsevier: St. Louis MI.

Schilling, K. (2000). *Ferrets for Dummies*. California, USA: IDG Books Worldwide Inc.

Schoemaker, N.J. (2009). Endocrine and neoplastic diseases. In: *BSAVA Manual of Rodents and Ferrets* (ed. A. Meredith and E. Keeble), 320–329. Gloucestershire: British Small Animal Veterinary Association.

Schoemaker, N.J. and van Zeeland, Y. (2013). Fret. In: *Diergeneeskundig memorandum Bijzondere gezelschapsdieren* (ed. F. Pasmans), 189–222. Oosterhout, the Netherlands: Leonard Strategische Communicatie bv.

Schoemaker, N.J., Schuurmans, M., Moorman, H., and Lumeij, J.T. (2000). Correlation between age at neutering and age at onset of hyperadrenocorticism in ferrets. *Journal of the American Veterinary Medical Association* 216: 195–197.

Schoemaker, N.J., Teerds, K.J., Mol, J.A. et al. (2002). The role of luteinizing hormone in the pathogenesis of hyperadrenocorticism in neutered ferrets. *Molecular and Cellular Endocrinology* 197: 117–125.

Solnick, J.V. and Schauer, D.B. (2001). Emergence of diverse Helicobacter species in the pathogenesis of gastric and enterohepatic diseases. *Clinical Microbiology Reviews* 14: 59–97.

Staton, V.W. and Crowell-Davis, S.L. (2003). Factors associated with aggression between pairs of domestic ferrets. *Journal of the American Veterinary Medical Association* 222 (12): 1709–1712.

Talbot, S., Freire, R., and Wassens, S. (2014). Effect of captivity and management on behaviour of the domestic ferret (*Mustela putorius furo*). *Applied Animal Behaviour Science* 151: 94–101.

Tetley, H. (1965). Notes on British polecats and ferrets. *Proceedings of the Zoological Society of London* 155 (1–2): 212–217. (published online 21 Aug 2009).

Thompson, A.D. (1951). A history of the ferret. *Journal of the History of Medicine and Allied Sciences* 6 (4): 471–480.

Vinke, C.M. and Schoemaker, N.J. (2012). The welfare of pet ferrets (*Mustela putorius furo* T). A review on the housing and management of pet ferrets. *Applied Animal Behaviour Science* 139: 155–168.

Vinke, C.M., van den Bos, R., and Spruijt, B.M. (2004). Anticipatory hyperactivity and stereotypical behaviour in American mink (*Mustela vison*) in three housing systems differing in the amount of enrichments. *Applied Animal Behaviour Science* 89: 145–161.

Wolf, P. and Hebeler, D. (2001). Characteristics of the digestive physiology in ferrets. *Kleintierpraxis* 46 (3): 161–164.

Woodley, S.K. and Baum, M.J. (2003). Effects of sex hormones and gender on attraction thresholds for volatile anal scent gland odours in ferrets. *Hormones and Behavior* 44: 110–118.

Rabbits and Rodents (*Glires*)

James Yeates and Vera Baumans

6.1 History and Context

6.1.1 Natural History

Glires is a mammalian clade that includes two mammalian orders – rodents and lagomorphs – and more than 2000 discovered species (Table 6.1). Glires are often categorised as 'small mammals' or 'small furries' because they are mammalian (and so warm-blooded), furry (which helps maintain body temperatures) and mostly of low body weight (with correspondingly high metabolic rates). Some wild glires are caught for food, research, or as pets, and many are killed using poisons, traps, introduced diseases, or predators. Currently, over 200 species are endangered or critically endangered (e.g. several species of kangaroo rat, IUCN 2014). However, humans have also spread several species as non-native wild populations, both accidentally (e.g. Siberian chipmunks [*Eutamias sibiricus*]) and deliberately (e.g. rabbits [*Oryctolagus cuniculus*]).

Glires live within habitats including rainforests, deserts, and tundra. Many species live on the ground or in burrows, although some are arboreal (e.g. tree squirrels) or semi-aquatic (e.g. muskrats [*Ondatra zibethicus*]). Several have adapted to live in urban or farming habitats (e.g. several species of rats and mice). Many glires are most

Companion Animal Care and Welfare: The UFAW Companion Animal Handbook,
First Edition. Edited by James Yeates.
© 2019 Universities Federation for Animal Welfare. Published 2019 by John Wiley & Sons Ltd.

Table 6.1 Examples of Glires kept as companion animals.

'Hare-like' (Lagomorpha)	'Porcupine-like' rodents (Hystricomopha)	'Mouse-like' rodents (Myomorpha)		'Squirrel-like' rodents (Sciuromorpha)
		Muridae	Cricetidea	
Rabbits (Oryctolagus cuniculus; Ch. 7)	Chinchillas (Chinchilla spp.; Ch. 8) Degus (Octodon degus; Ch. 8) Guinea pigs (Cavia porcellus; Ch. 8)	Brown Rat (Rattus norvegicus; Ch. 11) Domestic mouse (Mus musculus domesticus) Duprasi (Pachyuromys duprasi natronensis) Mongolian Gerbils (Meriones unguiculatus; Ch. 10)	Campbell's dwarf hamsters (Phodopus campbelli) Chinese hamsters (Cricetulus griseus) Golden Hamsters (Ch. 9) Roborovski hamsters (Phodopus roborovskii)	Cape ground squirrel (Xerus inauris) Richardson's ground squirrels (Urocitellus richardsonii) Siberian chipmunks (Eutamias sibiricus) Black-tailed prairie dogs (Cynomys ludovicianus)

active at night or at twilight. Many are highly active, travelling across wide ranges; for example, female striped mice (*Rhabdomys pumilio*) may range more than 80 000m² (Schradin et al. 2010) depending on resources, population density, and season. Dietary adaptations include teeth that continue to grow throughout life to balance out the wear from chewing and the use of forepaws to manipulate food. Many glires also naturally re-eat nutrient-rich pellets of partly digested cellulose ('caecotrophs'). The availability of foodstuffs such as plants or insects can be seasonal, so many glires are adapted to hibernate or store food (e.g. many species of hamsters).

Although some species may often be solitary (e.g. jerboas), many glires live in social groups (e.g. prairie dogs [*Cynomys ludovivianus*]), which can be complicated and cooperative. Breeding is rapid for many species as a result of short gestation periods and large litters. Glires are able to learn through both classical and operant conditioning, for example, about dangers and food locations and to manipulate their environments (e.g. Timberlake and Washburne 1989). In some species, family groups cooperate in raising offspring (e.g. gerbils, see Chapter 10); in others, the male does not participate in rearing young (e.g. Siberian dwarf hamsters, Wynne-Edwards 1995). Although rodents can have relatively good night vision, different species have different wavelength sensitivities, sometimes increased towards the ultraviolet range or reduced within the red part of the light spectrum (e.g. mice). Glires often have good hearing, including within ultrasonic frequencies, in which they can also vocalise. Glires also communicate through posture, foot drumming (e.g. kangaroo rats, Shier and Randall 2007), and smell from their urine and scent glands, including alarm signals that appear similar to predator scents (Brechbühl et al. 2013).

6.1.2 Domestic History

Glires as pets have been kept at least since 1100 BCE (Royer 2013). Many glires species were – and are – farmed for fur (e.g. chinchillas) or meat (e.g. rabbits and guinea pigs). Many are also used for scientific research and testing, so information about these pet species often involves extrapolating from laboratory contexts. Some may be bought for feeding to other pets such as reptiles. Most popular species are now largely captive-bred. When first domesticated, breeding initially selected primarily for meat or research models, such that domestic mice are now generally considered a subspecies of house mouse. Additional selection has also created 'fancy' varieties based on aesthetics. Selection has had some unintended changes; for example, albino varieties may have especially poor visual acuity (e.g. mice: Jennings et al. 1998). However, selection has had little effect on glires' basic needs and behaviour (e.g. mice, Dudek et al. 1983). There is also some hybridisation (e.g. between dwarf Campbell's and Djungarian hamsters), with the focus on developing novel coat patterns and colours rather than temperament.

6.2 Principles of Glires Care

6.2.1 Diets

Several are herbivorous, grazing, browsing, or chewing plant material (e.g. rabbits, guinea pigs); several are omnivorous (e.g. Siberian chipmunks [*Tamias sibericus*] and house mice [*Mus musculus*]). Many of the omnivores predominately eat one type or another, often eating mainly vegetation with the occasional insect (e.g. black-tailed prairie dogs [*Cynomys ludovicianus*]) or vice versa (e.g. Duprasi [*Pachyuromys duprasi natronensis*]). Owners should ensure they choose a diet that has been formulated for their specific species where possible.

All glires need adequate fibre for digestion and opportunity to chew their food. Indeed, rabbits and caviomorphs are often called 'fibrevores', and 'rodent' is from the *Latin* 'to gnaw' (Figure 6.1). Some species may also chew harder foods or nonfood items, such as gnawing blocks – or, harmfully, their cage bars. Teeth can otherwise become excessively long and deformed, causing discomfort, painful mouth injuries, difficulty in eating, and ultimately, starvation (Figure 6.2). However, many glires species enjoy eating other food with lower fibre and higher calories (Figure 6.3). Commercial concentrated foods may have high nutrition densities, especially if they are also suitable for growing, pregnant, and lactating animals. Excessive provision can lead to obesity, health problems, and reduced life spans. Obese animals may also be unable to eat their caecotrophs, leading to nutritional deficiencies or caecotroph accumulation (Figure 6.4). Glires can also suffer from nutritional deficiencies or excesses, particularly of calcium, phosphorus, and vitamin D, which can further affect tooth health.

Selective feeding can exacerbate dental and nutritional issues. Some animals may select certain parts of mixed diets that are high in energy and low in other necessary nutrients, so that even 'balanced diets' may lead to an imbalanced intake. In at least some glires, this risks tooth overgrowth, digestion problems, obesity, malnutrition, and boredom. In these cases, owners may need to limit their pets' access to the preferred foods to ensure they obtain a good balance or to use pellets, in which dietary components are combined, or allow the glire to graze or forage on its own. Glires are motivated to forage for food that has been scattered by their owners or to interact with puzzle-feeders (e.g. hiding food in chewable objects). Some species should be given opportunities to store food in 'larders' hygienically, away from toilet areas and with any rotten food regularly removed (e.g. some chipmunks, hamsters, and kangaroo rats).

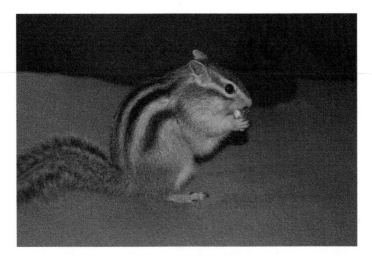

Figure 6.1 Chipmunk holding and gnawing food (*Source:* courtesy Yoann Prévert).

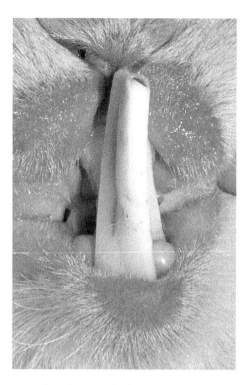

Figure 6.2 Severe overgrowth and mismatch of incisors (*Source:* courtesy Richard Saunders).

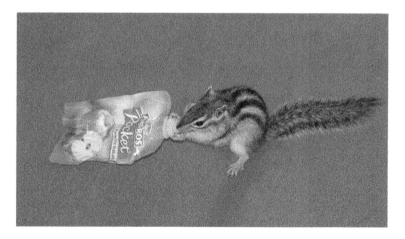

Figure 6.3 Chipmunk stealing food requiring less gnawing (*Source:* courtesy Yoann Prévert).

Fresh water should be provided ad libitum for all glires. Graduated water bottles can make measuring intake easier but may leak or block. Shallow bowls can avoid blockages but risk contamination by bedding and spillage, especially if they are turned upside down by the animal, so they should be raised above the bedding and located away from toilet areas.

(a)   (b)

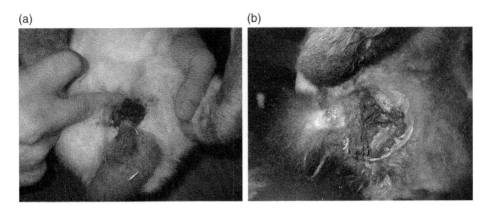

Figure 6.4 (a) Mild and (b) Severe caecotroph faecal pellet accumulation (*Source:* courtesy Richard Saunders).

6.2.2 Environment

Enclosures give some protection against external dangers and escape. However, they also limit animals' space and opportunities to explore, exercise, make choices, and avoid threats. Because different animals have different needs, owners should be particularly cautious about purchasing commercial housing labelled as suitable for a range of species. All glires species are active; some are highly athletic; and all need a large amount of three-dimensional space and environmental complexity for exercise, hiding, escape, climbing, and locomotory play. Many glires also prefer to compartmentalise their environment into separate places to sleep, toilet, and exercise. Consequently, more complex environments can reduce anxiety, stereotypical behaviour, and 'barbering' each other's hair (e.g. mice: Chamove 1989, Olsson and Sherwin 2006; Bechard et al. 2011; Gross et al. 2011). Additional complexity can come from platforms, hides, tubes, branches, ropes, and hammocks.

Noise and bright light within glires' sensitivity ranges can cause stress and retinal damage (Jennings et al. 1998; Burwell and Baldwin 2006). Man-made shelters, vertical barriers, and bedding can also allow animals to choose dimmer or quieter areas, although sometimes their motivation to gnaw chewable shelters is even stronger. Shelters and bedding can also help glires to avoid feeling exposed and to keep warm (Figure 6.5), and for some glires, to burrow. Insufficient substrate can cause cold stress, anxiety, aggression, or hibernation (Van Loo et al. 2003; Swoap et al. 2004; Kulesskaya et al. 2011). A variety of substrates allows animals to choose their preferences, which may be different for burrowing (e.g. cellulose chips) and nesting (e.g. tissue paper). Certain substrates should be avoided; for example, softwoods have been associated with cancers, and wood shavings or sawdust are associated with respiratory problems (Vesell 1967; Vaughan and Davis 1991).

Adequate ventilation and cleanliness are necessary to minimise respiratory and skin problems, but owners should minimise disruption and disturbance. Frequent spot cleaning should remove wet, dusty, unclean, or urine-soaked bedding, particularly from animals' toilet areas (and some glires can be toilet trained). Large-scale cleaning is needed less often. Owners should also minimise moving enclosure furniture around and human handing during cleaning, and they should maintain familiar smells by cleaning

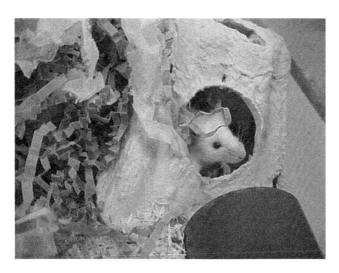

Figure 6.5 Mouse using shelter and bedding (*Source:* courtesy Vera Baumans).

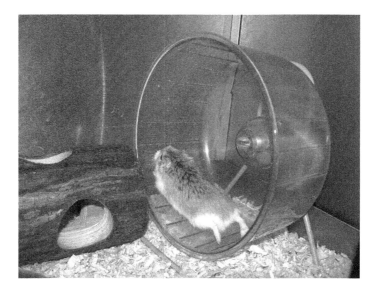

Figure 6.6 Roborovski hamster (*Phodopus roborovskii*) using a running wheel (*Source:* courtesy Bryan Howard).

separate areas or furniture at different times or by transferring some old nesting material to the clean enclosure, except in animals amongst whom it may increase aggression (e.g. in male mice; Van Loo et al. 2002).

Some glires are motivated to play with toys. Such play can help animals to cope with stressors, prompt endorphin release, and help development (e.g. Vanderschuren 2010; Pellis et al. 2014). In addition to ropes and obstacles to explore, owners can provide safe objects that glires can interact with and sometimes destroy. As a particular controversial enrichment, wheel use (Figure 6.6) may represent a strategy to cope with stress, a stereotypy, or an addiction (e.g. mice, Richter et al. 2014). Alternatively, it may simply be enjoyable, given that wild mice may use wheels spontaneously (Meijer and Robbers 2014), although this finding does not mean that wheel running is not ever, or even often, a sign of a welfare problem (Mason and Würbel 2016). Wheels should probably be provided to animals who use them but not as the only source of enrichment and only for limited 'exercise periods' if their use is causing problems and only alongside an exploration of potential welfare problems. Wheel sizes and designs should be solid to avoid injuries to their legs or tails in the rails or spokes and of large diameters to avoid excessive spine arching.

6.2.3 Animal Company

For many glires, group housing can allow positive social interactions such as grooming one another, sleeping in contact, and social play and allow shared vigilance (e.g. black-tailed prairie dogs, Hoogland 1979). In comparison, individual housing can increase glires' reactions to stressors and the risks of obesity (e.g. mice: Voikar et al. 2005; Nonogaki et al. 2007; Olsson and Westlund 2007). Related species may have different social needs; for example, golden hamsters are generally solitary animals (see Chapter 9), but this may not be the case for many popular dwarf species (*Phodopus* spp.). However, company can also cause problems even for social animals. Particular individuals may monopolise resources, show aggression, or pluck others' facial hairs, especially if there are limited resources. Mixing unfamiliar animals or disrupting scent markings may cause stress and aggression, and mixing unneutered animals can lead to accidental breeding and potential cannibalisation. For all animals, groups need adequate space and resources for all members – including at least one nest box per adult.

It can be difficult to work out whether to group house and what group sizes are best, and natural groupings may not always provide clear guidance for grouping in captivity. For example, wild chipmunks have solitary territories that overlap into loose colonies, but captive environments may not provide them with enough space to spread out, and pet chipmunks may be kept in small groups. Similarly, wild house mice live both solitarily and in groups (Frynta et al. 2005), whereas domestic mice appear to fare better in social housing (Van Loo et al. 2004), although they may have problems both in smaller groups (e.g. pairs, Jennings et al. 1998) and larger groups (e.g. five or eight, Van Loo et al. 2003). In many species, close relatives may form a more cohesive group than unfamiliar individuals.

Although some individuals may tolerate other species (Figure 6.7), in general, different glires species should not be kept together. Mixing species risks predation (e.g. rats and mice) or competition and bullying (e.g. rabbits and guinea pigs). Nonglires species can also cause injury or stress, and glires should be protected from both wild predators (e.g. foxes) and carnivore pets (e.g. cats, dogs, and birds of prey). Pet glires should be unable even to see or smell predators because this may be aversive (Apfelbach et al. 2005) or alarming (Brechbühl et al. 2013).

6.2.4 Human Interaction

All glires can suffer from human contact. Several rodents prefer to be inactive in the daytime when humans want to handle them (e.g. hamsters and duprasi). Many may perceive humans as predators (and indeed humans do eat several glires species), and

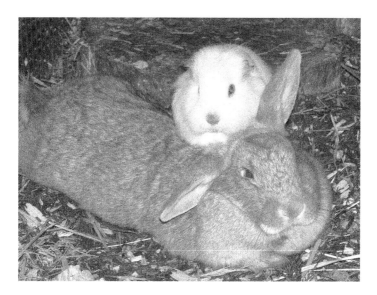

Figure 6.7 Rabbit and guinea pig showing some signs of social interaction (*Source*: courtesy Marit Emilie Buseth).

some may be particularly stressed by certain types of people (e.g. men, Sorge et al. 2014). For example, prairie dogs may produce different calls depending on humans' build and clothes (e.g. Gunnison's prairie dogs [*Cynomys gunnisoni*], Slobodchikoff et al. 1991; black-tailed prairie dogs, Frederiksen and Slobodchikoff 2007). Glires may show this fear through efforts to escape handling such as jumping, freezing, signs of stress such as hyperactivity, or defensive aggression such as biting. Notwithstanding glires' small sizes, speed, and jumping abilities, handlers must avoid overly forceful handling, which can be stressful or cause injury. For example, mice may be picked up in a tunnel or tube which they have entered voluntarily (Hurst and West 2010). Pet glires should never be picked up by their tails alone or lifted to altitudes many times their own height.

All animals should ideally be handled and their enclosures cleaned out by familiar humans in a quiet manner with consistent routines. Indeed, gentle or enjoyable handling can reduce glires' fear of humans. Owners can get new animals used to being brushed while eating, then to light hand contact, later to placing food items on their still, open palm and allowing the animal to approach, and progressing to handling. Owners can then train them to do this on cue and to perform other useful behaviours such as coming when called and sitting still on weighing scales. Where an animal is already showing fear of being handled, owners first need to understand and address the underlying reasons before retraining the animal to be comfortable around humans and being handled using rewards.

6.2.5 Health
Some diseases are common to several glires species. A few are potentially zoonotic, including monkeypox; *Salmonella*; bubonic plague (*Yersinia pestis*); Tularaemia (*Francisella tularensis*), and Lyme disease (*Borrelia* spp.). Glires can also act as

Table 6.2 Examples of veterinary specialisations relevant to Glires kept as companion animals (see also Chapter 1).

Recognising organisation	Example veterinary specialties
American Veterinary Medical Association	American Board of Veterinary Practitioners in Exotic Companion Mammal Practice
European Board of Veterinary Specialisation	European College of Zoological Medicine (Small Mammal)
United Kingdom (RCVS)	RCVS Recognised Specialists in Rabbit medicine and surgery

RCVS – Royal College of Veterinary Surgeons.

vectors for parasitic and other diseases in other species. Fly-strike can occur when flies lay eggs in damaged or dirty skin, for example around the anus after caecotroph accumulation. Glires' high metabolic rates can mean they can decline very rapidly when things start to go wrong. Because of the management and short life spans of some species, several conditions that might be considered 'geriatric' can also occur at ages of just 1 to 3 years. Because at least some of their teeth grow continuously, tooth damage or dental disease can lead to overgrowth and malocclusion.

All glires should receive regular health checks from specialist veterinary surgeons where possible and appropriate (Table 6.2). For most species, there are no annual vaccination programmes, but they should receive regular checks and may need treatment for overgrown or misshapen teeth or claws. Glires are also vulnerable to iatrogenic harm within veterinary care, through the stress of handling, inaccurate medical dosing, inappropriate procedures (such as teeth clipping that can shatter the teeth), hypothermia during or after anaesthesia because of their size (and more specifically, their high surface area-to-volume ratio), and anaesthetic complications resulting from undetected diseases (e.g. pneumonia). Veterinary surgeons should balance the risks and benefits of any intervention.

6.2.6 Euthanasia

The best methods of euthanasia of glires depend on the individual animal (Table 6.3). Although injecting an anaesthetic overdose into the vein can be best for some animals, many glires' small sizes make access to veins and restraint difficult. This small size can also make neck dislocation possible in smaller glires. Inhaled anaesthetics and low-oxygen levels can be aversive (Niel and Weary 2007; Makowska et al. 2009), and although glires are killed in laboratories using carbon dioxide overdose, this is also aversive and unsuitable for pets. Injecting an overdose of barbiturates into the abdomen can cause irritation if not adequately buffered, diluted, or combined with nonirritant local anaesthetic; particular dissociative anaesthetics (e.g. ketamine) and sedatives (e.g. xylazine) may be preferable in some rodents.

Table 6.3 Methods of euthanasia for (some) Glires kept as companion animals.

Method	Restraint required	Welfare benefits	Welfare risks
Intravenous or intraperitoneal injection of barbiturate	Secure handling Sedation advised (unless would require excessive handling)	Rapid loss of consciousness if intravenous; variable if intraperitoneal	Possible pain at injection site
Inhalation of volatile anaesthetics at increasing concentrations	Placement in chamber	Minimal handling	Chemical may be unpleasant
Neck dislocation	Secure handling	Immediate loss of consciousness and death as a result of physical damage to the brain stem	Pain if procedure done incorrectly. Injection or handling if sedation required
Brain trauma	Secure handling	Immediate unconsciousness resulting from brain destruction	Pain if performed incorrectly

Source: AVMA (2013).

6.3 Signs of Glires Welfare

6.3.1 Pathophysiological Signs

Pathological signs may be subtle and few, but general signs include ruffled fur, sunken eyes, and weight loss. Several diseases, such as example Tyzzer's disease, might suggest other underlying problems such as stress or poor husbandry. Acute stress can cause high heart rates (Burwell and Baldwin 2006), remembering that glires have normally high resting rates because of their small size and fast metabolisms. Increased corticosterone can also indicate stress, although this requires sampling. Chromodacryorrhea or 'red tears' may be excreted from the Harderian gland around the nose and eyes when the animal is ill or stressed (Richardson 1997; Lichtenberger and Hawkins 2009). Glires may quickly groom off the chromodacryorrhea, and it can be less visible in darker coloured animals, so its absence should not be relied on to indicate an absence of stress. Large amounts of chromodacryorrhea may also indicate that the animal is not self-grooming, suggesting severe, chronic stress, or illness.

6.3.2 Behavioural Signs

In general, most glires are not frequently expressive in ways that owners can perceive, although general signs can give some indications of welfare compromises (Table 6.4). Some may make distress vocalisations chatter their teeth, or make other audible noises (e.g. prairie dogs have a range of barks, Waring 1970, 2007; Smith et al. 1977), but glires often make ultrasonic vocalisations that, by definition, owners cannot hear except by using specialised equipment such as commercial bat detectors. Negative interactions between animals such as aggression and barbering may indicate inappropriate company, limited resources, or inadequate conditions. Abnormal behaviours include repetitive digging, circling, jumping up and down in a corner of the cage, wheel use, and bar chewing. These may be considered stereotypical or may reflect escape attempts. Not all glires show the same behavioural responses to the same stimuli; for example, rats may not show abnormal behaviours in situations in which mice might, perhaps because of them being more adaptable to different environments, tending to show a more passive response to stress, or because they are not given sufficient space to perform such abnormal behaviours.

6.4 Action Plan for Improving Glires Welfare Worldwide

Many glires are kept in enclosures. Priorities for improving care therefore include ensuring that their enclosures are sufficient, particularly in terms of space and substrates. Efforts should be made by both owners and the pet industry to move on from traditional housing and husbandry methods that were designed for short-lived glires intended for consumption, moving away from 'cages' (including hutches) towards larger enclosures with shelters included. For social glires, they need to be provided with adequate company of their own species, so that they do not suffer from isolation throughout their whole lives. Because glires in these cages do not share living space with their owners, and the owners need to make extra effort to give them enough attention to provide their needs and observe any problems. This attention needs to be gentle, enjoyable, and begun at an early age, so that they are not scared by handling and do not try to jump or bite and risk injury and further fear. Owners need to ensure that their glires will receive adequate attention throughout their lives, which can be many years if they are well cared for. In some cases, glires might be better off relinquished or even euthanised than left neglected.

There needs to be a recognition that glires are not all easy or 'children's' pets. There is no convincing evidence to conclude that they are any easier to care for adequately than, say, dogs, and cats. In addition, owners need to recognise that even if glires are cheap financially, their welfare is as important as other, larger pets'. In addition, although they are small animals, they do not necessarily therefore need less space or enrichment. Glires should not be bought as childrens' first pets to teach them how to look after animals (if they look after them well) or to teach them about death (especially if they look after them inadequately). They should be obtained only when children genuinely want a pet, when they are the right choice of pet for that child, and when the parent is confident that the child's enthusiasm will not wane over time or if the animal shows fear-based avoidance or aggression. Adults also need to ensure that they take responsibility for the animal's care assisted by their children.

Table 6.4 Key behavioural signs of possible welfare compromises in Glires kept as companion animals.

Aspect of behaviour	Specific responses
Altered activity or responsiveness	Increased vigilance or activity
	Attention to particular threats
	Startling
	Reaction on palpation or withdrawal of body part from contact
	Lethargy, immobility, decreased mobility (e.g. less movement or play)
	Unwillingness to leave their resting area
	Playing dead
Avoidance	Avoiding particular areas
	Hiding
	Immobility or 'freezing'
	Preparation for flight
	Escape attempts during handling
	Flight (jumping, running)
Altered posture or expression	Altered body or ear position
	Altered eye opening (e.g. wide or closed eyes)
	Looking 'smaller' or 'bigger'
Altered metabolic processes and maintenance or other common behaviour	Increased respiratory rate
	Altered appetite
	Increased drinking
	Altered urination or defaecation
	Altered toileting
	Altered grooming or bathing
	Altered time spent resting or sleeping
	Reduced time spent playing
	Reduced nest building
Altered interactions with the environment or other animals	Manipulating environmental objects
	Aggression
	Barbering
	Cannibalism
	Withdrawal from the group
Vocalisations	Social calls
	Alarm calls
Attack or preattack behaviours	Biting
Abnormal or repetitive movements	Repetitive digging
	Circling
	Jumping up and down in a corner of the cage
	Bar chewing
	Self-mutilation

(*Continued*)

Table 6.4 (Continued)

Aspect of behaviour	Specific responses
Specific local signs of local pain	Hunched or rigid posture Biting or scratching a specific area Lameness

All behavioural responses may also indicate other welfare issues than those listed; and the absence of any particular sign in any individual does not mean they are not experiencing that welfare compromise.

Another priority that applies to all glires is ensuring their health care. Owners, food manufacturers, and vendors should ensure glires have sufficient chewing opportunities to ensure their teeth are worn down enough and they cannot select foods that lead to imbalances. This may mean not selling 'muesli' foods for certain species. Veterinary surgeons need to ensure that they provide the same level of care for these animals as for other species. Owners may fail to notice problems or be unwilling to fund veterinary treatment because most rodents are small, cheap, cared for by children, and expected to be short-lived. Treatment may also be limited by size, stress responses, drug availability, and veterinary expertise (despite the amount of biomedical and pharmacological research and testing using these species). However, greater veterinary attention on in-practice research may help to fill these gaps. Indeed, many owners want, and expect, a high quality of veterinary care, and several drugs are now licensed for certain rabbit and rodent species in some countries.

Finally, as with other species, additional care needs to be taken to avoid taking wild-caught animals that are unsuited to being kept as pets. One driver for such changes may be attempts to reduce the risks of zoonotic disease, such as the monkeypox outbreak in the United States, with many humans catching the disease from prairie dogs after the importation of rope squirrels (*Funiscuirus* spp.), tree squirrels (*Heliosciurus* spp.), Gambian giant rats (*Cricetomys* spp.), brushtail porcupines (*Atherurus* spp.), dormice (*Graphiurus* spp.), and striped mice (*Hybomys* spp.) from Ghana (Centres for Disease Control and Prevention [CDC] 2003). At the very least, the importation and movement of such animals should be carefully controlled to limit disease spread and welfare compromises and allow diseases to be traced.

Bibliography

Apfelbach, R., Blanchard, C.D., Blanchard, R.J. et al. (2005). The effects of predator odors in mammalian prey species: a review of field and laboratory studies. *Neuroscience and Biobehavioral Reviews* 29: 1123–1144.

AVMA (American Veterinary Medical Association). (2013). AVMA Guidelines for the Euthanasia of Animals: 2013 Edition. Available at https://www.avma.org/KB/Policies/Pages/Euthanasia-Guidelines.aspx. Accessed 7 October 2015.

Baumans, V. (2005). Environmental enrichment for laboratory rodents and rabbits: requirements of rodents, rabbits and research. *ILAR Journal* 46: 162–170.

Baumans, V. and Van Loo, P.L.P. (2013). How to improve housing conditions of laboratory animals: the possibilities of environmental refinement. *The Veterinary Journal* 195: 24–32.

Bechard, A., Meagher, R., and Mason, G. (2011). Environmental enrichment reduces the likelihood of alopecia in adult C57BL/6J mice. *Journal of the American Association for Laboratory Animal Science* 50: 171–174.

Beery, A.K. and Kaufer, D. (2015). Stress, social behaviour and resilience: insights from rodents. *Neurobiology of Stress* 1: 116–127.

Brechbühl, J., Moine, F., Klaey, M. et al. (2013). Mouse alarm pheromone shares structural similarity with predator scents. *Proceedings of the National Academy of Sciences of the United States of America* 110 (12): 4762–4767.

Burwell, A.K. and Baldwin, A.L. (2006). Do audible and ultrasonic sounds of intensities common in animal facilities affect the autonomic nervous system of rodents? *Journal of Applied Animal Welfare Science* 9 (3): 179–200.

Centres for Disease Control and Prevention (CDC). (2003). Update: Multistate Outbreak of Monkeypox – Illinois, Indiana, Kansas, Missouri, Ohio, and Wisconsin. Available at http://www.cdc.gov/mmwr/preview/mmwrhtml/mm5227a5.htm. Accessed 12 August 2016.

Chamove, A.S. (1989). Cage design reduces emotionality in mice. *Laboratory Animals* 23 (3): 215–219.

Close, B., Banister, K., Baumans, V. et al. (1996). Recommendations for euthanasia of experimental animals. Part 1. *Laboratory Animals* 30 (4): 293–316.

Close, B., Banister, K., Baumans, V. et al. (1997). Recommendations for euthanasia of experimental animals. Part 2. *Laboratory Animals* 31 (1): 1–32.

Cloutier, S., Panksepp, J., and Newberry, R.C. (2012). Playful handling by caretakers reduces fear of humans in the laboratory rat. *Applied Animal Behaviour Science* 140: 161–171.

Cowley, J.J. and Widdowson, E.M. (1965). The effect of handling rats on their growth and behaviour. *British Journal of Nutrition* 19: 397–406. doi: 10.1079/BJN19650037.

Dudek, B.C., Adams, N., Boice, R., and Abbott, M.E. (1983). Genetic influences on digging behaviors in mice (Mus musculus) in laboratory and seminatural settings. *Journal of Comparative Psychology* 97 (3): 249.

Fitchett, A.E., Collins, S.A., Mason, H. et al. (2005). Urinary corticosterone measures: effects of strain and social rank in BKW and CD-1 mice. *Behavioural Processes* 70: 168–176.

Frederiksen, J.K. and Slobodchikoff, C.N. (2007). Referential specificity in the alarm calls of the black-tailed prairie dog. *Ethology Ecology and Evolution* 19 (2): 87–99.

Frynta, D., Slábová, M., Váchová, H. et al. (2005). Aggression and commensalism in house mouse: a comparative study across Europe and the near east. *Aggressive Behaviour* 31: 283–293.

Gaskill, B.N., Gordon, C.J., Pajor, E.A. et al. (2012). Heat or insulation: behavioral titration of mouse preference for warmth or access to a nest. *PLoS One* 7 (3): e32799.

Gross, A.N., Engel, A.K., Richter, S.H. et al. (2011). Cage-induced stereotypies in female ICR CD-1 mice do not correlate with recurrent perseveration. *Behavioral Brain Research* 216: 613–620.

Hoogland, J.L. (1979). The effect of colony size on individual alertness of prairie dogs (Sciuridae: *Cynomys* spp.). *Animal Behaviour* 27 (2): 394–407.

Howerton, C.L., Garner, J.P., and Mench, J.A. (2008). Effects of a running wheel-igloo enrichment on aggression, hierarchy linearity, and stereotypy in group-housed male CD-1 (ICR) mice. *Applied Animal Behaviour Science* 115: 90–103.

Hurst, J.L. and West, R.S. (2010). Taming anxiety in laboratory mice. *Nature Methods* 7 (10): 825–826.

International Union for Conservation of Nature (IUCN). (2014). The IUCN Red List of Threatened SpeciesTM. Available at www.iucnredlist.org. Accessed 27 September 2014.

Jennings, M., Batchelor, G.R., Brain, P.F. et al. (1998). Refining rodent husbandry: the mouse: report of the rodent refinement working party. *Laboratory Animals* 32 (3): 233–259.

Jirkof, P. (2014). Burrowing and nest building behavior as indicators of well-being in mice. *Journal of Neuroscience Methods* 30 (234): 139–146.

Keeble, E. and Meredith, A. (eds.) *BSAVA Manual of Rodents and Ferrets*. Gloucester, UK: BSAVA.

Kleiman, D.G., Thompson, K.V., and Baer, C.K. (2010). *Wild Mammals in Captivity: Principles and Techniques for Zoo Management*. Chicago, USA: University of Chicago Press.

Kohman, R.A., Rodriguez-Zas, S.L., Southey, B.R. et al. (2011). Voluntary wheel running reverses age-induced changes in hippocampal gene expression. *PLoS One* 6 (8): e22654.

Kulesskaya, N., Rauvala, H., and Voikar, V. (2011). Evaluation of social and physical enrichment in modulation of behavioural phenotype in C57BL/6J female mice. *PLoS One* 6: e24755.

Latham, N. and Würbel, H. (2006). Wheel-running: a common rodent stereotypy? In: *Stereotypic Animal Behaviour: Fundamentals and Applications to Welfare*, 2e (ed. G. Mason and J. Rushen), 91–92. Wallingford, England: CABI.

Lewis, R.S. and Hurst, J.L. (2004). The assessment of bar chewing as an escape behaviour in laboratory mice. *Animal Welfare* 13: 19–25.

Lichtenberger, M. and Hawkins, M.G. (2009). Rodents: physical examination and emergency care. In: *BSAVA Manual of Rodents and Ferrets* (ed. E. Keeble and A. Meredith), 18–31. Gloucester, UK: BSAVA.

Makowska, I.J., Vickers, L., Mancell, J. et al. (2009). Evaluating methods of gas euthanasia for laboratory mice. *Applied Animal Behaviour Science* 121: 230–235.

Mason, G. and Würbel, H. (2016). What can be learnt from wheel-running by wild mice and how can we identify when wheel-running is pathological? *Proceedings of the Royal Society B* 283: 1824.

Meijer, J.H. and Robbers, Y. (2014). Wheel running in the wild. *Proceedings of the Royal Society B* 281: 20140210.

Meredith, A. and Johnson-Delaney, C. (eds.) (2009). *BSAVA Manual of Exotic Pets*. Gloucester, UK: BSAVA.

Nichol, K.E., Parachikova, A.I., and Cotman, C.W. (2007). Three weeks of running wheel exposure improves cognitive performance in the aged Tg2576 mouse. *Behavioural Brain Research* 184 (2): 124–132.

Niel, L. and Weary, D.M. (2007). Rats avoid exposure to carbon dioxide and argon. *Applied Animal Behaviour Science* 107 (1–2): 100–109.

Nonogaki, K., Nozue, K., and Oka, Y. (2007). Social isolation affects the development of obesity and type 2 diabetes in mice. *Endocrinology* 148 (10): 4658–4666.

Olsson, I.A.S. and Dahlborn, K. (2002). Improving housing conditions for laboratory mice: a review of 'environmental enrichment'. *Laboratory Animals* 3: 243–270.

Olsson, I.A.S. and Sherwin, C.M. (2006). Behaviour of laboratory mice in different housing conditions when allowed to self-administer an anxiolytic. *Laboratory Animals* 40 (4): 392–399.

Olsson, I.A.S. and Westlund, K. (2007). More than numbers matter: the effect of social factors on behaviour and welfare of laboratory rodents and non-human primates. *Applied Animal Behaviour Science* 103: 229–254.

Pellis, S.M., Pellis, V.C., and Himmler, B.T. (2014). How play makes for a more adaptable brain: a comparative and neural perspective. *American Journal of Play* 7 (1): 73–98.

Richardson, V.C.G. (1997). *Diseases of Small Domestic Rodents*. Oxford, UK: Blackwell Science Ltd.

Richter, S.H., Gass, P., and Fuss, J. (2014). Resting is rusting: a critical view on rodent wheel-running behavior. *The Neuroscientist* 20 (4): 313–325.

Royer N 2013 The History of Fancy Mice. American Fancy Rat and Mouse Association. Available at http://www.afrma.org/historymse.htm. Accessed 17 December 2013.

Schradin, C., Schmohl, G., Rödel, H.G. et al. (2010). Female home range size is regulated by resource distribution and intraspecific competition: a long-term field study. *Animal Behaviour* 79 (1): 195–203.

Shier, D.M. and Randall, J.A. (2007). Use of different signalling modalities to communicate status by dominant and subordinate Heerman's kangaroo rats (*Dipodymus heermanni*). *Behavioural Ecology and Sociobiology* 61: 1023–1032.

Slobodchikoff, C.N., Kiriazis, J., Fischer, C., and Creef, E. (1991). Semantic information distinguishing individual predators in the alarm calls of Gunnison's prairie dogs. *Animal Behaviour* 42: 713–719.

Smith, W.J., Smith, S.L., Oppenheimer, E.C., and Devilla, J.G. (1977). Vocalizations of the black-tailed prairie dog, *Cynomys ludovicianus*. *Animal Behaviour* 25: 152–164.

Sorge, R.E., Martin, L.J., Isbester, K.A. et al. (2014). Olfactory exposure to males, including men, causes stress and related analgesia in rodents. *Nature Methods* 11 (6): 629–632.

Swoap, S.J., Overton, J.M., and Garber, G. (2004). Effect of ambient temperature on cardiovascular parameters in rats and mice: a comparative approach. *American Journal of Physiology-Regulatory, Integrative and Comparative Physiology* 287 (2): R391–R396.

Sztainberg, Y. and Chen, A. (2010). An environmental enrichment model for mice. *Nature Protocols* 5: 1535–1539.

Timberlake, W. and Washburne, D.L. (1989). Feeding ecology and laboratory predatory behavior toward live and artificial moving prey in seven rodent species. *Animal Learning & Behavior* 17 (1): 2–11.

Tynes, V.V. (2010). *Behaviour of Exotic Pets*. Oxford, UK: Wiley-Blackwell.

Van de Weerd, H.A., Van Loo, P.L.P., van Zutphen, L.F.M. et al. (1997). Preferences for nesting material as environmental enrichment for laboratory mice. *Laboratory Animals* 31: 133–143.

Van Loo, P.L.P., Kruitwagen, C.L.J.J., Koolhaas, J.M. et al. (2002). Influence of cage enrichment on aggressive behaviour and physiological parameters in male mice. *Applied Animal Behaviour Science* 76: 65–81.

Van Loo, P.L.P., Van Zutphen, L.F.M., and Baumans, V. (2003). Male management: coping with aggression problems in male laboratory mice. *Laboratory Animals* 37: 300–313.

Van Loo, P.L.P., Van der Meer, E., Kruitwagen, C.L.J.J. et al. (2004). Long-term effects of husbandry procedures on stress-related parameters in male mice of two strains. *Laboratory Animals* 38: 169–177.

Vanderschuren, L.J.M.J. (2010). How the brain makes play fun. *American Journal of Play* 2: 315–337.

Vaughan, T.L. and Davis, S. (1991). Wood dust exposure and squamous cell cancers of the upper respiratory tract. *American Journal of Epidemiology* 133 (6): 560–564.

Vesell, E.S. (1967). Induction of drug-metabolizing enzymes in liver Microsomes of mice and rats by softwood bedding. *Science* 157 (Sept. 1967): 1057–1058.

Voikar, V., Polus, A., Vasar, E., and Rauvala, H. (2005). Long-term individual housing in
C57BL/6J and DBA/2 mice: assessment of behavioral consequences. *Genes, Brain and
Behavior* 4 (4): 240–252.

Waring, G.H. (1970). Sound communications of black-tailed, white-tailed, and Gunnison's
prairie dogs. *American Midland Naturalist* 1: 167–185.

Waring, G. H. (2007). Sounds of black-tailed, white-tailed, and Gunnison's prairie dogs (Doctoral
dissertation, Colorado State University). Available at https://dspace.library.colostate.edu/
handle/10217/50534. Accessed 12 August 2016.

Wells, D.J., Playle, L.C., Enser, W.E.J. et al. (2006). Assessing the welfare of genetically altered
mice. *Laboratory Animals* 40 (2): 111–114.

Whittaker, A.L. and Howarth, G.S. (2014). Use of spontaneous behaviour measures to assess
pain in laboratory rats and mice: how are we progressing? *Applied Animal Behaviour
Science* 151: 1–12.

Würbel, H. (2001). Ideal homes? Housing effects on rodent brain and behaviour. *Trends in
Neurosciences* 24: 207–211.

Wynne-Edwards, K.E. (1995). Biparental care in Djungarian but not Siberian dwarf hamsters *(Phodopus)*. *Animal Behavior* 50: 1571–1585.

European Rabbits (*Oryctolagus cuniculus*)

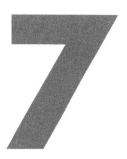

Siobhan Mullan and Richard Saunders

7.1 History and Context

7.1.1 Natural History

Rabbits (*Oryctolagus cuniculus*) are members of the class Mammalia, order Lagomorpha, and family Leporidae. European rabbits are native to Iberia and northwester Africa but were then introduced into other countries from around 3000 years ago. As examples, UK wild rabbits are descended from captive individuals who escaped from monasteries after approximately 1000 CE (McBride 1998), and the Australian wild rabbit population was introduced in the eighteenth century. The species is now well established in the wild in mainland Europe and Australia (Figure 7.1).

Wild European rabbits live in extensive networks of interconnected burrows with multiple entry points. These warrens branch, both horizontally and vertically, to confuse predators. Whilst generally narrow, they include various wider sections to allow meeting, resting, and nesting areas for individuals and groups (Kolb 1991; Serrano and Hidalgo de Trucios 2011). Warrens also provide consistent ambient temperatures in very hot or cold weather, so that rabbits have less need to regulate their body temperature in hot conditions.

Companion Animal Care and Welfare: The UFAW Companion Animal Handbook,
First Edition. Edited by James Yeates.
© 2019 Universities Federation for Animal Welfare. Published 2019 by John Wiley & Sons Ltd.

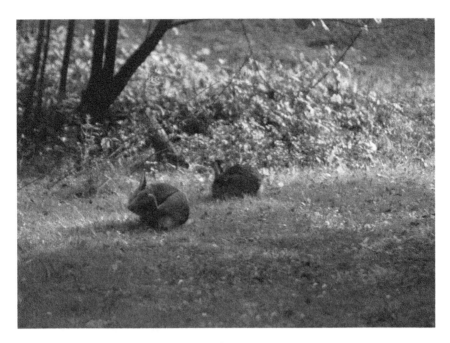

Figure 7.1 Wild rabbits (*Oryctolagus cuniculus*).

Wild rabbits emerge to eat in the early twilight, generally returning shortly after dawn (Mykytowycz and Rowley 1958). They are obligate herbivores, with teeth suited to a varied diet consisting predominantly of grasses, forbs, wild herbs, and leafy vegetation, with a small amount of buds, saplings, bark, and seeds (Marques and Mathias 2001; Martin et al. 2007). Both wild rabbits and pet rabbits placed in a semi-wild setting have large home ranges of approximately 2 km² (Stodart and Myers 1964). They then spend the majority of the daylight hours underground in their burrows, resting and ingesting caecotroph pellets (Lombardi et al. 2003).

Rabbits graze aboveground in groups, thereby improving vigilance against predators. Their laterally positioned eyes give them a wide visual field of almost 360 degrees (Harcourt Brown 2002), and their retinal anatomy and motivation for overhead scanning allow good perception of aerial predators (Tynes 2010). Rabbits signal alarm to one another by 'thumping' of the hind legs and the sight of the scut (the white underside of the tail) moving as they run. Loud vocalisations are extremely rare, and high-pitched screaming usually only occurs if a rabbit is caught by a predator. However they do make other noises, including grunting, growling, honking, and purring.

Wild rabbits live in social groups of up to several hundred individuals sharing a warren. Within these large colonies, individuals form strong and stable subgroups (Marsh et al. 2011). Subgroups of two to eight individuals defend territory within the warren, with males generally fighting one another for access to females, and females vying for access to nesting areas. Outside of the breeding season, rabbits (mainly the males) in a warren devote more effort to defending the warren against outside rabbit groups. Most digging is performed by the does (Southern 1948; Myers and Poole 1961; Lockley 1974; Cowan 1987).

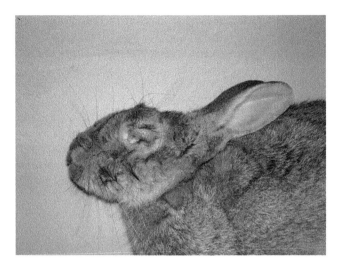

Figure 7.2 Deceased rabbit with myxomtosis.

Rabbits' gestation periods are only 29–35 days and their litter sizes often include 4–12 kittens. These factors can mean that large numbers of young are born from spring to mid-summer, with peak numbers born in late spring, early summer (Tablado et al. 2009). These provide an abundant food source for a range of predator species. In Iberia, the main predators are rabbit specialists such as the Iberian lynx (*Lynx pardina*) and the Spanish imperial eagle (*Aquila adalberti*) (Moreno et al. 2004). In Northern Europe, predators include birds such as the common buzzard (*Buteo buteo*) and mammals such as the stoat (*Mustela ermine*) and the red fox (*Vulpes vulpes*), with smaller juveniles also susceptible to smaller predators such as the weasel (*Mustela nivalis*).

Myxomatosis virus and strains of the calicivirus that cause Rabbit haemorrhagic disease (RHD) have been introduced as biological population control measures in countries such as Australia and the United Kingdom (Bartrip 2008; Wild 2011). Because of myxomatosis and habitat destruction, wild rabbits are categorised on the IUCN Red List as Near Threatened. Large numbers of of European rabbits have perished as a result of myxomatosis since the 1950s (Gibb 1990; Figure 7.2). RHD also caused the death of 55–75% of rabbits in the Iberian peninsula in the 1980s (Villafuerte et al. 1995).

7.1.2 Domestic History

Rabbits were kept as food and pelt animals until the middle of the nineteenth century. Companion rabbits were first reported in Renaissance Italy (Brown and Richardson 2004; Walker-Meikle 2012). Nowadays, rabbits continue to be kept for meat and fur and are an extremely common experimental animal species.

Selective breeding was carried out by monks from about 500 to 1000 CE. Meat breeds were predominantly selected for size, whereas wool breeds were selected for colour, length, and fineness of fur. From the sixteenth century, as rabbits started to be kept as pets, breeders began to experiment with different coat colours. Different breeds began to emerge, selected for size, facial shape, ear shape and fur colour, pattern, and length, with breeds now usually categorised as 'Fancy', 'Fur', 'Rex' (with short, dense, velvet-like fur, lacking guard hairs), and 'Lop' (downward pointing ears). In the United Kingdom, breed societies first emerged in the nineteenth century and breed standards were formally developed in 1946 (Whitman 2004; British Rabbit Council 2014b), with 81 breeds recognised as of 2010. In the United States, the American Rabbit Breeders Association was formed in 1953, and recognises 47 breeds.

Selective breeding has changed the basic body anatomy to a shorter legged, bulkier shape, with a usually longer and variably coloured coat. Compared to wild rabbits' weight of 1.5–2 kg, some breeds weigh around 1 kg (e.g. Polish) and other 'Giant' breeds around 6 kg (British Rabbit Council 2014a). Domestic rabbits are generally considered to be less nervous, although early, gentle handling is required to tame even domestic rabbits. They also have a more diurnal behaviour pattern than wild rabbits (Jilge 1991).

7.2 Principles of Rabbit Care

7.2.1 Diet

Rabbits are obligate herbivores (Table 7.1). An appropriate starting point is to base pet rabbits' diet on the high-fibre, low energy-density herbivorous diet that they have evolved to eat. Long fibre in the diet is essential for healthy peristalsis (Slade and Forbes 2014) and may promote healthy teeth by allowing optimal chewing movements and increased wear (Jekl and Redrobe 2013). This can be provided within grass, hay, or other fibrous vegetation (Figure 7.3). Energy-dense concentrated foods and seeds should rarely be fed in large quantities or for prolonged periods. When fed to excess, they do not allow an adequate amount of natural foraging behaviour and increase the likelihood of obesity (Sayers 2010). In addition, 'muesli' type foods lead to increased dental disease, probably partly because rabbits often select less nutritious parts and leave the pellets that include more vitamins and minerals (Harcourt-Brown 1996; Mullan and Main 2006).

Table 7.1 Nutritional requirements of adult, non-breeding rabbits.

Nutrient	Amount required, adult
Digestible energy	2100–2200 kcal kg^{-1} day^{-1}
Protein	12–13%
Indigestible fibre	at least 14–16%
Lipid	2–3%
Calcium	0.4–0.6%
Phosphorus	0.22–0.4%
Vitamin D	900 iu kg^{-1}
Water	50–100 mL kg^{-1} day^{-1}

All figures assume animals are of normal physiology, healthy, and non-breeding.
Source: NRC nutrient (1977), Lebas (1980), and Cheeke (1987).

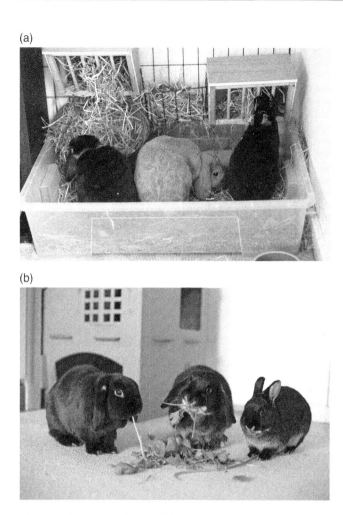

Figure 7.3 Rabbits (a) foraging on hay and (b) eating green vegetative material.

Inappropriate levels of calcium, phosphorous, and vitamin D can lead to metabolic bone disease, which is a major cause of dental disease in pet rabbits (Jekl and Redrobe 2013). Vitamin D can be provided in varied vegetation or can be synthesised by rabbits when exposed to sunlight (Fairham and Harcourt-Brown 1999; Emerson et al. 2014).

Foraging also provides rabbits with an occupation. Rabbits spend large proportions of their active time foraging if given the opportunity (Stodart and Myers 1964). Rabbits kept as pets forage less than wild or domestic rabbits in a semi-wild setting, and show more stereotypical behaviour (Schepers et al. 2009). Outdoors, rabbits should be allowed to graze and forage in contained lawns with a variety of suitable grassy and leafy plants. Indoors, rabbits should be given turf or other fibrous vegetation. Foraging may also be promoted by scattering favoured food items in areas which require digging, chewing, or other behaviours to access, such as within a mass of hay, ball feeders, or chewable toilet roll inners (James 2000; Dykes and Flack 2003).

Clean water should be available at all times. Rabbits may drink more from open bowls than nipple drinkers, similar to those used commonly as pet drinker bottles (Tschudin et al. 2011). Water intake is also greater in rabbits on higher fibre diets (Prebble and Meredith 2014). Increased voluntary water intake may help to prevent some urinary tract problems (Harcourt-Brown 2011).

7.2.2 Environment

Although pet houses cannot provide a wild rabbit's home range of 2 km², pet rabbits should be given enough space to move and exercise. This involves gaits ranging from slow walking and hopping to fast running, jumping and playing, non-locomotor alert behaviour, including standing on hind legs, and digging (Figure 7.4). Space should also allow rabbits to rest by lying flat out on their side and on their fronts, as well as foraging and social interactions. Restrictive environments significantly alter the behaviour of pet rabbits (Schepers et al. 2009), with rabbit pairs restricted to 0.73 m² plus access to 3 m² for 3 hours per day, showing high faecal corticosterone levels and significant 'rebound' increases in locomotor behaviour when allowed access to the 3 m² area (Held et al. 2018).

Many rabbits are kept permanently outdoors in a hutch, shed, partly enclosed run, or a restricted area of the garden, usually with a shelter provided. Others are kept permanently indoors, sometimes within a single room or cage. In each case, rabbits may be allowed temporary access to a larger area in the house or outdoors. The welfare effects of keeping rabbits indoors versus outdoors can depend on the foliage (for grazing and foraging), environment (e.g. climate), individual animal (e.g. prior experiences), presence of other animals (e.g. insects, wild rabbits, and predators), and the resources provided. In either case, owners need to ensure the rabbit's welfare needs are met.

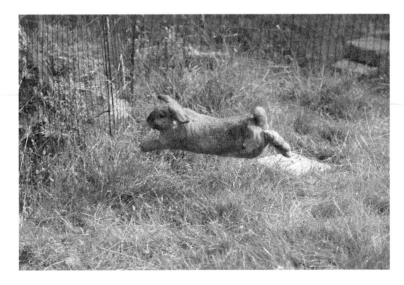

Figure 7.4 Rabbit exercising outdoors.

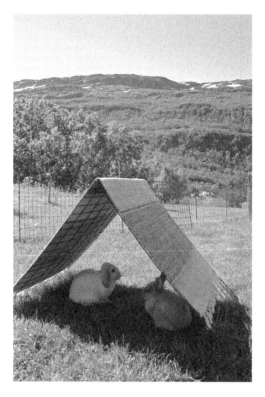

Figure 7.5 Outdoor shelter.

All rabbits need constant access to shelter to provide both security and protection from the elements (Figure 7.5), ideally within a tunnel or burrow. Rabbits can have particular difficulty regulating their body temperature in hot conditions, and the optimal climatic conditions for housed rabbits appears to be an air temperature of 13–20 °C (average 15 °C), relative humidity 55–65% (average 60%), and a moderate level of sunshine (Marai and Rashwan 2004). Domestic rabbits are strongly motivated to be near or under a cover, such as a platform, despite rarely sitting on it, suggesting they may be valuing it as a 'bolt-hole' (Seaman et al. 2008). Owners of pet rabbits should provide safe, complex, and unrestrictive environments that offer the choice to perform a variety of appropriate normal behaviours, either outdoors or indoors (Figure 7.6). Rabbits' natural daily rhythms of activity mean that that the highest motivations for activity are around dawn and dusk, so restrictive environments are likely to have greatest negative impacts during these times, and owners who provide intermittent access to wider spaces should prioritise doing so at these times.

Rabbits' normal behaviours may be carried out in areas or towards items which the owner would prefer they were not, such as urination in particular areas, damage to furniture, wallpaper, and so on by chewing and some sexual behaviour (McBride 1998; Magnus 2005). These can be reduced by providing suitable alternative substrates for them to interact with and a suitable social grouping (Isbell and Pavia 2009). Where owners are unable to provide a naturalistically rich environment, they should provide

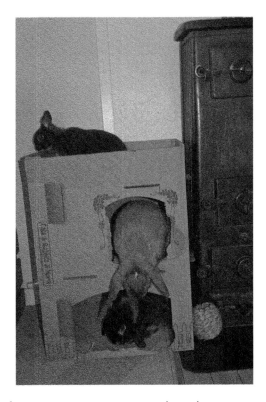

Figure 7.6 Indoor furniture to increase environmental complexity.

alternatives such as digging boxes full of earth. Rabbits also appear to enjoy interacting with a range of inanimate 'toys' (e.g. dried out pine cones, cardboard boxes, cat toys which can be tossed or rolled) and items which can be torn up, such as old telephone directories (James 2000; Dykes and Flack 2003). Rabbits can also be toilet-trained (RSPCA 2013a).

7.2.3 Animal Company

Individual housing has traditionally been seen as acceptable. Now, more knowledgeable and committed owners appear to value social housing (Edgar and Mullan 2011). Rabbits are social animals; their motivation for companionship is almost as high as that for food (Seaman et al. 2008). Pet rabbits kept socially appear to spend a large proportion of their time engaged in social interactions, and the majority of their rest time resting with a companion rather than alone (Mullan and Main 2007). Socially housing rabbits may reduce the development of abnormal behaviours such as digging, floor chewing, and bar biting and increase locomotion, as well as allowing social interactions (Chu et al. 2004). Owners also report very high levels of positive social behaviours displayed by pet rabbits housed with another rabbit, such as playing, grooming, and resting in contact with their companion (Figure 7.7). In comparison, owners report higher levels of negative behaviours and signs of ill health in pet rabbits kept on their own, such as matted fur or stained fur around the eyes (Rooney et al. 2014).

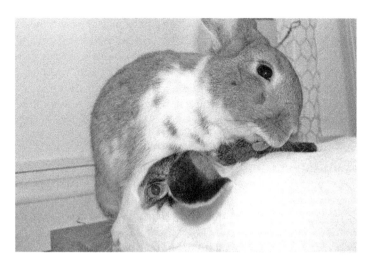

Figure 7.7 One rabbit engaging in grooming of another.

Some rabbits may bite one another or pull out each other's fur (Mullan and Main 2007; Rooney et al. 2014). Such incompatible relationships can be associated with greater fear of novel environments (Rooney et al. 2014). This suggests that they may be unpleasant, cause pain from injury, and also either increase or be caused by general anxiety or fear. Owners should carefully consider the choice of companions; managing introductions, only intervening if true aggression is seen; and providing large, varied environments in which to live.

Rabbits should be neutered before pairing or grouping. Unneutered rabbits may initially appear to get on, but problems will develop on reaching maturity or with the production of potentially unwanted litters. Entire male rabbits cannot be safely kept together past adolescence. Mixed-sex unneutered pairs or groups will lead to unwanted litters. Unneutered female rabbits kept together may fight or otherwise display negative behaviours. Neutered male and neutered female pairings are often considered, at least anecdotally, to be the most easily made and successful, but any combination is possible. Rabbits of similar size are often paired together, but this may have more to do with suitable enclosure sizes and life spans than compatibility. Pairing should take place in a neutral area, with some suggesting that the mild stress of a novel area is an enhancement to the ease of pairing. Greater stress environments are also sometimes suggested to enhance pairing, but this may involve significant welfare compromise. A full description of pairing is described by Buseth and Saunders (2014).

Owners should also neuter both sexes. Intact males and females may be distinguished by observing or palpating the external testes in the diverging male scrotum, which are visible when viewed from underneath. The penis has a more rounded, tubular appearance than the slitlike opening of the vulva. The dewlap – a flap under the chin which contains connective tissue and fat covered in furred skin – may also be significantly more pronounced in intact females than in males, but this is influenced also by body condition, with obese males often having a significant dewlap, and breed, with some rabbits of meat breed origin forming a dewlap more readily, even in males.

Rabbit relationships with other glires such as guinea pigs appear to be, at best, neutral (Mullan and Main 2007; Rooney et al. 2014) and can lead to fighting or the spread of some diseases. There are also welfare risks for those other species in such mixed groupings. In general, different glires species should not be kept together, except perhaps when an established relationship between individual animals is clearly better than isolation for both animals. Similarly, although some rabbits have been kept with dogs and cats, these may injure or prey on rabbits, with little warning, following changes in behaviour by either animal or external influences.

7.2.4 Human Interaction

Whether human contact can be enjoyable for rabbits is unclear, although some owners report that their rabbits follow them in the garden, indicating that rabbits are choosing to spend time with a human in that context (Mullan and Main 2007). The relative merits of human and rabbit companionship to a rabbit are also unknown but human companionship is unlikely to be an adequate substitute for compatible relationships with other rabbits.

However, all rabbits need to be handled occasionally for health and dental checks. Many owners also want and expect to handle their rabbit. However, handling, and especially lifting, is a fearful experience for a significant minority of pet rabbits (Mullan and Main 2007; Schepers et al. 2009; Rooney et al. 2014). Owners may persist in traumatic handling, given that they may not recognise signs of fear unless it is expressed as aggression (Mullan and Main 2007; Schepers et al. 2009; Rooney et al. 2014). Rabbits should be lifted by supporting the whole body and ensuring their hind legs are supported and restrained to avoid injuries associated with kicking out. In particular, inducing 'tonic immobility' (also known as 'trancing' or 'hypnosis') – for example by placing the rabbit on his or her back and repeatedly gently stroking from the chest to the stomach – may be stressful as it effectively causes the rabbit to respond as if to a predator. It should not be used for anything other than necessary, nonpainful procedures (Everitt 2013). According to a recent literature review, lifting rabbits from the ground is particularly stressful and should be avoided wherever possible, with other methods of handling and examination given a much greater priority (Bradbury and Dickens 2016). Good handling should reduce the stress of later human contact (Swennes et al. 2011) and make rabbits easier to handle (Mullan and Main 2007). In particular, gentle handling or exposure to human smells during the first week of life can significantly reduce later fear of humans (Bilko and Altbacker 2000; Ducs et al. 2009). Most owners obtain their rabbit after this time, although they can still have a role in getting young rabbits used to handling through gentle, progressive, positive handling. Breeders should therefore socialise kittens to people to ensure that future pets have every chance of becoming confident, friendly rabbits. Breeders may also select for a relaxed temperament and reduced aggression to humans, although it is difficult to separate the effect of breeding from that of early handling (Elliott and Lord 2014).

7.2.5 Health

Rabbits can suffer from several diseases, including many infectious agents (Table 7.2). Myxomatosis virus and RHD cause widespread suffering, and owners should vaccinate rabbits against both viruses in areas where they are found in local populations.

Table 7.2 Selected health problems in domestic rabbits.

Condition			Welfare effects
Infectious diseases	Bacterial	Pasteurellosis[a]	Respiratory distress; eye discomfort; abscesses; neurological problems
	Viral	Myxomatosis (V) Calicivirus (Rabbit Viral Haemorrhagic Disease) (V)	Prolonged suffering before death Acute death
	Fungal	Ringworm[a]	Minor skin itchiness
Parasitic	Internal parasites	*Encephalitizoon cuniculi* Coccidia (*Eimeria* spp.)	(No signs); head tilt, hindlimb paresis, urinary incontinence, death (No signs); loss of appetite; weight loss; lethargy; diarrhoea; dehydration
	External parasites	Fleas Lice Cheyletiella	Varying itchiness (ear mites usually being the most itchy)
Neoplastic		Uterine adenocarcinoma	Abdominal pain, bleeding, spread to lungs may be fatal
Inherited		Dental malocclusion Lop ears	Mouth pain, starvation Ear pain, infection
Degenerative or geriatric		Spondylosis	Spinal pain and stiffness affecting mobility and leading to flystrike, etc.
		Acquired dental disease	Mouth pain, starvation, death
Traumatic		Spinal damage from improper handling or being dropped Predation	Injury, paralysis, death
Gastrointestinal foreign body blockage			Abdominal pain, gut rupture, death

[a] (zoonotic); (V) = vaccine available.

Respiratory tract disease is common, particularly from *Pasteurella multocida* in breeding and rescue colonies. Control may require medication, good ventilation, and diets (Varga 2013). Gastrointestinal tract and urogenital tract disease are also common. They can cause chronic pain and may result in further health and welfare issues such as flystrike. Skeletal disease such as spondylosis and arthritis are chronic sources of pain and reduce mobility (Sayers 2010). Adrenal gland hyperplasia has been reported in male rabbits (Varga 2011), which may affect rabbits' behaviour towards previously amicably bonded rabbits and towards humans. Treponema is a common genital tract and dermatological infection in breeding and rescue situations. Zoonotic conditions include tularaemia (*Francisella tularensis*) and ringworm (van Praag et al. 2010).

Internal parasites are relatively uncommon in pet rabbits, with the exception of coccidia (*Eimeria* spp.) and *Encephalitizoon cuniculi* (Redrobe et al. 2010; Varga 2014). Levels of exposure to *E. cuniculi* can range from 7.4 to 100%, usually between 20 and 55%. Some authorities therefore propose routine treatment of all juvenile rabbits, although others suggest only treating affected animals (Keeble 2011). Because coccidia may be underdiagnosed, preventive treatment may be worthwhile in breeding production systems or in rescue situations (Redrobe et al. 2010). External parasites include *Cheyletiella parasitivorax*, which is the most common rabbit mite (Meredith 2006; Figure 7.8), and *Psoroptes cuniculi*, which are ear mites. Fly-strike, as a result, mainly of *Lucilia* serricata can be fatal. *Cheyletiella* and *E. cuniculi* are also potentially zoonotic, but other parasites are rarely passed from rabbits to humans (Mathis et al. 2005; Meredith 2006). Routine preventive measures against mites and fleas are usually unnecessary, unless they have been in contact with an animal in whom a parasite infestation has been diagnosed. However, rabbits should be given routine preventive treatment against fly-strike where they are at risk because it may be too late to treat rabbits by the time fly-strike is observed.

Inherited disorders include exaggeratedly large and downward hanging ears in breeds such as English lops (Castle and Reed 1936; Figure 7.9). This increases the risk of damage to the ears from injuries, soiling, or from frostbite. The bending of the ears

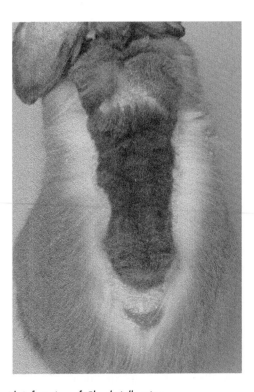

Figure 7.8   Rabbit with infestation of *Cheyletiella* mites.

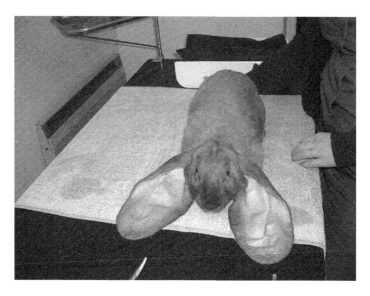

Figure 7.9 English lop with exaggerated physical features.

also makes the ear canals narrower and flattened, which can make them more likely to get bacterial ear infections and creates a weak point for normal aural secretions, with or without bacterial infection, to track from the ear canal to under the skin (Saunders and Shrubsole-Cockwill 2010). The size of the ears also reduces the rabbits' mobility and so increases the risk of obesity. Rex breeds have relatively bald hocks that are prone to ulcerating, whereas long-haired breeds such as Angoras, Cashmere, and Lionheads are prone to their fur becoming soaked with urine, leading to skin inflammation and fly-strike. Dwarf breeds such as the short-faced Netherland Dwarf and Lionheads commonly suffer from malocclusions between upper and lower incisors, leading to overgrowth, damage to the mouth, and if untreated, starvation (Huang et al. 1981; Lindsey and Fox 1994).

Dental disease is extremely common (Harcourt Brown 2009a, 2009b), affecting nearly 30% of pet rabbits in the United Kingdom (Mullan and Main 2006), although it may go unnoticed and untreated (Mullan and Main 2006; Rooney et al. 2014). Incisor ribbing may not have any negative impact at the time but may indicate a predisposition to more serious dental disease. In comparison, overgrowth of the incisors or cheek-tooth can cause ulceration, chronic oral pain, excessive drooling, and reduced food intake. Affected teeth may be treated by removal or regular shortening by a veterinary professional with appropriate equipment, often under general anaesthesia. Trimming incisors using inappropriate equipment can cause damage to the teeth or soft tissues (Cope et al. 2013). Another important preventative health measure is the neutering of female rabbits to reduce the risks of metritis, mammary neoplasia, and uterine cancer (Table 7.3). Uterine adenocarcinoma may affect 50–80% of intact does older than 3 years of age (Heatley and Smith 2004).

Table 7.3 Nontherapeutic elective surgical procedures performed on rabbits.

Mutilation	Reasons and possible benefits for the animal	Reasons and possible benefits for owners	Perioperative welfare risks	Behaviour prevented
Castration	Facilitation of social living Reduction of fighting with other unneutered males	Reduced urine spraying or sexual behaviour towards humans	Pain, distress Surgical complications (e.g. abdominal adhesions)	Breeding
Spaying	Facilitation of social living Prevention of uterine carcinomas Prevention of pregnancy if kept with unneutered males	May reduce aggression towards owners		

Table 7.4 Methods of euthanasia for pet rabbits kept as companion animals.

Method	Restraint required	Welfare benefits	Welfare risks
Intravenous pentobarbitone	Secure handling Sedation needed only if fractious	Rapid loss of consciousness	Possible pain at injection site Reversible at low dosages Needs restraint
Intraperitoneal pentobarbitone	Secure handling Sedation advised, unless already unresponsive because of disease process or trauma		Time to death can be considerable, although consciousness is lost first. Pain may be associated with the injection site

Source: Keller (1982), Dennis Jr et al. (1988), Flecknell et al. (1999), AVMA (2013).

7.2.6 Euthanasia

Acceptable methods of euthanasia of rabbits are listed in Table 7.4. The best method is usually sedation if needed, followed by the injection of an overdose of pentobarbitone ($100\,mg\,kg^{-1}$) into the marginal ear, cephalic, or saphenous vein. The use of local anaesthesia at the injection site and placement of an intravenous catheter may be helpful to avoid perivascular leakage of barbiturate, with subsequent pain. In very small individuals or those with poor peripheral perfusion, buffered pentobarbitone and local anaesthetic may be injected into the abdomen (or into the heart under general anaesthesia). Rabbits find many gases aversive and stressful (Flecknell et al. 1999; Richardson and Flecknell 2006), so these should not be used in conscious animals. Neck dislocation risks severe trauma to the head and spine without causing immediate death in rabbits more than 1 kg.

7.3 Signs of Welfare Problems

7.3.1 Pathophysiological Signs

A range of blood biochemical markers thought to be affected by stress have been used, including cortisol, lactate dehydrogenase, lactate, glucose, creatine kinase, packed cell volume, osmolarity, albumin and globulin concentrations, and white blood cell counts (e.g. de la Fuente et al. 2004; Liu et al. 2012). However, it is more practical and less invasive to use faecal cortisol metabolites, which can indicate the effects of both short-term stress and long-term poor conditions (e.g. Buijs et al. 2011a; Prola et al. 2013; Scarlata et al. 2013). Noninvasive physical examinations can also identify indications of poor welfare of pet rabbits (Mullan and Main 2006; Schepers et al. 2009; Rooney et al. 2014).

7.3.2 Behavioural Signs

Acute pain may prompt behaviours such as flexing their whole body, huddling tightly, and shuffling their hind legs, while reducing the occurrence of many normal behaviours (Farnworth et al. 2011). The 'Rabbit Grimace Scale' may be applied to assess acute pain (Keating et al. 2012), although the possibility of interindividual variations mean that treatment for pain should always be considered for a rabbit expected to be in pain, even if no grimace is detected. Apathy and stereotypies such as licking or pawing objects can be used as general indicators of poor welfare (Schepers et al. 2009).

Rabbits' level of anxiety or fear, and perhaps their overall emotional state, may be indicated by their behaviour in open spaces. For example, sitting up more and moving faster may indicate a stress such as solitary housing or incompatible company (Schepers et al. 2009; Rooney et al. 2014). Similarly, anxious or stressed rabbits' may react more fearfully to novel objects or sounds (Rooney et al. 2014) or to approach, handling, or restraint by people (Boissy et al. 2007; Mullan and Main 2007; Schepers et al. 2009). In particular, the ability to induce tonic immobility when handled may be used to assess rabbits' welfare (Zucca et al. 2012; Trocino et al. 2013), but the test itself may cause fear for those rabbits undergoing it (Boissy et al. 2007).

Signs of good welfare include relaxed posture and calm resting, for example, appearing positively interested in the environment, lying fully stretched out, social behaviours, and play (Mullan and Main 2007). A specific indicator of positive emotions may be 'binkying', which involves a jumping and twisting in the air movement and appears playful in origin (Figure 7.10). Purring can suggest contentment and should be differentiated from a similar, louder noise from teeth grinding that suggests pain. Growling can indicate aggressive or sexual behaviour; 'honking' may also suggest sexual behaviour.

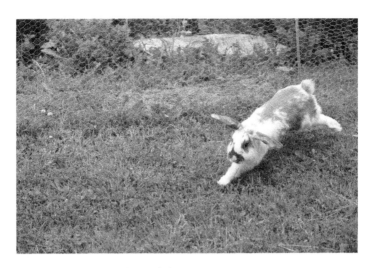

Figure 7.10 Rabbit showing 'binkying' behaviour.

Table 7.5 Most important welfare problems for pet rabbits in the United Kingdom, based on expert opinion and owner survey.

	Worst problems based on severity, duration, and numbers affected	Worst problems based on severity alone
1	Solitary living without company of other rabbits	Myxomatosis
2	Unpredictable daily routine (e.g. access to run varying with weather)	VHD
3	Lack of daily human contact for a friendly rabbit	Dental disease
4	No opportunity to dig	Living with an incompatible rabbit
5	No opportunity to graze	Fly strike

Source: Rooney et al. (2014).
VHD = Virtual haemorrhagic disease.

7.4 Worldwide Action Plan for Improving Rabbit Welfare

In terms of each problem's severity, duration, and numbers of rabbits affected, most important welfare problems probably mainly relate to poor environments and lack of company (Table 7.5). This suggests that the greatest impact is likely to occur when widespread changes are made to improve the day-to-day welfare of rabbits. Efforts should therefore be targeted at encouraging behaviour change amongst owners to ensure that all rabbits receive a varied, fibrous, and vegetation-based diet; a rich and stimulating environment; and a compatible rabbit companion. There is no information on how best to achieve this, and it probably requires a combination of owner and breeder education; strengthened legislation; and altered cultural norms, in particular to shake off traditional beliefs that the normal way to keep rabbits is alone in a hutch.

Some health problems have a shorter duration, largely because they are often acute and fatal. However, veterinary professionals need to do more to prevent infectious diseases such as myxomatosis, RHD, and *E. cuniculi*. Veterinary professional bodies in each country should encourage their memberships to reach out to rabbit owners, breeders, exhibitors, and rescue centres to advise on the correct health care, diet, and husbandry. The pet-food industry should take responsibility for ensuring that their products and advice are not contrary to animal health, working with leading clinicians and welfare scientists. Owners should be encouraged to vaccinate their rabbits (Cousquer 2013), especially for primary vaccination courses as soon as possible after owners obtain them. This also creates an opportunity to discuss other preventative healthcare issues. In some parts of the world, there may be a wider lack of veterinary education regarding vaccination, anaesthesia, and other veterinary care issues in rabbits and a lack of a suitable commercially available diets or awareness of suitable diets.

Large numbers of rabbits are abandoned or presented to rescue centres each year, for example, an estimated 67 000 rabbits in the United Kingdom (Todd and Mitchell 2012). A significant number of these are euthanised. Relinquishment may be for many reasons, for example, impulse buying (particularly around Easter in Western countries), errors in sexing paired individuals, or a desire by owners for the animals to have young. Owner education, accurate sexing, and neutering before or at sexual maturity are therefore important to help reduce the unwanted pet population.

The rabbit showing and breeding industries have a key role. They should ensure good welfare of rabbits during showing and breeding, including company and good environments. Once rabbits have reached adulthood, they may be more difficult to sell. Show breeders, commercial breeders, and pet shops may also euthanise ill, ex-breeding animals, or surplus rabbits or rehome them into the pet population directly or via pet shops, although commercial sensitivities make quantifying the numbers involved difficult. Professional breeders should also prioritise health, longevity, and temperament above show qualities such as size, shape, fur colour, and texture. All breeders should socialise breeding animals and kittens to people and other animals and familiarising them with common household or garden stimuli to ensure that in the future all rabbits have the chance of having good welfare as pets.

Bibliography

AVMA (American Veterinary Medical Association). (2013). AVMA Guidelines for the Euthanasia of Animals: 2013 Edition. Available at https://www.avma.org/KB/Policies/Pages/Euthanasia-Guidelines.aspx. Accessed 7 October 2015.

Bartrip, P.W.J. (2008). *Myxomatosis: A History of Pest Control and the Rabbit*. London: IB Taurus/Philip Wilson Publishers.

Batchelor, G.R. (1999). The laboratory rabbit. In: *The UFAW Handbook on the Care and Management of Laboratory Animals*, 7e (ed. T. Poole and P. English), 395–408. Oxford: Blackwell Science.

Bilko, A. and Altbacker, V. (2000). Regular handling early in the nursing period eliminates fear responses toward human beings in wild and domestic rabbits. *Developmental Psychobiology* 36: 78–87.

Boissy, A., Manteuffel, G., Jensen, M.B. et al. (2007). Assessment of positive emotions in animals to improve their welfare. *Physiology & Behavior* 92: 375–397.

Bradbury, A.G. and Dickens, G.J.E. (2016). Appropriate handling of pet rabbits: a literature review. *Journal of Small Animal Practice* 57 (10): 503–509.

British Rabbit Council (2014a). Breed standards. Available at http://thebritishrabbitcouncil. org/standards.htm. Accessed 24 August 2018.

British Rabbit Council (2014b). History. Available at http://thebritishrabbitcouncil.org/ history.htm. Accessed 24 August 2018.

Brown, M. and Richardson, V. (2004). *Rabbitlopaedia: a complete guide to rabbit care*. Dorking, UK: Interpet Publishing/Ringpress Books.

Buijs, S., Keeling, L.J., Rettenbacher, S. et al. (2011a). Glucocorticoid metabolites in rabbit faeces-influence of environmental enrichment and cage size. *Physiology & Behavior* 104: 469–473.

Buijs, S., Keeling, L.J., and Tuyttens, F.A.M. (2011b). Behaviour and use of space in fattening rabbits as influenced by cage size and enrichment. *Applied Animal Behaviour Science* 134: 229–238.

Buseth, M. and Saunders, R.A. (2014). *Rabbit Behaviour*. Publishing, Oxford, UK: Health and Care, CABI.

Campbell, F. (2010). *Bonding Rabbits*. Ipswich, UK: Coney Publications.

Castle, W.E. and Reed, S.C. (1936). Studies of inheritance in lop-eared rabbits. *Genetics* 21: 297–309.

Cheeke, P.R. (1987). *Rabbit Feeding and Nutrition*. Orlando: Academic Press.

Chu, L.R., Garner, J.P., and Mench, J.A. (2004). A behavioral comparison of New Zealand white rabbits (Oryctolagus cuniculus) housed individually or in pairs in conventional laboratory cages. *Applied Animal Behaviour Science* 85: 121–139.

Cope, I., Saunders, R., Crossley, D. et al. (2013). Clipping rabbits teeth. *Veterinary Record* 173: 252.

Cousquer, G. (2013). Rabbits: companion animals and arthropod Bourne diseases. *Veterinary Nursing Times*.

Cowan, D.P. (1987). Aspects of the social organisation of the European wild rabbit (Oryctolagus cuniculus). *Ethology: international journal of behavioural biology* 75 (3): 197–210.

Dennis, M.B. Jr., Dong, W.K., Weisbrod, K.A., and Elchlepp, C.A. (1988). Use of captive bolt as a method of euthanasia in larger laboratory animal species. *Laboratory Animal Science* 38 (4): 459–462.

Ducs, A., Bilko, A., and Altbaecker, V. (2009). Physical contact while handling is not necessary to reduce fearfulness in the rabbit. *Applied Animal Behaviour Science* 121: 51–54.

Dykes, L. and Flack, H. (2003). *Living with a House Rabbit*. Dorking, UK: Interpet Publishing/Ringpress Books.

Edgar, J.L. and Mullan, S.M. (2011). Knowledge and attitudes of 52 UK pet rabbit owners at the point of sale. *Veterinary Record* 168 (13): 353.

Elliott, S. and Lord, B. (2014). Breeding. In: *BSAVA Manual of Rabbit Medicine* (ed. A. Meredith and B. Lord), 36–44. Quedgely, UK: BSAVA Publications.

Emerson, J.A., Whittington, J.K., Allender, M.C., and Mitchell, M.A. (2014). Effects of ultra-violet radiation produced from artificial lights on serum 25-hydroxyvitamin D concentration in captive domestic rabbits (Oryctolagus cuniculi). *American Journal of Veterinary Research* 75 (4): 380–384. doi: 10.2460/ajvr.75.4.380.

Everitt, S. (2013). Dorsal immobility response in rabbits (appendix 4). In: *BSAVA Manual of Rabbit Surgery, Dentistry and Imaging* (ed. F. Harcourt-Brown and J. Chitty), 433. Quedgeley, UK: BSAVA Publications.

Fairham, J. and Harcourt-Brown, F.M. (1999). Preliminary investigation of the vitamin D status of pet rabbits. *Veterinary Record* 145: 452–454.

Farnworth, M.J., Walker, J.K., Schweizer, K.A. et al. (2011). Potential behavioural indicators of post-operative pain in male laboratory rabbits following abdominal surgery. *Animal Welfare* 20: 225–237.

Flecknell, P.A., Roughan, J.V., and Hedenqvist, P. (1999). Induction of anaesthesia with sevoflurane and isoflurane in the rabbit. *Laboratory Animals* 33: 41–46.

de la Fuente, J., Salazar, M.I., Ibanez, M., and de Chavarri, E.G. (2004). Effects of season and stocking density during transport on live weight and biochemical measurements of stress, dehydration and injury of rabbits at time of slaughter. *Animal Science* 78: 285–292.

Garner, M.G., Catton, M.G., Thomas, S. et al. (1998). Viral haemorrhagic disease of rabbits and human health. *Epidemiology and Infection* 121 (2): 409–418.

Gibb, J.A. (1990). The European Rabbit *Oryctolagus cuniculus*. In: *Rabbits, Hares and Pikas, Status Survey and Conservation Action Plan* (ed. J.A. Chapman and J.E.C. Flux), 116–120. Gland: International Union for Conservation of Nature and Natural Resources.

Gunn, D. and Morton, D.B. (1995). Inventory of the behaviour of New Zealand white rabbits in laboratory cages. *Applied Animal Behaviour Science* 45: 277–292.

Harcourt-Brown, F. (2002). Ophthalmic diseases. *The textbook of rabbit medicine*, 292–306. https://doi.org/10.1016/B978-075064002-2.50014-X.

Harcourt Brown, F. (2009a). Dental disease in pet rabbits. 1. Normal dentition, pathogenesis and aetiology. *In Practice* 31: 370–379.

Harcourt Brown, F. (2009b). Dental disease in pet rabbits. 2. Diagnosis and treatment. *In Practice* 31: 432–445.

Harcourt-Brown, F.M. (1996). Calcium deficiency, diet and dental disease in pet rabbits. *Veterinary Record* 139: 567–571.

Harcourt-Brown, F. (2011). Importance of water intake in rabbits. *Veterinary Record* 168: 185–186.

Hawkins, P., Hubrecht, R., Buckwell, E. et al. (2008). Refining rabbit care: A resource for those working with rabbits in research. RSPCA, West Sussex and UFAW, Hertfordshire.

Heatley, J. and Smith, A. (2004). Spontaneous neoplasms of lagomorphs. *Veterinary Clinics of North America: Exotic Animal Practice* 7: 561–577.

Held, S.D.E., Emily Blackwell, R Sanders. The science behind the housing recommendations for pairs of rabbits. RWAF Conference, Langford Vet School, Bristol, UK. 23-24 June 2018.

Huang, C., Mi, M., and Vogt, D. (1981). Mandibular prognathism in the rabbit: discrimination between single-locus and multifactoral models of inheritance. *Journal of Heredity* 72 (4): 296–298.

Isbell, C. and Pavia, A. (2009). *Rabbits for Dummies*, 2e. Indianapolis, USA: Wiley Publishing.

James, C. (2000). *The Complete House Rabbit. Kingdom Books*, 32–35. Dorking, UK: Interpet publishing.

Jekl, V. and Redrobe, S. (2013). Rabbit dental disease and calcium metabolism – the science behind divided opinions. *Journal of Small Animal Practice* 54: 481–490.

Jilge, B. (1991). The rabbit: a diurnal or nocturnal animal. *Journal of Experimental Animal Science* 34 (5-6): 170–183.

Keating, S.C.J., Thomas, A.A., Flecknell, P.A., and Leach, M.C. (2012). Evaluation of EMLA cream for preventing pain during tattooing of rabbits: changes in physiological, behavioural and facial expression responses. *PLoS One* 7 (9): e44437. doi: 10.1371/journal.pone.0044437.

Keeble, E. (2011). Encephalitizoonosis in rabbits-what we do and don't know. *In Practice* 33: 426–435.

Keller, G.L. (1982). Physical euthanasia methods. *Laboratory Animal* 11: 20–26.

Kolb, H.H. (1991). Use of burrows and movements by wild rabbits (Oryctolagus cuniculus) on an area of sand dunes. *Journal of Applied Ecology* 28: 879–891.

Lebas, F. (1980). Les recherches sur l'alimentation du lapin: Evolution au cours des 20 dernieres annees et perspectives d'avenir. *Proceedings of the 2nd World Rabbit Congress, Barcelona, Spain,* 2: 1–17.

Lindsey, J.R. and Fox, R.R. (1994). Inherited diseases and variations. In: *The Biology of the Laboratory Rabbit,* 2e (ed. P.J. Manning, D.H. Ringler and C.E. Newcomer), 293–320. London: Academic Press Limited.

Liu, H., Zhou, D., Tong, J., and Vaddella, V. (2012). Influence of chestnut tannins on welfare, carcass characteristics, meat quality, and lipid oxidation in rabbits under high ambient temperature. *Meat Science* 90: 164–169.

Lockley, R. (1974). *The Private Life of the Rabbit.* Company: MacMillan Publishing.

Lombardi, L., Fernandez, N., Moreno, S., and Villafuerte, R. (2003). Habitat-related differences in rabbit (Oryctolagus Cuniculus) abundance. *Distribution, and Activity Journal of Mammology* 84 (1): 26–36.

Magnus, E. (2005). Behaviour of the pet rabbit: what is normal and why do problems develop? *In Practice* 27 (10): 531–535.

Marai, I.F.M. and Rashwan, A.A. (2004). Rabbits behavioural response to climatic and managerial conditions – a review. *Archiv Tierzucht Dummerstorf* 47 (5): 469–482.

Marques, C. and Mathias, M.L. (2001). The diet of the European wild rabbit, Oryctolagus cuniculus (L.), on different coastal habitats of Central Portugal. *Mammalia* 65: 437–449.

Marsh, M.K., Hutchings, M.R., McLeod, S.R., and White, P.C.L. (2011). Spatial and temporal heterogeneities in the contact behaviour of rabbits. *Behavioral Ecology and Sociobiology* 65: 183–195.

Martin, G.R., Twigg, L.E., and Zampichelli, L. (2007). Seasonal changes in the diet of the European rabbit (Oryctolagus cuniculus) from three different Mediterranean habitats in south-western Australia. *Wildlife Research* 34: 25–42.

Martrenchar, A., Boilletot, E., Cotte, J.P., and Morisse, J.P. (2001). Wire-floor pens as an alternative to metallic cages in fattening rabbits: influence on some welfare traits. *Animal Welfare* 10: 153–161.

Mathis, A., Weber, R., and Deplazes, P. (2005). Zoonotic potential of the microsporidia. *Clinical Microbiology Reviews* 18: 423–445.

McBride, A. (1998). *Why Does my Rabbit....?* London: Souvenir Press.

McBride, E.A. (2013). *Rabbits and Hares.* Stansted, UK: Whittet Books Ltd.

McBride, E.A. (2014). Normal behaviour and behaviour problems. In: *BSAVA Manual of Rabbit Medicine* (ed. A. Meredith and B. Lord), 45–48. Gloucester, UK: BSAVA.

Meredith, A. (2006). Skin disease and treatment of rabbits. In: *Skin Diseases of Exotic Pets* (ed. S. Paterson), 288–311. Oxford: Blackwell Science.

Meredith, A. and Lord, B. (eds.) (2014). *BSAVA Manual of Rabbit Medicine.* UK: BSAVA: Gloucester.

Moreno, S., Villafuerte, R., Cabezas, S., and Lombardi, L. (2004). Wild rabbit restocking for predator conservation in Spain. *Biological Conservation* 118 (2): 183–193.

Mullan, S.M., 2006. A welfare assessment of pet rabbits, RCVS Diploma in Animal Welfare Science, Ethics and Law Thesis, Royal College of Veterinary Surgeons

Mullan, S.M. and Main, D.C.J. (2006). Survey of the husbandry, health and welfare of 102 pet rabbits. *Veterinary Record* 159: 103–109.

Mullan, S.M. and Main, D.C.J. (2007). Behaviour and personality of pet rabbits and their interactions with their owners. *Veterinary Record* 160: 516–520.

Myers, K. and Poole, W.E. (1961). A study of the biology of the wild rabbit, Oryctolagus cuniculus (L.), in confined populations. II. The effects of season and population increase on behaviour. *CSIRO Wildlife Research* 6 (1): 1–41.

Mykytowycz, R. and Rowley, I. (1958). Continuous observations of the activity of the wild rabbit during 24 hour periods. *CSIRO Wildlife Research* 3: 26–31.

National Research Council (NRC) (1977). *Nutrient Requirements of Rabbits*. Washington DC, USA: National Research Council.

Northern Ireland Government Website. (2013). Welfare of rabbits. Available at https://www.nidirect.gov.uk/articles/protecting-rabbits-pain-injury-and-disease. Accessed 11 July 2018.

Orr, J. and Lewin, T. (2005). *Getting Started: Clicking with your Rabbit*. Waltham, Mass USA: Sunshine Books.

van Praag, E., Maurer, A., and Saarony, T. (2010). *Skin Diseases of Rabbits*. Switzerland: MediRabbit.

Prebble, J.L. and Meredith, A.L. (2014). Food and water intake and selective feeding in rabbits on four feeding regimes. *Journal of Animal Physiology and Animal Nutrition* doi: 10.1111/jpn.12163.

Prola, L., Cornale, P., Renna, M. et al. (2013). Effect of breed, cage type, and reproductive phase on fecal corticosterone levels in doe rabbits. *Journal of Applied Animal Welfare Science* 16: 140–149.

Redrobe, S.P., Gakos, G., Elliott, S.C. et al. (2010). Comparison of Toltrazuril and sulphadimethoxine in the treatment of intestinal coccidiosis in pet rabbits. *The Veterinary Record* 167 (8): 287–290.

Richardson, C. and Flecknell, P. (2006). Routine neutering of rabbits and rodents. *In Practice* 28: 70–79.

Rooney, N.J., Blackwell, E.J., Mullan, S.M. et al. (2014). The current state of welfare, housing and husbandry of the English pet rabbit population. *BMC Research Notes* 7: 942.

RSPCA. (2013a). House rabbits. Available at www.rspca.org.uk/ImageLocator/LocateAsset?asset=document&assetId=1232734344469&mode=prd. Accessed 30 December 2016.

RSPCA. (2013b). *How to Take Care of Your Rabbits*. Horsham, UK: RSPCA.

Saunders, R. (2014). Husbandry. In: *The BSAVA Manual of Rabbit Medicine* (ed. A. Meredith and B. Lord), 13–26. Gloucester, UK: BSAVA.

Saunders, R. and Rees Davies, R. (2005). *Notes on Rabbit Internal Medicine*. Oxford: Blackwell Publishing.

Saunders, R. and Shrubsole-Cockwill, A. (2010). Vetstream Lapis: otitis externa. Available at https://www.vetstream.com/treat/lapis/freeform/otitis-externa. Accessed 24 August 2018.

Sayers, I. (2010). Approach to preventive health care and welfare in rabbits. *In Practice* 32: 190–198.

Scarlata, C.D., Elias, B.A., Godwin, J.R. et al. (2013). Influence of environmental conditions and facility on faecal glucocorticoid concentrations in captive pygmy rabbits (Brachylagus idahoensis). *Animal Welfare* 22: 357–368.

Schepers, F., Koene, P., and Beerda, B. (2009). Welfare assessment in pet rabbits. *Animal Welfare* 18: 477–485.

Seaman, S.C., Waran, N.K., Mason, G., and D'Eath, R.B. (2008). Animal economics: assessing the motivation of female laboratory rabbits to reach a platform, social contact and food. *Animal Behaviour* 75: 31–42.

Serrano, S. and Hidalgo de Trucios, S.J. (2011). Burrow types of the European wild rabbit in southwestern Spain. *Ethology Ecology & Evolution* 23: 81–90.

Slade, R. and Forbes, M. (2014). The importance of the source of fibre in the diet of the rabbit. *Veterinary Nursing Journal* 23 (3): 27–28. doi: 10.1080/17415349.2008.11013665.

Southern, H.N. (1948). Sexual and aggressive behaviour in the wild rabbit. *Behaviour* 1: 3/4.

Stodart, E. and Myers, K. (1964). A comparison of behaviour, reproduction, and mortality of wild and domestic rabbits in confined populations. *CSIRO Wildlife Research* 9: 144–159.

Swennes, A.G., Alworth, L.C., Harvey, S.B. et al. (2011). Human handling promotes compliant behavior in adult laboratory rabbits. *Journal of the American Association for Laboratory Animal Science* 50: 41–45.

Tablado, Z., Revilla, E., and Palomares, F. (2009). Breeding like rabbits: global patterns of variability and determinants of European wild rabbit reproduction. *Ecography* 32: 310–320.

Todd, R. and Mitchell, A. (2012). Survey of rabbit rescue and re-homing centres. Unpublished data.

Trocino, A., Majolini, D., Tazzoli, M. et al. (2013). Housing of growing rabbits in individual, bicellular and collective cages: fear level and behavioural patterns. *Animal* 7: 633–639.

Tschudin, A., Clauss, M., Codron, D., and Hatt, J.M. (2011). Preference of rabbits for drinking from open dishes versus nipple drinkers. *Veterinary Record* 168: 190–190.

Tynes, V.V. (2010). *Behavior of Exotic Pets*, 70. Oxford: Wiley Blackwell.

Varga, M. (2011). Hypersexuality in a castrated rabbit (Oryctolagus cuniculus). *Companion Animal* 16 (1): 48–51.

Varga, M. (2013). *Textbook of Rabbit Medicine 2nd Edition*. Oxford: Butterworth Heinemann.

Varga, M. (2014). Questions around Encephalitozoon cuniculi in rabbits. *Veterinary Record* 174: 347–348. doi: 10.1136/vr.g2494.

Verstraete, F. and Osofsky, A. (2005). Dentistry in pet rabbits. *Compendium of Continuing Education for the Practising Veterinarian* 27: 671–684.

Villafuerte, R., Calvete, C., Blanco, J.C., and Lucientes, J. (1995). Incidence of viral hemorrhagic disease in wild rabbit populations in Spain. *Mammalia* 59 (4): 651–659.

Walker-Meikle, K. (2012). *Medieval Pets*. Boydell press.

Welsh Assembly Government (2009). *Code of Practice for the Welfare of Rabbits*. Cardiff, UK: Welsh Assembly Government.

Whitman, B.D. (2004). *Domestic Rabbits & Their Histories: Breeds of the World*. Leawood, KS: Leathers Publishing.

Wild, A. (2011). Myxomatosis and Rabbits in Australia today. CSIRO Website: http://www.csiro.au/Outcomes/Safeguarding-Australia/Myxomatosis.aspx

Wolfensohn, S. (2010). Euthanasia and other fates for laboratory animals. In: *The UFAW Handbook on the Care and Management of Laboratory and Other Research Animals*, 8e (ed. R. Hubrech and J. Kirkwood), 222. Wiley-Blackwell.

Zucca, D., Redaelli, V., Marelli, S.P. et al. (2012). Effect of handling in pre-weaning rabbits. *World Rabbit Science* 20: 97–101.

Guinea Pigs, Chinchillas, and Degus (*Caviomorphs*)

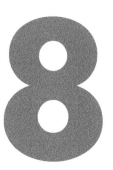

Anne McBride and Anna Meredith

8.1 History and Context

8.1.1 Natural History

Guinea pigs (*Cavia porcellus*), chinchillas (*Chinchilla* spp.), and degus (*Octodon degus*) are rodent members of the class Mammalia, order Rodentia, suborder of hystricomorphs, and parvorder of caviomorpha. They are members of the Caviidae, Chinchillidae, and Octodontidae families, respectively. All originate from the South American Andes.

Members of all three species are highly social. They use burrows and rock crevices to hide from birds and ground predators, rest, and maintain a comfortable body temperature when the outside is too hot, cold or wet. All are opportunistic herbivores and hind gut fermenters. Because of the seasonal availability of food, they are adapted to feed on a varied, high-fibre, low-quality diet of grasses, and herbs, with chinchillas also eating the fruit and leaves of some cacti. They spend the majority of their time when outside the burrow selectively foraging and feeding, which entails travelling substantial distances daily. To avoid being detected by predators, and as a result of spending

Companion Animal Care and Welfare: The UFAW Companion Animal Handbook,
First Edition. Edited by James Yeates.
© 2019 Universities Federation for Animal Welfare. Published 2019 by John Wiley & Sons Ltd.

much of the time in tunnel systems, they rely on vocalisations and scent more than visual signals.

Guinea pigs evolved in the grasslands of the lower slopes of the Andes. They are active mainly in the daytime, moving through the relatively tall grasses and creating tunnel-like runways over an estimated average area of 800m² (Asher et al. 2004). Rock crevices and burrows dug by other animals are used as resting and hiding places. They live in groups of 5 to 10 individuals, comprising several females and three or four males. They are not territorial and are generally tolerant of others, although adult males may fight when they first meet. The IUCN conservation status of the guinea pig (C. porcellus) is of Least Concern.

Chinchillas come from higher altitude, arid, rocky regions. They are active from the evening to early morning during periods of lower temperatures and dull light. Their home ranges vary from 1 to 100 ha. During the day they rest in rock crevices or simple burrows that they have dug. Group size varies in the wild from a few individuals to several hundred, depending on resource availability. The IUCN conservation status for both Short-tailed Chinchilla (Chinchilla chinchilla) and Long-tailed (Chinchilla lanigera) is Critically Endangered, with a decreasing population trend (IUCN Red List).

Degus live in harem groups of one or two males with two to four females in the semi-dry region of the Western Andes. The group cooperatively dig burrows that are used for resting, breeding, and for storage of food. They feed largely on grass, grains, seeds, and fruit. Depending on food availability, home ranges vary between 0.05 and 0.7 ha, with the average territory size estimated as 200 m² (Fulk 1976). Degus are usually active at dawn and dusk but become more active in the daytime on cool, dry days. In wet or cold weather, they may not emerge from their burrow at all but rely on food stored during the autumn. Male degus are territorial and likely to fight other males, especially during the breeding season. Victories are marked by adding to mounds built from pebbles, twigs, and dung that indicate territory boundaries. O. degus is classified as being of Least Concern, although related degu species are considered as threatened (Octodon lunatus) and vulnerable (Octodon bridgesi) (IUCN 2016).

8.1.2 Domestic History

All three species were originally kept for reasons other than as companions: the guinea pig for food, the chinchilla for fur, and the degu for laboratory use as a model for diabetes (because it is naturally unable to metabolise glucose). All are now popular laboratory and pet species. Although figures are unknown for degus and chinchillas, the UK Pet Food Manufacturers Association (PFMA 2017) estimates that 0.5 million pet guinea pigs are kept by 1% of UK households. Caviomorphs are bred and shown as 'fancy' animals. Chinchilla showing is sometimes associated with fur farming (Empress Chinchilla 2017). This breeding for appearance has led to in-breeding for a number of different coat colours and coat types (CAWC 2006). For example, the British Cavy Council (2017) list 50 breeds and the Mutation Chinchilla Breeders Association (2017) lists seven colours or 'mutations' of chinchillas.

8.2 Principles of Caviomorph Care

8.2.1 Diet

Although there are some differences in nutritional requirements, there are also significant similarities between the three species (Table 8.1). All are obligate herbivores and hind gut fermenters, adapted for a high-fibre, low-quality diet consisting of grasses and other plants, and are coprophagic. All three species have continually growing teeth that require a high degree of wear to maintain correct height and to occlude and function correctly. Acquired dental disease (overgrowth, malocclusion, tongue-trapping) is common in all three species because of low fibre intake, the feeding of sweet, sugary foods (e.g. dried fruits), and imbalances in calcium and phosphorus levels. Whilst there may be other causes such as trauma, in general, acquired dental problems can be minimised if a predominately hay based diet is fed supplemented with species-appropriate concentrates. Hereditary malocclusion may also be a primary factor in dental disease (Müller et al. 2015).

Good quality hay is therefore essential for all three species and must always be available, placed in hayracks to avoid being contaminated with faeces. However, satiety is governed more by gut fill and distension than metabolic energy need in guinea pigs (Cheeke 1987) and is likely to be similar in the chinchilla and degu. A hay-only diet is therefore insufficient and fresh leafy plants, fresh herbs, and concentrates must also be fed. Concentrate diets should be in the form of grass-based pellets or extruded nuggets. Coarse mixes are unsuitable because they allow selective feeding and are high in starch and sugars.

Table 8.1 Nutritional requirements of adult, nonbreeding caviomorphs.

Nutrient	Species	Amount required, adult
Protein	Guinea pigs	18–20%
	Chinchillas	15–20%
Fibre	Guinea pigs	12–16%
	Chinchillas	15–35%
Lipid	Guinea pigs	3–4%
	Chinchillas	2–5%
Calcium	All	0.8–1.0%
Phosphorus	All	0.4–0.7%
Calcium-to-phosphorus ratio	All	1.5–2:1
Vitamin C	Guinea pigs	10–30 mg kg^{-1} d^{-1} 200 mg kg^{-1} of diet or 200 mg l^{-1} drinking water
Water	All	100–200 mL kg^{-1}

All figures assume animals are of normal physiology, healthy, and non-breeding.
Source: Navia and Hunt (1976), Hoefer (1994), National Research Council (NRC 1995), Huerkamp et al. (1996), Keeble (2009), and Saunders (2009).

The recommended diet for guinea pigs is ad libitum grass hay and a limited amount of guinea pig pellets or extruded nuggets fed according to manufacturer's instructions, supplemented with leafy green vegetables (Cheeke 1987; Quesenberry and Carpenter 2004; Keeble 2009). Guinea pigs cannot synthesise vitamin C and their diet needs to provide adequate amounts, which can triple during pregnancy and lactation. Inadequate dietary vitamin C can rapidly cause weight loss, anorexia, reduced growth rate, stiff shuffling gait, lameness, gum haemorrhage, scaling of the pinnae, and salivation, with death ensuing within 21–28 days if it is completely absent (Harkness and Wagner 1989). This makes fresh plants especially important, and guinea pigs should be allowed daily access, ideally outdoors, to graze in suitably enclosed runs (Figure 8.1).

For pet chinchillas, the recommended diet is ad libitum good quality grass hay (e.g. Timothy) along with one or two tablespoons of commercial pellets (Quesenberry and Carpenter 2004; Johnson-Delaney 2009; Saunders 2009). Treats of approximately 1 teaspoon per day of fresh greens, fruit, root vegetables, or grains can also be offered, although items high in sugars should be avoided. The specific nutrient requirements for chinchillas are not known (Quesenberry and Carpenter 2004), but there are empirical formulas for protein and fibre (Table 8.1). Specific deficiencies in linoleic and arachidonic fatty acids are associated with flaking skin, reduced hair growth, fur loss, and

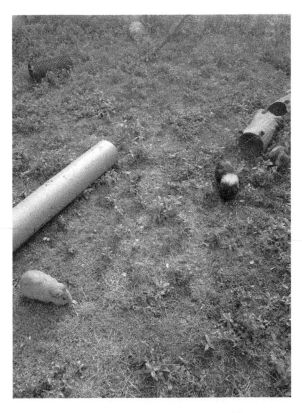

Figure 8.1 Guinea-pigs grazing in an outdoor pen with accessible cover.

cutaneous ulcers, and zinc deficiency is associated with scaling and alopecia (Hoefer 1994). Vitamin B_5 deficiency is associated with patchy alopecia, thickened scaly skin, anorexia, and hyperactivity, and a diet deficient in choline (part of the vitamin B complex), methionine (an amino acid), or vitamin E can lead to a condition known as 'yellow ears' or 'yellow fat' (Ellis and Mori 2001). Chinchillas sit on their haunches to feed and hold the food in their forepaws, and their diet must be of a suitable size and shape to allow this behaviour.

The exact dietary requirements of degus are not determined, but they may be fed in the same way as chinchillas. They are prone to type 2 diabetes, so the diet must be low in sugar and fat and high in fibre. Degus are motivated to hoard their food, and this should be permitted hygienically, with any rotting food regularly removed.

For all three species, opportunities for additional foraging, chewing, and mental stimulation also can be provided by a range of puzzle-feeders and items to chew. Caviomorphs have substantial cognitive abilities; for example, degus may use tools (Okanoya et al. 2008), and all three species are motivated to play with toys. Owners should provide some food in challenging ways to encourage active foraging behaviour and provide physical and mental exercise. Hay and greens can be stuffed into untreated paper bags or cardboard rolls. Concentrate food can be put in 'activity balls', scattered amongst the bedding (Figure 8.2), and for degu and chinchilla, can be provided in a heavy bowl covered with wire mesh whose holes are wide enough for paws and forelimbs but not heads.

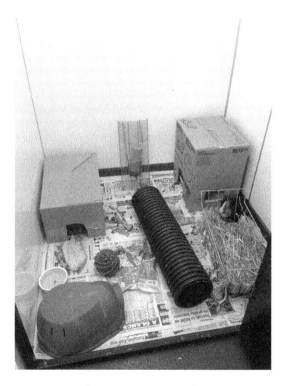

Figure 8.2 Indoor guinea-pig enclosure showing scatter feeding.

As with all cage furniture, there should be no sharp or pointed edges that could injure the animal. Commercial toys developed for rats or parrots that do not splinter when chewed are also suitable for these species. All three species can be given untreated twigs of birch, hazel, willow, beech, and apple, with their leaves removed.

All caviomorphs require ad libitum access to fresh, clean water from water bottles or no-spill water bowls. The latter should be slightly raised so that their bedding does not get damp (Figure 8.2).

8.2.2 Environment

Caviomorphs are very active, can move rapidly, with degu and chinchilla also being both agile and good climbers. All enclosures should therefore be as large as possible, including vertical space and escape-proof. All accommodation must be located so that animals remain in a comfortable ambient temperature and humidity range. All three species usually cope well with normal ambient household temperatures but cannot tolerate dampness, high heat, or bright light. Chinchillas need temperatures between 10 and 17°C with humidity less than 40% (Johnson-Delaney 2009). Degus require an environment similar to chinchillas (Keeble 2009). The ideal temperature range for guinea pigs is 16–24°C with humidity 30–70%, and guinea-pigs can therefore live outside in temperate regions if given suitable accommodation. Outside areas must be sheltered from direct sun, rain, and prevailing winds and contain a warm, dry place that is large enough for the whole group to rest comfortably. Indoor areas must be draught-proof and away from sunny windows and radiators. As low-light dwelling, prey species, all these animals are sensitive to bright lights, sudden movement, loud, or sudden sonic and ultrasonic noise. Their prime reaction to frightening and painful stimuli is to retreat at speed to a dark, small space, which means they are in danger of injury if they attempt to flee in accommodation that is of an inappropriate design or size.

Flooring should be solid and lined with suitable substrate and not be bare wire or metal. Degus and chinchillas also need access to dust baths of ground pumice stone or silver sand at least twice weekly, and more frequently if handled often. Dust should be at least 4–6 cm deep and the bath big enough to roll in (Figure 8.3). Using a box with 25 cm high sides, a covered cat litter tray, or commercially designed chinchilla sandbox can reduce sand scatter. Digging boxes should also be provided to chinchillas and degus in the form of a 1- to 2-m plastic box or fish tank, accessible via a ramp and filled with a mixture of sterilised sand (suitable for children's sandpits) and soil. Guinea pigs also use such sand and soil mixed substrate as a soft and cool resting place.

All caviomorphs need secure, comfortable resting places that are lined with suitable bedding such as hay and sufficient in number so that each individual can choose whether to be alone or with the others in their enclosure. Tiles can also provide cooler resting places. Additional hiding places, such as tubes or tunnels, should be dispersed around the accommodation, as should lookout items. If breeze blocks or bricks are used, these can also help wear down animals' nails as they walk over them. Both degu and chinchillas should also be provided with opportunities to climb and jump, including aerial pathways, ramps, raised sitting platforms, and hammocks. Degus may also use exercise wheels, which should be of solid design to avoid trapping limbs and of a suitable circumference to ensure the back is not arched. Caviomorphs should also be provided with novel objects to explore, such as cardboard boxes, sisal, and willow toys, as sold for rabbits.

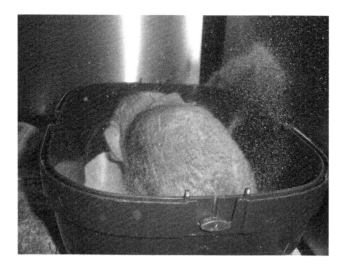

Figure 8.3   Chinchilla dustbathing.

8.2.3 Animal Company

These species all need the company of their own species. Living in social groups can provide better vigilance for predators and opportunities for play and mutual grooming, and caviomorphs are, generally, more stressed and anxious if kept alone. For both degus and guinea pigs, the best combination is one or more females and a neutered male, which mimics the natural harem society while avoiding unwanted breeding. For chinchillas, the most successful arrangement is to have a neutered male and a neutered female, although females can live together *if* they have been together since they were very young.

For all species, entire males are likely to fight on reaching maturity. Aggression to one another is also often a result of separating individuals, such as when one has been taken to the vet alone. The change in that animal's scent profile can lead to others reacting as if to an unfamiliar intruder. This can only be addressed through careful reintroduction. This should include scent swopping over a period of time before reintroduction, by rubbing a clean cloth over one animal and then over the other(s), and vice versa. It should also involve putting used bedding from each animal in the other's enclosure over a few days before reintroducing them. However, even this may not be successful. It is better to keep all group members together as much as possible, even on trips to the veterinarian (McBride 2017).

Breeding by pet owners is not recommended because of potential problems of homing offspring. Further, the male needs to be separated, if not before then immediately after the birth, to avoid the female being quickly re-inseminated and creating additional litters. However, this disruption can lead to serious fighting when the separated animal is re-introduced and may mean they have to be kept permanently apart. This is a reason for having pets neutered. If they are bred, the pups are precocial at birth and all group members take part in the rearing, so there is no need to separate pregnant females from the group. Nevertheless, they must be provided with the choice of giving birth in one of the current resting areas or in a separate box within the accommodation, with materials such as hay and shredded paper provided to make a nest.

Anatomical differences between mature male and females vary between species. Like other rodents, female caviomorphs have separate vaginal and urethral openings, with the former closed unless the female is in oestrus. Male caviomorphs do not have an obvious scrotal sac, and the testes lie in the abdomen or inguinal area but may be palpable. The male preputial orifice is round and the penis can be extruded by gentle pressure cranial to prepuce. The female guinea pig (sow) has a Y-shaped opening with V-shaped vagina forming the arms of the 'Y' and anal opening caudal to this. Both sexes of guinea pig have two inguinal nipples. In chinchillas and degus, the anogenital distance is greater in males. Female chinchillas and degus have a prominent cone shaped urogenital papilla (urethral process) that may resemble a penis.

As small prey species, these animals can attract unwanted and terrifying attention from dogs, cats, and ferrets. The odour and sound of predator species are also perceived as stressful (Apfelbach et al. 2005). Enclosures must be placed in secure places, and the animals should be outside the safety of their enclosure only in the absence of other species and have access to retreats at all times.

8.2.4 Human Interaction

Caviomorphs may find handling stressful, especially if they have had limited or negative experiences. It is not natural to be picked up and raised relatively high at speed with little or no warning, unless caught by a predator. This in itself can, therefore, trigger strong fear associations with human hands. In addition, animals may struggle and attempt to flee, and because of their small size and rapid movement, they may be easily dropped. This and their fragile bones increase the risk of injury. In chinchillas, areas of fur can also be lost (known as 'fur slip'). Fearful animals may try to avoid capture, and this can quickly progress to defensive biting when caught. Biting behaviour can lead to animals being neglected, 'effectively abandoned', rehomed, or euthanised. These risks mean that guinea pigs, chinchillas, and degus are not suitable as pets for young children.

Fear may be increased by humans approaching the enclosure in a startling and threatening manner, with quick or loud movements. Speaking softly or quietly whistling can be used to make the animals aware that someone is coming. Handling all these species should be by gentle but firm holding around the shoulders or under the thorax and supporting the animal's whole body with a hand under the rump, so the animal cannot escape or accidentally fall. Use of a thin cloth or towel to gently wrap the animal can help prevent fur slip in chinchillas. The young can be handled in a similar manner or cupped in the whole hand (Hurst and West 2010). Reward-based techniques such as clicker training can be used to train behaviours, reduce fear, provide mental stimulation, and improve the animal-human relationship. Gentle handing when young leads to more confident, less fearful adults (Figure 8.4).

8.2.5 Health

The basic measures and clinical standard of all three species are given in Tables 8.2–8.4. Caviomorphs can suffer from several diseases (Table 8.5). Poor ventilation and high ammonia levels predispose guinea pigs to respiratory disease from bacterial pathogens

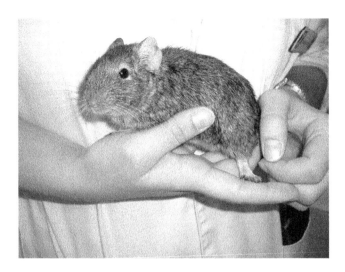

Figure 8.4 Handling of a confident, calm, and well-trained degu.

Table 8.2 Basic measures and clinical standards of guinea pigs (*Cavia porcellus*).

Parameter	Normal measures	
Life expectancy	4–7 years	
Mean weight	Males: 900–1200 g	Females: 700–900 g
Body temperature	37.2–39.5 °C	
Respiratory frequency	40–100 breaths/min	
Heart rate	230–380 beats/min	
Pubescence	Males: 90–120 days	Females: 60–90 days
Blood volume	75 mL kg^{-1}	
Haematocrit	35–45	

Source: Keeble (2009), Carpenter (2013).

Table 8.3 Basic measures and clinical standards of chinchilla (*Chinchilla* spps.)

Parameter	Normal measures	
Life expectancy	8–15 years	
Mean weight	Males: 450–600 g	Females: 550–800 g
Body temperature	36.1–37.8 °C	
Respiratory frequency	40–80 breaths/min	
Heart rate	100–150 beats/min	
Pubescence	Males: 240–540 days	Females: 240–540 days
Blood volume	70 mL kg^{-1}	
Haematocrit	27–54	

Source: Keeble (2009), Carpenter (2013).

Table 8.4 Basic measures and clinical standards of degu (*Octodon degus*).

Parameter	Normal measures	
Life expectancy	up to 10 years	
Mean weight	Males: 200–300 g	Females: 200–300 g
Body temperature	37.9 °C	
Respiratory frequency	No referenced value available	
Heart rate	No referenced value available	
Pubescence	Males: 90–180 days	Females: 90–180 days
Blood volume	70 mL kg^{-1}	
Haematocrit	No referenced value available	

Source: Keeble (2009), Carpenter (2013).

such as *Bordetella bronchiseptica*. Guinea pigs in pet stores or multipet households may also be housed with young rabbits or close to puppies that may carry the bacteria. Potential zoonoses from caviomorphs include leptospirosis, salmonellosis, yersiniosis, campylobacteriosis, monkeypox (*Orthopoxvirus*), *Trixacarus caviae* infection, and ringworm. Although transfer of zoonotic diseases from wild rodents is common, transfer from pet rodents is rare. Allergic reactions to guinea pigs are also reported.

Gastrointestinal disease is common in all three species, often linked to an inadequate diet. These species cannot vomit, and oesophageal choke can occur, frequently in association with dental disease or when animals swallow treats such as nuts or raisins whole (Saunders 2009). Bloat can occur with obstruction of the outflow from the stomach by ingested foreign bodies or rapid fermentation of food following a sudden change in diet. A lack of fibre and overfeeding of high-energy, high-protein concentrate diet may cause gastrointestinal stasis, constipation, and in severe cases, rectal prolapse. Diarrhoea is associated with the feeding of excessive amounts of fresh foods, poor-quality or mouldy foods, rapid changes in diet, or inappropriate antibiotic usage. Infectious and parasitic causes of gastrointestinal disease can occur, with young animals most susceptible (Donnelly and Brown 2004).

As their teeth grow continuously, dental disease leading to overgrowth and malocclusion is common (Jekl et al. 2008; Jekl 2009) and is a significant cause of pain and distress. Many causes are involved, including congenital defects (including conformation), diet (hypovitaminosis C, inadequate fibre, excess sugar), trauma (fractured teeth from falls, being dropped), oral abscessation, or systemic illness causing anorexia and secondary tooth overgrowth. Stress, including changes to the environment, diet, and ambient noise levels, can also alter eating habits and predispose to dental overgrowth. Clinical signs of dental disease generally include anorexia, weight loss, and salivation (Figure 8.5a–c). Guinea pigs are also prone to development of stones (uroliths) in the urinary tract, which are probably, at least partly, a result of diet and vitamin C intake.

Skin diseases such as sarcoptic mange and lice are common in guinea pigs, and ringworm can affect all species and can be spread via the dust bath in chinchillas and degus. Skin infections of the feet can occur with wire or rough flooring, obesity, or wet substrates. Fur chewing is widely reported in chinchillas (Kennedy 1952; Bowden 1962;

Table 8.5 Selected health problems in chinchillas (C), degus, and Guinea pigs (GP).

Condition			Welfare effects
Infectious or parasitic diseases	Viral	Cavian leukaemia (GP)	High mortality
	Bacterial	Pneumonia – various bacterial species esp. *Bordetella bronchiseptica* (GP)	Respiratory difficulty
		Yersiniosis (GP)	Weight loss, diarrhoea
	Fungal	Ringworm	
	Protozoal	Giardia (C)	
		Cryptosporidium wrairi (GP)	
	External parasites	Sarcoptic mange (GP) (*Trixacarus caviae*)	Severe itchiness
		Lice (GP)	
Metabolic or hormonal problems		Cystic ovarian disease (GP)	Abdominal pain
		Hyperadrenocorticism (GP)	Weight loss, urine scalding
		Diabetes mellitus	Cataracts, urine scalding
		Pregnancy toxaemia	Abortion, death
Nutritional		Hypovitaminosis C (GP)	Generalised joint and dental pain
		Dental disease	Oral pain, inability to eat
		Gastrointestinal stasis	Abdominal pain
		Urolithiasis (GP)	Dysuria; urinary obstruction
Neoplastic		Trichofolliculoma (GP)	Weight loss, debility
		Lymphoma or lymphosarcoma (GP)	
Inherited		Dental disease	Oral pain, inability to eat
Degenerative		Osteoarthritis	Pain, lameness
		Hepatic lipidosis	Depression, anorexia
		Chronic renal failure	Depression, weight loss, urine scalding
Toxic		Lead toxicity	Depression, neurological signs
Traumatic		Fur slip (C)	May affect thermoregulation if a large area is affected
		Pododermatitis	Pain, lameness

(a)   (b)

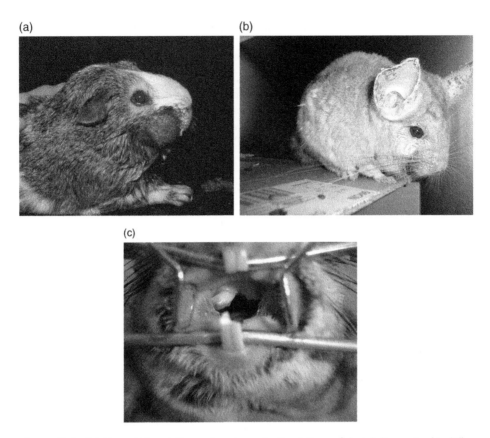

(c)

Figure 8.5   (a) Signs of dental disease in guinea-pig. (b–c) Signs of dental disease in chinchilla.

Vanjonack and Johnson 1973; Strake et al. 1996), and affected animals may have path-ological adrenal gland and skin changes consistent with hyperadrenocorticism (Tisljar et al. 2002). Fur chewing may also be seen in association with malocclusion and exces-sive salivation (Jekl 2009). Hairballs are often associated with fur chewing in chinchil-las (Donnelly and Brown 2004) and also associated with poor gut motility linked to lack of fibre. Male breeding chinchillas are prone to fur rings accumulating at the base of the penis.

There are no regular vaccination or worming programmes. However, post-purchase and annual examinations are advisable, especially in older or breeding animals, to check for dental disease and to review animals' husbandry and diet. Routine neutering is recommended for all three species to minimise the necessity for euthanasia as a result of unwanted litters (Table 8.6). Ovariohysterectomy, or more recently ovariectomy, is recommended both to prevent breeding and to prevent cystic ovarian disease in guinea pigs (Table 8.6), which is common in sows older than 1.5 years of age. If females are mated, dystocia and pregnancy toxaemia are reported in all three species, and because of the large young and the requirement for the pubic symphysis to separate widely to allow parturition, females should be mated shortly after reaching sexual maturity to minimise these potential problems.

Table 8.6 Nontherapeutic elective surgical procedures performed on guinea pigs.

Mutilation	Reasons (nonremedial) and benefits for the animal	Reasons and benefits for owners (or other humans)	Perioperative welfare risks	Welfare risks due to the behaviours prevented
Castration	May facilitate social housing		Pain; distress; anaesthetic complications	Loss of breeding and related behaviours
Spaying	Prevention of breeding and related risks Prevention of cystic ovarian disease May facilitate social housing			

Table 8.7 Methods of euthanasia for caviomorphs kept as companion animals.

Method	Restraint required	Welfare benefits	Welfare risks
Intravenous pentobarbitone	Secure handling Sedation advised when handling stressful	Rapid loss of consciousness	Possible pain at injection site Reversible at low dosages Needs restraint
Inhalation of volatile gas (e.g. isoflurane)	Placement in chamber and restraint for mask Sedation advised	Minimal handling	Aversive smell

Source: AVMA (2013) and BSAVA (2015).

8.2.6 Euthanasia

Acceptable methods of euthanasia of caviomorphs are listed in Table 8.7. The best method is usually sedation if needed, followed by the injection of an overdose of pentobarbitone (150 mg kg^{-1}) into a vein. Where restraint for intravenous injection would be stressful, or in a collapsed animal, pentobarbitone can be injected into a bone, the abdominal cavity, or heart but only after heavy sedation or anaesthesia because these methods are painful. Guinea pigs in particular may find volatile agents irritant. Neck dislocation is not recommended because it requires a high degree of skill.

8.3 Signs of Welfare Problems

8.3.1 Pathophysiological Signs

Pathophysiological signs of welfare problems are frequently linked to specific diseases (e.g. ocular and oral discharge is commonly associated with dental disease and oral pain). Excessive salivation can also be associated with heat stress, which, if severe, can also cause collapse, panting, cyanosis, and death. Decreased appetite and anorexia lead to weight loss and gastrointestinal stasis, resulting in a decrease in the number and size of faecal pellets.

8.3.2 Behavioural Signs

Caviomorphs often do not readily exhibit very clear signs of pain or stress. Stress-related behaviours and health conditions include over- or undereating, pica, over- or undergrooming, repetitive behaviours, and aggression either to other animals or humans. Animals experiencing pain may be quieter than normal, sit hunched with the limbs held tucked under the body, and stop eating. Teeth grinding is a sign of moderate to severe pain. Lack of grooming leads to an unkempt matted fur coat, which can also be an indicator of a health issue.

Although grooming one another is normal social behaviour, chewing of their own, or another's fur is an indicator of stress which may be caused by excessive or unfamiliar noise, overcrowding, excessive handling or sudden and marked changes in daily routine. For example, up to 15–20% of farmed chinchillas may show fur chewing, and it can develop in both sexes at 6 to 8 months of age (Tisjlar et al. 2002). In guinea pigs, it has also been linked to lack of dietary fibre. Another sign of stress is repetitive behaviour such as bar biting, repetitive pacing, back flipping (in chinchillas), or racing back and forth on the cage floor. These may be as a result of insufficient mental stimulation or physical space, including, for chinchillas and degus, lack of vertical height or perching platforms to enable jumping behaviour (Johnson 2006).

Caviomorphs also use a complex range of signals to communicate their emotional state and associated behavioural intentions. These include both large-scale and subtle body postures and movements; sonic and ultrasonic vocalisations, and the use of scent (Berryman 1976; Long 2007; Hunyady 2008). When relaxed, sounds denoting pleasure are of a lower frequency and volume and have been described as chirping and cooing noises. Animals in pain or fear when no escape is possible can make high-pitched, shrieking noises, and may bite. Chinchillas and degus can bark when alarmed, and the latter also drum their back feet, similar to rabbits. Aggressive behaviour to humans (Figure 8.6) or animals, particularly if it continues or if the individual changes from enjoyment or tolerance of interaction to aggression, can indicate several problems including health issues, environmental and social stressors, previous separation, changes in scent profiles, and learned responses to situations causing fear or frustration (Magnus and McBride 2019).

8.4 Worldwide Action Plan for Improving Caviomorph Welfare

Most health and welfare issues in caviomorphs are attributable to incorrect husbandry, including during early life. Prevention requires the education of all levels of commercial and fancy breeders, pet retailers, pet food and enclosure manufacturers, owners, and veterinary surgeons. The production of informed and regularly reviewed and updated guidelines and codes of practice for the various sectors regarding environmental, behavioural, dietary, and heath requirements is recommended. Owners and potential owners of these species must be made aware of their legal and moral responsibilities to animals

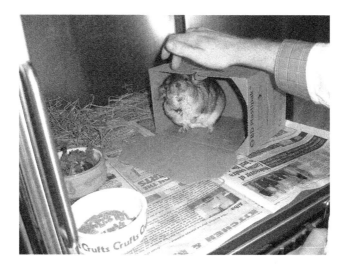

Figure 8.6 Chinchilla showing defensive behaviour against the perceived threat from the human hand.

they acquire and to ensure that they are both prepared for and can commit to these. This requires honest information to be provided to them about an animal's predicted life span and the associated costs of care, including veterinary check-ups, neutering, and treatment should an issue such as dental disease arise. Owners need to expect that, with appropriate care, these species should live for many years: 5 to 6 years for guinea-pigs, 5 to 8 for degus and 10 to 20 years for chinchillas.

There may be a public perception that these are 'cheap, easy to keep' species. Although cheaper than dogs or cats, this perception is not accurate and may be rein-forced, perpetuated, and exacerbated by the wide availability of unsuitable commercial cages, foods, and treats. This can lead to individual animals being kept by well-meaning pet owners in an inappropriate manner, potentially resulting in illness, stress, and pre-mature death. There is an urgent need to encourage cage manufacturers and suppliers of other products to take account of current welfare knowledge. All those involved in the companion animal industry need to lead by example, increase owner knowledge of these fascinating species, and thus change attitudes to stop them being thought of as 'easy to keep' or children's pets.

Understanding of the dietary and other physical needs of these species has increased dramatically through clinical research. Indeed, better understanding of their needs has improved their care in many progressive laboratory settings, leading to better research and more valuable and valid data. We are likewise becoming increasingly aware of the sentience and cognitive abilities of these animals, through both research and the expe-rience of empathetic keepers and clinical animal behaviourists. Unfortunately, to date, there is little direct research on how to meet the welfare needs of these species to underpin the clinical and experiential data. There is a need for further research into both their physiological needs and their cognitive abilities so that we can better provide for their social, environmental, and psychological welfare in all contexts, including when kept as pets.

Bibliography

Asher, M., Spinelli de Oliviera, E., and Sachser, N. (2004). Social system and spatial organization of wild Guinea pigs (Cavia aperea) in a natural population. *Journal of Mammalogy* 85 (4): 788–796.

Apfelbach, R., Blanchard, C.D., Blanchard, R.J. et al. (2005). The effects of predator odors in mammalian prey species: a review of field and laboratory studies. *Neuroscience & Biobehavioral Reviews* 29 (8): 1123–1144.

AVMA (American Veterinary Medical Association). (2013). AVMA Guidelines for the Euthanasia of Animals: 2013 Edition. Available at https://www.avma.org/KB/Policies/Pages/Euthanasia-Guidelines.aspx. Accessed 7 October 2015.

Berryman, J.C. (1976). Guinea-pig vocalisations: their structure, causation and function. *Zeitschrift fur Tierpsychologie* 41 (1): 80–106. doi: 10.1111/j.1439-0310.1976.tb00471.x.

Bowden, R.S.T. (1962). The nutrition of chinchillas – observation on pelleted diets, hay roughage, and fur chewing. *Journal of Small Animal Practice* 3: 141–149.

British Cavy Council (2017). Breeds of Cavy. Available at http://www.britishcavycouncil.org.uk/Breeds/. Accessed 26 May 2017.

BSAVA (2015). *Small Animal Formulary Part B: Exotic Pets*. Gloucester, UK: BSAVA.

Carpenter, J.W. (2013). *Exotic Animal Formulary*, 4e. Elsevier Saunders: St Louis, USA.

CAWC (2006). *Companion Animal Welfare Council Report: Welfare Aspects of Modifications, through Selective Breeding or Biotechnological Methods, to the Form, Function, or Behaviour of Companion Animals*. Cambridge, UK: Companion Animal Welfare Council.

Cheeke, P.R. (1987). Nutrition of Guinea pigs. In: *Rabbit Feeding and Nutrition* (ed. P.R. Cheeke), 344–353. Orlando, USA: Academic Press.

Donnelly, T.M. and Brown, C.J. (2004). Guinea pig and chinchilla care and husbandry. *Veterinary Clinics of North America: Exotic Animal Practice* 7 (2): 351–373.

Ellis, C. and Mori, M. (2001). Skin diseases of rodents and small exotic mammals. *Veterinary Clinics of North America: Exotic Animal Practice* 4 (2): 523–527.

Empress Chinchilla (2017). Empress Chinchilla. Available at https://empresschinchilla.org/about-us/. Accessed May 2017.

Fulk, G. (1976). Notes on the activity, reproduction, and social behavior of Octodon degus. *Journal of Mammalogy* 57 (3): 495–505.

Harkness, J.E. and Wagner, J.E. (1989). *The Biology and Medicine of Rabbits and Rodents*, 3e, 142–143. Philadelphia, USA: Lea and Febiger.

Hoefer, H.L. (1994). Chinchillas. *Veterinary Clinics of North America: Small Animal Practice* 24: 103–111.

Huerkamp, M.J., Murray, K.A., and Orosz, S.E. (1996). Guinea pigs. In: *Handbook of Rodent and Rabbit Medicine* (ed. K. Laber-Laird, M.M. Swindle and P. Flecknell), 91–149. Oxford, UK: Elsevier Science Ltd.

Hunyady H (2008). Vocal sounds of the chinchilla. MSc Thesis Bowling Green State University https://etd.ohiolink.edu/!etd.send_file%3Faccession%3Dbgsu1206318183%26disposition%3Dinline

Hurst, J.L. and West, R.S. (2010). Taming anxiety in laboratory mice. *Nature Methods* 7 (10): 825–826.

IUCN (International Union for the Conservation of Nature) (2016). The IUCN Red List of Threatened Species. Available at http://www.iucnredlist.org/. Accessed 22 August 2016.

Jekl, V. (2009). Rodents: dentistry. In: *BSAVA Manual of Rodents and Ferrets* (ed. E. Keeble and A. Meredith), 86–95. Gloucester, UK: BSAVA.

Jekl, V., Hauptman, K., and Knotek, Z. (2008). Quantitative and qualitative assessments of intraoral lesions in 180 small herbivorous mammals. *Veterinary Record* 162 (14): 442–149.

Johnson, D. (2006). Miscellaneous small mammal behaviour. In: *Exotic Pet Behaviour* (ed. T. Bradley Bays, T. Lightfoot and J. Mayer), 263–279. Saunders Elsevier: Missouri, USA.

Johnson-Delaney, C. (2009). Guinea pigs, chinchillas and degus. In: *BSAVA Manual of Exotic Pets*, 5e (ed. A. Meredith and C. Johnson-Delaney), 28–62. Gloucester, UK: BSAVA.

Keeble, E. (2009). Rodents: biology and husbandry. In: *BSAVA Manual of Rodents and Ferrets* (ed. E. Keeble and A. Meredith), 1–17. Gloucester, UK: BSAVA.

Kennedy, A.H. (1952). *Chinchilla Diseases and Ailments*. Bewdley, Ontario: Clay publishing.

Long, C. (2007). Vocalisations of the degu (Octodon degus), a social caviomorph rodent. *Bioacoustics* 16: 223–244. doi: 10.1080/09524622.2007.9753579.

Magnus, E. and McBride, E.A. (2019). Behavioural first aid: first aid advice for common behavioural signs: rabbits and rodents. In: *Companion Animal Behaviour Problems: Prevention and Management of Behaviour Problems in Veterinary Practice* (ed. R. Casey and S. Heath). Wallingford, UK: CABI.

McBride, A. (2010a). *Why Does My Rabbit....?* London, UK: Souvenir Press.

McBride, A. (2010b). *Guinea Pigs – Understanding and Caring for Your Pet*. Llandow: UK: Magnet and Steel.

McBride, A. (2014a). *Degus – Understanding and Caring for Your Pet*. Llandow, UK: Magnet and Steel.

McBride, A. (2014b). *Chinchillas – Understanding and Caring for Your Pet*. Llandow, UK: Magnet and Steel.

McBride, E.A. (2017). Small prey species' behaviour and welfare: implications for veterinary professionals. *Journal of Small Animal Practice* doi: 10.1111/jsap.12681.

Müller, J., Clauss, M., Codron, D. et al. (2015). Tooth length and incisal wear and growth in Guinea pigs (*Cavia porcellus*) fed diets of different abrasiveness. *Journal of Animal Physiology and Animal Nutrition* 99 (3): 591–604.

Mutation Chinchilla Breeders Association. (2017). Genetic information. Available at http://www.mutationchinchillas.com/genetics.htm. Accessed 26 May 2017.

National Research Council (NRC) (1995). Nutrient requirements of the guinea pig. In: *Nutrient Requirements of Laboratory Animals*, Fourth Revised Edition, 103–124. Washington DC: National Academy Press.

Navia, J.M. and Hunt, C.E. (1976). Nutrition, nutritional diseases and nutrition research applications. In: *The Biology of the Guinea Pig* (ed. J.E. Wagner and P.J. Manning), 235–267. New York NY: Academic Press.

Okanoya, K., Tokimoto, N., Kumazawa, N. et al. (2008). Tool-use training in a species of rodent: the emergence of an optimal motor strategy and functional understanding. *PLoS One* 3 (3): e1860.

PDSA (2013). Third Animal Wellbeing (PAW) report. Available at https://www.pdsa.org.uk/media/2579/paw_report_2013.pdf. Accessed 11 May 2018.

PFMA 2017 Pet Population (2017). Available at https://www.pfma.org.uk/pet-population-2017. Accessed 26 May 2017.

Quesenberry, K.E. and Carpenter, J.W. (2004). *Ferrets, Rabbits and Rodents: Clinical Medicine and Surgery*, 2e. St Louis, Missouri, USA: Saunders.

Saunders, R. (2009). Veterinary care of the chinchilla. *In Practice* 31 (6): 282–291.

Spotorno, A.E., Zuleta, C.A., Valladares, J.P. et al. (2004). Chinchilla laniger. *Mammalian Species* 758: 1–9. doi: 10.1644/758.

Strake, J.G., Davis, L.A., Laregina, M., and Boschert, K.R. (1996). Chinchillas. In: *Handbook of Rodent and Rabbit Medicine* (ed. K. Laber-Laird, M.M. Swindle and P. Flecknell), 151–181. Oxford, UK: Pergamon Elsevier Science.

Tisljar, M., Janić, D., Grabarević, Z. et al. (2002). Stress-induced cushing's syndrome in fur-chewing chinchillas. *Acta Veterinaria Hungarica* 50 (2): 133–142.

Vanjonack, W.J. and Johnson, H.D. (1973). Relationship of thyroid and adrenal function to 'fur chewing' in the chinchilla. *Comparative Biochemical Physiology* 45: 115–120.

The following websites demonstrate some of the vocalisation signals used by each species.
Degu: www.degutopia.co.uk/degusound.htm
Chinchilla: http://www.cheekychinchillas.com/chinsounds.html
http://www.chincare.com/HealthLifestyle/Chintelligence.htm#sounds
Guinea-pig: http://jackiesguineapiggies.com/guineapigsounds.html
www.guineapigcare.org.uk/language-guinea-pigs.htm

Golden Hamsters (*Mesocricetus auratus*)

Bryan Howard

9.1 History and Context

9.1 History and Context

9.1.1 Natural History

Syrian or Golden hamsters (*Mesocricetus auratus*) are rodents belonging to the class Mammalia, order Rodentia, family Cricetidae, and subfamily Cricetinae. There is a variety of other hamster species (Figure 9.1), although there is disagreement about the subdivision into genera and species (Neumann et al. 2006; Lebedev et al. 2008). This chapter is limited to *M. auratus*; other species may have different needs. Wild golden hamsters are found in a small area in the desert of Syria and Turkey (Figure 9.2), where the International Union for the Conservation of Nature (IUCN) has classified this species as 'Vulnerable' (IUCN 2013).

This habitat is dry, hot, and relatively barren. Movement during the daytime exposes the animals to potential predators and extremely high ambient temperatures. Golden hamsters therefore live in extensive and complex burrows, emerging at night or dawn and dusk to forage for their food. Conversely, temperatures may be low and food resources often scarce during winter. Hamsters therefore spend the winter in full or interrupted hibernation, triggered by short days, and low temperatures (Gumma and South 1970).

Companion Animal Care and Welfare: The UFAW Companion Animal Handbook,
First Edition. Edited by James Yeates.
© 2019 Universities Federation for Animal Welfare. Published 2019 by John Wiley & Sons Ltd.

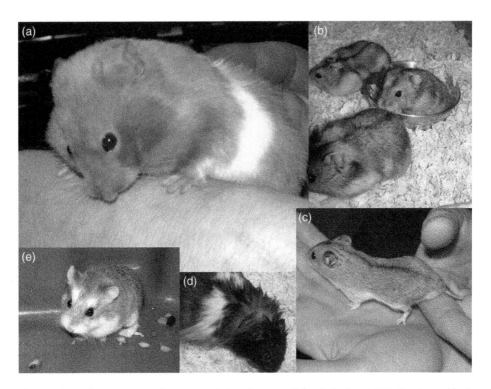

Figure 9.1 Some common hamster varieties. From top left, clockwise: (a) Syrian (or golden); (b) Russian dwarf; (c) Chinese dwarf; (d) long-haired (Syrian); (e) Roborovski.

They also hoard food in larders and have large cheek pouches for carrying food. Hamsters are also unusual amongst rodents, in that the stomach contains a keratinised pouch in which some food is fermented (Sakaguchi et al. 1987). Wild golden hamsters are largely solitary and territorial, except during mating (Murphy 1977). During the breeding season, the female may briefly allow the male into her burrow for mating. However, females may attack males during the early parts of their oestrus cycle (Takahashi and Lisk 1983). Male hamsters mark out their territory using pheromones secreted from a number of glands, principally the flank gland.

9.1.2 Domestic History

The golden hamster was first described in the eighteenth century (Russell and Russell 1797). However, there is no record of the animals being brought into captivity until 1930, when a small breeding colony of four littermates was founded. Hamsters are now commonly kept as pets and used in laboratory research. The original colony was the basis for most domestic golden hamsters (Henwood 2001; Bartlett 2003). Consequently, hamsters have lived in close contact with humans for around 90 years, during which there has been a dramatic genetic bottleneck, evidence of which can still be seen by back-crossing wild-trapped and domestic animals (Fritzsche et al. 2006). This has not prevented the formation of a large number of different breeds or types.

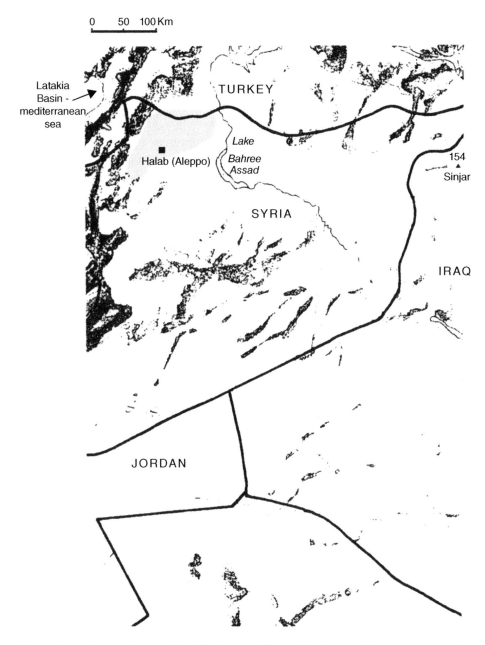

Figure 9.2 Estimated geographical distribution of the golden hamster (*Mesocricetus auratus*) in the wild. *Source:* After Gattermann et al. (2001).

9.2 Principles of Hamster Care

9.2.1 Diet

Hamsters are omnivores, with nutritional requirements as listed in Table 9.1. Commercial diets often consist of a mixture of cereals, pulses, and legumes, supplemented with minerals and vitamins, blended together and prepared as pellets. Golden hamsters can be fed standard commercial rodent pellets formulated for rats and mice. There are also unpelleted commercial hamster foods, which may often be rat or mouse diets with additions such as sunflower seeds, although the scientific rationale for these is not well evidenced.

Good quality commercial diets often have a high nutrient density, and excessive energy intake can lead to obesity, although the likelihood of this may be reduced by providing opportunity to exercise. Up to half of the dietary intake can be supplemented with titbits such as fresh fruit, green vegetables, seeds, and grains. These should first be washed and treated with a suitable dilute antiseptic solution such as sodium hypochlorite (with a chlorine activity of around 100 ppm) and rinsed, to remove any microorganisms or chemicals such as pesticides, especially for pregnant and lactating animals. Some of the food should have a hard texture to wear down their continually growing incisor teeth, and soft mashes or powders should generally be avoided because these may cause impaction of the cheek pouches.

Food can be mixed into dry clean litter to provide foraging opportunities. Hamsters frequently carry food to a 'larder' for storage. Food hoppers can be provided, but most hamsters remove food from these and transfer it to a larder of their own choosing (Sorensen et al. 2005). Allowing food to deteriorate or carelessness with hygiene may lead to diarrhoea. This makes it important for owners to ensure the bedding is not too moist, remove old food regularly, and provide food that does not rot quickly, such as dry pelleted food. Dry pellets may be especially useful to ensure that hibernating hamsters

Table 9.1 Nutritional requirements of adult, non-breeding golden hamsters.

Nutrient	Amount required, adult
Protein	15–25%[a]
Carbohydrate	35–60%
Fibre	5–12%
Lipid	4–20%
Calcium	Ca 0.6%; P 0.5%
Vitamin D	0.12 mg% (Cholecalciferol)
Water	5–15 mL/day[b]

Source: Clarke et al. (1977), Sakaguchi et al. (1987), Institute for Laboratory Animal Research (1995), and Suckow et al. (2012)
All figures assume animals are of normal physiology, healthy, and non-breeding.
[a] Declines in older ages.
[b] Depends on diet.

have food available if they wake for a short period while minimising disturbance, so long as the individual is accustomed to this food type before hibernation. There are also reports of hamsters eating caecotroph pellets, but the significance of this is also unclear.

All hamsters should receive adequate water, for example in a graduated water bottle. Constipation is generally related to ingestion of inappropriate materials such as sawdust and wood shavings or the inadequate provision of water. Again, during hibernation, it is important to ensure that hamsters have access to fresh water if they awaken.

9.2.2 Environment

Despite their rather stocky shape, hamsters are extremely active animals and should be provided with a sufficiently large enclosure to meet their needs. There is evidence that an area of $1\,m^2$ may not fully satisfy the animals' needs (Fischer et al. 2007; Figure 9.3). Enclosures should not have any gaps because hamsters are excellent escape artists or present any sharp or tight projections or angles that could cause injury or trap a hamster's digits.

Golden hamsters may choose to spend about half their time in areas where the temperature is around 26 °C, engaging in more active nest-building and food storage than at lower temperatures. Hamsters therefore appear to prefer a rather higher environmental temperature than that in which they are usually maintained, and the provision of nesting and burrowing material is also important to allow them to create a more suitable microclimate. Conversely, 80–90% of golden hamsters hibernate within about 3 weeks of being placed in an environment of 5 °C (Gumma and South 1970). If hamsters do hibernate, environmental conditions prevailing when they entered hibernation should be maintained as far as possible with minimal disturbances. High relative humidity should also be avoided because organisms that are normally commensal or of low pathogenicity may become a problem, particularly during periods of reduced metabolic

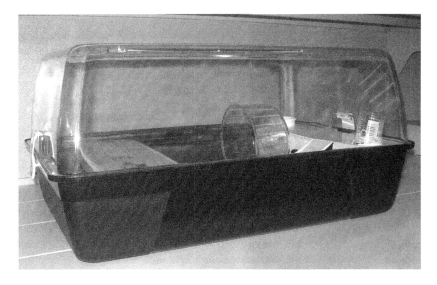

Figure 9.3 Typical cage kit sold by pet shops for housing hamsters of all breeds.

activity. Maintaining hamsters in high-humidity environments may lead to respiratory problems and skin lesions.

Golden hamsters' daily activity rhythms are strongly linked to the day-night cycle, and hamsters kept in captivity tend to show nocturnal behaviour with very little daytime activity (Gattermann et al. 2008). Each hamster should be provided with resting places that are dark and have two entrance passageways to simulate the burrows constructed in nature. Hamsters often use the roof of this as part of their living area, so it should not be slippery or unstable. Enclosures should have a solid floor covered with a deep layer of litter (Arnold and Estep 1994). The territorial instincts of the hamster are marked by pheromone deposits (Gattermann and Weinandy 1997). Removing these odours during cleaning can cause stress. This stress can be partially reduced by transferring a small amount of used litter material into the clean and freshly littered enclosure.

As well as sufficient space, pet hamsters may be given opportunities to exercise in running wheels in the enclosure, so the animal has should have free access to the wheel. Hamsters appear to be particularly motivated to use wheels, often for considerable periods of time. This may represent a stereotypy that helps them tolerate confinement (Sherwin 1998) and may reduce other abnormal behaviour such as stereotypical climbing activity and bar chewing (Gebhardt-Henrich et al. 2005). Hamsters run on wheels by extending and flexing the spine, with the fore feet providing traction and the rear feet providing propulsion. Consequently the inner surface of wheel should be sufficiently uneven to provide a grip for the feet but not so prominent as to damage the footpads, of a large enough diameter so hamsters do not need to run with their back strongly arched, strongly constructed, and well maintained (Reebs and St-Onge 2005). Poorly constructed wheels may cause abrasions or injuries to hamsters' hind feet, particularly in larger animals.

9.2.3 Animal Company

Keeping golden hamsters with other hamsters can be stressful (Lerwill and Makings 1971). Both sexes tend to be aggressive, particularly females. In one group of adult males, 40% had wounds on their bodies as a result of fighting (Arnold and Estep 1990). Golden hamsters should therefore be housed singly. Two or three littermates might be kept together after weaning if their environment is complex and positively challenging. However, hamsters may need to be separated after 4 to 12 weeks to prevent severe injuries (Gattermann and Weinandy 1997).

It is possible, although difficult, to maintain breeding pairs of golden hamsters (Suckow et al. 2012). Mating should be supervised. Because females can be aggressive and are generally larger than males (Figure 9.4), the latter are often cautious before and after copulation. When a female is sexually receptive, she will usually tolerate approaches by a male; at other times she is likely to attack him and may inflict severe injuries. The only consistent courtship behaviour by hamsters is the display of lordosis during oestrus (Figure 9.5), which appears to be a primary trigger for the male to attempt mating. The female will orient herself, generally facing away from the male, become immobile. and arch her back downward so that the abdomen almost touches the floor. Often she will stay in this position for 2 or 3 minutes and during this time the male will usually investigate her genitalia and mount her. Attempting to introduce a female hamster to a male at any other time requires careful supervision and the two

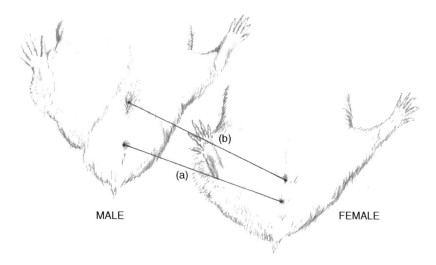

Figure 9.4 Differences between male (left) and female (right). Note the distance between rectum (above) and genital orifice (below) and the bulbous shape of the male perineum and that the mammary papillae are not always distinct.

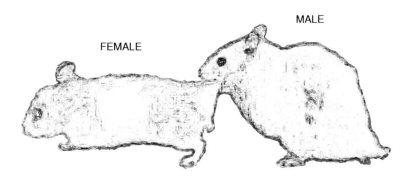

Figure 9.5 The only consistent courtship behaviour by hamsters is the display of lordosis during oestrus.

should be separated immediately if they start to fight. Imminent parturition is evidenced by the construction of a nest (Richards 1966). Male golden hamsters do not participate in rearing young. If litters are disturbed, the female may kill the young.

Hamsters should not usually be kept with other animals, including other hamster species. Pet hamsters should not be housed near potential predators such as ferrets or cats.

9.2.4 Human Interaction
Both male and female hamsters experience a degree of stress when handled (Gattermann and Weinandy 1997). In particular, handling may be stressful during their resting period (Gattermann and Weinandy 1997), such as during the daytime when owners may want

to interact. In addition, hamsters are small, active, and fragile, so they are easily injured during careless handling. Fearful hamsters may also bite their handler, causing them to be dropped. The pain and fear that such events cause may then increase hamsters' later fear of humans. However, hamsters can get used to regular gentle handling and relax sufficiently to voluntarily explore and accept food from human hands. It is, however, unlikely that they enjoy human company per se.

Hamsters can best be picked up by allowing them to come onto the hand and then cupping them in two hands. After a time, it may be possible to gently pick hamsters up by cradling them in one hand. Owners should handle hamsters more at night, or if hamsters are handled in daytime, they should be gently woken beforehand to minimise fear and reactions such as aggression. Hamsters should be allowed to undertake their typical waking routine, including stretching, yawning, and grooming (Kuhnen 2002) and to explore the surroundings before being handled. Any hamster who becomes nervous and anxious during handling should be returned to its familiar environment before any further attempts to pick it up again. Young hamsters should not be handled before they leave the nest unless completely necessary because this may lead the mother to neglect or even kill them.

9.2.5 Health

Hamsters can suffer from several diseases (Table 9.2). Naturally, they are susceptible to few infectious diseases. However, because of the considerable change in lifestyle imposed by captivity, they may develop a number of conditions resulting from imperfect husbandry. In the United States in 1975, the commonest illness appeared to be a type of enteric disorder often collectively called 'wet tail' (Renshaw and others 1975), and this still appears to be the case. This can be highly infectious and can cause severe diarrhoea, with soiling of the perineum and ventral abdomen. The microorganisms involved are uncertain, and although *Escherichia coli* and *Lawsonia intracellularis* have been implicated, the cause is probably multifactorial. Careful hygiene and prompt veterinary treatment is essential. Hamsters can also occasionally harbour infections that they can pass to humans, including salmonellosis, leptospirosis, hantavirus, rat bite fever, and lymphocytic choriomeningitis virus (Health Protection Agency 2013). These infections may have serious consequences for humans and may be acquired by hamsters through contact with wild rodents.

Abscesses often arise from infected bite wounds or other injuries sustained during fighting and appear as firm, painful lumps under the skin. Abscesses affecting the cheek pouch can arise from abrasions by harsh foods or bedding materials. Cancers, such as those of the female reproductive tract, can occur spontaneously and are more common in older animals. They are frequently benign, although if they affect hormone-producing organs such as the thyroid or adrenal glands, the resulting hormone imbalance can cause secondary effects such as hair loss and behavioural changes.

Routine check-up visits to the vet are probably inadvisable, unless there is a recurring problem that needs regular attention such as dental overgrowth because of the stresses of transport and the unfamiliar environment of the veterinary surgery. There are also no generally available vaccines for diseases of hamsters. However, if a hamster does develop a problem, then veterinary advice should be sought. Owners should not treat animals with unprescribed antibiotics, several of which can be fatal – for example

Table 9.2 Selected health problems in golden hamsters.

Condition			Welfare effects
Infectious or parasitic diseases	Viral	Lymphocytic Choriomeningitis*	Usually no symptoms
		Sendai virus; pneumonia virus of mice (PVM)	Generally no symptoms
		Hamster polyomavirus	Multicentric lymphoma in the organs of young animals or skin of adults
	Bacterial	Wet tail (*Escherichia coli* or *Lawsonia intracellularis*)	Severe dehydration, depression, not eating
		Salmonellosis*	Fever, lethargy, sometimes diarrhoea
		Tyzzer's disease	May cause severe diarrhoea and dehydration in weanling animals
		Pseudotuberculosis*	Weight loss and diarrhoea
		Pasteurella pneumotropica	Acute onset eye or nose discharge, not eating, and difficulty breathing
	Fungal	Ringworm*	Scaly red patches on skin – may itch if infected.
		Aspergillosis	Lethargy, difficulty breathing, blood in the urine, diarrhoea
	Protozoal	*Giardia muris, Spironucleus muris*	Usually no symptoms; wasting if severe
	Internal parasites	Cestodes. *Hymenolepis nana**	Mild to severe diarrhoea and loss of body condition
	External parasites	Demodectic mange	Hair-loss; dry, scaly skin
		Sarcoptic mange	Hair-loss; intense itchiness.
Metabolic or hormonal		Amyloidosis	Fluid in tissues or abdomen
Inflammatory		Age-related glomerulonephropathy	Progressive loss of body condition in older animals

(*Continued*)

Table 9.2   (Continued)

Condition		Welfare effects
Neoplastic	Adrenal cortical adenoma	Weight loss, lethargy, hair-loss
	Lymphosarcoma	Depression, dullness, loss of appetite
Inherited	Cardiomyopathy	Lethargy, difficulty breathing
Degenerative	Dental overgrowth	Difficulty eating
	Cholangiofibrosis	Older hamsters – unthriftiness and weight loss
Toxic	Inappropriate antibiotic administration	Acute dullness, diarrhoea, low temperature
Traumatic	infected bite wounds	Dullness, pain, loss of appetite

* Indicates that the condition is caused by an infection that can be passed on to humans (i.e., is a zoonosis).

ampicillin, penicillin, erythromycin, lincomycin, and streptomycin. Many hamsters object to having their teeth examined, although it is usually possible to check that the incisors are intact and that their surfaces meet. Dental problems may require intervention to improve the length and shape of the incisors. Otherwise, nontherapeutic surgery is rarely performed, with the occasional exception of vasectomy in males to prevent paired hamsters from mating, although an alternative is to keep the day length short (Morin and Zucker 1978).

9.2.6 Euthanasia
Acceptable methods of euthanasia of hamsters are listed in Table 9.3. The best method is usually the injection of an overdose of anaesthetic (such as ketamine or medetomidine) into the abdomen, followed by a method to ensure death. Injecting pentobarbitone into the abdomen or muscle can cause pain even if mixed with local anaesthetics and should only be used in anaesthetised animals. Cervical dislocation is difficult in hamsters and can cause considerable distress if inexpertly conducted, so should only be used as a last resort in emergencies. High concentrations of carbon dioxide gas appear to be highly stressful, particularly if the gas is of industrial quality which might contain contaminants.

9.3 Signs of Hamster Welfare

9.3.1 Pathophysiological Signs
Many signs are best observed from unobtrusive checks without handling. Sometimes evidence of illness may be observed in the hamster's surroundings – for example traces of blood in the litter material may indicate injury (e.g. if found in the vicinity of a

Table 9.3 Methods of euthanasia for hamsters kept as companion animals.

Method	Restraint required	Welfare benefits	Welfare risks
Intra-abdominal injection of a high dose of an anaesthetic agent	Secure handling or anaesthesia	Minimal handling	Possible pain at injection site
Intravenous injection of pentobarbitone	Secure handling or anaesthesia	Rapid loss of consciousness	Difficult to access a suitable vein and possible pain at injection site.
Inhalation of volatile anaesthesia	Placement in chamber Sedation not advised, as would involve more handling	Minimal handling	Possibly unpleasant smell

Source: AVMA (2013).

running wheel or the metal spout of a drinker) or medical problem (e.g. if associated with faeces or urine). Similarly, deposits of wet faecal material in the litter or on the walls of the hamster's enclosure may indicate an intestinal disorder. Normal hamster urine is thick and yellowish with a pH 8 and should not be mistaken for pus. Breathing is best assessed before a hamster is handled, including any changes in the pattern and depth or wheezing, which may indicate an underlying respiratory (or possibly cardiovascular) problem. Even occasional sneezing or coughing is abnormal unless there is an obvious one-off trigger.

Other pathophysiological signs are detected by handling of the animal. Failure to eat or drink can be indicated by a rapid loss of condition and dehydration because of their small body mass and high metabolic rate. This may appear as weight loss, changes in facial features such as dull or sunken eyes or prominent bony areas such as the spine and pelvis (which may be difficult to spot in long-haired hamsters). Food within the cheek pouches, which can cause considerable distortion of the side of the face and neck, does not reliably indicate eating because sick hamsters may stop eating but continue to hoard food. An increase in body weight may indicate normal growth of young animals, pregnancy, or underlying health problems such as inactivity, changes in metabolism, or neoplasia.

Eye protrusion may be a consequence of an underlying tumour, haemorrhage, or physical injury. Reddening of the sclera or discharge from the conjunctiva, which may appear as moist staining or a dried crusty area at the canthus of the eye or adherence of the eyelids, may indicate ocular damage or infection. A coat that is dull, uneven, coarse, or soiled may indicate reduced grooming. The presence of whitish-grey scaly deposits in the hairs may indicate infection by parasites and often accompanies depressed grooming activity. Soiling of the perineal area by wet faeces may be indicative of diarrhoea. A wound may indicate self-inflicted injuries consequent to it gnawing at a painful area; unsafe defects in the animal's enclosure walls or furniture; or fighting. Abnormal swellings may indicate abscesses, especially if there is evidence of penetration from the skin;

Table 9.4 Basic measures and clinical standards of the golden hamster (*Mesocricetus auratus*).

Parameter	Normal measures
Life expectancy	Mean about 2 years; Roborovski hamsters usually longer – about 3 years
Mean weight	Fully grown (6 m old) golden hamster 120–200 g; less if fed a controlled diet. Chinese, Russian dwarf and Siberian hamsters about 50 g.
Body temperature	37–38 °C
Respiratory frequency	40–130 breaths/min
Heart rate	280–500 beats/min
Pubescence	40–55 days
Blood volume	6.8–12 mL (6.5–8.0% of body mass)
Haematocrit	35–60

Source: Beynon and Cooper (1991), Field and Sibold (1998), Aiello and Moses (2016), Mitchell and Tully (2009), Suckow et al. (2012), Whittaker (2010).

an underlying disease such as cancer; normal swelling of the mammary glands before parturition; or the presence of stored materials in the cheek pouches.

Body temperature and oximetry may be useful for assessing stress (Gattermann and Weinandy 1997), although the former should be measured only by a veterinary surgeon, using a special thermocouple or high-performance noncontact thermometer. Blood samples taken for biochemical assessment can also indicate specific problems. Key measures of normal golden hamsters are given in Table 9.4.

9.3.2 Behavioural Signs

Some behavioural signs include changes in an individual hamster's normal daily routine or general temperament, such as altered grooming, use of furniture, or exploration. Other early signs of impaired welfare include changes in food and water intake, or where hamsters are given a mixed diet, a change in preference for particular foodstuffs. Ill hamsters may hide themselves more as an inherent response to the fear of predation. When concealment is impossible, they may become irritable and are more inclined to bite. If they are sharing an enclosure with other hamsters, there may also be a change in the social hierarchy or increased aggression.

However, inactivity during the day, when owners are more likely to observe them, is normal. Owners should observe their hamster at dawn or dusk. They may also hear changes in nighttime running-wheel activity. Alternatively, it is possible to attach a revolution counter to the wheel to accurately log the number of rotations. Decreased use may indicate lethargy; increased use may suggest the hamster is attempting to cope with a welfare problem. Repetitive bar biting may also indicate current or previous stress. Early detection of abnormal behaviour is also particularly difficult when days shorten and temperatures drop, and hamsters enter torpor or hibernation.

Very ill hamsters may be reluctant to move about the enclosure and when forced to move, their gait is often slow, unsteady, and stiff. A hunched back may suggest abdominal pain, as an attempt to relieve pressure on the abdominal organs. Altered movement may suggest limb pain, and it is usually possible to determine whether the source of pain is high in the limb or lower down, depending on the way that the animal moves, although drawing this distinction is complicated by hamsters' rather shuffling normal gait and relatively light body mass.

9.4 Action Plan for Improving Golden Hamster Welfare Worldwide

Although there is a considerable amount of anecdotal information about keeping pet hamsters, the advice offered to novices is often ambiguous or conflicting. The principal hamster interest groups should collaborate in the establishment of an open database for best practices for hamster owners, commercial interests, and veterinarians. For example, this could be a forum, with postings reviewed by an expert panel to build up an overall picture of successful care strategies. Website users could report their experiences of the recommended strategies, and modifications could be introduced to ensure the development of best practices. Such a forum could also foster debate about ethical issues such as castrating male hamsters to facilitate communal housing.

Additional scientific research is needed to improve our understanding of the basic biology of hamsters and of the interrelationship among husbandry, stress, and hamsters' behaviour. For example, studies could investigate the biological and psychological consequences of handling hamsters during the time when they would normally be sleeping. There also remains considerable uncertainty about the underlying motivation and the potential benefits of wheel running. If it were to be established that this running activity is a stereotypy, then strategies need to be developed to minimise the stress which the activity reveals. Scientific findings should inform laws, and legislative bodies such as the European Commission should press for common legal protections similar to or higher than the UK's Animal Welfare Act 2006.

Finally, the recent evolution of *Mesocricetus* species suggests that their genome is quite amenable to change (Neumann et al. 2006), and breeders should be encouraged to breed strains of hamster free of harmful genetic traits and tolerant of handling, company, and the variations in day length commonly associated with sharing domestic life with a human family.

Bibliography

Aiello, S.E. and Moses, M.A. (2016). *Merck Veterinary Manual*, 11e. Kenilworth, NJ: Merck. & Co.

Arnold, C.E. and Estep, D.Q. (1990). Effects of housing on social preference and behavior in male golden-hamsters (*Mesocriccius auratus*). *Applied Animal Behaviour Science* 27: 253–261.

Arnold, C.E. and Estep, D.Q. (1994). Laboratory caging preferences in golden hamsters (*Mesocricetus auratus*). *Laboratory Animals* 28: 232–238.

AVMA (American Veterinary Medical Association). (2013). AVMA Guidelines for the Euthanasia of Animals: 2013 Edition. Available at https://www.avma.org/KB/Policies/Pages/Euthanasia-Guidelines.aspx. Accessed 7 October 2015.

Bartlett, P.P. (2003). *The Hamster Handbook*. Hauppauge, US: Barron's Educational Series Inc.

Beynon, P.H. and Cooper, J.E. (1991). *Manual of Exotic Pets*. Cheltenham, UK: British Small Animal Veterinary Association.

Clarke, H.E., M Coates, E., Eva, J.K. et al. (1977). Dietary standards for laboratory animals: report of the laboratory animals Centre diets advisory committee. *Laboratory Animals* 11: 1–28.

Field, K.J. and Sibold, A.L. (1998). *The Laboratory Hamster and Gerbil*. Boca Raton, FL: CRC Press.

Fischer, K., Gebhardt-Henrich, S.G., and Steigert, A. (2007). Behaviour of golden hamsters (*Mesocricetus auratus*) kept in four different cage sizes. *Animal Welfare* 16: 85–93.

Fritzsche, P., Neumann, K., Nasdal, K., and Gattermann, R. (2006). Differences in reproductive success between laboratory and wild-derived golden hamsters (*Mesocricetus auratus*) as a consequence of inbreeding. *Behavioral Ecology and Sociobiology* 60: 220–226.

Gattermann, R. and Weinandy, R. (1997). Time of day and stress response to different stressors in experimental animals. Part I: Golden hamster (*Mesocricetus auratus* Waterhouse, 1839). *Journal of Experimental Animal Science* 38: 66–76.

Gattermann, R., Johnston, R.E., Yigit, N. et al. (2008). Golden hamsters are nocturnal in captivity but diurnal in nature. *Biology Letters* 4: 253–255.

Gattermann, R., Fritzscho, P., Neumann, K. et al. (2001). Notes on the current distribution and the ecology of wild golden hamsters *(Mesocricetus auratus)*. *Journal of Zoology* 254: 359–365.

Gebhardt-Henrich, S.G., Vonlanthen, E.M., and Steiger, A. (2005). How does the running wheel affect the behaviour and reproduction of golden hamsters kept as pets? *Applied Animal Behaviour Science* 95: 199–203.

Gumma, M.R. and South, F.E. (1970). Hypothermia and behavioural thermoregulation by the hamster (*Mesocricetus auratus*). *Animal Behaviour* 18: 504–511.

Health Protection Agency (2013). Reducing the risk of human infection from pet rodents. Available at http://webarchive.nationalarchives.gov.uk/20140714084352/www.hpa.org. uk/webc/HPAwebFile/HPAweb_C/1317138246716. Accessed 20 June 2016.

Henwood, C. (2001) The Discovery of the Syrian (Golden) Hamster, *Mesocricetus auratus*. *The Journal of the British Hamster Association* (39) [Online], Available at http://www. britishhamsterassociation.org.uk/get_article.php?fname=journal/discover_syrian.html. Accessed 24 July 2013.

Institute for Laboratory Animal Research (1995). *Nutrient Requirements of Laboratory Animals*, Fourth Revised Edition. Washington DC: The National Academies Press.

IUCN (2013). Red List of threatened species, [Online], Available at http://www.iucnredlist. org/details/13219/0. Accessed 23 July 2013.

Kuhnen, G. (2002). Comfortable quarters for hamsters in research institutions. In: *Comfortable Quarters for Laboratory Animals*, 9e (ed. V. Reinhardt and A. Reinhardt), 33–37. Washington, DC: Animal Welfare Institute Washington.

Lebedev, V.S., Bannikova, A.A., and Surov, A.V. (2008). Systematics of striped hamsters (*Cricetulus barabensis* group) from morphological and genetic viewpoints. In: *Cricetinae*, vol. 64 (5) (ed. E. Peschke and G. Moritz), 69–76. Leipzig: Abhandlungen der Stichsischen Akademie der Wissenschaften.

Lerwill, C.J. and Makings, P. (1971). The agonistic behaviour of the golden hamster *Mesocricetus auratus* (Waterhouse). *Animal Behaviour* 19: 714–721.

Mitchell, M.A. and Tully, T.N. Jr. (2009). *Manual of Exotic Pet Practice*. Philadelphia, PA: Saunders.

Morin, L.P. and Zucker, I. (1978). Photoperiodic regulation of copulatory behaviour in the male hamster. *The Journal of Endocrinology* 77: 249–258.

Murphy, M.R. (1977). Intraspecific sexual preferences of female hamsters. *Journal of Comparative and Physiological Psychology* 91: 1337–1346.

Neumann, K., Michaux, J., Lebedev, V. et al. (2006). Molecular phylogeny of the Cricetinae subfamily based on the mitochondrial cytochrome b and 12S rRNA genes and the nuclear vWF gene. *Molecular Phylogenetics and Evolution* 39: 135–148.

Reebs, S.G. and St-Onge, P. (2005). Running wheel choice by Syrian hamsters. *Laboratory Animals* 39: 442–451.

Renshaw, H.W., Van Hoosier, G.L. Jr., and Amend, N.K. (1975). A survey of naturally occurring diseases of the Syrian hamster. *Laboratory Animals* 9: 179–191.

Richards, M.P.M. (1966). Activity measured by running wheels and observation during the oestrous cycle, pregnancy and pseudopregnancy in the golden hamster. *Animal Behaviour* 14: 303–309.

RSPCA. (2016). Companion animals pet care. Available at https://www.rspca.org.uk/adviceandwelfare/pets/rodents/hamsters. Accessed 9 September 2018.

Russell, A. and Russell, P. (1797). *The Natural History of Aleppo*, 2nd edition. A. Millar, London.

Sakaguchi, E., Itoh, H., Uchida, S., and Horigome, T. (1987). Comparison of fibre digestion and digesta retention time between rabbits, Guinea-pigs, rats and hamsters. *British Journal of Nutrition* 58: 149–158.

Sherwin, C. (1998). Voluntary wheel running: a review and novel interpretation. *Animal Behaviour* 56: 11–27.

Sorensen, D.B.T., Krohn Hansen, H.N., Ottesen, J.L., and Hansen, A.K. (2005). An ethological approach to housing requirements of golden hamsters, Mongolian gerbils and fat sand rats in the laboratory – a review. *Applied Animal Behaviour Science* 94: 181–195.

Suckow, M.A., Stevens, K.A., and Wilson, R.P. (eds.) (2012). *The Laboratory Rabbit, Guinea Pig, Hamster, and Other Rodents*. London, UK: Academic Press, Elsevier.

Takahashi, L.K. and Lisk, R.D. (1983). Organization and expression f agonistic and socio-sexual behaviour in golden hamsters over the estrous cycle and after ovariectomy. *Physiology and Behaviour* 31: 477–482.

Whittaker, D. (1999). The Syrian hamster. In: *The UFAW Handbook on the Care and Management of Laboratory Animals*, (eds. R. Hubrecht and J. Kirkwood), 348–358. Wiley-Blackwell.

Mongolian Gerbils (*Meriones unguiculatus*)

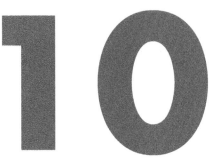

Elke Scheibler and Eva Waiblinger

10.1 History and Context

10.1.1 Natural History

Mongolian gerbils or jirds (*Meriones unguiculatus*) are rodent members of the class Mammalia, order Rodentia, and family Muridae. There are a variety of other gerbil species, including those in the genera *Gerbillus*, *Meriones*, *Rhombomys*, *Pachyuromys*, *Psammomys*, *Tatera*, and *Taterillus* (Chevret and Dobigny 2005). This chapter is limited to *M. unguiculatus*; other species, even within the same genus, may have different needs.

Wild Mongolian gerbils originate in the central Asian semi-deserts and steppes of Mongolia, inner Mongolia, and southern Siberia. These are arid regions with hot summers and very cold winters. Wild gerbils' usual habitats have short, sparse vegetation and dry, loose and sandy soil. Their diet consists of the green parts of plants and seeds, for example, of grasses and wormwood (*Artemisia* sp.). Occasionally insects or larvae are consumed as a source of water and protein (Bannikov 1954; Gulotta 1971; Agren et al. 1989a, 1989b). Gerbils hoard food extensively in their burrows. These are self-dug and widely branched (Figure 10.1) with depths of up to 1.2 m (Bannikov 1954; Naumov and

Companion Animal Care and Welfare: The UFAW Companion Animal Handbook,
First Edition. Edited by James Yeates.

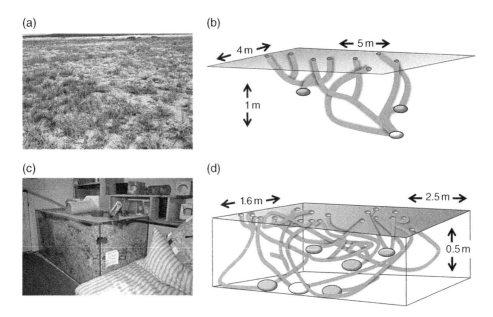

Figure 10.1   Gerbil burrows: (a) Gerbil burrow in Mongolia from above ground; (b) Wild gerbil burrow layout; (c) Pet gerbil housing in 120×50×50 cm terrarium; (d) Pet gerbil burrow layout in 160×150×50 cm terrarium. Grey circles indicate food store chambers and white ones indicate nest chamber.

Lobachev 1975; Scheibler et al. 2006b). Burrows are not only crucial for food storage and protecting the individual against predators and climate extremes. They also allow to raise the young in relative safety (Scheibler et al. 2006; Liu et al. 2007). In the wild, a burrowless gerbil is soon a dead gerbil.

Gerbils live in extended, territorial family groups of 2 to 17 animals comprised of one breeding pair and their offspring of several generations (Agren et al. 1989a, 1989b). Pups are naturally weaned when the next litter is born but remain with the family after puberty at 7 to 8 weeks of age (McManus 1972b). Only the dominant pair reproduces because the adult offspring are sexually suppressed by the presence of parents and siblings (Salo and French 1989; Clark and Galef 2001, 2002; Saltzman et al. 2006). They participate in digging the communal burrow, hoarding food, territorial defence, pup care, and vigilance for predators (Ostermeyer and Elwood 1984). This social organisation allows both sexes to acquire essential parental skills (French 1994). Natural emigration starts with the commencement of reproductive activity, which might be much later than 12–14 weeks.

10.1.2 Domestic History

Gerbils were first bred and used as laboratory animals. In 1935, the first breeding stock was established in Japan from animals caught in the Amur region (Rich 1968). In the 1960s, gerbils were first exported to the United States, later to Europe and around this time also found their way into the pet market. It has to be assumed that most pet gerbils today are descendants of this original laboratory stock.

Despite the short domestication period, there are pronounced differences between wild and captive-bred gerbils (Price 2002; Stuermer et al. 2003). Laboratory and pet gerbils show a lower brain weight, shorter intestine, and bigger litters of an average 5.6 pups in laboratory gerbils compared to 4 in wild gerbils (Norris and Adams 1982; Stuermer et al. 2003). There are several colour mutations from the original agouti. 'Black' and 'Spotted' pet gerbils appeared in the 1970s (Waring et al. 1978), and a wide variety of coat colours has since emerged. However, basic needs remain the same in all gerbils, in particular for intensive digging, a burrow, social contact, gnawing, and foraging activities.

10.2 Principles of Gerbil Care

10.2.1 Diet

Gerbils are omnivores, with nutritional maintenance requirements as listed in Table 10.1. For pet gerbils, these may be best met by commercial mouse or rat foods, so long as the protein content ranges between 16 and 20%, and fat content should be less than 5% to prevent the development of metabolic syndrome and obesity, which in turn compromise immune function (McManus 1972a; GV SOLAS 2009; Xu et al. 2011).

Food should be presented ad libitum as gerbils eat about 18 times during the day at random times, and time restrictions can impair growth in juveniles (Mulder et al. 2010). Food should be sprinkled in the bedding or mixed into fresh sand baths, allowing the gerbils to search for food and perform species-typical hoarding, which are rewarding occupations (Forkman 1993; Yang et al. 2011). Gerbils hoard food extensively (Roper and Polioudakis 1977), constructing food chambers in their burrows. Some of these contain dry food; others contain germinated grains (Brunner 1993). Substrates for burrowing should permit this behaviour.

Because gerbils are rodents with constantly growing incisors, they must be provided with nonpoisonous materials to gnaw and chew daily to wear down their teeth sufficiently. Examples include hay, straw, tissues, paper, cardboard, wood sticks and branches

Table 10.1 Nutritional requirements of adult, nonbreeding Mongolian gerbils.

Nutrient	Amount required, adult
Protein	16–20%
Carbohydrate	Unknown
Fibre	Unknown
Lipid	2–5% (or 1–2% if providing sufficient amounts of particular forms of omega 6 fatty acids)
Myo-Inositol	Males: If diet fat content is $2\,g\,kg^{-1}$ diet, no addition required Females: Generally $>20\,mg\,kg^{-1}$ diet, but if diet contains 20% saturated fat: $70\,mg\,kg^{-1}$ diet
Water	4–8 mL per 100 g body weight per day

All figures assume animals are of normal physiology, healthy, and non-breeding.
Source: Farm (1975), NRC (1995), and Field and Sibold (1999).

of hazel (*Corylus avellana*), beech (*Fagus* spp.), hornbeam (*Carpinus betulus*), and unsprayed fruit trees such as apple or pear (e.g. *Malus* spp. and *Pyrus* spp.). These also provide a necessary behavioural enrichment as gerbils are motivated to shred branches and cardboard.

As adaptations to dry climates, gerbils consume only 4–10 mL of water per day, excreting small amounts of urine (3–4 mL day^{-1}) and producing dry faecal pellets (Arringto and Ammerman 1969; McManus 1972a). Nevertheless, water-deprived gerbils may die, depending on the composition of their food (Thiessen and Yahr 1977). Ad libitum clean water should therefore always be provided via bottles or bowls. Additional water is provided by juicy greens, fruit, and vegetables such as dandelion leaves, cucumber, carrots, pumpkin, zucchini, fennel, apples, pears, or melon. However, excess provision can cause diarrhoea or can rot in the food chamber of the gerbils' burrows.

10.2.2 Environment

Gerbils should be kept in solid-sided 'terrariums' (from the Latin for earth) made of gnaw-resistant glass, metal, or plexiglass and covered with an escape-proof wire cover to allow for air circulation. Floorspace should be a minimum of 0.5 m² for two to five animals and 25 cm substrate depth (TSchV 2008). The terrarium's height should be at least 15 cm higher than the surface of the substrate so the animals can rear on their hind legs in their typical vigilance behaviour on top of the substrate. This requires a height of at least 55, preferably up to 135 cm. However, stability of the substrate and ventilation need to be considered. Smaller containers do not allow the gerbils to construct species-typical burrows and should therefore be avoided, whereas even bigger containers allow for more complex burrow construction and are recommended. There are no scientific indications that intragroup aggression is more pronounced in bigger terrariums.

Gerbils' optimal ambient temperature is between 20 and 24 °C. Juveniles are less temperature tolerant (19–24 °C) than adults (18–29 °C), and pups are unable to thermoregulate before the age of 12 days. Gerbils can tolerate a wider range of climatic temperatures as long as they can retreat underground into their burrows and can build insulated nests, humidity is low, and food is available ad libitum (Li et al. 2001). All pet gerbils should therefore be allowed to dig a burrow. However, commercially available beddings such as wood shavings have different insulating properties than soil. Pet gerbils given deep substrate can therefore compensate for lower temperatures but not higher ones (>30 °C). Because gerbils are motivated to sun themselves, terrariums should also offer both sunny and shady areas.

The ability to dig and inhabit a burrow is probably the most important resource for pet gerbils. It allows thermoregulation, security, and the storage of food. If gerbils are bred without a burrow, stereotypic digging can take up more than 22% of their active time (Wiedenmayer 1997a), although no adverse health effects from this behavioural abnormality have been observed so far and it is unknown whether stereotypic digging itself causes suffering (Würbel 2006). Gerbils should grow up in a burrow constructed by their parents in deep substrate or an adequate artificial burrow structure containing a dark nest box and a 20-cm access tunnel. This may also reduce stereotypic digging even in adult gerbils with an already fixed digging stereotypy. However, all pet gerbils should be provided with a deep layer of substrate to dig, maintain, and enlarge their own burrow. Depths of at least 40 cm are advisable. Substrates need to be absorbent, loose enough for digging, but still stable enough for constructing burrows, for example, wood shaving substrate mixed with hay, straw, branches, and cardboard items such as tubes and boxes.

If gerbils are given the opportunity to dig their own burrow in deep substrate, they do not need any added artificial shelters. But terrariums can be additionally structured with wooden platforms of different heights to add stability and to facilitate the safe placement of sand bath and water bowls. Running wheels are not a necessary provision for gerbils; there are very few positive and some negative effects (Sherwin 1998). If running wheels are used, they should be 30 cm in diameter and have a solid running surface. Letting gerbils run free in the home is not recommended because they may gnaw cables or slip behind bookshelves and other furniture from where they cannot be retrieved.

These desert animals need baths of bird or chinchilla sand to clean their fur of sebum and dirt. Low humidity is recommended in a range of 35–55% (McManus 1972a). If gerbils cannot groom themselves in sand or are kept at higher humidity, they develop a matted, ruffled fur because of the secretions of the Harderian gland (Thiessen and Yahr 1977). This disturbs thermoregulation at both higher (30 °C) and lower (5 °C) ambient temperatures. At lower temperatures, affected gerbils can only compensate by increasing metabolic rate or by maintaining a crouched body position during sleep and activity to reduce heat loss. A lack of sand-bathing also increases water loss and allows carcinogenic ultraviolet radiation to penetrate the fur (Pendergrass and Thiessen 1981, 1983). Sand bowls should be placed safely on a platform or be fixed to the container wall, so the gerbils cannot tunnel under it and be crushed. Gerbils first use sand for bathing and later as a latrine, so sand baths should be cleaned and replaced weekly or when they are soiled.

Mongolian gerbils structure their surroundings with a latrine and mark their territory with secretions from several scent glands, most typically the ventral sebaceous gland, which plays an important role in territorial behaviour and kin recognition (Tang Halpin 1975; Swanson and Lockley 1977; Thiessen and Yahr 1977; Shimozuru et al. 2006). As gerbils produce dry faecal pellets and very little urine, their bedding stays clean for quite a long time. A gerbil terrarium of 0.5 m² floor area with 40-cm deep bedding and only two occupants may need cleaning only every 2 to 3 months. Bedding should then be changed completely to remove food leftovers, parasites, fungal spores, dust, etc. As replacing the whole bedding and all scent marks is stressful for gerbils (Weinandy and Gattermann 1997), at least some old bedding and nesting material should be transferred to the cleaned terrarium.

10.2.3 Animal Company

As highly social animals, gerbils should never be kept alone but always in groups with other, compatible gerbils. Single housing might lead to depression-like symptoms (Starkey and Hendrie 1997; Hendrie and Starkey 1998; Hendrie and Pickles 2000). Gerbils should be kept in age-structured same-sex groups to promote a stable hierarchy.

Sudden outbreaks of aggression can occur in hitherto peaceful same-sex groups of gerbils. Sufficient hiding places, barriers, and burrows should therefore be provided so animals can hide and avoid each other. Owners should ensure that groups are constantly monitored. Unfortunately, there is a lack of recognisable signs of impending aggression (Scheibler et al. 2005b, 2006a). Even small bite wounds and chases between animals should therefore be taken seriously before attacks become more severe. Fighting animals should be separated and then not be reintroduced to one another. If a single gerbil remains, owners should try regrouping. This works best with newly weaned juveniles of 5 to 8 weeks before they become reproductive. Adult gerbils are difficult to regroup because they commonly do not tolerate other unfamiliar gerbils in their territory (other than subadults or mixing males with females during oestrus). The best methods are not scientifically studied, but owners should avoid forcing animals to endure each other's presence without the possibility to flee or interact species typically.

Breeding pairs should only be kept if offspring are explicitly wished. If gerbils are bred, fathers should be left with the mother. Both parents build a well-padded and insulated nest from available nesting material such as hay, straw, and tissues. From a few days after birth, the father and older siblings show parental behaviour such as warming the pups and retrieving them if they crawl away from the nest. The father's presence then increases pup activity and physical contact between pups and parents and speeds up maturation (Piovanotti and Vieira 2004). In rare cases, infanticide by any family member might occur. Both adults or subadults may hurt or kill newborn pups often because of inexperience in pup care. If the pups are eaten, especially only the head, malnutrition might be the cause (Elwood and Ostermeyer 1984; Saltzman et al. 2006).

Juveniles should be left with their parents at least until weaning is completed naturally, for example when the next litter is born. As offspring need to learn social skills, it is both possible and advisable to leave future breeding animals with their parents for this length of time and to mimic the natural situation as far as possible by separating animals late. Juveniles separated from their mother may show increased repetitive bar chewing (Waiblinger 2003), suggesting that they are motivated to escape to return to their mother. If gerbils are weaned early, they should be separated in same-sex groups by the age of 8–10 weeks.

In reproductive groups, social stress can sometimes increase when juveniles become reproductively active, although this is usually suppressed in subordinated family members. Competition for the reproductive position occasionally triggers aggression between females, forcing all fertile females but one to emigrate. Aggression usually originates from the breeding female (60%) and less commonly from the breeding male (13%; Scheibler et al. 2005b, 2006a). Possible causes include insufficient defendable resources, the illness or death of the top-ranking animal, or changes in the human household. With the inability to emigrate from terrariums in captivity, aggressive encounters between gerbils can often end with severe bite wounds or deaths.

As a rule, gerbils should not be mixed with other species of animals in the same housing unit. They might attack smaller rodents that are their natural competitors (e.g. Djungarian hamsters) or be attacked by bigger species. If carnivores such as cats or dogs are kept in the same household, gerbil terrariums need to be well locked to prevent the predator from accessing and killing the gerbils. Coexistence is only acceptable if the gerbils are able to cope with the situation in a species typical way (i.e. by fleeing into a burrow to hide and escape predator stimuli). That being the case, gerbils may even come to feed on the surface with a cat sitting near them, fleeing into their burrow if the cat pounces. The presence of such predators may therefore prompt natural vigilance and escape behaviours but risks potential stress.

10.2.4 Human Interactions

Humans are mostly perceived either as predators or as providers of food and other resources by gerbils. Most probably, humans are not viewed as a social partner and are not an acceptable substitute for the company of socially compatible gerbils. Allowing gerbils to dig their own burrow can also mean they interact less with their owner (Clark and Galef 1979; Hurst and West 2010) – although the advantages of providing burrowing opportunities far outweigh this disadvantage. Instead, gerbils should be encouraged to seek human interactions voluntarily, using rewards such as sunflower or pumpkin seeds.

Gerbils should be captured using a tube or tunnel (of around 20 cm length and 5 cm diameter and not a toilet paper roll), which they may readily enter (e.g. for cage cleaning). Children may often be unable to correctly catch gerbils because the animals are too quick for them, so using a tube is an excellent option. When handled, gerbils should not be picked up by their tail, and especially not by the tip of their tail, to prevent the tail degloving, which is a tactic used to escape predators. Gerbils' tail base may be held only if their bodies are constantly supported with the other hand (Figure 10.2).

10.2.5 Health

Gerbils may suffer a number of diseases and other health problems (Table 10.2). Tyzzer's disease is a *Clostridium* infection, and the prognosis is poor even with treatment. Keratitis can lead to blindness, although blind gerbils may show minimal behavioural changes in familiar surroundings. 'Red nose' may be caused by reduced grooming and accumulation of Harderian gland secretions or *Staphylococcus* spp. infection. These conditions may be often secondary to other diseases and exacerbated by social, physical, or handling stress. Contact with wild mice or outdoor resources can increase the risk of parasitic infestation, in which case regular treatment with a broad-spectrum antiparasitic drug may be advisable.

Regular health checks by the owner should include checking teeth, fur, and ventral gland. Claws and incisors should not need to be trimmed if animals are able to dig and provided with gnawing materials. However, if one incisor breaks, its counterpart continues to grow and needs to be filed down under anaesthesia to acceptable length every 2 weeks until its counterpart grows back. Neutering is possible, but there is a significant risk when using isoflurane as inhaled anaesthetic for respiratory arrest (about 10% probability).

(a)   (b)   (c)

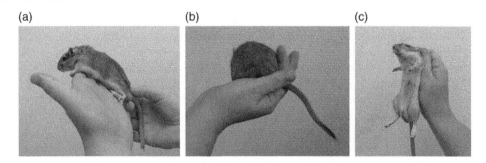

Figure 10.2 Handling options: (a) Fixation at the base of the tail, body supported with other hand; (b) one-handed fixation of gerbil at the base of the tail; (c) fixation of male gerbil at the neck.

Table 10.2 Selected health problems in gerbils.

Condition		Welfare effects
Infectious or inflammatory and parasitic diseases	Tyzzer's disease (*Clostridium piliformis*)	Hyperacute: Sudden death Subacute: Diarrhoea, weight loss, reduced water, and food intake, Lethargy Reduced autogrooming with perianal faecal staining
	Respiratory infections (Various pathogens)	Changed breathing rate Strained breathing Hunched posture Ruffled fur (May be associated with increased humidity)
	Erythema or conjuctivitis (e.g. *Staphylococcus* sp.)	'Red Nose' Reduced grooming Accumulation of Harderian gland secretions
	Keratitis	Blindness (with minimal behavioural changes in familiar surroundings)
	Protozoal (e.g. *Entamoeba*; *Spironucleus*; *Tritrichomonas*)	Diarrhoea Dehydration
	Mange (*Demodex* sp.)	Hair loss Parasites
	Nematodes (e.g. *Syphacia obvelata*; *Dentostomella translucida*; *Hymenolepis* spp.)	Diarrhoea Dehydration
Neurological	Epilepsy[a]	Seizures
Neoplastic	Cystic ovaries	Shape changes of flanks and abdomen May require surgery
	Scent gland tumours	Secondary bacterial infections if damaged during marking behaviour May require surgery[b]
Traumatic	Degloving of tail during handling	Pain Damage to tail skin Damage to tail muscles and bone Potential subsequent infections May require surgery
	Fractures due to accidents with equipment (running wheels) or animal being dropped during handling	Pain Potential infection in open fractures

[a]Cutler and Mackintosh 1989.
[b]Deutschland et al. 2011.

10.2.6 Euthanasia

Acceptable methods of euthanasia of gerbils are listed in Table 10.3. The best method is usually sedation or anaesthesia, followed by injection of an overdose of buffered pentobarbitone at two to three times the anaesthetic dose into the abdomen. The thickness and darkness of gerbils' skin increases the risk that intravenous injections miss the vein, causing pain, and irritation. Inhalational anaesthetics such as isoflurane or halothane appear aversive to gerbils. Neck dislocation risks error, and elevated pressure can cause degloving of the tail and tetraplegia without causing death and is especially unsuitable for gerbils of more than 20 g body weight.

10.3 Signs of Gerbil Welfare

10.3.1 Pathophysiological Signs

It is difficult for untrained or inexperienced persons to recognise many signs of reduced health in gerbils. Minor changes of body condition may be significant. Signs of reduced body condition include weight loss, sunken flanks, and palpable or visible pelvic bones. Dull eyes, laboured breathing or clicking sounds while breathing, decreased body temperature, and a rough or matted coat indicate serious health problems. The fur should instead have a silky shine and not be matted or stringy. Disturbed grooming can also be recognised by remains of reddish Harderian gland sebum on the fur of the face or faeces and urine sticking to the fur around the tail region, which is normally noticed before any altered behaviour is observed. Hair loss at the tail indicates long-term stress, irrespective of whether caused by a social or physical stressor (Figure 10.3).

Normal basic physiological measures are given in Table 10.4, which may change considerably during social stress. For example, white blood cell counts and cholesterol levels may increase as a result of intraspecific attacks (Scheibler et al. 2005a). Faecal levels of stress hormones, particularly corticosterone, can also be used to assess stress level. Social stress and intragroup aggression can be associated with an increase of corticosterone levels (Scheibler et al. 2004). Nevertheless, because of the metabolism in the gut and the impairment of food availability, digestion, and defecation, stress hormone levels exhibit strong variation and so data need to be carefully interpreted.

10.3.2 Behavioural Signs

Noticeable deviations from normal behaviour patterns are usually the first signs of reduced well-being that can be observed, long before any pathophysiological signs are detected. For example, increased or decreased activities, resting away from their social

Table 10.3 Methods of euthanasia for Mongolian gerbils.

Method	Restraint required	Welfare benefits	Welfare risks
Intraperitoneal injection of pentobarbitone	Secure handling Sedation or analgesia necessary, if fractious	Rapid loss of consciousness	Reversible at low dosages, needs restraint

Source: Schweigart (1995), and AVMA (2013).

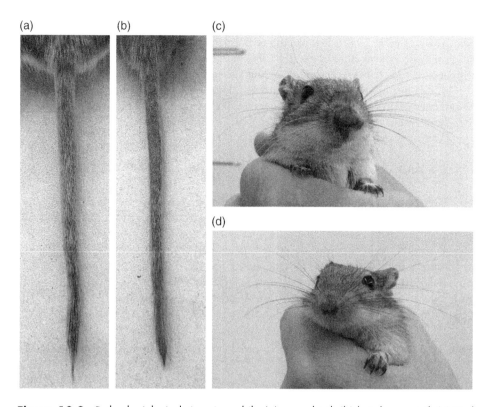

Figure 10.3 Pathophysiological signs in gerbils: (a) normal tail; (b) hair loss on tail; (c) 'Red nose', possibly paired with *Streptococcus* sp. infection; (d) healthy nose and face.

Table 10.4 Basic measures and clinical standards of gerbils (*Meriones unguiculatus*).

Parameter	Normal measures	
Life expectancy	up to 4.5 years, mean 3.5 years	
Mean weight	Males: 80–130 g	Females: 60–100 g
Body temperature	37–39 °C	
Respiratory frequency	70–130 breaths/min	
Heart rate	260–450 beats/min	
Pubescence	Males: 70–84 days	Females: 70–90 days
Gestation 24 to 28 days		
Blood volume	3.5–4.4 mL (6.5–8.0% of body mass)	
Haematocrit	41–52	

Sources: Marston and Chang (1965), Cheal (1983), and Field and Sibold (1999).

partners, a hunched posture, lethargy, or disturbed grooming are potential signs of severe health or other problems. Stereotypic digging is a frequently observed abnormal behaviour in gerbils and indicates a lack of a suitable burrow structure (Wiedenmayer 1997a). It can be recognised as lasting more than 12 seconds (Wiedenmayer 1997a) or as 'comprising more than seven front leg scratches that may be followed by hindleg kicks' (Moons et al. 2012). It is usually performed in the corners of the terrarium and takes up a large proportion of gerbils' time. Bar chewing or bar gnawing may develop from outside-directed exploratory behaviour such as rearing and sniffing (Wiedenmayer 1997b). It is not influenced by food hardness, location, or mode of presentation or by the presence of gnawing material and is more likely to indicate a motivation to escape or early weaning.

10.4 Worldwide Action Plan for Improving Gerbil Welfare

Free, high-quality, and scientifically based information for pet owners, current and future, is crucial to changing gerbil welfare for the better. These should focus firstly on enrichment, secondly on diet and health, and thirdly on social housing. In parallel, legislation should make appropriate care mandatory. Other countries could follow Switzerland's minimum legal requirements for pet gerbils since 2008, which make it compulsory to provide the company of other socially compatible gerbils, $0.5\,m^2$ floor space per two to five animals, $25\,cm$ substrate depth to allow for digging a burrow, and further other aspects of good care (Table 10.5).

Table 10.5 Minimum housing conditions for gerbils prescribed in selected European legislations.

Country	Switzerland	Austria
Legislation	TSchV (Swiss Animal Protection Ordinance, annex 2)	BGBl. II Nr. 486/2004 (2nd Ordinance – housing of vertebrates)
Type of gerbil	Gerbils as pets	Gerbils as pets
Minimum floor surface	$0.5\,m^2$	$60 \times 30 \times 40\,cm = 0.18\,m^2$ (cages) $80 \times 50 \times 50\,cm = 0.4\,m^2$ (terrariums)
Number of animals	2–5	not indicated
Floor surface per animal	0.1–$0.25\,m^2$	not indicated
Surface for each additional animal	$+ 0.05\,m^2$	$+ 0.036\,m^2$ $+ 0.08\,m^2$
Substrate depth	$25\,cm$	$10\,cm$
Enclosure height	not indicated	$40\,cm$ (cage) $50\,cm$ (terrarium)
Further provisions	One or several shelters that allow all animals to retreat, nesting material, hay, straw, grains as food, gnawing objects, sand bath, compulsory group housing	Occupation, gnawing material, airing slits at side of tank, three-dimensional structuring, fresh water daily, sand bath, free running outside cage or tank weekly; family or same-sex groups

   This progress could parallel improvements in laboratory gerbil care (which should match the requirements for pet care). After Switzerland made it compulsory to provide laboratory gerbils with either deep substrate or artificial burrows, large pharmaceutical companies headquartered in Switzerland had to find solutions for their laboratory gerbils, which they are beginning to implement in their animal facilities worldwide. One country has thereby acted as a role model for the rest of the world. Implementing such education and minimum requirements could help create international markets for adequately sized gerbil housing. For example, some rodent cage manufacturers in the European Union have begun to fabricate suitably large rodent terrariums to satisfy the Swiss and Austrian pet markets. These manufacturers are interested in recommendations from animal protection organisations that might provide a competitive edge as well as a clear animal welfare benefit.

Bibliography

Agren, G., Zhou, Q., and Zhong, W. (1989a). Ecology and social behaviour of Mongolian gerbils, *Meriones unguiculatus*, at Xilinhot, Inner Mongolia, China. *Animal Behaviour* 37: 11–27.

Agren, G., Zhou, Q., and Zhong, W. (1989b). Territoriality, cooperation and resource priority: hoarding in the Mongolian gerbil, *Meriones unguiculatus*. *Animal Behaviour* 37: 28–32.

Arringto, L.R. and Ammerman, C.B. (1969). Water requirements of gerbils. *Laboratory Animal Care* 19 (4): 503–504.

AVMA (American Veterinary Medical Association). (2013). AVMA Guidelines for the Euthanasia of Animals: 2013 Edition. Available at https://www.avma.org/KB/Policies/Pages/Euthanasia-Guidelines.aspx. Accessed 7 October 2015.

Bannikov, A.G. (1954). The places inhabited and natural history of *Meriones unguiculatus*. Mammals of the Mongolian Peoples Republic, USSR Academy of Sciences – Committee of the Mongolian Peoples Republic. *Trudy Mongol'skoi Komissii* 53: 410–415.

BGBl. II Nr. 486/2004 (2004). Verordnung der Bundesministerin für Gesundheit über die Haltung von Wirbeltieren, die nicht unter die 1. Tierhaltungsverordnung fallen, über Wildtiere, die besondere Anforderungen an die Haltung stellen und über Wildtierarten, deren Haltung aus Gründen des Tierschutzes verboten ist (2. Tierhaltungsverordnung) / Austrian Animal Housing Ordinance, (Online), Available at http://www.ris.bka.gv.at/GeltendeFassung.wxe?Abfrage=Bundesnormen&Gesetzesnummer=20003860. Accessed 28 September 2013.

Brunner, C. (1993). *The digging behaviour of the Mongolian gerbil (Meriones unguiculatus) in a semi-natural enclosure.* Unpublished Thesis. Ethology and Wildlife Research, Zoological Institute, University of Zürich.

Cheal, M. (1983). Lifespan ontogeny of breeding and reproductive success in Mongolian gerbils. *Laboratory Animals* 17: 240–245.

Chevret, P. and Dobigny, G. (2005). Systematics and evolution of the subfamily Gerbillinae (Mammalia, Rodentia, Muridae). *Molecular Phylogenetics and Evolution* 35: 674–688.

Clark, M.M. and Galef, B.G. (1979). A sensitive period for the maintenance of emotionality in Mongolian gerbils. *Journal of Comparative and Physiological Psychology* 93 (2): 200–210.

Clark, M.M. and Galef, B.G. (2001). Socially-induced infertility: familial effects on reproductive development of female Mongolian gerbils. *Animal Behaviour* 62: 897–903.

Clark, M.M. and Galef, B.G. (2002). Socially induced delayed reproduction in female Mongolian gerbils *(Meriones unguiculatus)*: is there anything special about dominant females? *Journal of Comparative Psychology* 116 (4): 363–368.

Cutler, M.G. and Mackintosh, J.H. (1989). Epilepsy and behaviour of the Mongolian gerbil – an ethological study. *Physiology and Behavior* 46 (4): 561–566.

Deutschland, M., Denk, D., Skerritt, G., and Hetzel, U. (2011). Surgical excision and morphological evaluation of altered abdominal scent glands in Mongolian gerbils *(Meriones unguiculatus)*. *Veterinary Record* 169: 636–641.

Elwood, R.W. and Ostermeyer, M.C. (1984). The effects of food deprivation, aggression, and isolation on infanticide in the male Mongolian gerbil. *Aggressive Behavior* 10 (4): 293–301.

European Convention for the Protection of Pet Animals (ETS 125). (1987). Available at http://www.conventions.coe.int/treaty/en/treaties/html/125.htm. Accessed 11 June 2015.

Farm, T. (1975). Gerbil care and maintenance. *The Gerbil Digest* 2 (2): 2.

FELASA (2007). Euroguide: On the accommodation and care of animals used for experimental and other scientific purposes. Based on the revised Appendix A of the European Convention ETS 123. (Online), Available: http://www.felasa.eu/?ACT=43&file_id=3febF EIR0u7CQrFxJjuEQ0huckeOB8jyGR%2BwLatdmSQ%3D&access=mrP8h0aXi3WGD OsOUE59J7u6%2F%2F6lXaGBbUeqEcuq2hc%3D. Accessed 29 May 2018.

Field, K.J. and Sibold, A.L. (1999). *The Laboratory Hamster and Gerbil*. Washington, DC: CRC Press Ltd.

Forkman, B.A. (1993). Self-reinforced behavior does not explain contra-freeloading in the Mongolian gerbil. *Ethology* 94 (2): 109–112.

French, J.A. (1994). Alloparents in the Mongolian gerbil: impact on long-term reproductive performance of breeders and opportunities for independent reproduction. *Behavioral Ecology* 5 (3): 273–279.

Gulotta, E.F. (1971). Meriones unguiculatus. *Mammalian Species* 3: 1–5.

GV SOLAS (2009). Fütterungskonzepte und -methoden in der Versuchstierhaltung und im Tierversuch: Mongolische Wüstenrennmaus *(Meriones unguiculatus)*, (Online), Available: www.gv-solas.de/assets/files/PDFs/pdf_PUBLIKATION/ern_fuetterung_rennmaus.pdf. Accessed 28 September 2013.

Hendrie, C.A. and Pickles, A.R. (2000). Short-term individual housing in female gerbils as a putative model of depression. *Society for Neuroscience – Abstracts* 26 (1–2): Abstract 103.12.

Hendrie, C.A. and Starkey, N.J. (1998). Pair-bond distruption in Mongolian gerbils: effects on subsequent social behaviour. *Physiology and Behavior* 63 (5): 895–901.

Hurst, J.L. and West, R.S. (2010). Taming anxiety in laboratory mice. *Nature Methods* 7: 825–826.

Li, Q., Sun, R., Huang, C. et al. (2001). Cold adaptive thermogenesis in small mammals from different geographical zones of China. *Comparative Biochemistry and Physiology Part A* 129: 949–961.

Liu, W., Wan, X., and Zhong, W. (2007). Population dynamics of the Mongolian gerbils: seasonal patterns and interactions among density, reproduction and climate. *Journal of Arid Environments* 68 (3): 383–397.

Marston, J.H. and Chang, M.C. (1965). The breeding, management and reproductive physiology of the Mongolian gerbil *(Meriones unguiculatus)*. *Laboratory Animal Care* 15 (1): 34–48.

McManus, J.J. (1972a). Water relations and food consumption of the Mongolian gerbil, *Meriones unguiculatus*. *Comparative Biochemistry and Physiology* 43A: 959–967.

McManus, J.J. (1972b). Early postnatal growth and development of temperature regulation in Mongolian gerbils, *Meriones unguiculatus*. *Journal Of Mammology* 51 (4): 782.

Moons, C.P.H., Breugelmann, S., Cassiman, N. et al. (2012). The effect of differing working definitions on behavioural research involving stereotypies in Mongolian gerbils (*Meriones unguiculatus*). *Journal of the American Association for Laboratory Animal Science* 51 (2): 170–176.

Mulder, G.B., Pritchett-Corning, K.R., Gramlich, M.A., and Crocker, A.E. (2010). Method of food presentation affects the growth of Mongolian gerbils (*Meriones unguiculatus*). *Journal of the American Association for Laboratory Animal Science* 49 (1): 36–39.

Naumov, N.P. and Lobachev, S.V. (1975). Ecology of the desert rodents of the USSR (Jerboas and Gerbils). In: *Rodents in Desert Environments* (ed. I. Prakash and P.K. Gosh), 529–536. The Hague: Dr. W. Junk b.v. Publishers.

Norris, M.L. and Adams, C.E. (1981). Mating post partum and length of gestation in the Mongolian gerbil (*Meriones unguiculatus*). *Laboratory Animals* 15: 189–191.

Norris, M.L. and Adams, C.E. (1982). Lifetime reproductive performance of Mongolian gerbil (*Meriones unguiculatus*). *Laboratory Animals* 16: 146–150.

NRC (1995). Nutrient Requirements of Laboratory Animals, Fourth Revised Edition 1995, Subcommittee on Laboratory Animal Nutrition; Committee on Animal Nutrition; Board on Agriculture; National Research Council. The National Academies Press, Washington, DC.

Ostermeyer, M.C. and Elwood, R.W. (1984). Helpers (?) at the nest in the Mongolian gerbil, *Meriones unguiculatus*. *Behaviour* 91: 61–77.

Pendergrass, M. and Thiessen, D.D. (1981). Body temperature and autogrooming in the Mongolian gerbil, *Meriones unguiculatus*. *Behavioural and Neural Biology* 33: 524–528.

Pendergrass, M. and Thiessen, D.D. (1983). Sandbathing is thermoregulatory in the gerbil, *Meriones unguiculatus*. *Behavioural and Neural Biology* 37 (1): 125–133.

Piovanotti, M.R.A. and Vieira, L.M. (2004). Presence of the father and parental experience have differentiated effects on pup development in Mongolian gerbils (*Meriones unguiculatus*). *Behavioural Processes* 66 (2): 107–117.

Price, E.O. (2002). Morphological and physiological traits. In: *Animal Domestication and Behaviour* (ed. E.O. Price), 83–94. CABI Publishing.

Rich, S.T. (1968). The Mongolian gerbil (*Meriones unguiculatus*) in research. *Laboratory Animal Care* 18 (2): 235–243.

Roper, T.J. and Polioudakis, E. (1977). The behaviour of Mongolian gerbils in a semi-natural environment, with special reference to ventral marking, dominance and sociability. *Behaviour* 61 (3–4): 205–237.

Salo, A.A. and French, J.A. (1989). Early experience, reproductive success, and development of parental behaviour in Mongolian gerbils. *Animal Behaviour* 38: 693–702.

Saltzman, W., Ahmeda, S., Fahimi, A. et al. (2006). Social suppression of female reproductive maturation and infanticidal behavior in cooperatively breeding Mongolian gerbils. *Hormones and Behavior* 49: 527–537.

Scheibler, E., Weinandy, R., and Gattermann, R. (2004). Social categories in families of Mongolian gerbils. *Physiology and Behavior* 81 (3): 455–464.

Scheibler, E., Weinandy, R., and Gattermann, R. (2005a). Intra-family aggression modulates physiological features of the Mongolian gerbil *Meriones unguiculatus*. *Acta Zoologica Sinica* 51 (6): 989–997.

Scheibler, E., Weinandy, R., and Gattermann, R. (2005b). Intra-family aggression and offspring expulsion in Mongolian gerbils (*Meriones unguiculatus*) under restricted environments. *Mammalian Biology – Zeitschrift für Säugetierkunde* 70 (3): 137–146.

Scheibler, E., Weinandy, R., and Gattermann, R. (2006a). Male expulsion in cooperative Mongolian gerbils (*Meriones unguiculatus*). *Physiology and Behavior* 87 (1): 24–30.

Scheibler, E., Liu, W., Weinandy, R., and Gattermann, R. (2006b). Burrow systems of the Mongolian gerbil (*Meriones unguiculatus* Milne Edwards, 1867). *Mammalian Biology – Zeitschrift für Säugetierkunde* 71 (3): 178–182.

Schweigart, G. (1995). *Chinchilla – Heimtier und Patient*. Stuttgart, Germany: Gustav Fischer Verlag.

Sherwin, C.M. (1998). Voluntary wheel running: a review and novel interpretation. *Animal Behaviour* 56: 11–27.

Shimozuru, M., Kikusui, T., Takeuchi, Y., and Mori, Y. (2006). Scent-marking and sexual activity may reflect social hierarchy among group-living male Mongolian gerbils (*Meriones unguiculatus*). *Physiology and Behavior* 89 (5): 644–649.

Starkey, N.J. and Hendrie, C.A. (1997). Parallels between pairbond disruption in gerbils and human depression. *Behavioural Pharmacology* 8: 663–664.

Stuermer, I.W., Plotz, K., Leybold, A. et al. (2003). Intraspecific allometric comparison of laboratory gerbils with Mongolian gerbils trapped in the wild indicates domestication in *Meriones unguiculatus* (Milne-Edwards, 1867) (Rodentia: Gerbillinae). *Zoologischer Anzeiger* 242: 249–266.

Swanson, H.H. and Lockley, R.M. (1977). Population growth and social structure of confined colonies of Mongolian gerbils: scent gland size and marking behaviour as indices of social status. *Aggressive Behaviour* 4: 57–89.

Tang Halpin, Z. (1975). The role of individual recognition by odours in the social interactions of the Mongolian gerbil (*Meriones unguiculatus*). *Behaviour* 58 (1–2): 117–129.

Thiessen, D.D. and Yahr, P. (1977). *The Gerbil in Behavioral Investigations*. Austin, Texas: University of Texas Press.

TSchV (2008) Tierschutzverordnung / Animal Protection Ordinance, annex 2 (Wild animals), gerbils as pets, and annex 3, laboratory gerbils (Online), Available: https://www.admin.ch/opc/de/classified-compilation/20080796/index.html. Accessed 29 May 2018.

Waiblinger E. 2003 Behavioural stereotypies in laboratory gerbils (*Meriones unguiculatus*): Causes and solutions. PhD thesis, University of Zurich, Switzerland.

Waiblinger, E. (2010). The laboratory gerbil. In: *The UFAW Handbook on the Care and Management of Laboratory and Other Research Animals*, 8e (ed. R. Hubrecht and J. Kirkwood), 327–347. Chichester: Wiley-Blackwell.

Waring, A.D., Poole, T.W., and Perper, T. (1978). White spotting in the Mongolian gerbil. *Journal of Heredity* 69: 347–349.

Weinandy, R. and Gattermann, R. (1997). Time of day and stress response to different stressors in experimental animals. 2. Mongolian gerbil (*Meriones unguiculatus* Milne Edwards, 1867). *Journal of Experimental Animal Science* 38 (3): 109–122.

Wiedenmayer, C. (1997a). Causation of the ontogenetic development of stereotypic digging in gerbils. *Animal Behaviour* 53: 461–470.

Wiedenmayer, C. (1997b). The early ontogeny of bar-gnawing in laboratory gerbils. *Animal Welfare* 6: 273–277.

Würbel, H. (2006). The motivational basis of caged rodents' stereotypies. In: *Stereotypic Animal Behaviour*, 2e (ed. G. Mason and J. Rushen), 86–120. Wallingford: CAB International.

Xu, D.L., Liu, X.Y., and Wang, D.H. (2011). Impairment of cellular and humoral immunity in overweight Mongolian gerbils (*Meriones unguiculatus*). *Integrative Zoology* 6 (4): 352–365.

Yang, H.D., Wang, Q., Wang, Z., and Wang, D.H. (2011). Food hoarding and associated neuronal activation in brain reward circuitry in Mongolian gerbils. *Physiology and Behavior* 104: 429–436.

Domestic Rats (*Rattus norvegicus*)

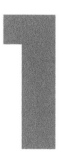

Oliver Burman

11.1.1 Natural History

Domestic rats (*Rattus norvegicus*) are rodent members of the class Mammalia, order Rodentia, and family Muridae. They are thought to have evolved from the Norway or brown rat (*R. norvegicus Berkenhout*). Their original location is unclear, but they now cover a range of habitats across many continents, particularly associated with human habitations and dispersal. *R. norvegicus* is classified as being of Least Concern (IUCN 2016).

Wild brown rats are highly social animals and live for about 2 to 3 years. When resources are limited or dispersed, they live in small social units of a male with several females and their offspring, typically based around an underground burrow. When resources are more readily available, they can live in large, interconnected colonies. Wild rats can recognise related individuals and colony members and may be aggressive towards unfamiliar individuals. Territories are marked using scent, usually in urine or faeces. Rats also communicate by emitting vocalisations of audible and ultrasonic frequencies. Their hearing range is around 0.2–80 kHz (Kelly and Masterton 1977),

Companion Animal Care and Welfare: The UFAW Companion Animal Handbook,
First Edition. Edited by James Yeates.
© 2019 Universities Federation for Animal Welfare. Published 2019 by John Wiley & Sons Ltd.

encompassing ultrasonic frequencies beyond the typical human hearing range (i.e. >20 kHz). Rats are more active at night, with peak activity exhibited at dawn and dusk, using a network of pathways to get around their territory. Wild rats forage for a wide variety of food types, including seeds, nuts, fruits, eggs, invertebrates, and young animals such as chicks, often carrying food back to the security of their burrow. Rats use their highly sensitive whiskers for discrimination, detection, to maintain balance, and to guide them around complex spaces and their footpads and toe tips are also particularly sensitive to tactile cues.

11.1.2 Domestic History

In the eighteenth century, rat catchers would sell caught rats for use in the blood sport of rat baiting (Hilscher-Conklin 1996). In the nineteenth century, the greatest phase of rat domestication began with the advent of systematic scientific investigation, and some unusually coloured rats were also bred for sale as pets (Royer 2015). In the twentieth century, rat showing began in England and later in the century, in the United States. More recently, the increase in reptile keeping has prompted increased rat breeding for feeding. Pet rats are increasingly popular (Williams 2002), with an estimated 0.1 million rats kept as pets in the United Kingdom (PFMA 2018).

During artificial selection, different colour types appeared, possibly genetically linked to temperament (Trut et al. 1997). Selective breeding, for personal interest and for exhibiting at rat shows, has resulted in a wide range of 'fancy rat' varieties based on coat colour (Siamese), curly coats (Rex), hairlessness (Sphinx), absence of a tail (Manx), or low-positioned ears (Dumbo). Compared to wild rats, domestic rats are often less fearful of novelty, quicker to interact with humans, and less aggressive towards one another. Despite these differences, even domestic rats exhibit a variety of wild-type behaviours if given the opportunity (Berdoy 2002, www.ratlife.org).

11.2 Principles of Rat Care

11.2.1 Diet

Rats are omnivores, with nutritional maintenance requirements as listed in Table 11.1. Some vitamins (e.g. vitamins D, C, K, folic acid, and biotin) can be synthesised by the rats themselves; others (e.g. vitamins A, E, B1, B_2, B_6, B_{12}) must be obtained from external food sources. Complete pelleted rat diets should have all these included. Owners should also give small quantities of unprocessed food types such as seeds, grains, fresh fruit and vegetables, and of cooked egg or meat. However, owners do not need to give supplementary fibrous material such as alfalfa or hay. Although rats need adequate calcium, excessive calcium (relative to phosphorus) can lead to kidney calcium deposits. A balanced diet is most easily achieved by providing a complete pelleted diet specifically formulated for rats. It is particularly important to avoid pelleted diets formulated for herbivorous glires species. Many human foods may be toxic or indigestible, such as dairy products, chocolate, and orange juice (Burn 2008).

Ad libitum balanced food is suitable for most active rats and can reduce competition between rats. The amount rats eat depends on their social status and age, with growing

Table 11.1 Nutritional requirements of adult, nonbreeding rats.

Nutrient	Amount required
Protein (including essential amino acids, e.g. lysine)	c.15% of daily intake
Carbohydrate	c.75% of daily intake
Fibre	c.5% of daily intake
Lipids including essential fatty acids (e.g. arachidonic acid)	c.5% of daily intake
Minerals	Trace amounts
Water	c.10 mL /100 g body weight day^{-1}

Source: Himsel (1991), McGivern et al. (1996), McIntyre et al. (1993), Rao et al. (1959), Reddy and Maeura (1984), Reeves (1997), and Richardson (1997).
All figures assume animals are of normal physiology, healthy, and non-breeding.

rats requiring more food. Rats grow at different rates according to their diet, age, strain, and sex, with the most rapid growth occurring during early life. Pregnant and nursing females need more nutrients, which can usually be provided through increased amounts of the normal diet. Inadequate nutrition can result in lethargy, weight loss or low growth, hair loss, a predisposition towards infections, muscle and skeletal problems, flaky or scaly skin, poor coat condition, or dull eyes. Body weight, body condition, feeding rate, and growth rate are key indicators that should be monitored daily or weekly as rats can lose weight very quickly. Conversely, excessive fat and sugar, especially alongside a sedentary lifestyle, commonly leads to obesity, which can be associated with reduced exercise levels, hypertension, tumour development, liver disease, osteoarthritis, tumours, and shorter life spans. Balanced, calorie-controlled diets and sufficient exercise can prevent or treat obesity. Rats may select foods that are sweet (e.g. sugar coated cereals) or fatty (e.g. nuts), and these should be given only sparingly.

Some individual rats may show preferences for particular foods and require gradual introduction to new foods. However, rats enjoy a variety in their diet and may avoid their favourite food if they have been fed it for several days (Galef and Whiskin 2003). Rats should be given both easily-accessible food (e.g. from an open bowl) and regular opportunities to forage. Foraging activity can be encouraged by hiding food around the enclosure and placing treats in hard to reach spots, such as buried in sand or gravel trays, hidden in cardboard tubes, or placed in water (Figure 11.1). Scattering food can also enable all rats to access treats without competition. Occasional whole food items, such as nuts, sunflower seeds, or eggs in shells can encourage rats to manipulate food with their paws. Materials such as wood blocks and low-calorie dog biscuits can encourage gnawing behaviour, thereby helping to wear the teeth down naturally and prevent overgrowth. Rats feed most at dusk and dawn (Burton et al. 1981), although dominant individuals may exclude subordinates to less preferable feeding times, which should be taken into account when judging food intake.

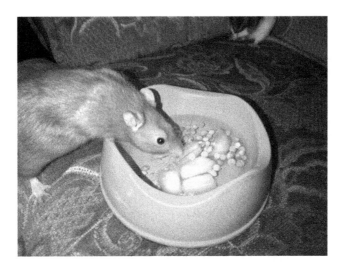

Figure 11.1 Food placed in water for the rat to 'fish' for it (*Source:* courtesy of Karen Brady).

Fresh, clean water should always be available. Rats have higher water requirements when fed dry pelleted food or lactating. Water should be provided in bottle drinkers to avoid contamination, with enough drinkers to allow all rats to drink simultaneously (i.e. one at each drinker), although rats may choose to share drinkers.

11.2.2 Environment

Large enclosures are necessary to give pet rats sufficient opportunity to explore and exercise. However, rats dislike open spaces (Valle 1970), so it is important that this space contains plenty of shelter and three-dimensional complexity including platforms, hammocks, and tubes (Figure 11.2). Each rat should be able to have access to their own area and plenty of bedding to form a nest. This is particularly important for pregnant females (Denenberg et al. 1969).

Enclosures should usually have a solid base and wire sides. Wire floors may lead to foot injuries and subsequent infection from bacteria present in soiled bedding material, such as round, red swelling or ulcers on the bottom or heel of the foot (Richardson 1997; Davidson et al. 2000). Rats are able to squeeze through very small gaps, so this must be taken into account when selecting an enclosure. However, owners should avoid using enclosed cages with high, nonperforated sides to ensure sufficient ventilation.

Rats should be kept within a temperature range of around 19–23 °C and a humidity of around 40–70% (Wolfensohn 1998). A shelter, bedding material, and company let rats raise their body temperature (e.g. by huddling in a nest), whereas access to a shallow tray of water can allow rats to cool themselves down. Rats use their hair and tails to thermoregulate, so hairless varieties are particularly vulnerable to cold, and tail-less varieties to overheating. Low humidity can occur as a result of overabsorbent bedding materials, such as corncob beddings (Burn and Mason 2005), and may cause ringtail, especially in young rats. Humidity should be monitored and can be raised using a water mister and reduced with dehumidifiers or the enclosure can be relocated to a more suitable location.

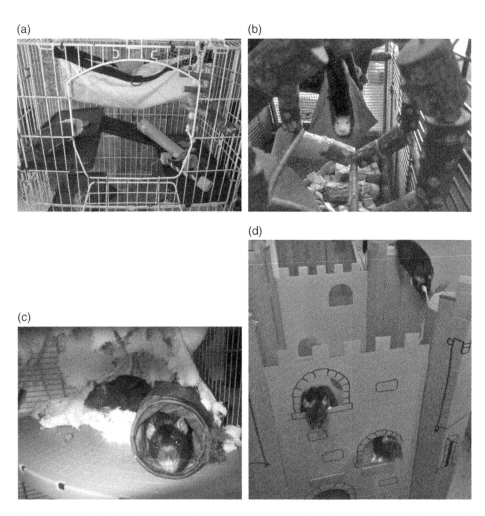

Figure 11.2 (a) A small but complex cage environment; (b) a hammock created from an old jumper; (c) rats utilising a tunnel; (d) a 'castle' to create three-dimensional complexity (*Source:* courtesy of Karen Brady).

Rat enclosures should also not be exposed to draughts, which may lead to pneumonia. However, insufficient ventilation and hygiene can result in the build-up of ammonia from urine and faeces and dust from bedding materials, which can also lead to respiratory infections, as well as to unacceptable levels of carbon dioxide. Rat enclosures should therefore be cleaned out regularly enough to maintain bedding and air quality, while leaving a handful of unsoiled nesting material behind to maintain familiar smells that may help maintain social cohesion (Van Loo et al. 2000). Cleaning should be completely avoided in the few days before and after birth to prevent infanticide (Burn and Mason 2008).

Rats are especially sensitive to light and find it aversive. Long-term exposure to moderate-light intensities or short-term exposure to high-light intensities can also result in retinal degeneration, especially in albino rats (Wasowicz et al. 2002).

Pet rats should therefore be kept away from bright light, including direct sunlight, and always have access to a dark shelter or hiding place. Similarly, unpredictable short- and long-term noise can be stressful (Gesi et al. 2002), and rats need to be kept away from disruptive sources of both nonultrasonic (e.g. building work) and ultrasonic (e.g. some televisions and computer monitors) noise (Sales et al. 1988). Strong scents such as air fresheners or cleaners can also be disruptive.

Rats must be kept mentally as well as physically active. Young rats can climb by 20 days of age and, because of their light body weight, jump and climb around their enclosure, often hanging upside down. Enclosures should include ropes, platforms, ladders, and hammocks. Relaxed and well-handled rats should also be given supervised 'free-range' exploration outside their enclosure in a large exercise pen or room. This area should be safe, inescapable, and filled with objects to explore and space to run and climb. The inclusion of a foraging tray (e.g. a sand-filled tray containing buried treats), a digging arena, and a water bath provide opportunities to express natural behaviours, such as the building of burrows and swimming, helping to maintain physical and mental activity.

11.2.3 Animal Company

Rats seek out and actively demand contact with other rats (Patterson Kane et al. 2002; Figure 11.3), which allows grooming one another, social investigation, huddling, and play, even amongst adults. In comparison, isolation can lead to stress and a more pronounced response to other stressors (Sharp et al. 2002). Manipulating or chasing their own tail is also a form of self-directed behaviour typically only observed in singly housed rats (Hurst et al. 1997). It is thought to be a redirection of social behaviour, with the tail acting as a company surrogate as a way of coping with social isolation (Baenninger 1967).

However, some rats may be anxious in the presence of other individuals. Some rats may 'barber' (bite off) the whiskers of other rats. Barbering can be painful, reduce sensory perception, and lead to bald patches. Aggression can include behaviour such as stand-up 'boxing', wrestling, standing over (by the 'winner'), lying upside down (by the 'loser'), vocalisations, biting, and chasing. Barbering and aggression may be avoided or reduced by providing sufficient resources for all individuals to gain access at the same

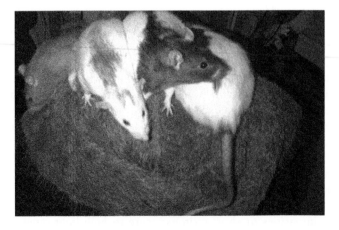

Figure 11.3 Compatible rats engaging in close contact (*Source:* courtesy of Karen Brady).

time, more things to do such as foraging for food and areas for digging, and multiple shelters, bolt holes and visual barriers so that animals can withdraw from unwanted attention (Baumans 2005). If levels of aggression or barbering remain or become high in an established group, then this may indicate that those particular individuals cannot be housed together or a health problem that should be investigated further.

Genuine aggression most commonly occurs between unfamiliar individuals (Wurbel et al. 2009). After an initial period of aggression, a settled social group should show little aggression because each individual knows how to behave appropriately. Rats investigate one another by sniffing others' heads, faces, anogential regions, and urine, particularly when familiar individuals are reintroduced (Meaney and Stewart 1981; Burman and Mendl 1999). This behaviour enables rats to gather a wide range of up-to-date information about other individuals' gender, age, social status, health, diet, oestrus, familiarity, and relatedness (Thom and Hurst 2004). Owners should therefore avoid doing anything that changes a rat's smell. Ideally, individuals should be housed together from a young age so that they grow up together, and disruption of stable social groups should be avoided where possible. Any later introductions should be done over several days under supervision, in a neutral environment (i.e. not introducing one rat into the home enclosure of another) with plenty of hiding places and barriers so that the rats can easily avoid each other. It may help to start off an introduction with an exchange of scent (i.e. a small amount of bedding), before progressing to the actual meeting.

Rat groups should be all of the same sex, after weaning. Differences between males and females are visually identifiable at an early age, with a bigger gap between the urethra and anus in the male than in the female. By sexual maturity after 6 weeks of age, these differences are increasingly obvious, with clearly descended testicles in the males. If bred, breeding pairs should usually be left together after birth because the female releases pheromones that make the father tolerate the pups and show paternal behaviour. If they are separated, it might also be hard to reintroduce them again. Dams may lick, groom, nurse (in various positions), and carry the pups. Pups who stray too far vocalise at ultrasonic frequencies until they are carried back to the nest. Some females show aggression towards other rats or human intruders during the first week after birth (Flannelly and Flannelly 1987), so nests should be disturbed as little as possible.

Other species may be predators. Exposure to the smell or presence of other companion animal species (e.g. dogs, cats) should be avoided because of the likely induction of fear and anxiety (Blanchard et al. 2003). Some other species may be preyed on by rats, such as mice.

11.2.4 Human Interaction

Human company can never substitute for company of rats' own kind. Rats are active at night and sleeping rats are motivated to huddle with another rat for warmth. However, many rats do appear to enjoy 'tickling' in which humans simulate play with their hand, involving repeated gentle pinning and small, rapid finger movements (Burgdorf and Panksepp 2001; see also https://www.youtube.com/watch?v=j-admRGFVNM). Rats may seek, encourage, and initiate tickling bouts and emit large numbers of ultrasonic vocalisations that are believed to indicate pleasure during it. Tickling can be attempted with pet rats, allowing each rat to choose whether to engage in it by actively approaching and seeking it out; it should not be forced on them.

Rats can find handling and restraint stressful, particularly if not used to it or after unpleasant experiences. Owners should encourage rats to approach and then climb onto their hand by using treats, allowing the rat to sniff the hand for a few seconds before being picked up. (Conversely, rough handling can make handling more aversive.) Rats can then be lifted loosely around the middle of the body, just behind the front legs, using the thumb and fingers of one hand while always supporting the body with the other hand. Rats should never be picked up by the tail. Even rats who are relaxed when handled by one person may not be confident when handled by another. Rats may respond differently to different handlers and can remember familiar people for many months (Davis et al. 1997). Rats may also respond differently to being picked up, for example vocalising strongly, when in pain, discomfort, or distress.

Rats are quick learners with excellent memories. They are therefore highly trainable (Davis 1996). For example, they can be trained to climb onto weighing scales, with such interactions under the rat's control. More complex training such as 'rat agility' may also be used as a means of forming a relationship with a pet rat and keeping it mentally occupied. All training should only involve well-timed rewards such as food treats and 'tickling'. The most easily trainable behaviours are usually those that most closely relate to the animal's natural behaviour. It is also impossible to train rats to stop engaging in natural behaviours such as gnawing or scent marking.

11.2.5 Health

Rats can suffer from several diseases (Table 11.2). Respiratory problems are common, particularly mycoplasmal or multibacteria infections caught from other animals through the air, transmitted in the womb or at birth, or passed by humans carrying microorganisms on their hands and clothes (Nicklas et al. 2002). Once infected, rats may remain infected, and disease can be triggered by unsuitable environments (e.g. poor ventilation, inappropriate company, or vitamin deficiencies). Prevention therefore involves good hygiene and quarantine, minimising stress, good ventilation, and appropriate bedding such as compressed paper. Problems are likely to reoccur after treatment unless the underlying triggers are identified and rectified.

Rats can also suffer diarrhoea resulting from bacteria, internal parasites, severe stress, or diet, and severe stresses such as high temperatures and overcrowding can precipitate infections. The disease can lead to rapid dehydration, and treatment should usually include rehydration and veterinary attention. Wild rats can transmit a variety of zoonotic diseases that could be transmitted to pet rats, such as leptospirosis, which may cause no signs in the rats. Good hygiene practice should be followed at all times (i.e. washing hands before and after touching rats or their enclosures). However, the most likely risks to human health from pet rats are probably bites and allergies.

Rats' incisors can overgrow, grow out of line, or grow unevenly because of tooth damage, inappropriate nutrition, bar chewing, and genetic predispositions (Moore 2000), resulting in difficulties with feeding and subsequent weight loss. As well as providing gnawing materials, teeth should be regularly inspected and trimmed by a veterinary surgeon if necessary. Tumours, particularly of the mammary glands, are common in older rats and appear as large lumps beneath the skin. Tumour formation is linked to high dietary fat intake and obesity (Freedman et al. 1990). Although the tumours are usually benign, their rapid growth and location can restrict movement and other behaviour. They can be surgically removed but are often quick to recur.

Table 11.2 Selected health problems in rats.

Condition			Welfare effects
Infectious or parasitic	Viral	Lymphocytic choriomeningitis virus[a]	Malcoordination; paralysis
		Corona-viruses (Parker's rat coronavirus; Sialodacryoadenitis virus)	Possibly no effects or Decreased growth; eye inflammation; photophobia; chromodacryorrhoea; swollen salivary glands; discomfort; difficulty breathing; sneezing
		Infectious diarrhoea of infant rats (IDIR)[a]	Diarrhoea; gastrointestinal ulcers; reduced growth
		Parvovirus	Decreased immunity; infections
		Mice pneumonia virus	Difficulty breathing Decreased immunity; infections
		Reovirus-3	Poor skin or coat condition; damage to multiple organ systems
		RNS-paramyxovirus (Sendai virus)	Decreased immunity; infections Reduced healing Difficulty breathing
		Toolan's and Kilham's rat virus	Decreased immunity; infections; bone problems; liver disease
	Bacterial	*Corynebacterium kutscheri* *Streptobacillis moniliformis*[a]	Joint pain; decreased mobility; respiratory distress
		Mycoplasma pulmonis Cilia-associated respiratory bacillus *(CAR)*	Difficulty breathing; abscesses; neurological signs
		Pasteurella pneumotropica *Streptococcus pneurmoniae*	
		Salmonella typhimurium[a]	Diarrhoea
		Clostridium pitiforme (Tyzzer's disease)	Diarrhoea; malaise; dehydration; neurological problems
		Staphylococcus aureus	Skin ulcers; itchiness; self-mutilation; pain
	Internal parasites	Protozoa *Giardia muris*	No effects or Diarrhoea; weight loss; rectal prolapse
		Spironucleus muris Nematodes (*Aspicularis* spp.; *Syphacia muris*; *S.obvelata*)	
		Tapeworms (*Hymenolepis diminuta*; *Rodentolepis nana*)	
	External parasites	Mites (*Notoedres muris*; *Radfordia affinis*)	Itchiness; pain from self-trauma

(*Continued*)

Table 11.2 (Continued)

Condition		Welfare effects
Neoplastic	Mammary fibroadenomas	Often benign but may cause impaired mobility; skin ulceration and infection
	Pituitary tumours	Depression; loss of appetite; weight loss; malcoordination; seizures; increased thirst (due to diabetes mellitus)
Degenerative or geriatric conditions	Dental disease	Pain; inappetance; weight loss
	Retinal atrophy	Reduced vision; head weaning
	Chronic progressive nephropathy	Weight loss;
Traumatic	Gnawing on cage bars	Tooth damage; dental disease

[a] Zoonotic.

Rats are not normally neutered because they live happily in same-sex social groups, but if rats live in mixed-sex groups, then neutering is necessary to prevent unwanted litters (Table 11.3). Neutering may also reduce the risks of mammary and pituitary tumours (Hotchkiss 1995) and kidney stones (Johnson-Delaney 1998). Given the sensitivity and usefulness of whiskers, trimming of rats' whiskers or selective breeding for whisker deformities (e.g. curly vibrissae in Rex and hairless Sphinx fancy rats) should be avoided, as should harmful mutations, such as the Sphinx and Manx, which can affect the rat's abilities to regulate their body temperatures.

11.2.6 Euthanasia
Acceptable methods of euthanasia of rats are listed in Table 11.4. The best method is usually an overdose of inhaled or intravenously injected anaesthetic. The injection of pentobarbitone into the abdomen may be painful (Svendsen et al. 2007). Rats find carbon dioxide, nitrogen, and argon aversive, so these gases should be avoided for euthanasia (Niel et al. 2008; AVMA 2013). For rats less than 500 g in body weight, neck dislocation can result in an immediate loss of consciousness (Cartner et al. 2007). For rats less than 1 kg, brain concussion can cause immediate unconsciousness, through either striking the head with a blunt instrument or against a solid object with enough force, but because it is not necessarily fatal, neck dislocation should always be carried out subsequently to ensure death.

11.3 Signs of Welfare Problems

11.3.1 Pathophysiological Signs
Chromodacryorrhea (i.e. 'red tears') can be a sign of stress or illness (Mason et al. 2004), with the nasal secretion appearing almost immediately, and ocular secretion generally about 15–30 minutes after the onset of the stressful event (Harkness and

Table 11.3 Nontherapeutic elective surgical procedures performed on rats.

Procedure	Possible animal benefits	Possible owner benefits	Perioperative risks	Behaviour reduced
Castration	Facilitation of social living; Reduction of fighting with other unneutered males	Reduced scent marking; reduced smell	Pain, distress	Breeding; aggression
Spaying	Facilitation of social living Prevention of pregnancy if kept with unneutered males Reduced likelihood of mammary and pituitary tumours and kidney stones	Altered behaviour to humans during oestrus		

Table 11.4 Methods of euthanasia for rats kept as companion animals.

Method	Restraint required	Welfare benefits	Welfare risks
Intravenous or intraperitoneal injection of barbiturate	Secure handling	Rapid loss of consciousness if intravenous	Possible pain at injection site
Inhalation of volatile anaesthetic agent at increasing concentrations	Placement in chamber	Minimal handling No injection	Aversiveness of chemical
Cervical (neck) dislocation (manually or with the use of a rod or bar)[a]	Secure handling	Immediate loss of consciousness and death resulting from physical damage to the brain stem	Pain if procedure done incorrectly Injection or handling if sedation required
Brain concussion using blunt instrument or solid object	Secure handling	Immediate unconsciousness due to brain destruction	Pain if performed incorrectly

Source: AVMA (2013), Cartner et al. (2007), Niel et al. (2008), Svendsen et al. (2007), and Working Party (1997).
[a] Not suitable for rats more than 500 g body weight.

Ridgway 1980). Chromodacryorrhea may also be produced during normal social inter-actions as well as during illness (e.g. respiratory infection). If a small amount is detected, further attention should therefore be paid to see if it reoccurs. Other general physical signs of poor health or welfare include a rough, clumped 'starey' coat, and diarrhoea. Bald patches may indicate barbering behaviour or conditions such as mange. Loss of body weight in an adult rat, slow growth, or reduced food intake can suggest various problems. In fully grown adult rats, unexpected increases in body weight may also be used to monitor potential obesity and tumour formation.

11.3.2 Behavioural Signs

Signs of anxiety include a hesitancy to emerge from secure or familiar environments, increased wall-hugging, increased fear of new things, or exaggerated escape or hiding responses. Continued signs of anxiety suggest recurrent stressors rather than just fear of novelty. Signs of pain or infections such as *Corynebacterium kutscheri* include a hunched or stiff body posture, reduced activity, decreased grooming or reduced appe-tite, abnormal gait, malcoordination, guarding of a body part, or increased aggression (Roughan and Flecknell 2003). However, aggression needs to be differentiated from play. In general, aggression is usually unidirectional and unwanted by the victim, whereas during play encounters, both rats appear to actively seek out, approach, and engage in play behaviour. Rats playing usually target the nape of the neck, with the fur remaining sleek and flat, unlike genuine aggression when the target is the rump and the fur may be raised (Pellis and Pellis 1987). True aggression may reflect underlying stress-ors for the aggressor or barber, particularly an unsuitable environment or company.

Audible vocalisations can be emitted in response to pain and anxiety. Hence, if a well-handled and usually quiet rat were to vocalise strongly when picked up, then it may suggest that the animal is in some discomfort or distress. Ultrasonic vocalisations may be of two main types. Vocalisations of around 50 kHz may indicate pleasure (Knutson et al. 2002). Vocalisations of around 22 kHz may indicate an unpleasant emotional state and tend to be produced in situations such as aggression, predator presence, startle, and pain (Litvin et al. 2007). For humans to hear these vocalisations requires the use of special-ised – but often affordable – equipment such as bat detectors.

Barbering of themselves or others may suggest social incompatibility, insufficient hiding places, nesting material, resting sites, or enrichments. Tail manipulation may sug-gest a lack of social interaction (Hurst et al. 1998). Bar biting or chewing may represent a frustrated attempt to escape the home cage (Hurst et al. 1999), thereby indicating an underlying social or environmental problem. These behaviours may occur mostly at night (although some owners may indirectly notice differences in cage bar appearance). The absence of abnormal behaviour therefore does not necessarily imply that all is sat-isfactory in terms of health and welfare.

11.4 Worldwide Action Plan for Improving Rat Welfare

Rats are highly intelligent, sociable, and interactive animals, and provided that their needs are met, they can form close human-animal relationships. Potential owners should be educated about the range of rats' needs, and rats should not be sold as individuals but rather as established single-sex pairs or groups. Breeders should also be educated and encouraged to ensure that new 'fancy rat' varieties should not be promoted unless they have excellent general health and welfare and that selective breeding should focus on improving long-term rat health (e.g. targeting the reduction of tumour formation in aged rats) and educating their customers about the full range of pet rat needs. Owners should also be encouraged to keep a close eye on the behaviour of their pet rats to identify any problems and seek veterinary or other assistance early on.

Bibliography

AVMA (American Veterinary Medical Association). (2013). AVMA Guidelines for the Euthanasia of Animals: 2013 Edition. Available at https://www.avma.org/KB/Policies/Pages/Euthanasia-Guidelines.aspx. Accessed 7 October 2015.

Baenninger, L.P. (1967). Comparison of behavioural development in socially isolated and grouped rats. *Animal Behaviour* 15: 312–323.

Baumans, V. (2005). Environmental enrichment for laboratory rodents and rabbits: requirements of rodents, rabbits, and research. *ILAR Journal* 46: 162–170.

Berdoy, M. (2002). The Laboratory Rat: A Natural History. Film. 27 minutes. www.ratlife.org.

Blanchard, D.C., Griebel, G., and Blanchard, R.J. (2003). Conditioning and residual emotionality effects of predator stimuli: some reflections on stress and emotion. *Progress in Neuro-Psychopharmacology and Biological Psychiatry* 27: 1177–1185.

Burgdorf, J. and Panksepp, J. (2001). Tickling induces reward in adolescent rats. *Physiology & Behavior* 72: 167–173.

Burman, O.H.P. and Mendl, M. (1999). The effects of environmental context on laboratory rat social recognition. *Animal Behaviour* 58: 629–634.

Burn, C.C. (2008). What is it like to be a rat? Rat sensory perception and its implications for experimental design and rat welfare. *Applied Animal Behaviour Science* 112: 1–32.

Burn, C.C. and Mason, G.J. (2005). Absorbencies of six different rodent beddings: commercially advertised absorbencies are potentially misleading. *Laboratory Animals* 39: 68–74.

Burn, C.C. and Mason, G.J. (2008). Effects of cage-cleaning frequencies on rat reproductive performance, infanticide, and welfare. *Applied Animal Behaviour Science* 114: 235–247.

Burton, M.J., Cooper, S.J., and Popplewell, D.A. (1981). The effect of fenfluramine on the microstructure of feeding and drinking in the rat. *British Journal of Pharmacology* 72: 621–633.

Cartner, S., Barlow, S., and Ness, T. (2007). Loss of cortical function in mice after decapitation, cervical dislocation, potassium chloride injection, and CO2 inhalation. *Comparative Medicine* 57: 570–573.

Davidson, M. K., Schoeb, T. R., & Davis, J. K. (2000). Rats and mice: Bacterial and mycotic diseases.

Davis, H. (1996). Underestimating the rat's intelligence. *Cognitive Brain Research* 3: 291–298.

Davis, H., Talor, A.A., and Norris, C. (1997). Preference for familiar humans by rats. *Psychonomic Bulletin and Review* 4: 118–120.

Denenberg, V.H., Taylor, R.E., and Zarrow, M.X. (1969). Maternal behavior in the rat: an investigation and quantification of nest building. *Behaviour* 34: 1–16.

Flannelly, K.J. and Flannelly, L. (1987). Time course of postpartum aggression in rats (rattus norvegicus). *Journal of Comparative Psychology* 101: 101–103.

Freedman, L.S., Clifford, C., and Messina, M. (1990). Analysis of dietary fat, calories, body weight, and the development of mammary tumors in rats and mice: a review. *Cancer Research* 50: 5710–5719.

Galef, B.G. Jr. and Whiskin, E.E. (2003). Preference for novel flavors in adult Norway rats (Rattus norvegicus). *Journal of Comparative Psychology* 117: 96–100.

Gesi, M., Lenzi, P., Alessandri, M.G. et al. (2002). Brief and repeated noise exposure produces different morphological and biochemical effects in noradrenaline and adrenaline cells of adrenal medulla. *Journal of Anatomy* 200: 159–168.

Harkness, J.E. and Ridgway, M.D. (1980). Chromodacryorrhea in laboratory rats (Rattus norvegicus): etiologic considerations. *Laboratory Animal Science* 30: 841–844.

Hilscher-Conklin, C. (1996). Rattus biologicus: The Dometication of the Rat. Rat and Mouse Gazette (July/August). Available at http://www.rmca.org/Articles/domestication.htm. Accessed 18 November 2015.

Himsel, C.A. (1991). *Rats – a Complete Pet Owner's Manual*. Barron's Educational Series, Inc.

Hotchkiss, C.E. (1995). Effect of surgical removal of subcutaneous tumors on survival of rats. *Journal of the American Veterinary Medical Association* 206 (10): 1575–1579.

Hurst, J.L., Barnard, C.J., Nevison, C.M., and West, C.D. (1997). Housing and welfare in laboratory rats: welfare implications of isolation and social contact among caged males. *Animal Welfare* 6: 329–347.

Hurst, J.L., Barnard, C.J., Nevison, C.M., and West, C.D. (1998). Housing and welfare in laboratory rats: the welfare implications of social isolation and social contact among females. *Animal Welfare* 7: 121–136.

Hurst, J.L., Barnard, C.J., Tolladay, U. et al. (1999). Housing and welfare in laboratory rats: effects of cage stocking density and behavioural predictors of welfare. *Animal Behaviour* 58: 563–586.

IUCN (2016). IUCN Red List of Threatened Species. Available at https://www.iucn.org/theme/species/our-work/iucn-red-list-threatened-species. Accessed 22 August 2016.

Johnson-Delaney, C.A. (1998). Diseases of the urinary system of rats and mice. *Exotic Pet Practice* 3 (9): 65–68.

Kelly, J.B. and Masterton, B. (1977). Auditory sensitivity of the albino rat. *Journal of Comparative and Physiological Psychology* 91: 930–936.

Knutson, B., Burgdorf, J., and Panksepp, J. (2002). Ultrasonic vocalizations as indices of affective states in rats. *Psychological Bulletin* 128: 961–977.

Litvin, Y., Blanchard, D.C., and Blanchard, R.J. (2007). Rat 22kHz ultrasonic vocalizations as alarm cries. *Behavioural Brain Research* 182: 166–172.

Mason, G., Wilson, D., Hampton, C., and Wurbel, H. (2004). Non-invasively assessing disturbance and stress in laboratory rats by scoring chromodacryorrhoea. *Alternatives to Laboratory Animals* 32: 153–159.

McGivern, R.F., Henschel, D., Hutcheson, M., and Pangburn, T. (1996). Sex difference in daily consumption of water by rats: effect of housing and hormones. *Physiology and Behaviour* 59: 653–658.

McIntyre, A., Gibson, P.R., and Young, G.P. (1993). Butyrate production from dietary fibre and protection against large bowel cancer in a rat model. *Gut* 34: 386–391.

Meaney, M.J. and Stewart, J. (1981). A descriptive study of social-development in the rat (rattus-norvegicus). *Animal Behaviour* 29: 34–45.

Moore, D.M. (2000). *Rats and mice: Biology, Laboratory Animal Medicine and Science, Series II*. University of Washington.

Nicklas, W., Baneux, P., Boot, R. et al. (2002). Recommendations for the health monitoring of rodent and rabbit colonies in breeding and experimental units. *Laboratory Animals* 36: 20–42.

Niel, L., Stewart, S., and Weary, D. (2008). Effect of flow rate on aversion to gradual-fill carbon dioxide exposure in rats. *Applied Animal Behaviour Science* 109: 77–84.

Patterson Kane, E.G., Hunt, M., and Harper, D.N. (2002). Rats demand social contact. *Animal Welfare* 11: 327–332.

Pellis, S.M. and Pellis, V.C. (1987). Play-fighting differs from serious fighting in both target of attack and tactics of fighting in the laboratory rat Rattus-norvegicus. *Aggressive Behavior* 13: 227–242.

Pet Food Manufacturers' Association (PFMA). (2018). Pet population 2018. Available at https://www.pfma.org.uk/pet-population-2018. Accessed 2 July 2018.

Rao, P.B., Metta, V.C., and Johnson, B.C. (1959). The amino acid composition and the nutritive value of proteins. I. Essential amino acid requirements of the growing rat. *The Journal of Nutrition* 69: 387–391.

Reddy, B.S. and Maeura, Y. (1984). Tumor formation by dietary fat in Azoxymethane-induced colon carcinogensis in female F344 rats: influence of amount and source of dietary fat. *Journal of the National Cancer Institute* 72: 745–750.

Reeves, P. (1997). Components of the AIN-93 diets as improvements in the AIN-76A diet. *Journal of Nutrition* 127: 838S–841S.

Richardson, V.C.G. (1997). *Diseases of Small Domestic Rodents*. Blackwell Science Ltd.

Roughan, J.V. and Flecknell, P.A. (2003). Evaluation of a short duration behaviour-based post-operative pain scoring system in rats. *European Journal of Pain* 7: 397–406.

Royer, N. (2015). The History of Fancy Rats. American Fancy Rat & Mouse Association. Available at http://www.afrma.org/historyrat.htm. Accessed 24 August 2018.

Sales, G.D., Wilson, K.J., Spencer, K.E., and Milligan, S.R. (1988). Environmental ultrasound in laboratories and animal houses: a possible cause for concern in the welfare and use of laboratory animals. *Laboratory Animals* 22: 369–375.

Sharp, J.L., Zammit, T.G., Azar, T.A., and Lawson, D.M. (2002). Stress-like responses to common procedures in male rats housed alone or with other rats. *Contemporary Topics in Laboratory Animal Science* 41: 8–14.

Svendsen, O., Kok, L., and Lauritzenã, B. (2007). Nociception after intraperitoneal injection of a sodium pentobarbitone formulation with and without lidocaine in rats quantified by expression of neuronal c-Fos in the spinal cord – a preliminary study. *Laboratory Animals* 41: 197–203.

Thom, M.D. and Hurst, J.L. (2004). Individual recognition by scent. *Annales Zoologici Fennici* 41: 756–787.

Trut, L.N., Iliushina, I.Z., Prasolova, L.A., and Kim, A.A. (1997). The hooded allele and selection of wild Norway rats rattus norvegicus for behavior. *Genetika* 33: 1155–1161.

Valle, F.P. (1970). Effects of strain, sex, and illumination on open-field behavior of rats. *American Journal of Psychology* 83: 103–111.

Van Loo, P.L.P., Kruitwagen, C.L.J.J., Van Zutphen, L.F.M. et al. (2000). Modulation of aggression in male mice: influence of cage cleaning regime and scent marks. *Animal Welfare* 9: 281–295.

Wasowicz, M., Morice, C., Ferrari, P. et al. (2002). Long-term effects of light damage on the retina of albino and pigmented rats. *Investigative Ophthalmology and Visual Science* 43: 813–820.

Williams, D.L. (2002). Ocular disease in rats: a review. *Veterinary Ophthalmology* 5: 183–191.

Wolfensohn, S. (1998). *Handbook of Laboratory Animal Management and Welfare*, 2e. London; Malden, MA: Blackwell Science.

Working Party (1997). Recommendations for euthanasia of experimental animals: working party report. *Laboratory Animals* 31: 1–32.

Wurbel, H., Burn, C.C., and Latham, N.R. (2009). The behaviour of laboratory mice and rats. In: *The Ethology of Domestic Animals* (ed. P. Jensen), 217. CABI.

Ungulates (*Ungulata*)

12

James Yeates and Paul McGreevy

12.1 History and Context

12.1.1 Natural History

Ungulata is a mammalian group that includes the two orders of the odd-toed and even-toed ungulates (Table 12.1). 'Ungulates' means 'hooved', and pet species all have hooves of some form. Most are therefore ground dwelling, occupying a range of terrestrial habitats including high altitude mountains, forests, and deserts and often covering large distances.

Most pet ungulate species are herbivorous. Odd-toed ungulates are usually hind-gut fermenters, whereas even-toed ungulates are usually fore-gut fermenters (e.g. ruminants). In both cases, large proportions of their diet are usually made up of grasses (e.g. sheep and cows), shrubs and leaves (e.g. goats and deer), nuts and roots (e.g. boar). A few species are omnivorous (e.g. boar). Their hooves make manual manipulation difficult, and many have prehensile tongues and lips with which to select and consume foods, as well as to manipulate other objects. They spend many hours each day foraging. For example, goats spend considerable time browsing, whereas sheep may spend more time grazing. Some are particularly active at dawn and dusk; others are more active by day.

Companion Animal Care and Welfare: The UFAW Companion Animal Handbook,
First Edition. Edited by James Yeates.
© 2019 Universities Federation for Animal Welfare. Published 2019 by John Wiley & Sons Ltd.

Table 12.1 Examples of ungulate species.

Order	Family	Examples
Odd-toed (Perissodactyla)	Equidae	Horse (*Equus caballus*; Chapter 13)
		Donkey (*Equus africanus asinus*)
Even-toed (Arteriodactyla)	Bovidae	Domestic cattle (*Bos taurus*)
		Domestic zebu (*Bos indicus*)
		Domestic goat (*Capra aegagrus hircus*)
		Domestic sheep (*Ovis aries*)
	Camelidae	Alpaca (*Vicugna pacos*)[a]
		Llama (*Lama glama*)
		Bactrian (*Camelus bactrianus*)
		Dromedary (*Camelus dromedarius*)
	Cervidae	Muntjac deer (*Muntiacus puntoensis*)
		Reindeer (*Rangifer tarandus*)
	Suidae	Domestic pig (*Sus scrofa domesticus*)
		Collared peccary (*Pecari tajacu*)

[a] Alpacas are sometimes categories within the Lama genus.

All ungulates are naturally prey species, often with keen senses of smell, vision, and hearing, although the key senses vary (e.g. pigs use vision relatively little). Many ungulates are naturally social, which can help in protection from predators (Estevez et al. 2007). For example, pigs' wild counterparts live in small family groups, bachelor groups or single males; and feral goats live in groups ranging from a few individuals up to several hundreds (Shackleton and Shank 1984; Miranda-de la Lama and Mattiello 2010). Offspring may stay with their mother for significant periods (e.g. kids until around 1 year old; Miranda-de la Lama and Mattiello 2010). Although pigs and goats are sometimes characterised as active and inquisitive (and 'capricious') and cattle and sheep as more passive (and 'sheepish'), individuals vary in personality, and the young of many species are quite active, inquisitive, and playful.

Communication can involve visible posturing, noises such as foot stamping, smells from scent marking and musk glands, and pheromones, which are particularly sensed during the 'flehmen' behaviour in many male ungulates. Many ungulates also have horns (usually permanent) or antlers (usually shed annually), which may be used in defence and fighting. However, social structures limit conflicts outside of meetings between unfamiliar animals.

12.1.2 Domestic History

Several ungulate species were probably amongst the earliest domesticated, perhaps because of their sociability, large sizes, and reproductive successfulness. For example, goats may have been first kept around 8000 to 9000 BCE and perhaps in both Asia and the Middle East (Zeder and Hesse 2000; Luikart et al. 2001). Most domestic species have been farmed for meat (e.g. pork and lamb), milk (e.g. goats' and cows'), leather, and fibre (e.g. wool, mohair, and cashmere). Some ungulates are also used for traction and transportation (e.g. cattle and camelids), particularly in agriculture, commerce, and leisure and a small number in laboratory research.

Ungulates are generally bred in captivity. Within the farming sector, traditional breeding has selected for tameness and productivity, in particular greater yields of milk, fibre, or offspring, faster growth, and larger body weights. The wild relatives of some ungulates may now be considered as different strains or species; for example, domestic pigs are probably descended from the European wild boar (*Sus scrofa*) and donkeys from the African wild ass (*Equus africanus*). Selection for farming, traction, and research has also created some hybrids (e.g. mules), variations such as hornless breeds (e.g. polled goats). and local traditional breeds of many species. Although mainstream agriculture uses a more restricted genepool, many traditional breeds are kept for particular products or showing. In a few cases, there has been some selection for pet varieties, often in smaller sizes (e.g. pygmy goats). Using pigs as an example: the normal adult pig body weight of farmed pigs is around 200–300 kg; traditional selection has also bred 'miniature' breeds such as the Vietnamese Pot-Bellied weighing around 35–70 kg; laboratory research has bred strains such as Goettingen pigs weighing around 40 kg; and pet breeders have recently bred so-called 'minipigs'.

12.2 Principles of Ungulates Care

12.2.1 Diets

Pet ungulates may be herbivorous or omnivorous, although both usually obtain the majority of their nutrition from plant sources. Insufficient nutrition may occur when pasture is overgrazed (Figure 12.1) or indoor animals are not provided with enough food.

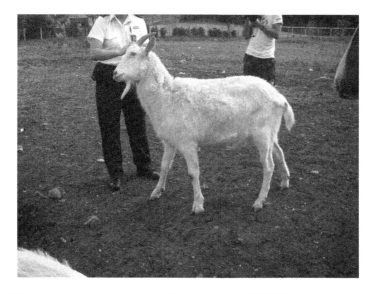

Figure 12.1 Goat in overgrazed pasture (*Source:* courtesy RSPCA).

(b)

(a)

(c)

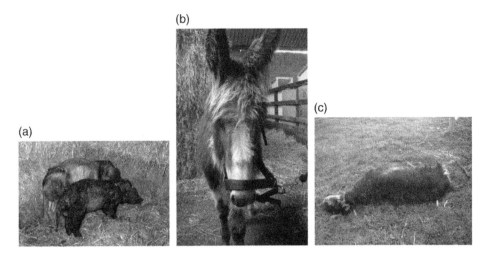

Figure 12.2 Emaciated (a) pigs; (b) donkey, and (c) goat (deceased) (*Source:* courtesy RSPCA).

This can lead to starvation (Figure 12.2), ketosis or acidosis, which can also sometimes occur when pregnancy reduces how much space there is for food in the rumen. Different species may also be susceptible to deficiencies, for example of calcium, cobalt, copper, iodine, magnesium, selenium, zinc, and vitamins A, B, and E. Although much plant material may contain limited energy, many ungulates can extract enough nutrition from low-energy plants or forage, if they are provided with sufficient quantities and allowed to select preferred foods and waste the rest (e.g. goats).

Additional concentrated foods are not normally necessary but may be beneficial during periods of increased nutritional demands. For example, breeds selected for high milk production may need additional protein and calcium during lactation. However, excessive nutrients can lead to obesity, acidosis, metabolic syndromes, or intestinal problems. Large or ruminant ungulates' are difficult to accurately weigh because of their size and because the weight of the rumen's contents can vary enormously. Owners should monitor each animal's body condition by sight and by feeling the animal's muscle and fat deposits, particular around the body prominences of the spine and pelvis.

Many ungulates spend considerable parts of their day (and night) engaged in foraging. For example, pigs may spend 54% of daylight hours foraging (Rodríguez-Estévez et al. 2009) and some overnight (Hyun et al. 1997). Without adequate opportunities to forage, some ungulates may chew nonfood items such as household objects (and, in commercial settings, one another's tails). This motivation may be increased by curiosity, a lack of stimulation, poor nutrition (e.g. insufficient protein or salt), genetic predispositions, frustration from lack of access to food or water, or a lack of material for foraging or rooting. Owners should ensure animals spend plenty of time foraging and feeding. Many need a large proportion of their diet to be provided by grazing, browsing, or foraging long-fibre plant material such as live or cut grass. Fibre can increase animals' feeding time (Meunier-Salaün et al. 2001) and satiety (Rushen et al. 1999; Ramonet et al. 2000).

Ungulates should also be allowed to perform feeding behaviour suitable for their species. This may include both grazing from the floor and browsing from higher food (e.g. goats and llamas). It may also include rooting and moving food around (e.g. pigs: Stolba and Woodgush 1989), and owners should ensure such animals have sufficient substrates such as earth or straw in which to forage and root (e.g. pigs, Fraser et al. 1991; Beattie et al. 1998; Hulbert and McGlone 2006). Some ungulates may also use puzzle-feeders such as balls filled with food (e.g. pigs, Ernst et al. 2005). At the same time, care should be taken to ensure that ungulates are not able to reach anything that may be poisonous (e.g. poisonous plants) or damaging (e.g. goats may eat twine).

Inadequate water provision can lead to problems such as salt poisoning. Although minimum water requirements have been formulated for several species in farm conditions, all ungulates should be given free unlimited access to fresh, clean water.

12.2.2 Environments

Ungulates need adequately large and complex spaces to allow each to meet their basic biological needs (Figure 12.3), including both basic behaviour (e.g. lying down) and behaviour needing much larger areas to explore, play, engage in social interactions, and escape threats, which is likely to require a large area of many metres width and length. Many ungulates also need sufficient height to rise up fully and to climb and jump when motivated (e.g. goats).

Ungulates usually need to be kept contained and provided with shelter, and different methods have advantages and disadvantages. Ungulates should not be tethered as an

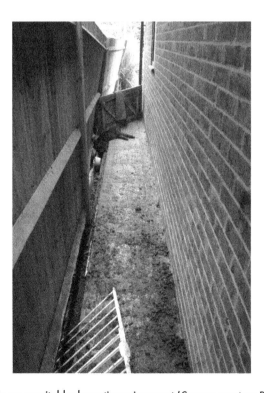

Figure 12.3 Pig in an unsuitable domestic environment (*Source:* courtesy RSPCA).

alternative to fencing, particularly because it limits animals' ability to interact socially and avoid threats (e.g. dogs) and risks entanglement. Throughout the year, ungulates need sheltered areas to avoid inclement weather, sunlight, and insects. Shelters should have adequate ventilation and bedding for comfort and should be located to avoid excessive poaching of the ground. They should provide enough space for all animals to lie down together or multiple shelters to allow animals to lie separately, depending on the animals' preferences and to avoid competition for resources. Pigs should also be provided with showers or the opportunity to wallow to cool off. Unsuitable flooring, especially if too rough or slippery, can lead to bursitis (Mouttotou et al. 1998; Gillman et al. 2008) and lameness (Jorgensen 2003). Several ungulates may also be motivated to roll on the floor (e.g. camelids) or scratch, for example on brushes or plants (e.g. cows).

Bedding can provide additional thermal comfort when animals are lying down (Tuyttens 2005), although some animals may prefer less insulating floors in warmer ambient temperatures (e.g. pigs: Fraser 1985). Bedding can also reduce injuries and unwanted behaviours (e.g. pigs: Gentry et al. 2002; Guy et al. 2002; Van de Weerd et al. 2006) or lameness (e.g. pigs, Kilbride et al. 2007). Bedding should be of good quality and mould-free, and both bedding and pasture need to be managed to avoid a build-up of pathogens or parasites. Ungulates may choose a particular area to use for toileting, which should usually be separate from their feeding area.

Ungulates are often motivated to explore, interact with their environment, and play. Insufficient opportunities may lead to frustration or boredom (e.g. pigs, Fraser et al. 1991) or to exploratory behaviour being redirected to the environment or to injuring one another (e.g. pigs: Wood-gush and Vestergaard 1993; Petersen et al. 1995). Opportunities should therefore be provided by more complex environments (e.g. raised areas for goats), substrates for exploration, toys, and objects to manipulate or destroy. Providing such opportunities can mean animals are more active (e.g. pigs: Guy et al. 2002; Scott et al. 2006) and improve their resilience to stress (Hillman et al. 2003). Toys may be less attractive if they are damaged, dirty, or older (e.g. pigs, Grandin and Curtis 1984a, 1984b; Blackshaw et al. 1997; Scott et al. 2006; Docking et al. 2008), although ungulates can also be fearful of some unfamiliar objects (e.g. pigs: Murphy et al. 2014; lambs, Désiré et al. 2004, 2006).

Transportation can cause stress (e.g. pigs, Warriss 1998; Von Borell and Schäffer 2005; Johnson et al. 2013), especially at the start and during longer journeys. Pigs appear to be particularly sensitive to travel sickness and should not be transported within four hours after eating.

12.2.3 Animal Company

Many ungulates are social animals. They may form particular bonds with specific individuals, grooming, nosing, licking, and staying close to one another. Such positive social interactions may 'buffer' against stress (e.g. sheep, Porter et al. 1995; cows, Mounier et al. 2006). In comparison, social isolation (Figure 12.4) can lead to increased cortisol concentrations and vocalisations (e.g. goats, Boivin and Braadstad 1996; Kannan et al. 2002). In many cases, ungulates should be kept with the company of their own kind, in groups that are appropriately sized, well structured, and stable.

However, incompatible company can also cause bullying, competition, aggression, and injuries from hooves, horns, antlers, or teeth. Some behaviours such as mouthing or

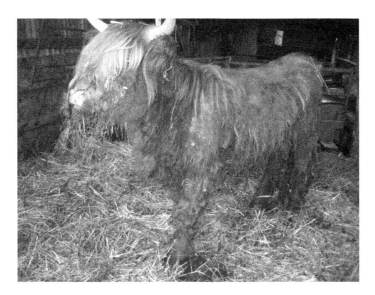

Figure 12.4   Isolated highland cow (*Source:* courtesy RSPCA).

mounting one another may be normal (e.g. pigs and cows) but can cause injuries if excessive. Risks of competition and aggression are likely to be higher if ungulates are overcrowded, underresourced, unable to escape, unfamiliar, or poorly introduced (e.g. the first week for pigs, Arey 1999). Owners should therefore ensure animals are adequately socialised and compatible (e.g. not mixing horned and hornless animals). Groups need enough resources, spaced out to reduce competition and poaching of the ground, as well as escape routes and barriers to avoid one another or during any confrontations. In some cases, unfamiliar animals may accept one another better if they are younger (e.g. crias – young camelids) or by the use of maternal pheromones (e.g. pigs: McGlone and Anderson 2002).

Some ungulates may choose to interact with animals of different species (e.g. llamas with sheep, Cavalcanti and Knowleton 1998). However, consideration should be given to the risk that species might bully or injure one another, carry infections, or parasites that can be transmitted between them. Ungulates should usually be separated from predator animals whose presence can cause fear or injury, such as dogs.

12.2.4 Human Interactions

Some ungulates may form positive relationships with humans, especially if they are hand-reared (e.g. pigs, Terlouw and Porcher 2005). However, human presence and handling can cause acute and chronic fear (Hemsworth et al. 1981; Coleman et al. 1998; Waiblinger et al. 2006). Deer can suffer fatal muscle degeneration, respiratory distress, and hyperthermia. Fearful ungulates can also injure humans or themselves, risk factors including their size, hooves, horns, and antlers. Individual ungulates can react to humans very differently (e.g. cows and pigs, Hemsworth et al. 1994, 1996a, 1996b; Marchant et al. 2001), depending on the animals' early life experiences (e.g. sheep, Hargreaves and Huston 1990; cows, Boivin et al. 1994), genetics (e.g. some dairy cow bloodlines appear very quiet and tolerant of humans), reproductive status, whether the animals have been castrated (e.g. llamas, Grossman an Kutzler 2007), and on the humans' behaviour.

Owners should be consistent and confident and provide positive interactions wherever possible (e.g. pigs, Gonyou et al. 1986; Hemsworth et al. 1986, 1987; Tanida et al. 1995). They should avoid fast, unexpected movements; hitting, slapping, or pushing (Hemsworth et al. 1989; Coleman et al. 1998); shouting (e.g. cows, Pajor et al. 2000) and lifting animals by the coat, horns, ears, legs, or tail. Some ungulates can be trained to tolerate halters, stocks, 'crushes' or chutes. Pigs may pull back on a rope placed behind their canines, and so remain still, although this may be aversive and minpigs may often instead jump or turn. Ungulates may be more willing to move along corridors without any unfamiliar objects or dark areas, or if they are following another animal, their social group, or a familiar human carrying food.

12.2.5 Health

Some diseases are common to several ungulate species, many of which affect their hooves, teeth, gastrointestinal tracts, or mammary glands. Infections include viruses (e.g. Foot and Mouth Disease and Maedi-visna); bacteria (e.g. *Clostridium* spp., *Mycobacteria,* and *Pastuerella*); internal parasites (e.g. intestinal worms, flukes, lungworms, and protozoa); and external parasites (e.g. lice and mites), some of which may transmit other diseases (e.g. tick-borne Anaplasmosis and insect-borne bluetongue). Some conditions are potentially zoonotic conditions spread through faeces, pasteurised milk, or aborted material, such as borelliosis, brucellosis, campylobacter, colibacillosis (*Escherichia coli*), cryptosporidiosis, enzootic abortion, leptospirosis, listeriosis, louping ill, orf, pox virus, ringworm, salmonellosis, toxoplasmosis, and tuberculosis. Anecdotally, some pet breeds are predisposed to certain conditions; for example, Vietnamese pot-bellied pigs to dry skin and inverted eyelids, and pygmy goats to a particular skin disease. All new pets should be checked, quarantined, and given preventative parasite control and vaccination where appropriate and legally permitted.

All ungulates should receive regular health checks, from specialist veterinary surgeons where possible and appropriate (Table 12.2). Some ungulates may need their hooves trimmed if they are not subject to sufficient wear during locomotion (Figure 12.5). They should be identified using microchipping or tagging (and in compliance with local laws). Castration may improve handling and avoid unwanted litters. Other procedures, such as disbudding, tail docking, teeth clipping, and nose ringing may reduce damage to humans, property, or other animals. However, such procedures can cause considerable distress, pain, and later problems including tail neuromas (e.g. pigs), damage to the scent glands behind the horns (e.g. goats), or meningoencephalitis if done badly (e.g. calves). Good pet husbandry, handling, and company should mean these procedures are unnecessary, except for hoof and dental care, identification, castration, and disbudding (where appropriate). All should be performed only by veterinary surgeons on pet animals under anaesthesia and with adequate, safe painkillers.

12.2.6 Euthanasia

The best methods of euthanasia of ungulates are usually sedation if needed, followed by either intravenous anaesthetic overdose (e.g. pentobarbitone into the jugular vein) or brain trauma, such as shooting or using a captive bolt (Table 12.3). All methods should

Table 12.2 Examples of veterinary specialisations relevant to ungulates kept as companion animals (see also Chapter 1).

Recognising organisation	Example veterinary specialties
American Veterinary Medical Association	American Board of Veterinary Practitioners in Equine Practice
European Board of Veterinary Specialisation	European College of Equine Internal Medicine
	European College of Veterinary Surgeons (Large Animal Surgery)
	European College of Porcine Health Management
	European College of Small Ruminant Health Management
Australian and New Zealand College of Veterinary Scientists	Australian and New Zealand College of Veterinary Scientists: Equine Chapter
United Kingdom (RCVS)	RCVS Recognised Specialists in Camelid health and production
	RCVS Recognised Specialists in Cattle Health and Production
	RCVS Recognised Specialists in Equine Surgery/Medicine/Gastroenterology
	RCVS Recognised Specialists in Pig Medicine
	RCVS Recognised Specialists in Sheep health and production

RCVS, Royal College of Veterinary Surgeons.

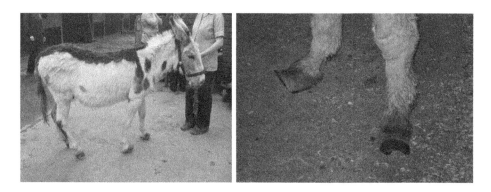

Figure 12.5 Donkey with overgrown and misshapen hooves (Source: courtesy RSPCA).

Table 12.3 Methods of euthanasia for (some) ungulates kept as companion animals.

Method	Restraint required	Welfare benefits	Welfare risks
Anaesthetic overdose injected into a vein	Restraint or handling for vein access Sedation advised	Fast	Minor pain of injection Pain from chemical in tissues if vein missed
Head or brain trauma (e.g. captive bolt or free bullet)	Restraint of head and body to ensure accuracy (where possible)	Instantaneous prevention of any experiences	Severe pain if inaccurate

avoid injury to humans or others, particularly from ricocheting free bullets or struggling or falling ungulates. Some ungulates may be killed for meat, which may involve transport and slaughter.

12.3 Signs of Ungulate Welfare

12.3.1 Pathophysiological signs
Stress hormones are used commonly to test animal's stress responses in experimental situations, but are less useful for routine assessment of pets' welfare. Similarly, on-farm welfare assessments use measures such as mortality, productivity, growth rate, and particular health problems that commonly occur in farming, but these may not be useful for individual pets kept in very different circumstances. Nevertheless, body weight and body condition can still be useful measures of general condition. Skin lesions towards the front of the body and flanks may indicate aggression (Geverink et al. 1996; Turner et al. 2006). Other measures such as heart and respiration rate, urination, and defaecation may also indicate stress or excitement.

12.3.2 Behavioural Signs
Many types of behaviour observed in farmed animals may be useful indicators in pet ungulates (Table 12.4). For example, excessive nosing or sucking one another, mounting, fighting, biting the environment, or drinking may indicate a lack of enrichment or stress either at the time of during earlier development (e.g. early weaning). Escape attempts, freezing, kicking, spitting, and elimination may indicate distress. A lack of activity or engagement may indicate apathy as a result poor environmental conditions (e.g. dog sitting in pigs, Guy et al. 2002). Owners might also assess ungulates' overall welfare qualitatively (e.g. pigs: Wemelsfelder et al. 2000).

Ungulates may also vocalise to express a variety of feelings, including grunting, barking (e.g. pigs), squealing, snorting, bleating, sneezing (e.g. goats), braying (e.g. donkeys), humming, clicking, screeching, and orgling (e.g. alpacas). Some ungulates also stamp as an alarm or threat. Signs of social or environmental disruption may include altered

Table 12.4 Key behavioural signs of possible welfare compromises in ungulates.

Aspect of behaviour	Specific responses	Example potential welfare issues
Altered activity or responsiveness	Increased vigilance or activity Attention to particular threats Startling Reaction on palpation or withdrawal of body part from contact Lethargy, immobility, decreased mobility (e.g. less movement or play)	Fear, agitation, pain, illness
Avoidance	Standing still or 'freezing' Escape attempts during handling Flight (running) Avoiding particular areas	Fear, uncertainty, previous unpleasant experiences
Altered posture or expression	Altered head, neck, body, tail, or ear position Tail flicks	Fear, pain, irritation, aggression
Altered metabolic processes and maintenance or other common behaviour	Increased respiratory rate Reduced appetite Trembling Wide pupils or showing white parts of the eyes Increased urination or defecation Increased grooming Altered time spent resting or sleeping	Fear, distress, stress, heat, fatigue, pain, itchiness, illness
Altered interactions with the environment	Manipulating environmental objects Altered social interactions (e.g. increased nosing or sucking one another, mounting and aggression)	Stress, lack of stimulation, hunger, social stress
Vocalisations	Social calls (e.g. lowing, bleats, whinnying) Stamping	Fear or threats, signalling, social separation
Attack or preattack behaviours	Biting, kicking, or spitting	Fear, pain, aggression
Specific local signs of local pain	Hunched back or tucked up abdomen Rigid posture Biting or scratching a specific area Lameness	Pain

All behavioural responses may also indicate other welfare issues than those listed; and the absence of any particular sign in any individual does not mean they are not experiencing that welfare compromise.

social interactions, such as increased mounting, decreased play, and aggression (e.g. pigs: De Jong et al. 1996; Haskell et al. 1996; Colson et al. 2012; Hintze et al. 2013; Rydhmer et al. 2013). Play may be indicated by waving or tossing of the head, scampering, jumping, hopping, pawing, pivots, flops, gambolling, shaking, or carrying an object and, for social play, pushing another pig, biting or lifting another pig, and self-handicapping postures (e.g. pigs: Murphy et al. 2014).

12.4 Action Plan for Improving Ungulate Welfare Worldwide

Many ungulate species are large, social herbivores, making adequate space, foraging, and company high priorities. Especially where ungulates are kept in climates very different from their native countries'; other priorities include good ground quality and adequate shelter from high temperatures and flies. Owners need to ensure they have the space and resources to provide for these needs, especially where this requires providing for multiple animals of social species. There is no evidence that human company is a substitute for company of their own species, and some species may not easily adapt to pet lifestyles. In some cases, ungulates that are hand-reared may be amenable, small, and good human companions as juveniles but show behaviour such as aggression when adult (by which time they are significantly larger). These changes may lead owners to regret obtaining them. It can then be difficult to rehome ungulates, especially as owners may be unwilling to rehome them into commercial farming settings.

Many ungulates are bred and used in farming, and animal welfare scientific research has focused on commercial farm settings and strains. Applying ideas from farming contexts to pet ungulates needs careful extrapolation. Some owners may lack the knowledge to safely keep ungulates in ways that rely on good stockmanship and careful management. Also, some owners may keep ungulates beyond their 'productive' lives. Older animals may experience geriatric problems rarely seen on farms, especially because some commercial strains of ungulates have been bred for use in systems where they do not reach very high ages and may undergo degenerative changes at relatively young ages. In such cases, a priority is to ensure owners have enough knowledge and provide ungulates with adequate treatment, including euthanasia, when necessary.

Bibliography

Aba, M.A., Bianchi, C., and Cavilla, V. (2010). South American camelids. In: *Behaviour of Exotic Pets* (ed. V.V. Tynes), 157–167. Oxford: Wiley-Blackwell.

Arey, D.S. (1999). Time course for the formation and disruption of social organisation in group-housed sows. *Applied Animal Behaviour Science* 62: 199–207.

Beattie, V.E., Walker, N., and Sneddon, I.A. (1998). Preference testing of substrates by growing pigs. *Animal Welfare* 7: 27–34.

Blackshaw, J.K., Thomas, F.J., and Lee, J. (1997). The effect of a fixed or free toy on the growth rate and aggressive behaviour of weaned pigs and the influence of hierarchy on initial investigation of the toys. *Applied Animal Behaviour Science* 53: 203–212.

Boivin, X. and Braadstad, B.O. (1996). Effects of handling during temporary isolation after early weaning on goat kid's later response to humans. *Applied Animal Behaviour Science* 48: 61–71.

Boivin, P., Le Neindre, J.P., Garel, J.M., and Chupin, J.M. (1994). Influence of breed and rearing management on cattle reactions during human handling. *Applied Animal Behaviour Science* 39: 115–122.

Bracke, M.B.M. and Spoolder, H.A.M. (2011). Review of wallowing in pigs: implications for animal welfare. *Animal Welfare* 20: 347–363.

Buttle, H., Mowlem, A., and Mews, A. (1986). Disbudding and dehorning goats. *In Practice* 8: 63–65.

Cavalcanti, S.M.C. and Knowleton, F.F. (1998). Evaluation of physical and behavioural traits of llamas associated with aggressiveness towards sheep-threatening canids. *Applied Animal Behaviour Science* 61: 143–158.

Coleman, G.J., Hemsworth, P.H., and Hay, M. (1998). Predicting stockperson behaviour towards pigs from attitudinal and job-related variables and empathy. *Applied Animal Behaviour Science* 58 (1): 63–75.

Colson, V., Martin, E., and Orgeur, P. (2012). Prunier a 2012 influence of housing and social changes on growth, behaviour and cortisol in piglets at weaning. *Physiology & Behavior* 107: 59–64.

De Jong, F.H., Bokkers, E.A.M., Schouten, W.G.P., and Helmon, F.A. (1996). Rearing piglets in apoor environment: developmental aspects of social stress in pigs. *Physiology and Behaviour* 60: 389–396.

Désiré, L., Veissier, I., Després, G., and Boissy, A. (2004). On the way to assess emotions in animals: do lambs (*Ovis aries*) evaluate an event through its suddenness, novelty, or unpredictability? *Journal of Comparative Psychology* 118: 363–374.

Désiré, L., Veissier, I., Després, G. et al. (2006). Boissy a 2006 appraisal process in sheep (*Ovis aries*): interactive effect of suddenness and unfamiliarity on cardiac and behavioral responses. *Journal of Comparative Psychology* 120: 280–287.

Docking, C.M., Van de Weerd, H.A., Day, J.E.L., and Edwards, S.A. (2008). The influence of age on the use of potential enrichment objects and synchronisation of behaviour of pigs. *Applied Animal Behaviour Science* 110: 244–257.

Düpjan, S., Schön, P., Puppe, B. et al. (2008). Differential vocal responses to physical and mental stressors in domestic pigs (*Sus scrofa*). *Applied Animal Behaviour Science* 114 (2008): 105–115.

Ernst, K., Puppe, B., Schön, P.C., and Manteuffel, G. (2005). A complex automatic feeding system for pigs aimed to induce successful behavioural coping by cognitive adaptation. *Applied Animal Behaviour Science* 91: 205–218.

Estevez, I., Andersen, I.L., and Nævdal, E. (2007). Group size, density and social dynamics in farm animals. *Applied Animal Behaviour Science* 103: 185–204.

Faucitano, L. and Schaefer, A.L. (eds.) (2008). *Welfare of Pigs from Birth to Slaughter*. Wageningen: Wageningen Publishers.

Fisher, T.F. (1993). Miniature swine in biomedical research – applications and husbandry considerations. *Lab Animal* 22: 47–50.

Forkman, B., Boissy, A., Meunier-Salauen, M.C. et al. (2007). A critical review of fear tests used on cattle, pigs, sheep, poultry and horses. *Physiology & Behavior* 92: 340–374.

Fraser, D. (1985). Selection of bedded and unbedded areas by pigs in relation to environmental temperature and behaviour. *Applied Animal Behaviour Science* 14: 117–126.

Fraser, D., Phillips, P.A., Thompson, B.K., and Tennessen, T. (1991). The effect of straw on the behaviour of growing pigs. *Applied Animal Behaviour Science* 30: 307–318.

Gentry, J.G., McGlone, J.J., Blanton, J.R., and Miller, M.F. (2002). Alternative housing systems for pigs: influences on growth, composition and pork quality. *Journal of Animal Science* 80: 1781–1790.

Geverink, N.A., Engel, B., Lambooij, E., and Wiegant, V.M. (1996). Observations on behaviour and skin damage of slaughter pigs and treatment during lairage. *Applied Animal Behaviour Science* 50: 1–13.

Gillman, C.E., Killride, A.L., Ossent, P., and Green, L.E. (2008). A cross-sectional study of the prevalence and associated risk factors for bursitis in weaner, grower and finisher pigs from 93 commercial farms in England. *Preventive Veterinary Medicine* 83: 308–322.

Gonyou, H.W., Hemsworth, P.H., and Barnett, J.L. (1986). Effects od frequent interactions with humans on growing pigs. *Applied Animal Behaviour Science* 16: 269–278.

Grandin, T. and Curtis, S.E. (1984a). Material affected cloth-toy touching and biting by pigs. *Journal of Animal Science* 59 (Suppl. 1): 150.

Grandin, T. and Curtis, S.E. (1984b). Toy preferences in young pigs. *Journal of Animal Science* 59 (Suppl. 1): 85.

Grossman, J.L. and Kutzler, M.A. (2007). Effects of castration in male llamas (*Lama glama*) on human-directed aggression. *Theriogenology* 68: 511.

Guy, J.H., Rowlinson, P., Chadwick, J.P., and Ellis, M. (2002). Behaviour of two genotypes of growing-finishing pig in three different housing systems. *Applied Animal Behaviour Science* 75 (3): 193–206.

Hargreaves, A.L. and Huston, G.D. (1990). Some effects of repeated handling on stress responses in sheep. *Applied Animal Behaviour Science* 26: 253–256.

Harwood, D. (2006). *Goat Health and Welfare – A Veterinary Guide*. The Crowood Press.

Haskell, M.J., Wemelsfelder, F., Mendl, M.T. et al. (1996). The effect of substrate-enriched and substrate-impoverished housing environments on the diversity of behaviour in pigs. *Behaviour* 133: 741–761.

Hemsworth, P.H., Barnett, J.L., and Hansen, C. (1981). The influence of handling by humans on the behavior, growth, and corticosteroids in the juvenile female pig. *Hormones and Behavior* 15: 396–403.

Hemsworth, P.H., Barnett, J.L., and Hansen, C. (1986). The influence of handling by humans on the behaviour, reproduction and corticosteroids of male and female pigs. *Applied Animal Behaviour Science* 15: 303–314.

Hemsworth, P.H., Barnett, J.L., and Hansen, C. (1987). The influence of inconsistent handling on the behaviour, growth and corticosteroids of young pigs. *Applied Animal Behaviour Science* 17: 245–252.

Hemsworth, P.H., Barnett, J.L., Coleman, G.J., and Hansen, C. (1989). A study of the relationships between the attitudinal and behavioural profiles of stockpeople and the level of fear of humans and the reproductive performance of commercial pigs. *Applied Animal Behaviour Science* 23: 301–314.

Hemsworth, P.H., Coleman, G.J., Cox, M., and Barnett, J.L. (1994). Stimulus generalization: the inability of pigs to discriminate between humans on the basis of their previous handling experience. *Applied Animal Behaviour Science* 40 (1994): 129–142.

Hemsworth, P.H., Verge, J., and Coleman, G.J. (1996a). Conditioned approach-avoidance responses to humans: the ability of pigs to associate feeding and aversive social experiences in the presence of humans with humans. *Applied Animal Behaviour Science* 50 (1996): 71–82.

Hemsworth, P.H., Price, E.O., and Borgwardt, R. (1996b). Behavioural responses of domestic pigs and cattle to humans and novel stimuli. *Applied Animal Behaviour Science* 50 (1996): 43–56.

Hillman, E., Von Hollen, F., Bünger, B. et al. (2003). Farrowing condition affect the reaction of piglets toward novel enrichment and social confrontation at weaning. *Applied Animal Behaviour Science* 89: 99–109.

Hintze, S., Scott, D., Turner, S. et al. (2013). Mounting behaviour in finishing pigs: stable individual differences are not due to dominance or stage of sexual development. *Applied Animal Behaviour Science* 147 (1–2): 69–80.

Horrell, I., Ness, P.A., Edwards, S.A., and Eddison, J. (2001). The use of nose ringing in pigs: consequences for rooting, other functional activities, and welfare. *Animal Welfare* 10: 3–22.

Hulbert, L.E. and McGlone, J.J. (2006). Health and well-being: evaluation of drop versus trickle-feeding systems for crated or grouppenned gestating sows. *Journal of Animal Science* 84: 1004–1014.

Hunter, L.T.B. and Skinner, J.D. (1998). Vigilance behaviour in African ungulates: the role of predation pressure. *Behavior* 135: 195–211.

Hyun, Y., Ellis, M., McKeith, F.K., and Wilson, E.R. (1997). Feed intake pattern of group-housed growing-finishing pigs monitored using a computerized feed intake recording system. *Journal of Animal Science* 75: 1443–1451.

Imfeld-Mueller, S., Van Wezemael, L., Stauffacher, M. et al. (2011). Do pigs distinguish between situations of different emotional valences during anticipation? *Applied Animal Behaviour Science* 131 (2011): 86–93.

Johnson, A.K., Gesing, L.M., Ellis, M. et al. (2013). Farm and pig factors affecting welfare during the marketing process. *Journal of Animal Science* 91 (6): 2481–2491.

Jorgensen, B. (2003). Influence of floor type and stocking density on leg weakness, osteochondrosis and claw disorders in slaughter pigs. *Animal Science* 77: 439–449.

Kannan, G., Terrill, T.H., Kouakou, B. et al. (2002). Simulated preslaughter holding and isolation effects on stress responses and live weight shrinkage in meat goats. *Journal of Animal Science* 80: 1771–1780.

Keeling, L. and Gonyou, H. (eds.) (2001). *Social Behaviour in Farm Animals*. Wallingford, Oxon: CABI Publishing.

KilBride, A.L., Gillman, C.E., and Green, L.E. (2007). A cross-sectional study of the prevalence of lameness in finishing pigs, gilts and pregnant sows and associations with limb lesions and floor types on commercial farms in England. *Animal Welfare* 18 (3): 215–224.

Luikart, G., Gielly, L., Excoffier, L. et al. (2001). Multiple maternal origins and weak phylogeographic structure in domestic goats. *Proceedings of the National Academy of Sciences* 98 (10): 5927–5932.

Manteuffel, G., Puppe, B., and Schön, P.C. (2004). Vocalization of farm animals as a measure of welfare. *Applied Animal Behaviour Science* 88 (2004): 163–182.

Marchant, J.N., Whittaker, X., and Broom, D.M. (2001). Vocalisations of the adult female domestic pig during a standard human approach test and their relationships with behavioural and heart rate measures. *Applied Animal Behaviour Science* 72 (1): 23–39.

McGlone, J.J. and Anderson, D.L. (2002). Synthetic maternal pheromone stimulates feeding behaviour and weight gain in weaned pigs. *Journal of Animal Science* 80: 3179–3183.

Meunier-Salaün, M.C., Edwards, S.A., and Robert, S. (2001). Effect of dietary fibre on the behaviour and health of the restricted fed sow. *Animal Feed Science an Technlogy* 90: 53–69.

Miranda-de la Lama, G.C. and Mattiello, S. (2010). The importance of social behaviour for goat welfare in livestock farming. *Small Ruminant Research* 90 (2010): 1–10.

Mounier, L., Veissier, I., Andanson, S. et al. (2006). Mixing at the beginning of fattening moderates social buffering in beef bulls. *Applied Animal Behaviour Science* 96: 185–200.

Mouttotou, N., Hatchell, F.M., and Green, L.E. (1998). Adventitious bursitis of the hock in finishing pigs: prevalence, distribution and association with floor type and foot lesions. *Veterinary Record* 142: 109–114.

Murphy, E., Nordquist, R.E., and van der Staay, F.J. (2014). A review of behavioural methods to study emotion and mood in pigs, *Sus scrofa*. *Applied Animal Behaviour Science* 159: 9–28.

O'Connor, E.A., Parker, M.O., McLeman, M.A. et al. (2010). The impact of chronic environmental stressors on growing pigs, *Sus scrofa* (part 1): stress physiology, production and play behaviour. *Animal* 4: 1899–1909.

Pajor, E.A., Rushen, J., and de Passillé, A.M.B. (2000). Aversion learning techniques to evaluate dairy cattle handling practices. *Applied Animal Behaviour Science* 69: 89–102.

Petersen, V., Simonsen, H.B., and Lawson, L.G. (1995). The effect of environmental enrichment on the development of behaviours in pigs. *Applied Animal Behaviour Science* 45: 215–224.

Petherick, J.C. and Phillips, C.J.C. (2009). Space allowances for confined livestock and their determination from allometric principles. *Applied Animal Behaviour Science* 117: 1–12.

Porter, R.H., Nowak, R., and Orgeur, P. (1995). Influence of a conspecific agemate on distress bleating by lambs. *Applied Animal Behaviour Science* 45: 239–244.

Ramonet, Y., Robert, S., Aumaître, A. et al. (2000). Influence of the nature of dietary fibre on digestive utilization, some metabolite and hormone profiles and the behaviour of pregnant sows. *Animal Science* 70: 275–286.

Rodríguez-Estévez, V., García, A., Pena, F., and Gómez, A.G. (2009). Foraging of Iberian fattening pigs grazing natural pasture in the dehesa. *Livestock Science* 120: 135–143.

Ross, S. and Berg, J. (1956). Stability of food dominance relationships in a flock of goats. *Journal of Mammalogy* 37: 129–131.

Rushen, J., Robert, S., and Farmer, C. (1999). Effects of an oat-based high-fibre diet on insulin, glucose, cortisol and free fatty acid concentrations in gilts. *Animal Science* 69: 395–401.

Rydhmer, L., Hansson, M., Lundström, K. et al. (2013). Welfare of entire male pigs is improved by socialising piglets and keeping intact groups until slaughter. *Animal* 7 (9): 1532–1541.

Shackleton, D.M. and Shank, C.C. (1984). A review of the social behavior of feral and wild sheep and goats 1. *Journal of Animal Science* 58 (2): 500–509.

Scott, K., Taylor, L., Gill, B.P., and Edwards, S.A. (2006). Influence of different types of environmental enrichment on the behaviour of finishing pigs in two different housing systems: 1. Hanging toy v. rootable substrate. *Applied Animal Behaviour Science* 99 (3–4): 222–229.

Stolba, A. and Woodgush, D.G.M. (1989). The behaviour of pigs in a semi-natural environment. *Animal Production* 48: 419–425.

Tanida, H., Miura, A., Tanaka, T., and Yoshimoto, T. (1995). Behavioural response to humans in individually handled weanling pigs. *Applied Animal Behaviour Science* 42: 249–259.

Terlouw, E.M.C. and Porcher, J. (2005). Repeated handling of pigs during rearing. I. Refusal of contact by the handler and reactivity to familiar and unfamiliar humans. *Journal of Animal Science* 83: 1653–1663.

Turner, S.P.F., White, M.J., Brotherstone, I.M.S. et al. (2006). The accumulation of skin lesions and their use as a predictor of individual aggressiveness in pigs. *Applied Animal Behaviour Science* 96: 245–259.

Tuyttens, F.A.M. (2005). The importance of straw for pig and cattle welfare: a review. *Applied Animal Behaviour Science* 92 (3): 261–282.

Van de Weerd, H.A., Docking, C.M., Day, J.E.L. et al. (2006). Effects of species relevant environmental enrichment on the behaviour and productivity of finishing pigs. *Applied Animal Behaviour Science* 99 (3–4): 230–247.

Von Borell, E. and Schäffer, D. (2005). Legal requirements and assessment of stress and welfare during transportation and preslaughter handling of pigs. *Livestock Production Science* 97 (2–3): 81–87.

Waiblinger, S., Boivin, X., Perdersen, V. et al. (2006). Assessing the human animal relationship in farmed species: a critical review. *Applied Animal Behaviour Science* 101: 185–242.

Warriss, P.D. (1998). The welfare of slaughter pigs during transport. *Animal Welfare* 7 (4): 365–381.

Wemelsfelder, F., Hunter, E.A., Mendl, M.T., and Lawrence, A.B. (2000). The spontaneous qualitative assessment of behavioural expressions in pigs: first explorations of a novel methodology for integrative animal welfare measurement. *Applied Animal Behaviour Science* 67: 193–215.

Wood-Gush, D.G.M. and Vestergaard, K. (1993). Inquisitive exploration in pigs. *Animal Behaviour* 45: 185–187.

Wood-Gush, D.G.M., Jensen, P., and Algers, B. (1990a). Behaviour of pigs in a novel semi-natural environment. *Biology of Behaviour* 15 (1990): 62–73.

Wood-Gush, D.G.M., Vestergaard, K., and Petersen, H.V. (1990b). The significance of motivation and environment in the development of exploration in pigs. *Biology of Behaviour* 15: 39–52.

Zeder, M.A. and Hesse, B. (2000). The initial domestication of goats (Capra hircus) in the Zagros mountains 10 000 years ago. *Science* 28 (7): 2254–2257.

Horses (*Equus caballus*)

13

Paul McGreevy and James Yeates

13.1 History and Context

13.1.1 Natural History

Domestic horses (*Equus caballus*) are equid members of the class Mammalia, order Perissodactyla, and family Equidae. The ancestors of the domestic horse are probably now extinct. However, there are modern feral populations, living in a range of habitats from deserts to woods, subject to varying degrees of human management. *E. caballus* has not been included in the IUCN Red List.

Horses are a prey species, avoiding predation by vigilance, bunching together, and fleeing, often at the first sight of a threat. To be ready for flight, their lower legs feature anatomical structures known as reciprocal apparatuses that allow them to doze while standing and often divide sentry duty amongst different band members (Fraser 1992; McGreevy 1996). They often live in reproductive or bachelor groups (Figure 13.1). These bands are relatively stable except for the movements of adults for breeding purposes (Monard et al. 1996; Goodloe et al. 2000; Linklater et al. 2000). Within these groups, individuals can form particularly close relationships (Feh 1999, 2001; Linklater and Cameron 2000). These groups occupy large, overlapping home ranges of up to

Companion Animal Care and Welfare: The UFAW Companion Animal Handbook,
First Edition. Edited by James Yeates.
© 2019 Universities Federation for Animal Welfare. Published 2019 by John Wiley & Sons Ltd.

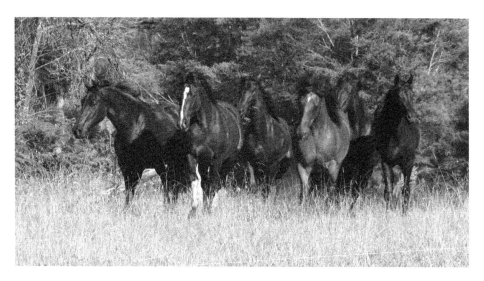

Figure 13.1   Horses in a social group at pasture.

78 km² (Boyd and Keiper 2005). Such wide ranges allow extensive grazing or foraging large quantities of low-quality food for the majority of each day.

13.1.2 Domestic History

The first human-horse interactions would have been as predator and prey as depicted in cave paintings. Horses were first kept around 5000–6000 years ago (Lippold et al. 2011) and have since been kept for transport, traction, meat, hunting, and war. As expensive animals to buy and keep, their ownership has often been associated with people of higher social status (Anthony 1996; Diamond 1997). Nowadays, horses are also kept both for leisure and for sports competition, although estimates of total horse populations (Table 13.1) usually include companion, working, and semi-feral animals (Waran 2007).

Domestic horses are bred using both 'natural' mating and artificial insemination. Selection has created nearly seven hundred recognised breeds, which vary in size (e.g. Falabellas and Shire horses), shape (e.g. cobs and Arabians), and characteristics such as reactivity (e.g. draught breeds are considered to generally have a smaller flight and critical distances than Thoroughbreds; McGreevy and McLean 2010). Despite this selection, horses remain behaviourally similar to their feral counterparts (Clutton-Brock 1999; Goodwin 1999); their various uses and management make use of their behavioural flexibility rather than their ethological origins.

13.2 Principles of Horse Care

13.2.1 Diet

Horses are obligate herbivores, with nutritional requirements as described in Table 13.2. These needs are usually best met by allowing horses to eat growing vegetation. Pasture allows horses to forage, browse, choose from a variety of foods and chew. It should

Table 13.1 2012 Horse population estimates for various countries or areas to nearest thousand.

Country	Estimated Population '000s
European Union	3618
Argentina	3650
Australia	265
Brazil	5363
China	8301
Ethiopia	1907
India	525
Indonesia	422
Japan	16
Kenya	2
Mexico	6356
New Zealand	57
Russian Federation	1362
United States	10250
Worldwide	c59000

Source: Food and Agricultural Organisation of the United Nations (FAO 2014).

Table 13.2 Nutritional requirements of adult, nonbreedinghorses.

Nutrient	Amount required for 500-kg adult
Energy	30–36 kcal kg^{-1}
Protein	630 g
Fibre	1.5–3% body weight/day
Calcium	20 g
Phosphorus	14 g
Calcium-to-potassium ratio	1.5 : 1
Salt	1.7 g, plus compensation for sweat losses
Vitamin A	1500 IU
Vitamin D	0 (if adequate sunlight)
Water	At least 5% body weight/day

All figures assume animals are of normal physiology, healthy, non-breeding, and non-working.
Source: Merck Veterinary Manual (2015), National Research Council (NRC 2007).

also provide sufficient fibre and grazing fills large amounts of horses' time budgets. Nevertheless, where there is a shortage of grazing, owners may need to provide 'forage' such as hay. Ad libitum natural forages should provide all nutritional needs and avoid the risks of imbalances from inappropriate supplements. One possible exception is when horses excrete large amounts of salt and other minerals during exercise. Many horses offered salt blocks may alter their salt intake to compensate for their losses.

In some cases, supplementary oil or 'concentrates' (e.g. cereals and sugar beet) may provide additional nutrients to unthrifty or highly active horses. Manufacturers have produced a range of commercial formulations to meet hypothesised needs or to regulate horses' temperament or performance. Although these are usually focused on benefits to their owner, some food choices may affect horses' emotional states. For example, there is some evidence that alpha-casozepine supplementation may reduce fear during handling (McDonnell et al. 2013).

However, feeding significant amounts of concentrates can have several effects. Excessive energy can predispose horses to conditions such as being overweight or obese, metabolic syndrome, and laminitis (although these conditions can have multiple interacting causes and may occur in non-obese horses). Laminitis can affect up to 14% of horses in some countries and can cause severe pain (Bailey et al. 2004; Carter et al. 2009). Animals at particular risk of obesity or laminitis should have strictly restricted exposure to concentrates and lush grass, especially in spring and summer and at dawn and dusk (Becvarova and Pleasant 2012). These restrictions may lead to hunger and frustration, but this may be justified by avoiding the severe suffering involved in laminitis for horses at particular risk.

Low-forage, high-concentrate rations can also lead to conditions such as gastric hyperacidity or ulceration and hind-gut acidosis. They may also be associated with the development of crib biting (McGreevy et al. 1995) or wood chewing. These may cause incisor erosion (Hothersall and Nicol 2009; Wickens and Heleski 2010), intestinal wood impactions (Krzak et al. 1991), or prompt owners to use inappropriate anti-cribbing straps that cause further stress (McGreevy et al. 1995). The precise interactions of causes and effects are complicated and still unclear, but it is clear that feeding excessive concentrates is far from ideal. Some competition horses appear to thrive on a predominantly forage-based feed supplemented with oil, rather than a high concentrate feed.

Factors that alter the flow of food through the intestines can precipitate colic, including feeding highly fermentable foods (e.g. grass clippings), some high concentrate feeds, poor quality hay, insufficient water, or sudden dietary changes, as well as underlying problems such as worm damage, oral stereotypies, and poor dental health (Davidson and Harris 2002; Mills and Clarke 2002; Archer et al. 2004; Archer and Proudman 2006). Any dietary changes should also be made gradually to allow changes in gut flora.

The best feeding enrichment is ad libitum grazing or forage and forage should usually comprise 40–100% of dry matter intake for all horses (Davidson and Harris 2002). Horses kept indoors are motivated to spend around 60% of their time eating forage if available and rarely stop foraging for longer than 4 hours (Davidson and Harris 2002). In comparison, horses may eat pelleted rations within 2 hours, leaving long periods of inactivity and the potential for frustration (Hintz and Loy 1966). Some horses may eat straw bedding, and although this may avoid behaviour problems, it can risk intestinal impactions (Hunter and Houpt 1989; McGreevy et al. 1995; Mills et al. 2000; Cooper and Albentosa 2005; Thorne et al. 2005). Some horses appear to prefer forage on the ground and may deliberately spread their hay around (Sweeting et al. 1985). Some may interact with puzzle-feeders (e.g. Winskill et al. 1996; Henderson and Waran 2001; Goodwin et al. 2002).

Owners should prevent horses eating large amounts of sand, foreign bodies, or toxic plants (e.g. ergot alkaloids, ragwort, bracken, rye grass, locoweed, flatweed), many of which cause intestinal or liver damage. Such risks may be greater on overgrazed pastures or drought (as some toxic plants are more resistant). Cut forage such as hay can also contain particles that can cause inflammatory airway disease (Davidson and Harris 2002; Berndt et al. 2008). Owners can reduce this risk by soaking or steaming hay for 10–30 minutes (Blackman and Moore-Colyer 1998) or by placing hay on the ground so that gravity helps to clear the upper airway (Racklyeft and Love 1990; Mills and Clarke 2002), although this can increase food wastage and contamination with soiled bedding. Both pasture and forage should be kept clean and uncontaminated by faeces to reduce parasites and bacteria. In large enough pastures, horses can separate their feeding and toilet areas, but this may not be possible in stables.

The daily water intake of stabled horses is in the range 2–4 L kg^{-1} of dry-matter food consumed (Houpt 1987). This variation reflects the amount of chewing, and therefore salivation, required for hay versus, for example, concentrates (Harris 1999). Meanwhile, for working horses, water intake also relates to workload and can push daily requirements up to 90 L (Hinton 1978). Ideally, all horses should have ad libitum water at all times, except when providing water during transportation would make the floor too wet and slippery. Automated water provision can be restricted by technical failures or by freezing and so needs to be checked regularly.

13.2.2 Environment

Adequate space is necessary for exercise, exploration, flight, sharing resources, play, and rolling. Horses are motivated to access space at least for short periods, especially after spatial restriction or isolation (Houpt and Houpt 1988; Chaya et al. 2006, Freire et al. 2010) and if they are unused to stabling (Houpt et al. 2001). Space restrictions can be associated with weaving and stall walking (McGreevy et al. 1995; Cooper and Mason 1998; Nicol 1999; Bachmann et al. 2003a; Christie et al. 2006). Being ridden can provide some exercise but is no substitute for free movement. All horses should be kept out permanently or at least turned out every day, although there is little evidence for any specific minimum length of time.

Horses need shelter from natural (e.g. trees) or man-made (e.g. field-shelters) cover. In summer, it is needed to help horses stay within their critical temperature of below 20–30 °C (Holcomb et al. 2013) and to escape the irritation of insects. In winter, healthy and well-fed horses can generally tolerate dry cold weather, but rain can increase heat loss and contribute to the risk of conditions such as rain-scald and mud fever. Rugs can provide some protection from the elements and flies, although inappropriate rugging can be uncomfortable, dangerous, and unnecessary. Conversely, clipping may be aversive (Yarnell et al. 2013) and reduces thermal insulation, depending on the ambient temperature, housing and rugging.

Stabling restricts visual exploration, vigilance, and movement and increases the risk of airway disease (Table 13.3). Stabled horses may show increased plasma cortisol concentration (Houpt et al. 2001), haemoglobin concentration (Mal et al. 1991a), and signs of agitation (Harewood and McGowan 2005). When horses show stereotypies, owners may then close upper stable doors or install anti-weave bars, which reduce the visibility of the behaviours while the horse's welfare remains unimproved or even worsened

Table 13.3 Benefits of indoor versus outdoor housing.

Indoor stabling (individual stables in group yard)	Outdoor paddock (group, with outdoor shelter)
Easier dietary management by owners	Better foraging, particularly grass
Reduced risk of aggression or injury from other horses	Physical access to other horses
Reduced exposure to inclement weather and insects	Better ventilation
Easier catching and observation by owner	Decreased risk of some infectious diseases
Decreased risk of sand impaction	Decreased risk of straw impaction
	Opportunities for safe rolling and recumbent sleep
	Increased environmental complexity and visual range
	Opportunities for exercise and play
	Opportunities for flight

(McBride and Cuddeford 2001). Outdoor tethering may improve ventilation but has unacceptable additional risks of entanglement, overturned buckets, and exposure. Outdoor pasture should be the preferred method of 'housing' horses wherever possible.

Adult horses may sleep for 5 to 7 hours per day (Dallaire 1986). Although they can drowse standing up, lying down is necessary for deeper REM. sleep (during which horses appear to dream). Horses may be unwilling to lie down in new environments, in confined spaces, if tied, or if not given comfortable bedding (Ruckebusch 1975; Hunter and Houpt 1989; Houpt et al. 2001). Indoors, many horses prefer straw bedding, which some may also eat. All bedding should be clean and fresh because damp or mouldy bedding can increase the likelihood of thrush or airway disease, especially if ventilation is less than six air changes per hour (Berndt et al. 2008).

Toys may be provided to offset any presumed boredom from confinement and insufficient forage and may be especially valued by young horses (McDonnell and Poulin 2002). However, unfamiliar or moving objects or environments may be stressful for some horses (Le Scolan et al. 1997; Wolff et al. 1997; Seaman et al. 2002). Handlers and riders should avoid unnecessary stresses and be mindful that horses' likely motivation in such situations is avoidance and, if necessary, flight.

Transportation can be especially stressful, potentially causing distress, urine retention, muscle metabolism, and dehydration. It may also predispose horses to diseases such as Pasteurellosis, particularly during long journeys. Horses' preferences to avoid transportation can often be seen in their reluctance to load. Loading may be particularly stressful for horses who have not been properly trained to load, who are used to another type of transporter (e.g. horsebox versus trailer), or if loaders deliberately cause fear to motivate the horse to move into the vehicle. Owners should minimise this stress through sympathetic loading, driving, and using rewards to make entering the trailer or horsebox a positive experience.

13.2.3 Animal Company

Company is essential for all horses, including stallions. Company provides opportunities for mutual grooming and play and allows horses to stand head-to-tail to remove flies (McDonnell and Poulin 2002). Horses are motivated to be with other horses (Christensen et al. 2002; Hartmann et al. 2012). Isolated horses can show signs of frustration and loneliness (Table 13.4), including rebound effects on social activities (Christensen et al. 2002). If horses need to be isolated, for example for short-term veterinary treatment, horse images or mirrors may reduce feelings of isolation and can reduce weaving behaviour (McAfee et al. 2002; Mills and Riezebos 2005; Figure 13.2).

However, horses may also occasionally chase, bite, or kick one another. Owners should avoid restricting company completely through fear of such injuries because they are relatively uncommon and usually minor, even in stallion groups. Nevertheless, owners should try to ensure horses are compatible, particularly by observing their behaviour (Table 13.5). Herds with a broad range of ages and heights may also be associated with less aggression than those of a homogenous composition (Giles et al. 2015). Owners should also provide groups with sufficient space to allow individuals to escape from one other and minimise competition by providing more feeding sites than there are horses in the group.

It is important to avoid disrupting established groups. Horses can recognise other individuals after several months (Berger and Cunningham 1987; Feh 1999; Lemasson et al. 2009; Proops et al. 2009; Krueger et al. 2011) and can form personal relationships (Wolski et al. 1980; Feh 1999; Linklater and Cameron 2000). Horses separated from other familiar horses may show behaviours such as nickering, stalling, and napping. On the other hand, horses introduced into groups with high social flux may suffer chronic stress (Alexander et al. 1988). Such groups need to establish a new social structure (Monard and Duncan 1996; Monard et al. 1996), and stress can occur when animals move up or

Table 13.4 Potential effects of isolation.

Pathophysiological measures	Behavioural measures
Increased blood cortisol	Increased sleep
Desensitised cortisol responses	Increased stress-related behaviours
Decreased body condition	Increased stereotypies (e.g. weaving)
	Increased difficulty to catch
	Increased difficulty to train
	Increased aggression to handlers
	Rebound effects on social activities
	Self-mutilations (e.g. rubbing, biting, kicking, and lunging into fixed objects)

Source: Alexander et al. (1988), McGreevy et al. (1995), Cooper and Mason (1998), Christensen et al. (2002), Søndergaard and Ladewig (2004), McDonnell (2008), and Visser et al. (2008).

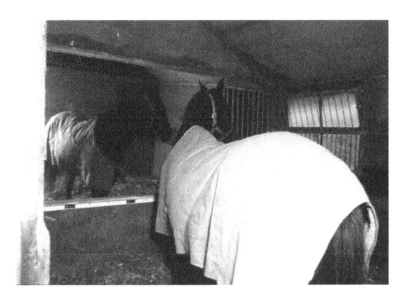

Figure 13.2 Isolated horse with mirror.

Table 13.5 Behavioural assessments of suitability of horse company.

Initial interactions	Threatening behaviours	Affiliative behaviours
'Greetings' through close nasal proximity	Tail swishing	Maintaining proximity
	Displacement	Allogrooming
'Greetings' through nasal contact	Aggressive chasing	Standing with necks overlapping
	Physical aggression	Standing head to tail
Agonistic behaviours	Responses to threats	Following one another
	'Snapping' – clapping the teeth with the lips drawn back	Rubbing the side of the face on another horse
	Avoiding the protagonist through non-approach	Rubbing the underneath of the face on another horse
	Avoiding the protagonist through flight	Social play
		Play initiating behaviours such as nipping, 'prancing' 'High blowing'

Source: McDonnell and Poulin (2002) and van Dierendonck et al. (2004).

down the social scale. When owners change liveries (also known as agistment or board-ing facilities) or transfer ownership, the movement of horses both fractures established relationships and creates new groups of unfamiliar animals.

Managed mating methods usually minimise contact between the mare and stallion, largely for easier management and to avoid expensive injuries to valuable animals. However, these methods restrict courtship and post-mating bonding behaviours of both mares and stallions (McDonnell 2000). After birth, maternal contact is important for foal development and probably pleasurable for both mare and foal, although some mares may reject some foals or show maternal aggression (Houpt and Olm 1984). Foals are naturally weaned at around 9 months, and separating young foals from their mother (e.g. for training or for remating of the mare during the foal heat) can damage their relationships with their dam and other horses (Henry et al. 2009) and possibly predispose to stereotypies. Foals also appear motivated to interact with one another (Crowell-Davis 1986), and a lack of socialisation may lead to subsequent inappropriate social behaviours towards other horses or humans.

Some horses may tolerate or form bonds with animals of other species, such as familiar herbivorous ungulates. However, there are also rare reports of horses attacking cows and sheep (Fraser 1992; Giles and Tupper 2006) and anecdotal reports of horses showing fear response to pig odours. Dogs may be perceived as predators, prompting escape or defence behaviours, although horses can learn to tolerate them.

13.2.4 Human Interactions

Unhandled horses may respond to humans as they would to predators, whereas handled horses' responses depend on their previous interactions with humans (Fureix et al. 2009; Sankey et al. 2010a, 2010b), particularly early life experiences (Diehl et al. 2002; Henry et al. 2009). Previous unpleasant experiences (such as pain or maternal separation) can increase fear and responses such as aggression or becoming 'head-shy' (Pritchard et al. 2005; Sankey et al. 2010a). Previous pleasant experiences can make horses less fearful (Birke et al. 2011), and some horses may learn to enjoy human company, perhaps associating it with stroking or grooming (Figure 13.3) or food (McGreevy et al. 2012).

Human company is no substitute for equine company. Human-horse relations are only superficially similar to human-human or horse-horse relationships. Humans can, to some extent, understand and be understood by horses, and good horsemanship should be based on good communication between horses and humans. On the one hand, humans need to be able to accurately interpret horses' responses. On the other, they should also help horses interpret human actions through predictable, calm movements, and consistent cues.

Such communication is particularly difficult during riding, when horses are largely reliant on specific, unnatural nonvisual stimuli. Many horses appear to enjoy being ridden, and it provides opportunities for exercise, company, environmental exploration, and perhaps a form of interspecific social play. Riding and training should be based on the use of subtle cues, minimal pressures, appropriate rewards, and natural behaviour. However, riding can risk fatigue, azoturia (equine rhabdomyolysis syndrome (ERS) – similar to severe cramp), and injury. In addition, *bad* riding can involve punishment; continuous and inescapable pressures; conflicting signals (e.g. acceleration and deceleration cues at the same time); inaccurate, inconsistent, or poorly timed cues; and poor rider balance. These may cause confusion, pain, discomfort, or learned helplessness.

In particular, many items of riding equipment can cause discomfort or pain, including whips, spurs, curb bits, curb chains, bitless bridles, nosebands, balancing reins, or side reins (Evans and McGreevy 2011; McLean and McGreevy 2010; McGreevy 2012; McGreevy et al. 2012). Any use of relentless pressure while training a horse must be avoided because it may lead to habituation (McLean and McGreevy 2010). For example,

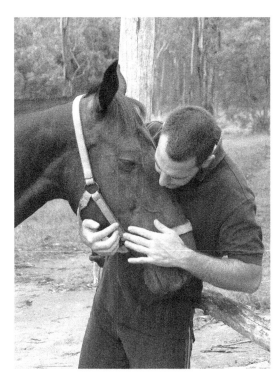

Figure 13.3 Horse appearing to enjoy stroking.

tightened nosebands have recently found favour amongst many equestrians because they can mask oral responses that are regarded as resistances and evasions and which emerge as a result of rough riding (McGreevy 2015). Doherty et al. (2016) found that tightened nosebands were used in at least half the population in a large sample of completion horses. However, the practice prevents normal behaviour including yawning, chewing, and licking and is difficult to defend on ethical grounds because riding without a tight noseband is entirely possible (Fenner et al. 2016).

Riding and training can also suppress horses' own normal motivations (e.g. to flee threats) and promote behaviours that are unnatural or decontextualised from their natural stimuli. As examples, humans acting as 'alpha mares' or 'leaders' in chasing a horse in a pen from which it cannot escape may cause fear; backing can stimulate anti-predator responses and then fatigue; and exaggerated hyperflexion of the neck (rollkur), which could compromise breathing and cause pain or discomfort (von Borstel et al. 2009; Cehak et al. 2010; Go et al. 2014a, 2014b, 2014c). Horses' responses, such as head shaking and bolting, can then result in even harsher control or punishment (or the horse being relinquished or euthanised).

13.2.5 Health
Horses can suffer from several diseases (Table 13.6). Their management and sociability make them prone to infections spread by shared airspaces, contaminated bedding, human contact, or biting insects. Clostridial bacteria can also produce toxins causing

Table 13.6 Selected health problems in horses.

Condition		Key Welfare effects
Infectious or parasitic diseases	Viral	African Horse Sickness (V)	Fever, extreme respiratory distress (sometimes colic)
		Equine Herpes Virus (V)	Fever; upper respiratory tract inflammation, loss of appetite Neurological problems (EHV-1);
		Equine Infectious Anaemia	Fever, depression, weakness, weight loss Can be unaffected carriers
		Equine Viral Arteritis (V)	Fever, depression, loss of appetite, swelling, conjunctivitis, respiratory distress
		Equine (Arbo)viral encephalitis, e.g. West Nile Disease (alphaviruses and flaviviruses) (V)	Depression Neurological problems: disorientation; impaired vision; difficulty swallowing and moving; seizures; paralysis
		Hendra Virus (V)	Fever; depression Respiratory distress Neurological problems: difficulty moving; weakness; collapse; muscle spasms; impaired vision
		Influenza (V)	Fever; depression Mild to severe respiratory inflammation and coughing
	Bacterial	Glanders (*Burkholderia mallei*)	Chronic respiratory difficulty; upper respiratory tract inflammation; skin pain or discomfort
		Salmonella; *Clostridium difficile*; *C. perfringens*; *Neorickettsia risticii*	Acute: Fever; depression; coughing; loss of condition; respiratory distress Diarrhoea; dehydration; depression; abdominal pain; fever; malaise; (laminitis)
		Strangles (*Streptococcus equi equi*)	Some horses have no effects Fever; depression; loss of appetite; loss of condition Pain or discomfort from abscesses; respiratory inflammation; difficulty breathing; painful guttural pouch; skin damage

Fungal Oomycetes	Ringworm; Malassezia Pythiosis (*Pythium insidiosum*)	Itchiness (during active infection) Itchiness; (lameness if infects joints)
Protozoal	Equine protozoal myencephalitis (*Sarcocystis neurona*)	Malcoordination; weakness; disorientation
Internal parasites	Large or small redworms (Strongyles)	Mild diarrhoea; poor condition; depression; intestinal impaction: pain; anxiety
	Roundworms (Ascarids)	Poor body condition; lethargy; colic
	Tapeworms (esp. *Anoplocephala perfoliata*)	May have no effect; colic
External parasites	Mites; lice; fly larvae (warbles, blow-flies); ticks	Itchiness; loss of condition
Metabolic or hormonal	Equine Metabolic Syndrome	Obesity; increased thirst; laminitis; secondary infections
	Hyperlip(id)aemia	Loss of appetite; diarrhoea; depression; weakness; malcoordination; disorientation; head-pressing
	Fatty liver syndrome	Loss of appetite; depression; disorientation
	Laminitis	Pain (usually both forefeet); reluctance to move
Inflammatory	Insect hypersensitivity (Sweet itch or Queensland itch)	Itchiness
	Sarcoidosis	Skin damage
Neoplastic or paraneoplastic	Pedunculated lipoma	If wraps around intestine: severe acute abdominal pain; malaise; distress
Degenerative	Navicular disease[a]	Chronic, insidious pain, and lameness in both forelimbs
	Osteoarthritis	Chronic, progressive lameness (often on both limbs)
Toxic	Tetanus (V)	Stiffness and muscle spasms; light sensitivity; difficulty eating and drinking (i.e. 'lockjaw'); respiratory distress

(*Continued*)

Table 13.6 (Continued)

Condition		Key Welfare effects
	Botulism	Shaking (foals); difficulty eating; malcoordination; weakness; respiratory distress; paralysis (adults)
	Pyrrolizidine alkaloid, saponin	Poor body condition; loss of appetite; diarrhoea; depression; sensitivity to light; (malcoordination and other neurological signs for some toxins); can be acute or chronic
	Mycotoxins	
	Monensin, urea, ammonium salts	Malcoordination and weakness
Traumatic	Road accidents and fencing injuries	Pain; distress
	Tendon injury	Pain; altered movement

[a] Current hypotheses support navicular being a degenerative condition, although its causation is complex and unclear.

botulism (from intestinal bacteria) and tetanus (from wounds). Internal parasites can cause colic and diarrhoea, as well as additional problems as larvae migrate. External parasites can cause irritation or pain, and some horses develop severe 'sweet itch' reactions to midge bites which can cause intense irritation. Several infections are zoonotic, including Hendra virus, salmonellosis, ringworm, and rabies.

Horses are at risk of conditions such as bone fractures and tendon defects, and certain riding gear can also cause injury, for example, restrictive nosebands and standing martingales. External wounds can be particularly problematic for horses because of complications in healing and high susceptibility to tetanus. Horses may also suffer chronic and geriatric conditions such as arthritis, metabolic disorders (e.g. excessive cortisol production and insulin resistance) and dental disease. Some conditions may be more common in particular breeds or bloodlines. For example, navicular disease may be more common in American Quarter Horses and Thoroughbreds with particular foot conformations. Azoturia is also predisposed in some bloodlines, including Quarter Horses (Valberg et al. 1996) and some other breeds (Stanley et al. 2009).

Hygiene, ventilation, biosecurity, quarantining, monitoring, and health checks are all important, especially when moving horses to new livery yards. Horses should receive core vaccinations, in particular against tetanus and H7N7/H3N8 influenza strains. Parasites can be controlled by good pasture management, faecal testing, and deworming drugs. Unfortunately, many worm populations have developed resistance to particular drugs through overuse, poor drug selection, and underdosing. All horses require regular dental care and regular foot trimming (and be shod as necessary). However, inappropriate dentistry and farriery may cause footsoreness, altered foot balance, abscesses, or pain.

Horses may undergo various surgical procedures (Table 13.7). Myectomy, buccostomy, and neurectomy to address stereotypies (e.g. the Forssell procedure) are painful, ineffective, and fail to address the inappropriate conditions that cause them (Fraser 1992; Broom and Kennedy 1993; Fjeldborg 1993). Other archaic, painful, and largely unjustified surgeries include tail docking, tendon firing, and other procedures when aimed at improving performance rather than for a particular clinical need. For identification, hot branding and ear notching can cause significant pain and inflammation (Lindegaard et al. 2009; Erber et al. 2012), whereas microchipping appears to cause only mild short-term inflammation (Gerber et al. 2012). Males are usually castrated for the effects on temperament and to avoid unwanted breeding, but this procedure may also reduce frustration for the horse from unsatisfied sexual motivations. In contrast, mares are rarely spayed, although competition mares' hormones are commonly manipulated (Paul et al. 1995).

Some horses may be distressed by veterinary, farriery, or other procedures (Van Sommeren and Van Dierendonck 2010). Rather than relying on physical restraint, horses should be habituated to nonpainful procedures where possible, or where this is not possible, they should be sedated. 'Twitching' should be avoided because it causes a stress response (Thompson et al. 1988; Minero et al. 1999) and may work either by promoting analgesic endorphin release (Lagerweij et al. 1984) or by diverting attention to an additional pain. Twitching the ear is entirely unacceptable. Twitching the lip is an approach that should be adopted only when chemical restraint is not available and is best regarded as a last resort method of restraint justified only to help inject a psychotropic drug (McGreevy 2012). Local anaesthesia and systemic analgesia should be provided for all painful procedures such as tooth removal, castration, and other surgeries. Sedation may also decrease behavioural responses, although potentially without

Table 13.7 Non-therapeutic elective surgical procedures performed on horses.

Procedure	Reasons and benefits for the animal	Reasons and benefits for owners	Perioperative welfare risks	Welfare risks due to the behaviours prevented
Castration	Reduce sexual frustration Some health benefits	Ease of handling or management	Pain Infection	Inability to perform sexual behaviour
Vulval remodelling (Caslick's procedure)	Can reduce infections because of vulval conformation	Improved fertility	Pain; may require repeated surgery	Risks at birth if not corrected May allow mating of mares with inheritable vulval conformational problems
Surgical procedures to improve respiration (e.g. Hobday)	Perhaps reduced respiratory distress during extreme exercise	Improved performance?	Pain	
Wolf teeth removal	Reduced discomfort from bit	Improved responses to bit pressure	Severe pain	

reducing distress, depending on the drugs and dosages used. General anaesthesia for surgery risks musculoskeletal damage, myopathies, colic, and increased postoperative cortisol concentrations, perhaps as a result of distress or vertigo during anaesthetic recovery (Taylor 1989; Senior 2013).

13.2.6 Euthanasia

Acceptable methods of euthanasia of horses are listed in Table 13.8. The best method is usually sedation followed by either cranial shooting or the injection of an overdose of pentobarbitone into the jugular vein, usually alongside intravenous local anaesthetic or potassium chloride to achieve cardiac arrest. Horses may be slaughtered by head trauma using a captive bolt, followed by bleeding out, at an abattoir (but transportation to an abattoir should be avoided).

13.3 Signs of Horse Welfare

13.3.1 Pathophysiological Signs

Signs of acute pain or stress (or perhaps excitement) include heart rate, heart-rate variability and respiratory rate, glucose, adrenocorticotropic hormone (ACTH) concentrations, noradrenaline, cortisol, and its metabolites (Table 13.9), although, conversely,

Table 13.8 Methods of euthanasia for horses kept as companion animals.

Method	Restraint required	Welfare benefits	Welfare risks
Intravenous barbiturate (combined with local anaesthetic or potassium chloride to cause cardiac arrest)	Secure handling Sedation advised	Rapid loss of consciousness	Possible pain at injection site Reversible at low dosages Needs restraint
Free bullet	Secure handling Sedation advised	Immediate loss of consciousness	Intense pain if inaccurate shot Risk of bullet ricochet

Table 13.9 Selected conditions in which increased cortisol concentration has been observed in horses.

Context	Possible associated feelings
Isolation	Distress
Exercise	Activity, excitement
Sex	Excitement
Transportation	Distress, fear, physiological challenge
Twitching	Pain
Colic, grass-sickness, and laminitis	Pain, malaise, physiological challenge
Orthopaedic conditions	Pain
Surgery	Pain, distress, dysphoria

Source: Hoffsis and Murdick (1970), Kirkpatrick et al. (1979), Alexander et al. (1988), Colborn et al. (1991), Mal et al. 1991a; Mills et al. (1997), Rivera et al. (2002), Shanahan (2003), Pritchett et al. (2003), Snow and Rose (1981), Thompson et al. (1988), Niinistö et al. (2010), Ayala et al. (2012).

decreased cortisol concentration may indicate chronic stress. Low body-condition score may suggest not only poor nutrition but also health problems including parasites, cachexic diseases, grass sickness, chronic infections, pain, or dental disease. Gastric ulceration may suggest poor diet or stress, for example, associated with training, transportation, confinement, or social isolation (McGreevy et al. 1995; Murray and Eichorn 1996; McClure et al. 2005). All generic equine pathophysiological welfare measures should be interpreted cautiously (Table 13.10). Some appear unreliable (e.g. Mal et al. 1991a; Mills et al. 1997), and several seem to be evidence of horses' coping abilities more than of their suffering (McGreevy and Nicol 1998; Bachmann et al. 2003b). Many parameters can also vary without representing any change in welfare at all as a result of horses' age, temperament, season, and time of the day, although differences in such variations can themselves be used as a sign of stress (Leal et al. 2011).

Table 13.10 Basic measures and clinical standards of horses (*Equus caballus*).

Parameter	Normal measures	
Life expectancy	up to 62 years, mean 20 years	
Mean weight	Males: Breed dependent	Females: Breed dependent
Body temperature	37.2–38.3 °C	
Respiratory frequency	8–16 breaths/min	
Heart rate	36–40 beats/min	
Pubescence	Males: 56–97 weeks	Females: 31–148 weeks
Blood volume	10.31 (Thoroughbred)	
Haematocrit	41–52	

Source: Marcilese et al. (1964), Hayes (1968), Javic and Conroy (2003), and McKinnon et al. (2011).

13.3.2 Behavioural Signs

Horses in pain or illness may appear depressed (Pritchard et al. 2005) or unresponsive (Ashley et al. 2005; Burn et al. 2010b). Conversely, they may show signs of restlessness or discomfort such as pinning down the ears, flicking the tail, restlessness or snorting, rearing or stomping, aggression, and pawing on the floor (Ashley et al. 2005; Lindgaard et al. 2009). Particular sources of pain may be indicated by locally directed behaviours, for example, orthopaedic pain by lameness and colic by kicking at the abdomen. Several pain scoring systems and a 'Horse Grimace Scale' have been developed (e.g., Dalla Costa et al. 2014), although there can be differences in pain expression between individuals (Ijichi et al. 2014), and lack of a grimace response does not necessarily indicate lack of pain.

Behavioural signs of distress can include increased locomotory activity, vigilance behaviours, neighing, snorting, pawing, nibbling walls and buckets, defaecation, rearing, flehmen responses, kicking stable walls or doors, 'high blowing' through the nose, and high-stepping 'prancing' (Wolff et al. 1997; McDonnell and Poulin 2002; Harewood and McGowan 2005; Visser et al. 2008). Aggression can indicate unsuitable company, pain, insufficient resources, or other stresses. However, it can be difficult to distinguish social play and aggression; the former can involve circling, chasing, and 'mock' bites and kicks, which owners could misinterpret as aggression. The development of stereotypies can also suggest some environmental or other stressor with which the horse is otherwise unable to cope (Sarrafchi and Blokhuis 2013; Figure 13.4).

13.4 Action Plan for Improving Animal Welfare in this Species Worldwide

There have been relatively few studies to determine key priorities for improving horse welfare (exception are Collins et al. 2009, 2010a and McGreevy et al. 2018). Nevertheless, it is possible to identify several broad priorities for action. The first is to ensure owners are adequately prepared for looking after a horse, purchase appropriate animals, and appreciate the knowledge, costs, space, time, and effort required for several decades over a horse's life.

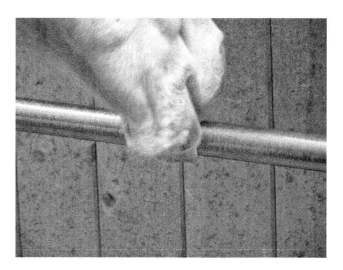

Figure 13.4   Oral stereotypy in a horse.

Owners' unawareness of the common challenges and how to tackle them may be compounded by difficulty in identifying genuine experts from self-styled authorities. Owners' difficulties are compounded by particular beliefs and attitudes that may include an unquestioning respect for traditional, outdated practices, 'fads', and the belief that, unlike most other pets, horses need to be used (as when owners are unwilling to retire injured horses from work). Some problems are hard to tackle because they are so common that owners are unlikely to question them or to explore alternatives (e.g. whipping).

Owners need to be encouraged to house horses in social, outdoor pasture wherever possible. The main benefits of stabling and tethering are for ease of management and reduced land requirements, so owners need to expect and plan for keeping horses at pasture. Isolation in either tethering or permanent stabling is also sufficiently common that many owners may not consider alternatives. Some owners may be anxious that their horse will be injured if given adequate space or company; education needs to inform them that, in fact, restrictions may actually increase those risks. Owners should also be encouraged to minimise changes in horse social groups.

Owners also need to be encouraged to use humane and rewarding methods of training, and should be taught to ride with an understanding of learning theory (McLean and McGreevy 2010). However, there is a lack of understanding about ethology and the principles of humane training. For example some riders worry that hand-feeding rewards may prompt biting or erroneously think they already mainly use reward-based methods (Warren-Smith and McGreevy 2008; Hockenhull and Creighton 2010). Many 'aids' such as whips and spurs are common. Riders and trainers may also feel that horses are being 'disobedient', forgetting that they are asking horses to overcome their own natural preferences. Elite global organisations need to promote training practices that are based on horses' cognitive abilities, learning, and ethology. This requires overcoming some current sports rules that actually mandate the use of potentially harmful equipment (e.g. the *Fédération Equestre Internationale*'s mandate on double bridles in elite dressage). Elite organisations need to regularly review their rules using ethical guidelines such as those produced by the International Society for Equitation Science. Organisations that teach riding and sport governing bodies can then take a leadership role in improving horse welfare.

Those who are breeding and selling horses also have a role in improving horse welfare. They should avoid breeding from horses with heritable health conditions or predispositions to diseases and should avoid breeding horses unless there is a good prospect of ensuring that they go to responsible and informed owners. Horse owners who transfer ownership should also take reasonable steps to ensure the long-term welfare of their horses, including in minimising harms from irresponsible ownership, live transportation, or slaughter. Owners may instead loan their horses to new keepers instead of selling them, thereby retaining some control and reducing the risk of the horse being abandoned, sold, or neglected. Live transportation of horses to slaughter has no clear benefit and has the potential for severe welfare compromises. Where it is not prohibited, long-distance – or any – transport should be carried out in ways that ensure the welfare of the horses involved.

Improvements will require research into the effects of husbandry, training, and riding methods. There is already sufficient scientific evidence to stop many common practices that result in poor welfare such as single housing, tethering, and insufficient forage. For these issues, research should focus on how to use those data to effect change amongst owners. Further research is needed to identify how horses respond, develop, and learn, particularly during training and riding, to work out the best training methods and debunk traditional myths or new fads. These issues are increasingly being addressed by the new discipline of equitation science (McGreevy 2007; Goodwin et al. 2009). Although there is increasing amount of research in equine veterinary medicine, research is needed in the epidemiology of diseases spread by biting insects, when climate change may spread these insect vectors to other areas. There is little scientific evidence for some areas of 'paraprofessional' work. This makes it important that paraprofessionals do not stray beyond their competence or deter owners from seeking genuine veterinary care.

Bibliography

Alexander, S.L., Irvine, C.H.G., Livesey, J.H., and Donald, R.A. (1988). Effect of isolation stress on concentrations of arginine, vasopressin, a -melanocyte-stimulating hormone and ACTH in the pituitary venous effluent of the normal horse. *Journal of Endocrinology* 116: 325–334.

Anthony, D.W. (1996). Bridling horse power: the domestication of the horse. In: *Horses Through Time* (ed. S.L. Olsen), 57–82. Dublin: Roberts Rinehart.

Archer, D.C., Freeman, D.E., Doyle, A.J. et al. (2004). Association between cribbing and entrapment of the small intestine in the epiploic foramen in horses: 68 cases (1991–2002). *Journal of the American Veterinary Medical Association* 224 (4): 562–564.

Archer, D.C. and Proudman, C.J. (2006). Epidemiological clues to preventing colic. *The Veterinary Journal* 172: 29–39.

Ashley, F.H., Waterman-Pearson, A.E., and Whay, H.R. (2005). Behavioural assessment of pain in horses and donkeys: application to clinical practice and future studies. *Equine Veterinary Journal* 37: 565–575.

AWIN (Horse Grimace Scale App). (2014). Available at https://play.google.com/store/apps/details?id=info.awinhub.HorseGrimacePainScale. Accessed 1 June 2014.

Ayala, I., Martos, N.F., Silvan, G. et al. (2012). Cortisol, adrenocorticotropic hormone, serotonin, adrenaline and noradrenaline serum concentrations in relation to disease and stress in the horse. *Research in Veterinary Science* 93: 103–107.

Bachmann, I., Audige, L., and Stauffacher, M. (2003a). Risk factors associated with behavioural disorders of crib-biting, weaving and box-walking in Swiss horses. *Equine Veterinary Journal* 35 (2): 158–163.

Bachmann, I., Bermasconi, P., Herrmann, R. et al. (2003b). Behavioural and physiological responses to an acute stressor in crib-biting and control horses. *Applied Animal Behaviour Science* 82: 297–311.

Bailey, S.R., Marr, C.M., and Elliott, J. (2004). Current research and theories on the pathogenesis of acute laminitis in the horse. *The Veterinary Journal* 167: 129–142.

Becvarova, I. and Pleasant, R.S. (2012). Managing obesity in pasture-based horses. *Compendium: Continuing Education for Veterinarians* 34 (4): E1–E4.

Berger, J. and Cunningham, C. (1987). Influence of familiarity on frequency of inbreeding in wild horses. *Evolution* 41 (1): 229–231.

Berndt, A., Derksen, F.J., and Edward Robinson, N. (2008). Endotoxin concentrations within the breathing zone of horses are higher in stables than on pasture. *The Veterinary Journal* 183 (1): 54–57.

Birke, L., Hockenhull, J., Creighton, E. et al. (2011). Horses' responses to variation in human approach. *Applied Animal Behaviour Science* 134: 56–63.

Blackman, M. and Moore-Colyer, M.J.S. (1998). Hay for horses: the effects of three different wetting treatments on dust and nutrient content. *Animal Science* 66: 745–750.

Boyd, L. and Keiper, R. (2005). Behavioural ecology of feral horses. In: *The Domestic Horse, the Evolution, Development and Management of Its Behaviour* (ed. D.S. Mills and S.M. McDonnell), 55–82. Cambridge: Cambridge University Press, Cambridge.

Broom, D.M. and Kennedy, M.J. (1993). Stereotypies in horses: their relevance to welfare and causation. *Equine Veterinary Education* 5 (3): 151–154.

Burn, C.C., Dennisonb, T.L., and Whay, H.R. (2010a). Environmental and demographic risk factors for poor welfare in working horses, donkeys and mules in developing countries. *The Veterinary Journal* 186: 385–392.

Burn, C.C., Dennisonb, T.L., and Whay, H.R. (2010b). Relationships between behaviour and health in working horses, donkeys, and mules in developing countries. *Applied Animal Behaviour Science* 126: 109–118.

Carter, R.A., Treiber, K.H., Geor, R.J. et al. (2009). Prediction of incipient pasture-associated laminitis from hyperinsulinaemia, hyperleptinaemia and generalized and localised obesity in a cohort of ponies. *Equine Veterinary Journal* 41 (2): 171–178.

Cehak, A., Rohn, K., Barton, A.-K. et al. (2010). Effect of head and neck position on pharyngeal diameter in horses. *Veterinary Radiology & Ultrasound* 51: 491–497.

Chaya, L., Cowan, E., and McGuire, B. (2006). A note on the relationship between time spent in turnout and behaviour during turnout in horses (Equus caballus). *Applied Animal Behaviour Science* 98: 155–160.

Christensen, J.W., Ladewig, J., Søndergaard, E., and Malmkvist, J. (2002). Effects of individual versus group stabling on social behaviour in domestic stallions. *Applied Animal Behaviour Science* 75: 233–248.

Christie, J.L., Hewson, C.J., Riley, C.B. et al. (2006). Management factors affecting stereotypies and body condition score in nonracing horses in Prince Edward Island. *Canadian Veterinary Journal* 47: 136–143.

Clutton-Brock, J. (1999). *A Natural History of Domesticated Mammals*, 2e. Cambridge: Cambridge University Press.

Colborn, D.R., Thompson, D.L.J., Roth, T.L. et al. (1991). Responses of cortisol and prolactin to sexual excitement and stress in stallions and geldings. *Journal of Animal Science* 69: 2556–2562.

Collins, J., Hanlon, A., More, S.J., and Duggan, V. (2009). Policy Delphi with vignette methodology as a tool to evaluate the perception of equine welfare. *Veterinary Journal* 181: 63–69.

Collins, J.A., Hanlon, A., More, S.J. et al. (2010a). Causes, desirability, feasibility and means of raising standards. *Equine Veterinary Journal* 42 (2): 105–113.

Collins, S.N., Pollitt, C., Wylie, C.E., and Matiasek, K. (2010b). Laminitic pain: parallels with pain states in humans and other species. *Veterinary Clinics of North America: Equine Practice* 26 (2010): 643–671.

Cooper, J.J. and Albentosa, M.J. (2005). Behavioural adaptation in the domestic horse: potential role of apparently abnormal responses including stereotypic behaviour. *Livestock Production Science* 92: 177–182.

Cooper, J.J. and Mason, G.J. (1998). The identification of abnormal behaviour and behavioural problems in stabled horses and their relationship to horse welfare: a comparative review. *Equine Veterinary Journal. Supplement* 27: 5–9.

Crowell-Davis, S.L. (1986). Development behavior. *The Veterinary Clinics of North America. Equine Practice* 2: 573–590.

Dalla Costa, E., Minero, M., Lebelt, D. et al. (2014). Development of the Horse Grimace Scale (HGS) as a pain assessment tool in horses undergoing routine castration. *PLoS One* 9 (3): e92281.

Dallaire, A. (1986). Rest behavior. *Veterinary Clinics of North America: Equine Practice* 2 (3): 591–607.

Davidson, N. and Harris, P. (2002). Nutrition and welfare. In: *The Welfare of Horses* (ed. N. Waran), 45–76. Dordrecht: Kluwer Academic Publishers.

Diamond, J. (1997). *Guns Germs and Steel: The Fates of Human Societies*. London, UK: Vintage.

Diehl, N.K., Egan, B. and Tozer, P. (2002). Intensive, early handling of neonatal foals: mare–foal interactions. *Havemeyer Workshop on Horse Behavior and Welfare*, Holar, Iceland, Pp. 40–46.

Doherty, O., Casey, V., McGreevy, P., Arkins, S. (2016). An investigation into noseband tightness levels on competition horses. Proceedings of the 12th International Conference of International Society for Equitation Science. Eds: M. Cressent, M. Renault, H. Randle, A. Bailey. June 23–25, 2016, French National Riding School, Saumur, France, Page 53.

Donaldson, M.T., McDonnell, S.M., Schanbacher, B.J. et al. (2005). Variation in plasma adrenocorticotropic hormone concentration and dexamethasone suppression test results with season, age, and sex in healthy ponies and horses. *Journal of Veterinary Internal Medicine* 19: 217–222.

Dugdale, A.H.A. (2014). Progress in equine pain assessment? *The Veterinary Journal* 200: 210–211.

Erber, R., Wulf, M., Becker-Birck, M. et al. (2012). Physiological and behavioural responses of young horses to hot iron branding and microchip implantation. *The Veterinary Journal* 191 (2): 171–175.

Evans, D.L. and McGreevy, P.D. (2011). An investigation of racing performance and whip use by jockeys in Thoroughbred races. *PLoS One* 6 (1): e15622. doi: 10.1371/journal.pone.0015622.

Evans, K.E. and McGreevy, P.D. (2006). The distribution of ganglion cells in the equine retina and its relationship to skull morphology. *Anatomia, Histologia, Embryologia* 35: 1–6.

Feh, C. (1999). Alliances and reproductive success in Camargue stallions. *Animal Behaviour* 57: 705–713.

Feh, C. (2001). Alliances between stallions are more than just multi-male groups: reply to Linklater & Cameron. *Animal Behaviour* 61: 27–30.

Fenner, K., Yoon, S., White, P. et al. (2016). The effect of noseband tightening on horses' behavior, eye temperature, and cardiac responses. *PLoS One* 11 (5): e0154179. doi: 10.1371/journal.pone.0154179.

Fjeldborg, J. (1993). Results of surgical treatment of cribbing by neurectomy and myectomy. *Equine Practice* 15 (7): 34–36.

Food and Agriculture Organisation of the United Nations (FAO). (2014). FAOSTAT. Available at http://faostat3.fao.org/faostat-gateway/go/to/download/Q/QA/E. Accessed 24 May 2018.

Fraser, A.F. (1992). *The Behaviour of the Horse*. Wallingford, UK: CABI.

Freire, R., Buckley, P., and Cooper, J.J. (2010). Effects of different forms of exercise on post inhibitory rebound and unwanted behaviour in stabled horses. *Equine Veterinary Journal* 41 (5): 487–492.

Fureix, C., Jego, P., Sankey, C., and Hausberger, M. (2009). How horses (Equus caballus) see the world: humans as significant "objects". *Animal Cognition* 12: 643–654.

Gerber, M.I., Swinker, A.M., Staniar, W.B. et al. (2012). Health factors associated with microchip insertion in horses. *Journal of Equine Veterinary Science* 32: 177–182.

Giles, N. and Tupper, J. (2006). Letter: equine interspecies aggression. *Veterinary Record* 159 (22): 756.

Giles, S.L., Nicol, C.J., Harris, P.A., and Rands, S.A. (2015). Dominance rank is associated with body condition in outdoor-living domestic horses (Equus caballus). *Applied Animal Behaviour Science* 166: 71–79.

Go, L., Barton, A.K., and Ohnesorge, B. (2014a). Pharyngeal diameter in various head and neck positions during exercise in sport horses. *Veterinary Research 2014* 10: 117.

Go, L., Barton, A.K., and Ohnesorge, B. (2014b). Objective classification of different head and neck positions and their influence on the radiographic pharyngeal diameter in sport horses. *Veterinary Research* 10: 118.

Go, L., Barton, A.K., and Ohnesorge, B. (2014c). Evaluation of laryngeal function under the influence of various head and neck positions during exercise in 58 performance horses. *Equine Veterinary Education* 26 (1): 41–47.

Goodloe, R.B., Warren, R.J., Osborn, D.A., and Hall, C. (2000). Population characteristics of feral horses on Cumberland island, Georgia and their management implications. *Journal of Wildlife Management* 64 (1): 114–121.

Goodwin, D. (1999). The importance of ethology in understanding the behaviour of the horse. *Equine Veterinary Journal* 28 (S): 15–19.

Goodwin, D., Davidson, H.P.B., and Harris, P. (2002). Foraging enrichment for stabled horses: effects on behaviour and selection. *Equine Veterinary Journal* 34 (7): 686–691.

Goodwin, D., McGreevy, P., Waran, N., and McLean, A. (2009). How equitation science can elucidate and refine horsemanship techniques. *The Veterinary Journal* 181 (1): 5–11.

Harewood, E.J. and McGowan, C.M. (2005). Behavioural and physiological responses to stabling in naïve horses. *Journal of Equine Veterinary Science* 25 (4): 164–170.

Harris, P.A. (1999). How understanding the digestive process can help minimise digestive disturbances due to diet and feeding practices. In: *Proceedings of the BEVA specialist days on behaviour and nutrition* (ed. P.A. Harris, G. Gomarsall, H.P.B. Davidson and R. Green), 45–49. Newmarket, UK: Equine Veterinary Journals.

Hartmann, E., Søndergaard, E., and Keeling, L.J. (2012). Keeping horses in groups: a review. *Applied Animal Behaviour Science* 136 (2012): 77–87.

Hayes, M.H. (1968). *Veterinary Notes for Horse Owners*. London: Stanley Paul.

Henderson, J.V. and Waran, N.K. (2001). Reducing equine stereotypies using an equiball. *Animal Welfare* 10: 73–80.

Hennessy, K.D., Quinn, K.M., and Murphy, J. (2008). Producer or purchaser: different expectations may lead to equine wastage and welfare concerns. *Journal of Applied Animal Welfare Science* 11 (3): 232–235.

Henry, S., Richard-Yris, M.-A., Tordjman, S., and Hausberger, M. (2009). Neonatal handling affects durably bonding and social development. *PLoS One* 4 (4): e5216.

Hinton, H. (1978). On the watering of horses – a review. *Equine Veterinary Journal* 10: 27–31.

Hintz, H.F. and Loy, R.G. (1966). Effects of pelleting on the nutritive value of horse rations. *Journal of Animal Science* 25: 1059–1062.

Hockenhull, J. and Creighton, E. (2010). Unwanted oral investigative behaviour in horses: a note on the relationship between mugging behaviour, hand-feeding titbits and clicker training. *Applied Animal Behaviour Science* 127 (2010): 104–107.

Hoffsis, G.F. and Murdick, P.W. (1970). The plasma concentrations of corticosteroids in normal and diseased horses. *Journal of the American Veterinary Medical Association* 157: 1590–1594.

Holcomb, K.E., Tucker, C.B., and Stull, C.L. (2013). Physiological, behavioral, and serological responses of horses to shaded or unshaded pens in a hot, sunny environment. *Journal of Animal Science* 91 (12): 5926–5936. doi: 10.2527/jas.2013-6497.

Holcomb, K.E., Tucker, C.B., and Stull, C.L. (2014). Preference of domestic horses for shade in a hot, sunny environment. *Journal of Animal Science* jas.2013-7386; published ahead of print February 3, 2014 doi: 10.2527/jas.2013-7386.

Hothersall, B. and Nicol, C. (2009). Role of diet and feeding in normal and stereotypic behaviors in horses. *Veterinary Clinics of North America: Equine Practice* 25 (2009): 167–181.

Houpt, K.A. (1987). Thirst of horses: the physiological and psychological causes. *Equine Practice* 9: 28–30.

Houpt, K.A. and Houpt, T.R. (1988). Social and illumination preferences of mares. *Journal of Animal Science* 66: 2159–2164.

Houpt, K.A. and Olm, D. (1984). Foal rejection: a review of 23 cases. *Equine Practice* 6: 38.

Houpt, K., Houpt, T.R., Johnson, J.L. et al. (2001). The effect of exercise deprivation on the behaviour and physiology of straight stall confined pregnant mares. *Animal Welfare* 10: 257–267.

Hunter, L. and Houpt, K.A. (1989). Bedding material preferences of ponies. *Journal of Animal Science* 67: 1986–1991.

Ijichi, C., Collins, L.M., and Elwood, R.W. (2014). Pain expression is linked to personality in horses. *Applied Animal Behaviour Science* 152 (2014): 38–43.

Javic, K. and Conroy, C.N. (2003). Equine clinical pathology normal values. New bolton center Field service department. Available at http://cal.vet.upenn.edu/projects/fieldservice/Equine/EQCLPATH.htm. Accessed 30 December 2016.

Kirkpatrick, J.F., Baker, C.B., Turner, J.W. Jr. et al. (1979). Plasma corticosteroids as an index of stress in captive feral horses. *The Journal of Wildlife Management* 43 (3): 801–804.

Krueger, K., Flauger, B., Farmer, K., and Maros, K. (2011). Horses (Equus caballus) use human local enhancement cues and adjust to human attention. *Animal Cognition* 14: 187–201.

Krzak, W.E., Gonyou, H.W., and Lawrence, L.M. (1991). Wood chewing by stabled horses: diurnal pattern and effects of exercise. *Journal of Animal Science* 69: 1053–1058.

Lagerweij, E., PC Nelis, P.C., Wiegant, V.M., and van Ree, J.M. (1984). The twitch in horses: a variant of acupuncture. *Science* 225 (4667): 1172–1174.

Leal, B.B., Alves, G.E.S., Douglas, R.H. et al. (2011). Cortisol circadian rhythm ratio: a simple method to detect stressed horses at higher risk of colic? *Journal of Equine Veterinary Science* 31 (2011): 188–190.

Lemasson, A., Boutin, A., Boivin, S. et al. (2009). Horse (Equus caballus) whinnies: a source of social information. *Animal Cognition* 12: 693–704.

Le Scolan, N., Hausberger, M., and Wolff, A. (1997). Stability over situations in temperamental traits of horses as revealed by experimental and scoring approaches. *Behavioural Processes* 41 (3): 257–266.

Lindegaard, C., Vaabengaard, D., Christophersen, M.T. et al. (2009). Evaluation of pain and inflammation associated with hot iron branding and microchip transponder injection in horses. *American Journal of Veterinary Research* 70: 840–847.

Linklater, W.L. and Cameron, E.Z. (2000). Tests for cooperative behaviour between stallions. *Animal Behaviour* 60: 731–743.

Linklater, W.L., Cameron, E.Z., Stafford, K.J., and Veltman, C.J. (2000). Social and spatial structure and range use by Kaimanawa wild horses (*Equus caballus: Equidae*). *New Zealand Journal of Ecology* 24 (2): 139–152.

Lippold, S., Matzke, N.J., Reissmann, M., and Hofreiter, M. (2011). Whole mitochondrial genome sequencing of domestic horses reveals incorporation of extensive wild horse diversity during domestication. *BMC Evolutionary Biology* 11 (1): 328.

Mal, M.E., Friend, T.H., Lay, D.C. et al. (1991a). Physiological responses of mares to short term confinement and isolation. *Journal of Equine Veterinary Science* 11: 96–102.

Mal, M.E., Friend, T., Lay, D. et al. (1991b). Behavioral responses of mares to short-term confinement and social isolation. *Applied Animal Behaviour Science* 31: 13–24.

Marcilese, N.A., Valsecchi, R.M., Figueiras, H.D. et al. (1964). Normal blood volumes in the horse. *The American Journal of Physiology* 207: 223–227.

McAfee, L.M., Mills, D.S., and Cooper, J.J. (2002). The use of mirrors for the control of stereotypic weaving behaviour in the stabled horse. *Applied Animal Behaviour Science* 78 (2–4): 159–173.

McBride, S.D. and Cuddeford, D. (2001). The putative welfare-reducing effects of preventing equine stereotypic behaviour. *Animal Welfare* 10: 173–189.

McClure SR, Carithers DS, Gross SJ, Murray MJ (2005). Gastric ulcer development in horses in a simulated show or training environment.

McDonnell, S.M. (2008). Practical review of self-mutilation in horses. *Animal Reproduction Science* 107: 219–228.

McDonnell, S.M. (2000). Reproductive behaviour of stallions and mares: comparison of free-running and domestic in-hand breeding. *Animal Reproduction Science* 60–61: 211–219.

McDonnell, S.M. and Poulin, A. (2002). Equid play ethogram. *Applied Animal Behaviour Science* 78: 263–295.

McDonnell, S.M., Miller, J., and Vaala, W. (2013). Calming benefit of short-term alpha-casozepine supplementation during acclimation to domestic environment and basic ground training of adult semi-feral ponies. *Journal of Equine Veterinary Science* 33 (2): 101–106.

McGreevy, P. (1996). *Why Does My Horse…?* London: Souvenir Press.

McGreevy, P.D. (2007). The advent of equitation science. *The Veterinary Journal* 174 (3): 492–500.

McGreevy, P.D.A. (2012). *Equine Behavior – Guide for Veterinarians and Equine Scientists.* London: W.B. Saunders.

McGreevy, P.D. (2015). Right under our noses. *Equine Veterinary Education.* 27 (10): 503–504.

McGreevy, P., Warren-Smith, A., and Guisard, Y. (2012). The effect of double bridles and jaw-clamping crank nosebands on facial cutaneous and ocular temperature in horses. *Journal of Veterinary Behavior: Clinical Applications and Research.* 7: 142–148.

McGreevy, P.D. and Nicol, C.J. (1998). Behavioural and physiological consequences associated with the short-term prevention of crib-biting in horses. *Physiology and Behaviour* 65 (1): 15–23.

McGreevy, P.D., Cripps, P.J., French, N.P. et al. (1995). Management factors associated with stereotypic and redirected behaviour in the thoroughbred horse. *Equine Veterinary Journal* 27 (2): 86–91.

McGreevy, P.D., Berger, J., de Brauwere, N. et al. (2018). Using the five domains model to assess the adverse impacts of husbandry, veterinary and equitation interventions on horse welfare. *Animals* 8: 71.

McGreevy, P.D. and McLean, A.N. (2010). *Equitation Science.* Oxford, UK: Wiley-Blackwell.

McIlwraith, C.W. and Rollin, B.E. (2011). *Equine Welfare.* Oxford, UK: UFAW/Wiley-Blackwell.

McKinnon, A., Squires, E., Vaala, W., and Varner, D. (2011). *Equine Reproduction.* Ames, Iowa: Blackwell.

McLean, A.N. and McGreevy, P.D. (2010). Horse-training techniques that may defy the principles of learning theory. *Journal of Veterinary Behavior: Clinical Applications and Research.* 5: 187–195.

Merck Veterinary Manual (2015). Nutritional Requirements of Horses. Available at https://www.merckvetmanual.com/management-and-nutrition/nutrition-horses/ nutritional-requirements-of-horses. Accessed 17 September 2015.

Mills, D.S. and Riezebos, M. (2005). The role of the image of a conspecific in the regulation of stereotypic head movements in the horse. *Applied Animal Behaviour Science* 91 (1–2): 155–165.

Mills, P.C., Ng, J.C., Kramer, H., and Auer, D.E. (1997). Stress response to chronic inflammation in the horse. *Equine Veterinary Journal* 29: 483–486.

Mills, D.S. and Clarke, A. (2002). Housing, management and welfare. In: *The Welfare of Horses* (ed. N. Waran), 77–97. Dordrecht: Kluwer Academic Publishers.

Mills, D.S., Eckley, S., and Cooper, J.J. (2000). Thoroughbred bedding preferences, associated behaviour differences and their implications for equine welfare. *Animal Science* 70 (1): 95–106.

Minero, M., Canali, E., Ferrante, V. et al. (1999). Heart rate and behavioural responses of crib-biting horses to two acute stressors. *Veterinary Record* 145: 430–433.

Monard, A.-M. and Duncan, P. (1996). Consequences of natal dispersal in female horses. *Animal Behaviour* 52: 565–579.

Monard, A.-M., Duncan, P., and Boy, V. (1996). The proximate mechanisms of natal dispersal in female horses. *Behaviour* 133: 1095–1024.

Murray, M.J. and Eichorn, E.S. (1996). Effects of intermittent feed deprivation, intermittent feed deprivation with ranitidine administration, and stall confinement with ad libitum access to hay on gastric ulceration in horses. *American Journal of Veterinary Research* 57: 1599–1603.

Niinistö, K.E., Korolainen, R.V., Raekallio, M.R. et al. (2010). Plasma levels of heat shock protein 72 (HSP72) and β-endorphin as indicators of stress, pain and prognosis in horses with colic. *The Veterinary Journal* 184 (1): 100–104.

National Research Council (NRC) (2007). *Nutrient Requirements of Horses*, 6e. Washington, USA: National Academies Press.

Nicol, C. (1999). Understanding equine stereotypies. *Equine Veterinary Journal. Supplement* 28: 20–25.

Parker, R.A. and Yeates, J. (2011). Assessment of quality of life in equine patients. *Equine Veterinary Journal* 44: 244–249.

Paul, J.W., Rains, J.R., and Lehman, F.D. (1995). The use and misuse of progestins in the mare. *Equine Practice* 17 (3): 21–22.

Pritchard, J.C., Lindberg, A.C., Main, D.C.J., and Whay, H.R. (2005). Assessment of the welfare of working horses, mules and donkeys, using health and behaviour parameters. *Preventive Veterinary Medicine* 69: 265–283.

Pritchett, L.C., Ulibarri, C., Roberts, M.C. et al. (2003). Identification of potential physiological and behavioural indicators of postoperative pain in horses after exploratory celiotomy for colic. *Applied Animal Behaviour Science* 80: 31–43.

Proops, L., McComb, K., and Reby, D. (2009). Cross-modal individual recognition in domestic horses (Equus caballus). *Proceedings of the National Academy of Sciences (USA)* 106 (3): 947–951.

Racklyeft, D.J. and Love, D.N. (1990). Influence of head posture on the respiratory tract of healthy horses. *Australian Veterinary Journal* 67 (11): 402–405.

Rivera, E., Benjamin, S., Nielsen, B. et al. (2002). Behavioral and physiological responses of horses to initial training: the comparison between pastured versus stalled horses. *Applied Animal Behaviour Science* 78 (2): 235–252.

Ruckebusch, Y. (1975). The hypnogram as an index of adaptation of farm animals to change their environment. *Applied Animal Ethology* 2: 3–18.

Sankey, C., Richard-Yris, M.-A., Leroy, H. et al. (2010a). Positive interactions lead to lasting positive memories in horses, Equus caballus. *Animal Behaviour* 79: 869–875.

Sankey, C., Richard-Yris, M.A., Henry, S. et al. (2010b). Reinforcement as a mediator of the perception of humans by horses (Equus caballus). *Animal Cognition* 13: 753–764.

Sarrafchi, A. and Blokhuis, H.J. (2013). Equine stereotypic behaviors: causation, occurrence, and prevention. *Journal of Veterinary Behavior* 8 (2013): 386–394.

Seaman, S.C., Davidson, H.P.B., and Waran, N.K. (2002). How reliable is temperament assessment in the domestic horse (*Equus caballus*)? *Applied Animal Behaviour Science* 78 (2): 175–191.

Senior, J.M. (2013). Morbidity, mortality, and risk of general anesthesia in horses. *Veterinary Clinics of North America: Equine Practice* 29 (2013): 1–18.

Shanahan, S. (2003). Trailer loading stress in horses: behavioral and physiological effects of nonaversive training (TTEAM). *Journal of Applied Animal Welfare Science* 6 (4): 263–274.

Smith, B.L., Jones, J.H., Hornof, W.J. et al. (1996). Effects of road transport on indices of stress in horses. *Equine Veterinary Journal* 28 (6): 446–454.

Snow, D.H. and Rose, R.J. (1981). Hormonal changes associated with long distance exercise. *Equine Veterinary Journal* 13 (3): 195–197.

Søndergaard, E. and Ladewig, J. (2004). Group housing exerts a positive effect on the behaviour of young horses during training. *Applied Animal Behaviour Science* 87 (1): 105–118.

Stanley, R.L., McCue, M.E., Valberg, S.J. et al. (2009). A glycogen synthase 1 mutation associated with equine polysaccharide storage myopathy and exertional rhabdomyolysis occurs in a variety of UK breeds. *Equine Veterinary Journal* 41: 597–601.

Sweeting, M.P., Houpt, C.E., and Houpt, K.A. (1985). Social facilitation of feeding and time budgets in stabled ponies. *Journal of Animal Science* 160: 369–374.

Taylor, P.M. (1989). Equine stress responses to anesthesia. *British Journal of Anaesthesia* 63: 702–709.

Thompson, D.L., Garza, F., Mitchell, P.S., and St. George, R.L. (1988). Effects of short-term stress, xylazine tranquilization and anesthetization with xylacine plus ketamine on plasma concentrations of cortisol, luteinizing hormone, follicle stimulating hormone and prolactin in ovariectomized pony mares. *Theriogenology* 30: 937–946.

Thorne, J.B., Goodwin, D., Kennedy, M.J. et al. (2005). Foraging enrichment for individually housed horses: practicality and effects on behaviour. *Applied Animal Behaviour Science* 94: 149–164.

Valberg, S.J., Geyer, C., Sorum, S.A., and Cardinet, G.H. (1996). Familial basis of exertional rhabdomyolysis in quarter horse-related breeds. *American Journal of Veterinary Research* 57: 286–290.

Van Dierendonck, M.C., Sigurjónsdóttir, H., Colenbrander, B., and Thorhallsdóttir, A.G. (2004). Differences in social behaviour between late pregnant, post-partum and barren mares in a herd of Icelandic horses. *Applied Animal Behaviour Science* 89 (3): 283–297.

Van Sommeren, A. and Van Dierendonck, M. (2010). The use of equine appeasing pheromone to reduce ethological and physiological stress symptoms in horses. *Journal of Veterinary Behavior* 5 (4): 213–214.

Visser, E.K., Ellis, A.D., and Van Reenen, C.G. (2008). The effect of two different housing conditions on the welfare of young horses stabled for the first time. *Applied Animal Behaviour Science* 114: 521–533.

Von Borstel, U.U., Duncan, I.J.H., Shoveller, A.K. et al. (2009). Impact of riding in a coercively obtained Rollkur posture on welfare and fear of performance horses. *Applied Animal Behaviour Science* 116: 228–236.

Waran, N. (ed.) (2007). *The Welfare of Horses*. Dordrecht, The Netherlands: Kluwer Academic Publishers.

Warren-Smith, A.K. and McGreevy, P.D. (2008). Equestrian coaches' understanding and application of learning theory in horse training. *Anthrozoös* 21 (2): 153–162.

Wickens, C.L. and Heleski, C.R. (2010). Crib-biting behavior in horses: a review. *Applied Animal Behaviour Science* 128 (2010): 1–9.

Winskill, L.C., Waran, N.K., and Young, R.J. (1996). The effect of a foraging device (a modified Edinburgh Foodball) on the behaviour of the stabled horse. *Applied Animal Behaviour Science* 48: 25–35.

Wolff, A., Hausberger, M., and Le Scolan, N. (1997). Experimental tests to assess emotionality in horses. *Behavioural Processes* 40 (3): 209–221.

Wolski, T.R., Houpt, K.A., and Aronson, R. (1980). The role of the senses in mare-foal recognition. *Applied Animal Ethology* 6: 121–138.

Yarnell, K., Hall, C., and Billett, E. (2013). An assessment of the aversive nature of an animal management procedure (clipping) using behavioral and physiological measures. *Physiology & Behavior* 118 (2013): 32–39.

Birds (*Avia*)

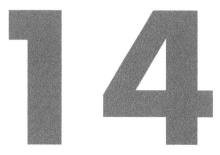

John Chitty and James Yeates

14.1 History and Context

14.1.1 Natural History

Birds include over 10 000 species, about half of which are passerine or 'perching' birds (Table 14.1). They span all continents, including Antarctica, and a variety of habitats, including desert, polar, tropical, and aquatic niches. Many bird species are now critically threatened or endangered and some have recently become extinct (e.g. Carolina parakeets [*Conuropsis carolinensis*]).

Birds are warm-blooded animals, and most, particularly small birds, have high metabolic rates. All modern birds have wings, which most use for flying and many populations migrate across significant distances. Flight is assisted by feathers, which also provide insulation, waterproofing, and visual displays, and by complex respiratory systems involving bellows-like air sacs and air-filled bones, which both reduce body weight and allow highly efficient gaseous exchange. Feathers also allow displays and colours, often with significant differences between males and females of the same species (e.g. peafowl) and some variations in colours (e.g. Gouldian finches' head colours can be red, black, or yellow). The anatomy of birds' legs and digits allow a

Companion Animal Care and Welfare: The UFAW Companion Animal Handbook,
First Edition. Edited by James Yeates.
© 2019 Universities Federation for Animal Welfare. Published 2019 by John Wiley & Sons Ltd.

Table 14.1 Examples of bird groups.

Order	Family	Species
Anseriormes	Anatidae	Mallard (*Anas platyrhynchos*) Muscovy duck (*Cairina moschata*) Domestic Grey Geese (*Anser anser domesticus*) Chinese goose (*Anser cygnoides*) Greylag goose (*Anser anser*) (Domestic forms usually categorised as *Anser cygnoides domesticus* or *Anser anser domesticus or hybrids*)
Columbiformes	Columbidae	Domestic pigeon (*Columba livia*; Chapter 17) Diamond dove (*Geopelia cuneata*) Eurasian collared dove (*Streptopelia decaocto*)
Falconiformes	Falconidae	Harris Hawk (*Parabuteo unicinctus*) Northern Goshawk (*Accipiter gentilis*) Peregine falcons (*Falco peregrinus*)
Galliformes	Phasianidae	Chickens (*Gallus gallus domesticus*) Indian peafowl (*Pavo cristatus*)
Passeriformes	Estrildidae	Zebra finches (*Taeniopygia guttata*; Chapter 15) White rumped munia (*Lonchura striata*) Bengalese/Society finch (*Lonchura domestica*) Gouldian finch (*Erythrura gouldiae*) Java sparrow *(Lonchura oryzivora)*
	Fringillidae	Domestic canaries (*Serinus canaria domestica*) American goldfinches (*Spinus tristis*) European goldfinches (*Carduelis carduelis*) Eurasian bullfinch (*Pyrrhula pyrrhula*) European greenfinch (*Chloris chloris*)
	Sturnidea	European starlings (*Sturnus vulgaris*)
	Corvidae	Pied crows (*Corvus albus*) White-necked ravens (*Corvus albicollis*)
Piciformes	Ramphastidea	Collared aracaris (*Pteroglossus torquatus*) Green aracaris (*Pteroglossus virdis*) Emerald toucanets (*Aulacorhynchus prasinus*) Guyana toucanets (*Selenidera culik*)

Table 14.1   (Continued)

Order	Family	Species
Psittaciformes (Chapter 16)	Cacatuidae	Cockatiels (*Nymphicus hollandicus*)
		White Cockatoos (*Cacatua alba*)
		Sulphur-crested cockatoos (*Cacatua galerita*)
		Long-billed corellas (*Cacatua tenuirostris*)
		Little corellas (*Cacatua sanguinea*)
		Red-tailed black cockatoos (*Calyptorhynchus banksii*)
		Palm Cockatoos (*Probosciger aterrimus*)
	Psittaculidae[a]	Fischer's lovebirds (*Agapornis fischeri*)
		Budgerigars (*Melopsittacus undulatus*)
		Goldie's lorikeets (*Psitteuteles goldiei*)
		Olive-headed lorikeets (*Trichoglossus euteles*)
		Rainbow lorikeets (*Trichoglossus moluccanus*)
		Red lories (*Eos bornea* or *Eos rubra*)
		Rose-ringed parakeets (*Psittacula krameri*)
	Psittacidae[a]	Pacific parrotlet (*Forpus coelestis*)
		Black-headed parrot (*Pionites melanocephalus*)
		Blue-crowned conures (*Thectocercus acuticaudatus*)
		Green-cheeked conure (*Pyrrhura molinae*)
		Jenday conures (*Aratinga jandaya*)
		Red-masked parakeets (*Psittacara erythrogenys*)
		Sun conures (*Aratinga solstitialis*)
		Blue-headed parrots (*Pionus menstruus*)
		Scaly-headed parrots (*Pionus maximiliani*)
		White-headed parrots (*Pionus seniloides*)

[a] Psittacidea, Psittaculidae and Psittrichasiidae are collectively in the infraorder Psittacoidea (Chapter 16).

variety of behaviours, including perching on trees or plants (Figure 14.1), swimming, and obtaining and manipulating food.

Birds may be carnivorous, omnivorous, or herbivorous, with a variety of adaptations in their anatomy (e.g. beak shapes), behaviours (e.g. hunting methods), and cognitive abilities (e.g. several species using tools in the wild). Many passerine and other species are omnivores, primarily eating certain types of foods. Estreldid finches and buntings primarily eat grain and may also eat insects. Mockingbirds, mynah-birds, and starlings primarily eat insects and fruit. Ducks generally eat a more varied diet, including

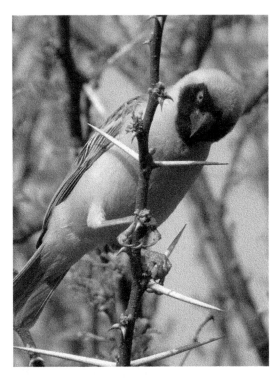

Figure 14.1 Masked weaver bird in Kwalata Game reserve, South Africa (*Source:* courtesy Graham Law).

algae, plants, seeds, berries, molluscs, crustaceans, fish eggs, small fish, and amphibians, depending on the species. Many wild birds' diets will change by season and age, depending on reproduction and migration.

Vision is an important sense for many birds, and some have excellent binocular vision (e.g. birds of prey), can detect ultraviolet light (e.g. many falconiformes, psittaciformes, and passeriformes such as starlings: Greenwood et al. 2002), or can sense magnetic fields (e.g. many migratory birds: Mourtizen and Ritz 2005; Heyers et al. 2007). They communicate using body language and sounds, including postures, gestures, colour, wing flapping, beak tapping, song, and other vocalisations. Birds live in a variety of social structures, including being largely solitary (e.g. many birds of prey), relatively unstructured flocks (e.g. starlings), and small structured groups (e.g. Red jungle fowl and Japanese quails). Large flocks provide some protection from predators by increased vigilance, confusing predators, defensive 'mobbing', or reducing each individual's risk of being caught. Relationships are maintained by behaviours such as proximity, grooming, mutual feeding, and cooperation. Some birds develop relationships between particular individuals (e.g. Japanese quail, Cheng et al. 2010; barnacle geese, Choudhury and Black 1994), and many remain with particular reproductive partners for many years. Reproductive relationships can also involve a variety of courtship, prelaying exploration, and nest-building behaviours, often with both parents caring for the chicks who may 'imprint' onto their parents while very young (depending on the speed of the development in the species).

14.1.2 Domestic History

The first birds were kept more than 2000 years ago. Since then, they have been used for communication, zoological exhibition, entertainment, sport, hunting, pest control, poisonous-gas detection, scientific research, and products such as feathers (for bedding, quills, arrows, and costumes), guano (for fertiliser), and of course, eggs. As pets, various birds have been popular in many different cultures, socioeconomic groups, and countries. For example, java sparrows were prominent in seventeenth-century Japanese culture, and canaries were the most popular caged bird in the United States in the 1930s (Anon 2013). Birds are still popular amongst various East Asian communities, where they are often associated with good luck. Birds can be used socially to provide companionship for people, and some species can be taught to mimic human speech. Birds can also be appreciated because of their attractive appearance and their ability to sing complex songs, and bird showing now involves thousands of birds internationally.

Domestic breeding of many species is relatively unsuccessful (e.g. starlings), and many are still caught from the wild, either for keeping as pets or as breeding stock for captive breeding. For example, most of the tropical birds that are captured as part of either the legal or illegal wildlife trade are destined for the pet markets, with the European Union the major importing region (Sodhi et al. 2011). In recent times, the popularity of caged birds, alongside habitat loss, has deleteriously reduced wild populations (Owen et al. 2014).

Other birds have been bred in captivity for use as pets. Some have been changed in that process, for example Bengalese or society finches (*Lonchura striata domestica*) are probably the product of selective breeding from white-rumped munias. Some hybrids have also been created (e.g. between canaries and red siskins [*Spinus cucullate*]). Fancy show birds have been bred into a variety of shapes and postures (e.g. canaries: berner, gibber italicus, gloster, Norwich, Belgian fancy, and Parisian frill), feathering (e.g. bronze, satinette, mosaic colours), and songs (e.g. Spanish Timbrado, Hartz Mountain rollers, Waterslager). Often such types are a result of recessive genes (i.e. their expression requires some degree of in-breeding). In fact, many changes are seen in other bird species in the wild, such as feathered feet (e.g. rock ptarmigans [*Lagopus mutus*] and snowy owls [*Nyctea scandiaca*]), feathered crests and ornamental feathers in many species – but these traits are not seen in the wild relatives of these fancy breeds (Bartels 2003). Indeed, wild-types of some pet species are rare in captivity (e.g. canaries). In all cases, many or all of the birds' wild needs remain unchanged, with some exceptions (e.g. the reduced feathering of chickens' necks that may help them avoid overheating in hot, domestic environments).

14.2 Principles of Bird Care

14.2.1 Diets

Birds may be carnivores (e.g. insects or small vertebrates), omnivores, or herbivores (e.g. nectar, fruit, grains, or foliage). Each needs an appropriate level of energy, proteins, vitamins (e.g. A, D_3, E, K, and various B vitamins), minerals (e.g. calcium, phosphorus, sodium, selenium, iron, copper), essential amino acids (e.g. lysine and methionine), fatty acids (e.g. omega 3 and 6), and fibre (soluble and insoluble), as well as pigments such as chlorophyll and canthaxanthin. Owners should ensure they provide the right nutrition for the bird's species, age, health, activity, and any processes such as reproduction.

Insufficient energy provision can lead to starvation; excess energy can lead to problems such as obesity, arteriosclerosis, liver, kidney, and heart disease. Birds should be assessed for their body condition, which is often best achieved by touch rather than by eye, particularly feeling around the breast bone, pectoral muscles, and near the cloaca (PFMA 2014). In fact, many birds self-regulate their intake to match their energy requirements. In doing so, they may limit their intake of high-calorie foods (e.g. fatty seeds or high-energy invertebrates), and thereby also limit their intake of essential proteins, vitamins, minerals, and fibre. More generally, some diets can be low in particular nutrients, for example invertebrate foods can be low in thiamine or calcium. Insufficient or poor quality protein can lead to beak and nail problems; insufficient vitamin A (or vitamin B in raptors) can lead to respiratory, skin, and urinary problems; and insufficient calcium can lead to problems laying eggs or osteoporosis, especially when birds are in lay. Birds' metabolic rates mean that dietary deficiencies can have rapid effects.

Birds' precise requirements for micronutrients can vary. For example, the genetic defect that makes some canaries white or yellow can also affect their need for beta-carotene or vitamin A (Wolf et al. 2000), although some diets might meet the needs of both groups (Preuss et al. 2007). Micronutrient supplementation is generally unnecessary for birds given a balanced diet (Chitty 2008), and excessive supplements can cause problems (e.g. vitamin A and vitamin D_3). Some birds may also be susceptible to iron-storage disease and some diets can alter the uptake of iron (e.g. collared aracanis, Jennings 1996; mynahs, Mete et al. 2001). Some species (e.g. several gallinaceous birds, Beer and Tidyman 1942) may also deliberately consume insoluble grit to aid digestion or soluble grit as a source of minerals.

The best method of feeding differs considerably. Many birds are motivated to forage or browse, sometimes even in the presence of freely available food (e.g. Inglis and Ferguson 1986; Bean et al. 1999), and insufficient opportunities to forage may be linked to feather-pecking, presumably because of underlying boredom or frustration (Duncan 1999). Food can be of types that require manipulation such as millet twigs, pinecones, nuts or whole grains, scattered or buried in clean litter or grass, or placed in "puzzle feeders" such as pipes, hanging baskets or fruit (Mendoza 1996). Allowing birds outdoors may allow them to eat extra food such as vegetation, seeds, and invertebrates (e.g. geese and chickens, Clark and Gage 1996, 1997; Mwalusanya et al. 2002). This may help provide particular nutrients such as lysine, methionine, and calcium (Horsted et al. 2006; Horsted and Hermansen 2007), but it is unlikely to meet all pet birds' needs. Outdoor environments also need management to ensure everything present is suitable for the birds to avoid health problems (e.g. grass crop compaction in chickens, Christensen 1998) and that the nutrients are not overforaged.

For carnivorous or omnivorous species, live food (usually invertebrates for most birds) can allow birds to perform motivated feeding behaviours, but it also carries some risks of injury to the bird and can severely compromise the welfare of the animal eaten unless death is instantaneous. Some invertebrate feeds can also carry gapeworms (*Syngamus trachea*), botulism (if raised badly) or cause crop or gizzard impactions, especially in young chicks. Some vertebrate prey items for raptors may also carry zoonotic bacteria such as Campylobacter, *Escherichia coli*, and Salmonella. Commercial producers can reduce some risks of disease, and prekilled prey may provide adequate nutrition for some birds (e.g. day-old chicks for raptors, Chitty 2008). Owners should also ensure that vegetative feed is free from high levels of bacteria or fungi that can cause diarrhoea (e.g. if seeds are soaked to improve their nutritional value) or toxins (e.g. biocidal products on unwashed fresh fruit and vegetables).

All birds, including raptors, need constant access to fresh drinking water. Some birds may consume more water than they biologically require (Koutsos et al. 2001), but excess water should be excreted without problems. Most birds normally drink by scooping or sucking water and drinking water can be provided in dishes such as troughs and bell drinkers. However, some birds can also learn to 'peck' at nipple drinkers, which may reduce spillage and contamination, so long as they are trained to do so and the nipples are placed at an appropriate height.

14.2.2 Environments

Birds should have space to stretch out, and the dimensions required to stretch out and flap their wings can be greater than the actual anatomical width suggests (Bradshaw and Bubier 1991). Nearly all adult birds should also be given adequate vertical and horizontal space for meaningful flight, both as a motivated behaviour in itself and to maintain fitness. Some birds may not voluntarily spend much time flying (e.g. some falcons when not in work), but the opportunities should still be given. Other birds may need space to move around on foot (e.g. chickens) or swim (e.g. ducks). As a rule of thumb, enclosures should be at least large enough to be termed 'aviaries', rather than smaller 'cages' or tethers (Figure 14.2). Birds kept in a house may be given an indoor enclosure and allowed to fly freely in the house. The exact distances required depend on the species. Birds who show physiological and behavioural preparations for migration in captivity (see Landys et al. 2004; Styrsky et al. 2004) should be kept only when the lack of migration does not lead to any welfare compromises, which may depend on the motivational drivers for migration in the wild.

Birds should be encouraged to use the space by ensuring they feel safe throughout the range. In particular, birds may not use particular areas (e.g. outdoors) if they are not adequately sheltered (e.g. chickens: Newberry and Shackleton 1992; Dawkins et al. 2003; Hegelund et al. 2005; Jones et al. 2007). All birds need somewhere to hide from perceived threats, for example, by being given naturalistic foliage or man-made barriers and cover (situated above perches for birds who prefer to perch); this can reduce anxiety (e.g. in starlings, Lazarus and Symonds 1992). Some birds may feel more secure under dappled lighting similar to sunlight through trees (e.g. hens, Newberry and Shackleton 1997) and may prefer to lie down more in covered, shady areas (Mirabito and Lubac 2001). It can also be important for some resources such as food to be located in safe areas, so that birds do not feel too nervous to access them. Breeders should also acclimatise chicks to their future environments, for example, allowing young chicks to go outdoors – at least when breeding for the pet market.

All birds need sufficient light, including ultraviolet (UV) ranges, for vision and calcium metabolism. Insufficient UV light can also lead to increased cortisol levels (e.g. young starlings, Maddocks et al. 2002) and risks metabolic bone conditions

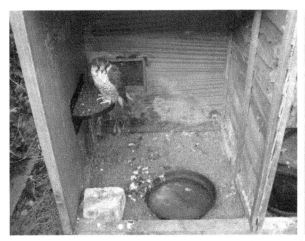
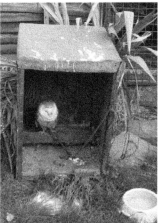
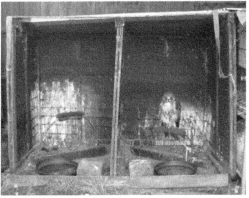

Figure 14.2   Birds in unsuitable conditions (*Source:* courtesy RSPCA).

(e.g. chickens). Lighting routines, and in particular 'daylight' length and 'twilight' periods, (or their artificial equivalents) can affect many aspects of birds' motivations, including roosting, sleeping, migration, moulting, singing, aggression, breeding, and egg-laying, and continuous light, or darkness can cause eye problems (e.g. chickens, Lauber and Kinnear 1979; Li et al. 1995, 2000). Often, naturalistic light schedules should be used, although one group of broilers trained to turn lights on and off chose to spend around 80% of the day in daylight (Savory and Duncan 1982). Cage covers can be used to provide dark periods, so long as they do not overly reduce ventilation; ensuring the room's lights are turned off overnight is preferable. Many birds can also see flickering from fluorescent lights, and although some may seem unaffected (e.g. chickens, Widowski and Duncan 1996), others may show lower activity, increased cortisol levels or muscle spasms (e.g. starlings, Smith et al. 2005a, 2005b).

Ambient temperature and humidity should mirror the birds' natural habitat. High metabolic rates can mean birds suffer from hypothermia rapidly, and outdoor or metal enclosures can be colder in the winter (Inglis and Hudson 1999). Birds kept indoors can have poor quality plumage as a result of an environment that is too dry as a result of central heating, which in turn encourages feather plucking. This may be lessened by providing water for bathing or misting the bird with a water spray. Ventilation should be enough to avoid build-up of dust (e.g. at least 12 air changes per hour, Hawkins 2010), although unguarded fans should not be used because of the risk of injury if birds fly into them. Birds' feathers can produce large amounts of dust, and their respiratory systems make them susceptible to environmental pathogens (e.g. Aspergillus). They are similarly vulnerable to respiratory toxins such as tobacco smoke and polytetrafluoroethylene, which is found in nonstick cookware, irons, ironing board covers, and heat lamps and which can emit toxic gases when heated above 280 °C (Lightfoot and Yeager 2008).

Enclosures should be safe and clean. Round aviaries can help avoid flying injuries in aviary corners. Outer walls and roofs can be made of soft nylon mesh to reduce the risks of injuries from wire mesh (Hawkins 2010), zinc poisoning from galvanised metal bars, unhygienic materials (e.g. wood), or the risks of impact (e.g. clear glass). Such mesh should be of sufficient size and tension to prevent birds becoming entangled (Kirkwood 1999). Floors should always be solid, well-drained and non-abrasive, so sandpaper, rough concrete, and wire are not usually suitable. Birds' droppings may not be malodorous, but cleaning is needed to avoid a build-up of bacteria and parasites. Lining enclosure floors with nontoxic, nonabrasive paper, or clean, dry substrate (e.g. shavings or sand) may facilitate cleaning, so long as it is suitable for the species and itself clean (e.g. free from cat faeces or other sources of toxoplasmosis). Floors can be cleaned daily with minimal interference, while the bird is elsewhere or on a perch.

Floors should also usually be covered with an appropriate natural or man-made substrate for the species, and many birds may dig or peck at litter (or other objects such as string) as a form of exploration. Insufficient substrate for such exploration may mean birds peck instead at other birds' feathers (Jones et al. 2000; Huber-Eicher and Sebö 2001; Nicol et al. 2001; McAdie and Keeling 2002). Substrate should be kept clean because wet litter and ammonia may lead to skin problems, including on the foot pads (e.g. chickens: Ekstrand et al. 1997).

Most birds enjoy bathing in fine substrates such as 'dust' (e.g. hens, Widowski and Duncan 2000) or water (e.g. starlings, Brilot et al. 2009). This can help remove fats, contaminants, and potentially parasites in the feathers, although birds may retain this motivation even if genetic changes have made the behaviour less functionally valuable (e.g. in scaleless or featherless chickens, Vestergaard et al. 1999). Bathing areas should be large enough to allow the birds to spread their wings out fully and include space for multiple birds where they are motivated to bathe communally. Without adequate bathing areas, birds may otherwise bathe in their drinking water (e.g. starlings, Bateson and Asher 2010). Some birds use sprinklers, misting, or dampened plants to walk through and rub their feathers on. Aquatic and semi-aquatic birds need clean water to safely immerse their bodies, as well as to swim and dive as appropriate. Many birds also use water for cleaning, feeding, defaecation, exercise, and play. Unclean water can reduce feather waterproofing, risking chilling, or drowning (Hawkins 2010).

Nesting birds may be highly motivated to make a nest, often well before their point of lay (e.g. chickens, Struelens et al. 2005). Birds' nesting needs can vary significantly; some may use premade structures (e.g. nesting bowls or boxes), substrate materials (e.g. linear vegetation), or both. Some birds may prefer to nest high up; others low down. Some birds may be motivated to make very neat or elaborate structures, and others more messy forms; some may even create two separate nests for the male and female (e.g. some Estrildid finches). All nesting provisions should be clean to avoid the build-up of harmful organisms such as *Aspergillus* spp.

Perches (and, for some birds, ledges) can make birds feel more secure, strengthen legs, promote exercise, provide destinations for escaping predators or other birds, and help maintain social hierarchies. The right perch designs and locations depend on the species and group composition and the individual's experiences (e.g. chickens, Gunnarsson et al. 2000). But in general, perches should be of suitable diameters, shapes, materials, rigidities, heights, horizontal distances, and locations so that they are safe, nontoxic, and used. Suitable living plants can often provide both suitable perches and good cover. Perches should be located to avoid food or water contamination and where birds feel thermally comfortable, secure (e.g. high perches, particularly at night), and are able to fly to other perches unobstructed. Inappropriate perches or locations can lead to flying injuries, contamination of food and water from faeces, aggression and feather pecking, overgrown nails, and foot problems. Birds' feet can also be damaged by standing for too long on similar perches, so owners should offer a variety of perches of different diameters and shapes, and birds should also not have to choose between a comfortable perch or one in the right location.

'Toys' can allow climbing, chewing, hiding, object manipulation, exploration, and mental stimulation. Some enrichment may increase activity (e.g. strings and sand trays in chickens, Arnould et al. 2001), whereas impoverished cages may be linked to stereotypies such as repeated somersaulting or to negative 'pessimistic' moods (e.g. starlings: Bateson and Matheson 2007). However, birds need the right toys. All toys should be safe if chewed, particularly to prevent toxicity or ingestion; toys should be indestructible unless they are specifically designed to be destroyed. Some birds are scared by close moving objects, particularly isolated birds in small cages (Bateson and Asher 2010). Some birds may interact with mirrors, although this is not a sufficient substitute for companionship in social species. Some birds may show repetitive behaviours that look like play, and these should not usually be prevented without addressing any underlying problems.

14.2.3 Animal Company

Many birds are generally social. Some appear motivated to come together in large flocks that are hard to recreate in human homes (e.g. starlings, Vasquez and Kacelnik 2000). Others may form pairs or may move away from a 'flock' for breeding and rearing. Company may help birds to learn (e.g. hens, Nicol and Pope 1999; corvids, Fritz and Kotrschal 1999; Cornell et al. 2012) and to cope with other stresses (e.g. Edgar et al. 2015). Some birds may even have some capacity to empathise with other birds (e.g. hens with chicks, although they may not show the same responses to adults in distress, Edgar et al. 2011, 2012, 2013). Social birds should be given company and never be isolated for long periods. Where social birds are physically isolated, the sight and sound of others may reduce welfare compromises and stereotypical behaviour (e.g. canaries: Keiper 1970).

Grouped birds may also show aggression, bullying, or defend resources against one another, and this may be more pronounced during breeding or chick-rearing. Aggressive behaviours may include bill gaping, bill fencing, flying at, chasing, and supplanting one another. Gently pecking at other birds' feathers may be normal behaviour, particularly towards unfamiliar animals (e.g. hens, Riedstra and Groothuis 2002), but it can become excessive and injurious. Some birds may have social hierarchies (e.g. Harris hawks), which may be linked to their size, behaviour, or plumage. For example, Gouldian finches' positions may depend partly on their head colour: with red being higher than black, which is in turn above yellow, and even the tone of redness may affect social position (Pryke and Griffin 2006). Some birds may be much less social and aggressive to one another (e.g. many raptors) or less social or more aggressive at particular times (e.g. pairing up for only breeding and raising chicks).

For any grouped birds, sufficient accessible resources need to be provided, including multiple feeding and nesting sites, to minimise competition, and sufficient litter or string, which may make birds peck those instead of other birds' feathers (Jones et al. 2000; Huber-Eicher and Sebö 2001; Nicol et al. 2001; McAdie and Keeling 2002). Group size may be more important than space per bird (Bateson and Asher 2010), although birds still need enough space each (e.g. for hens, Keeling and Duncan 1989; Channing et al. 2001). Bird groups should be kept as stable as possible, with introductions made gradually and carefully, although there is limited evidence for some social birds having specific 'friends' within their group (e.g. hens, Abeyesinghe et al. 2013).

Breeding allows natural group composition and reproductive behaviours. Birds show a variety of species-specific courtship behaviours, including songs, colouration, and physical displays. However, the fate of the hatchlings should also be considered. Dietary or environmental manipulation may reduce the motivation to breed in some animals (so long as this does not cause any other welfare problems). Otherwise, eggs can be injected with anaesthetic overdose and left, where this is safe (in particular so long as they will not be eaten), or removed for destruction and perhaps replaced with fake 'dummy' eggs. Where birds are bred, the young often benefit from contact with other birds of the same species (i.e. the parents or siblings); this can help them interact appropriately with other birds when older, and this is important even for solitary birds intended to be used for breeding.

Some birds can be kept in mixed-species aviaries, and a rule of thumb might be to mix only birds who flock together in the wild (e.g. zenaida doves [*Zenaida aurita*] and carib grackles [*Quiscalus lugubris*], Griffin et al. 2005). Some birds may also rear chicks of other species (e.g. Bengalese finches). In some cases, birds may tolerate other herbivorous species (Figure 14.3). Other animals, such as raptors or cats, may well be seen by other birds as predators – often correctly – and birds should be kept out of sight or smell of predators. For outdoor birds, fencing can help protect birds, especially at night, although some predators may attack outdoor birds despite electric fencing (Moberley et al. 2004). In chickens, having a cockerel may improve vigilance, as he may warn the hens if predators approach.

14.2.4 Human Interaction

Humans may be seen as predators, and their presence may cause significant stress. However, familiar humans may be tolerated by hand-reared individuals of domesticated species, who may then choose not to escape when given the chance. Other birds do appear to be motivated to interact with humans, although some cases may involve

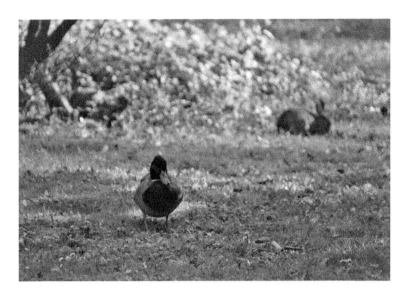

Figure 14.3 Duck cohabiting with a rabbit (*Source:* courtesy Richard Saunders).

the humans 'substituting' for company of the same species or learned associations with other rewards such as food. Some birds may see humans as potential sexual partners (e.g. some hand-reared birds), which can lead to frustration and behaviours that are problematic for the owner (although it can also facilitate artificial reproduction). However, there is little evidence that most birds (including most finches) enjoy the company of humans per se.

All birds should be able to hide and escape from humans, for example through low cover and high perches (ideally usually above human reach), and many birds may be better kept without regular interaction. All birds should also be given adequate positive contact with humans while young to get used to them (e.g. chickens, Murphy and Duncan 1978; Jones and Faure 1981). Although isolating birds from their parents may even lead to them imprinting onto human caregivers instead of their parents, such hand-rearing can lead to later screaming, aggression, and food-begging that damages the human-animal relationship (e.g. birds of prey). This behaviour can then be reinforced by the carer giving food to get the bird to stop. Methods of hand-rearing that involve food restriction, visual restriction, or social isolation can cause welfare compromises such as hunger and weight loss or fear or poor social interactions later in life.

Handling can also cause injury, especially if birds are handled by their wings alone, or respiratory distress if restricted around the chest, as well as hyperthermia or hypothermia because restraint can affect birds' abilities to regulate their body temperatures. Catching and handling may be made safer, shorter, and so presumably less stressful and fatiguing by using nets or dimming the lights (as many birds will not fly in dim light) and holding the legs, wings, and head still to avoid injury to the bird and handler from claws or bites (Figure 14.4). Birds should be released on the floor or onto a perch, rather than in midair. Many birds can be trained to 'step up' onto a finger or to perform other behaviours. Such training should be achieved by positively rewarding the desired

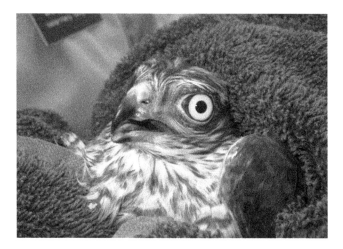

Figure 14.4 Handling of a sparrowhawk for examination using a towel (*Source:* courtesy RSPCA).

behaviour (e.g. food treats) and avoid causing unnecessary stress or suffering (e.g. starving hawks so they take food from humans' hands). Occasionally, birds may show aggressive behaviour towards humans, particularly because of defensive fear or when soliciting food.

14.2.5 Health

Some diseases are common to a variety of bird species, several of which affect their respiratory systems. *Chlamydia psittaci* bacteria can be inhaled or eaten from infected faeces, feathers, or eggs and can cause chlamydiosis in many bird species (it is also known as psittacosis but is does not only affect psittacines), causing respiratory distress and more generalised conditions, general malaise, and potentially death. The fungal disease aspergillosis can commonly affect the respiratory tract or lead to less specific weight loss or depression, with chronic infections sometimes triggered by stress. Internal parasites (e.g. intestine or throat worms) and external parasites (e.g. lice, ticks, and mites) can cause anaemia, skin problems, coughing, or weight loss, although they should have limited effect if their health and husbandry is otherwise good. Avian pox viruses can cause raised skin lumps, particularly in wild-caught juveniles. Yeast infections can cause crop infections.

Zoonotic conditions include respiratory, gastrointestinal, and other conditions such as psittacosis, avian influenza (including H5-N1 strains), Campylobacter, *E. coli*, Giardia, histoplasmosis, Newcastle disease, pasteurellosis, Q fever, Salmonella, tuberculosis due to *Mcobacterium avium*, West Nile fever, and Yersinia. New flock members should be quarantined for at least 2 weeks, ideally in pre-established groups. During this time, birds should be monitored, tested, and treated as appropriate. Vaccination is possible for some conditions. Infected birds should be removed if they pose a risk to other birds (balancing this risk with the stress of isolation and relocation) and treated, ensuring good hygiene to prevent human infections. Treatment in birds can be made more difficult by their small size, difficult handling, high metabolic rates, limited

Table 14.2 Examples of veterinary specialisations specifically relevant to birds kept as companion animals (see also Chapter 1).

Recognising organisation	Example veterinary specialties
American Veterinary Medical Association	American Board of Veterinary Practitioners in Avian Practice
European Board of Veterinary Specialisation	European College of Zoological Medicine (Avian Medicine and Surgery)
Australian and New Zealand College of Veterinary Scientists	Australian and New Zealand College of Veterinary Scientists: Avian Health Chapter

licensed products, and limited expertise, although there are increasing opportunities for veterinary surgeons to specialise in avian medicine (Table 14.2).

Breeding can also alter birds' susceptibility to diseases, including nutritional problems (e.g. chickens, Kjaer et al. 2001; Knierim 2006). Some 'fancy' breeds also have inherent genetic diseases or exaggerated characteristics (Bartels 2003). In some cases, colours may be associated with variations in hormone levels, stress responses, or immune function; for example, red-headed Goudlian finches appear more susceptible to stress (Pryke et al. 2007). Genetics may also be associated with feather pecking injuries (e.g. hens: Brunberg et al. 2011). Changes in feather structure may affect birds' abilities to fly (e.g. silky feathering in chickens), control their temperature (e.g. frizzle-feathering in chickens), see (e.g. feather crests), or communicate (e.g. reduced wattles). Some feather changes are also linked to other genetic problems, often requiring birds to have two recessive genes (e.g. ear tufts in chickens and feather crests in canaries and ducks). Whether genetic problems are seen as 'hereditary defects' or desirable types depends upon breeders' aesthetic tastes, but some breeds are now described as 'Qualzucht', which roughly translates as 'Torment breeds' (Bartels 2003).

Moulting is a normal process, although it is a significant impact on birds' physiology, sometimes involving the replacement of 10% of smaller birds' body weight and often lasting many weeks (e.g. canaries). Feather problems can be the result of various diseases (e.g. viruses, parasites, malnutrition, hyperkeratosis, and liver disease) or behavioural causes (i.e. damage by the individual animal or other animals). Wings can be injured or deformed (Figure 14.5). Birds are sometimes prevented from flying by clipping (Figure 14.6) or altering feathers, pulling feathers out ('feather-pulling'), cutting tendons ('tenotomy'), removing bones ('pinioning'), or tying wings down ('brailing'). These cause varying degrees of pain (Zhang et al. 2011), frequent handling (e.g. from repeated clipping), prevention of locomotion (especially in birds who are not good beak climbers), injury ('crash landing'), frustration of various other forms of behaviour (e.g. courtship and balance), and fear (because of an inability to escape by flight). Keeping de-flighted birds outdoors may be better than impoverished indoor captivity (Hestermann et al. 2001), but birds who cannot be kept adequately without undergoing a mutilation should not be kept as pets at all.

Foot infections may be linked to poor environments (e.g. unclean litter, badly shaped perches, or spending too long on the same diameter perches) or diet (e.g. vitamin A deficiency). Beaks and claws have hard keratin sheaths that grow continuously and

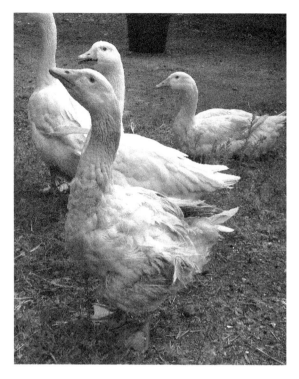

Figure 14.5 Domestic duck with deformed wing (*Source:* courtesy RSPCA).

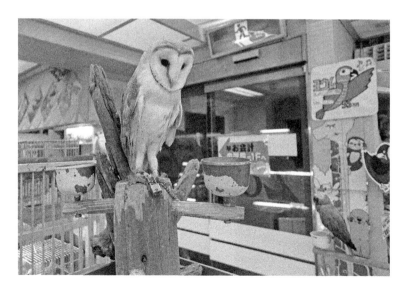

Figure 14.6 Owl in pet shop appearing to have one wing clipped (*Source:* courtesy Phil Wilson).

need to be worn down. Birds therefore need resources on which to scratch their claws (Tauson 1998) and wipe their beaks (Cuthill et al. 1992). Where beaks and claws do grow too long or become deformed, birds can be trained to let owners gently file their beak or nails with an emery board (Heidenreich 2007). Birds can be restrained or sedated for sanding or clipping, but this risks injury to the underlying bone or nerves, and mechanical rotary tools are often safer and therefore preferred for larger species. Debeaking should never be performed because damage to the sensitive nerves can cause considerable acute pain during the operation, deformation, and chronically painful granulomas (Gentle 2011).

Birds should be identified through microchipping, ringing, or dying (or noting descriptions), rather than toe clipping or web punching (Hawkins 2010), and rings should be monitored for damage or tightening. The risks of surgical neutering in both sexes and the limited availability of analgesic drugs and validated pain-relief regimes for birds may mean that the risks may outweigh the benefits for the individual birds, except in social birds where the only other option is social isolation. Surgical interventions to prevent crowing are not acceptable (e.g. in roosters or crows).

14.2.6 Euthanasia

The best methods of euthanasia of birds are usually sedation or anaesthesia if needed, followed by the injection of an overdose of pentobarbitone into a vein (Table 14.3). Head trauma or neck dislocation may also be used where necessary, although neck dislocation may not lead to immediate unconsciousness (Gregory and Wotton 1990; Erasmus et al. 2010). Pentobarbitone should not be injected into the air sacs because this can cause irritation or drowning. Birds often show convulsive movements after some physical methods, so rapid brain death should always be ensured and confirmed. Fertilised eggs should also be destroyed instantaneously and completely or injected with an anaesthetic overdose.

Table 14.3 Methods of euthanasia for (some) birds kept as companion animals.

Method	Restraint required	Welfare benefits	Welfare risks
Injection of anaesthetic overdose into a vein	Secure handling	Rapid loss of consciousness	Pain from injection
Inhalation of anaesthetic overdose	Confinement within sealed chamber	Minimal or no handling	Confinement
Neck dislocation	Secure handling	Rapid loss of consciousness	Momentary pain, distress / Severe pain if performed incorrectly
Instantaneous head trauma or destruction	Secure handling	Immediate loss of consciousness	Severe pain if performed incorrectly

14.3 Signs of Bird Welfare

14.3.1 Pathophysiological signs

Clinical measures include body temperature, pulse, and respiration, as well as changes in droppings' consistency, colour, volume, and frequency. Specific conditions may be indicated by particular biochemical and haematological measures. Poor feather condition, loss, or damage may represent disease, bullying, wire mesh cages, normal moulting, or brooding. Body fat may reflect food intake or disease, may relate to ambient temperature (e.g. starlings: Cuthill et al. 2000), or may reflect preparation for migration (Styrsky et al. 2004). Although there is an argument that bright plumage in males suggests they are otherwise healthy (e.g. house finch, [*Carpodacus mexicanus*], Hill 1991), that is not applicable to birds bred by human selection. Severe welfare compromises may be indicated by mortality or by decreased reproductive performance, particularly measuring egg quality and quantity (although these can also vary between seasons, breeds, ages, and individuals). In socially housed birds, some signs may be at the flock level, making it difficult to identify which individuals are affected.

14.3.2 Behavioural signs

It is usually valuable to first observe birds at a distance and ideally without being seen by them, as some birds' behaviour may change in the presence of the human observer because they are unsettled, afraid, or interested (Hawkins 2010). Behavioural signs may be observed at the flock level (e.g. flocking itself) or performed by individuals (Table 14.4). However, signs of illness and suffering can be subtle and generic in birds. Adult birds may rarely show signs of suffering overtly because doing so can risk attracting predators (Gentle 1992), and birds do not have particularly mobile faces, mouths, or facial muscular structures.

Birds' vocalisations can indicate social motivations or threats. Many birds produce alarm calls in response to threats; and some alarm calls may differentiate terrestrial versus aerial predators (e.g. chickens, Evans et al. 1993; Evans and Evans 1999) or characteristics of the predators (e.g. tufted titmice [*Baeolophus bicolour*], Courter and Ritchison 2010). Birds may also produce vocalisations and other behaviour related to soliciting food from parents (e.g. raptors). In juveniles, such behaviour may simply represent normal behaviour, including when directed towards humans on whom they have imprinted. Continuing such behaviours in later life may indicate that the bird has learned to associate humans with food (e.g. through hand-rearing). However, similar behaviour in adult birds can also suggest problems such as mal-imprinting, stress from recent captivity, or frustration from restricted hunting and may progress to aggression.

However, many vocalisations can be misleading, and their functions in birds are often different from those of humans (e.g. singing and speaking). Some song qualities (e.g. complexity, length, and tempo) may indicate fitness to potential mates (e.g. canaries, Drăgănoiu et al. 2002; Pasteau et al. 2004, 2009; Wright et al. 2004), insofar as some songs are harder to produce and require well-developed brains (Gil and Gahr 2002) that may be affected by earlier parasites (e.g. canaries, Spencer et al. 2005); developmental stress (e.g. starlings, Buchanan et al. 2003), or nutrition (e.g. Bengalese finches, Soma et al. 2006; swamp sparrows [*Melospiza georgiana*] Nowicki et al. 2002).

Table 14.4 Key behavioural signs of possible welfare compromises in individual birds.

Aspects of behaviour	Specific responses
Reduction in overall activity	Reduced locomotion
Reductions in maintenance behaviours	Reduced eating
	Reduced drinking
	Reduced grooming
	Reduced bathing
Reduced responsiveness	Poor righting reflex
	Tonic immobility
Particular vocalisations	Distress calls
	Screeching for attention
Avoidance	Hiding
	Escape attempts
Huddling	Feathers fluffed up, closed eyes
Increase in particular behaviours	Increased head movements
	Excessive feather-pecking
Specific indicators of local disease or injury	Lameness
	Wing drop
Abnormal repetitive movements	Repetitive circling
	Pacing
	Pecking at particular spots
	Somersaulting, flipping, feather plucking, and regurgitation
Altered interactions	Increased aggression to other birds
	Increased aggression to humans
	Inattention
Altered performance	Poor flight, song production or hunting

However, a bird's song quality may also be affected by a variety of other factors that make it an unreliable indicator of welfare for owners to use (e.g. canaries, Müller et al. 2010).

Some birds may stop or subtly change their normal behaviour; for example passerine birds may spend approximately 9% of their time in maintenance activities such as grooming (Cotgreave and Clayton 1994), so reductions or increases in grooming may be a subtle indicator of a problem and not just a sign of feather cleanliness; indeed, preening may not increase when birds are dirtier (e.g. canaries, Lenouvel et al. 2009). Pulling feathers from themselves can suggest sources of chronic stress, boredom, or frustration such as social problems and long-term captivity (as well as some medical problems, although these may be combined with other causes of stress). Pecking at other birds' feathers may also be normal behaviour – exploration towards unfamiliar animals (e.g. hens, Riedstra and Groothuis 2002). However, it can also represent insufficient litter, imperfect social grouping, or other wider problems. Abnormal, repetitive behaviour may be also noticeable but misinterpreted as normal displays, including somersaulting and rocking.

14.4 Action Plan for Improving Bird Welfare Worldwide

Birds' needs can be as complex across all domains as other species'. One priority is to educate owners on feeding of captive birds because they are unable to select their own food choices. Social birds also need adequate company of their own kind, and owners should not deliberately restrict birds' access to company to enhance their performance. Other priorities for all birds are to provide adequate space to exercise, avoiding any permanent or long-term restrictions on their ability to fly (except for short-term reasons such as transportation and rehabilitation), and to provide an adequate complex environment for foraging and mental stimulation. However, these two priorities may conflict when owners will provide adequate foraging opportunities only if their birds are de-flighted, in which case the best advice to them should address whichever is more important for those animals.

Captive breeding for the pet trade has the potential to reduce some of the harms of wild capture and international transportation. Purchasers can ask traders about the origins of their birds, sometimes using closed rings as supportive evidence that birds are captive bred (as the rings have to be placed on young birds). Commercially, owners' desire for unnatural colours, patterns, and songs may also favour buying captive bred over wild-caught birds. However, although many captive breeding programmes are in relatively early stages, those responsible should take steps to avoid issues of inherited disorders, by ensuring that use of a wide gene pool and by avoiding overly selecting for features such as song and appearance.

More generally, birds need to be recognised as sentient animals and not just valued for the aesthetics of their song or plumage or kept for luck. Increased research on welfare needs is also needed across all bird species. A lot of good research has focused on birds known for higher cognitive function (e.g. larger psittacines and starlings) or been focussed on improving the welfare of certain species used in research (e.g. some finches). However, research is also needed on the welfare of common pet birds within the home setting.

Bibliography

Abeyesinghe, S.M., Drewe, J.A., Asher, L. et al. (2013). Do hens have friends? *Applied Animal Behaviour Science* 143 (1): 61–66.

Anon. (2013). A secret history of pets: why humans have kept animals as pets since ancient times. Available at https://www.express.co.uk/news/weird/417324/A-secret-history-of-pets-Why-humans-have-kept-animals-as-pets-since-ancient-times. Accessed 2 December 2014.

Appleby, M.C., Mench, J.A., and Hughes, B.O. (2004). *Poultry Behaviour and Welfare*. Wallingford, UK: CABI.

Arnould, C., Bizeray, D. and Leterrier, C. (2001). Influence of environmental enrichment on the use of pen space and activity of chickens. *Proceedings 6th European Symposium Poultry Welfare*, Zollikofen, Switzerland, 1–4 September: 335–337.

Bartels, T. (2003). Variations in the morphology, distribution and arrangement of feathers in domesticated birds. *Journal of Experimental Zoology* 298B: 91–108.

Bateson, M. and Asher, L. (2010). The European starling. In: *The UFAW Handbook on the Care and Management of Laboratory and Other Research Animals* (ed. R. Hubrecht and J. Kirkwood), 697–705. Oxford, UK: UFAW/Wiley-Blackwell.

Bateson, M. and Feenders, G. (2010). The use of passerine bird species in laboratory research: implications of basic biology for husbandry and welfare. *ILAR Journal* 51: 394–408.

Bateson, M. and Matheson, S.M. (2007). Performance on a categorisation test suggests that removal of environmental enrichment induces 'pessimism' in captive European starlings (*Sturnus vulgaris*). *Animal Welfare* 16: 33–36.

Bean, D., Mason, G.J., and Bateson, M. (1999). Contrafreeloading in starlings: testing the information hypothesis. *Behaviour* 136: 1267–1282.

Beer, B. and Tidyman, W. (1942). The substitution of hard seeds for grit. *The Journal of Wildlife Management* 6 (1): 70–82.

Beynon, P.H., Forbes, N.A., and Harcourt-Brown, N.H. (1996). *BSAVA Manual of Raptors, Pigeons and Waterfowl*. Gloucester, UK: BSAVA.

Bradshaw, R.H. and Bubier, B.E. (1991). The effect of spatial restriction on the duration and frequency of wing flapping in the domestic hen. *Applied Animal Behaviour Science* 28: 298.

Brilot, B.O., Asher, L., and Bateson, M. (2009). Water bathing in European starlings improves escape flight performance. *Animal Behaviour* 78: 801–807.

Brunberg, E., Jensen, P., Isaksson, A., and Keeling, L. (2011). Feather pecking behavior in laying hens: hypothalamic gene expression in birds performing and receiving pecks. *Poultry Science* 90 (6): 1145–1152.

Buchanan, K.L., Spencer, K.A., Goldsmith, A.R., and Catchpole, C.K. (2003). Song as an honest signal of past developmental stress in the European starling (Sturnus vulgaris). *Proceedings of the Royal Society of London B: Biological Sciences* 270: 1149–1156.

Channing, C.E., Hughes, B.O., and Walker, A.W. (2001). Spatial distribution and behaviour of laying hends housed in an alternative system. *Applied Animal Behaviour Science* 72: 335–345.

Cheng, K.M., Bennett, D.C., and Mills, A.D. (2010). The Japanese quail. In: *The UFAW Handbook on the Care and Management of Laboratory and Other Research Animals* (ed. R. Hubrecht and J. Kirkwood), 655–673. Oxford, UK: UFAW/Wiley-Blackwell.

Chitty, J. (2008). Raptors: Nutrition. In: *BSAVA Manual of Raptors* (ed. J. Chitty and M. Lierz), 190–201. Gloucester UK: *Pigeons and Passerine birds*. BSAVA.

Chitty, J. and Lierz, M. (eds.) (2008). *BSAVA Manual of Raptors, Pigeons and Passerine Birds*. Gloucester, UK: BSAVA.

Choudhury, S. and Black, J.M. (1994). Barnacle geese preferentially pair with familiar associates from early life. *Animal Behaviour* 48: 81–88.

Christensen, N.H. (1998). Alleviation of grass impaction in a flock of free-range hens. *Veterinary Record* 143: 397.

Clark, M.S. and Gage, S.H. (1996). Effects of domestic chickens and geese on insect pests and weeds in an agroecosystem. *American Journal of Alternative Agriculture* 11: 39–47.

Clark, M.S. and Gage, S.H. (1997). The effects of free-range domestic birds on the abundance of epigeic predators and earthworms. *Applied Soil Ecology* 11 (1): 255–260.

Cornell, H., Marzluff, I., and Pecorano, S. (2012). Social learning spreads knowledge about dangerous humans among American crows. *Proceedings of the Royal Society* B279: 499–508.

Cotgreave, P. and Clayton, D.H. (1994). Comparative analysis of time spent grooming by birds in relation to parasite load. *Behaviour* 131: 171–187.

Courter, J.R. and Ritchison, G. (2010). Alarm calls of tufted titmice convey information about predator size and threat. *Behavioral Ecology* 21: 936–942.

Cuthill, I.C., Witten, M., and Clarke, L. (1992). The function of bill-wiping. *Animal Behaviour* 43: 103–115.

Cuthill, I.C., Maddocks, S.A., Weall, C.V., and EKM, J. (2000). Body mass regulation in response to changes in feeding predictability and overnight energy expenditure. *Behavioural Ecology* 11: 189–195.

Dawkins, M.S., Cook, P.A., Whittingham, M.J. et al. (2003). What makes free range broiler chickens range? *In situ* measurement of habitat preference. *Animal Behaviour* 66: 151–160.

Drăgănoiu, T.I., Nagle, L., and Kreutzer, M. (2002). Directional female preference for an exaggerated male trait in canary (Serinusanaria) song. *Proceedings of the Royal Society of London B: Biological Sciences* 269 (1509): 2525–2531.

Duncan, I.J.H. (1999). The domestic fow. In: *The UFAW Handbook on the Care and Management of Laboratory Animals* (ed. T. Poole and P. English), 677–696. Oxford, UK: UFAW/Blackwell.

Duncan, I.J.H. and Hawkins, P. (eds.) (2010). *The Welfare of Domestic Fowl and Other Captive Birds*. New York, USA: Springer.

Edgar, J.L., Lowe, J.C., Paul, E.S., and Nicol, C.J. (2011). Avian maternal response to chick distress. *Proceedings of the Royal Society of London B: Biological Sciences* 278 (1721): 3129–3134.

Edgar, J.L., Paul, E.S., Harris, L. et al. (2012). No evidence for emotional empathy in chickens observing familiar adult conspecifics. *PLoS One* 7 (2): e31542.

Edgar, J.L., Paul, E.S., and Nicol, C.J. (2013). Protective mother hens: cognitive influences on the avian maternal response. *Animal Behaviour* 86 (2): 223–229.

Edgar, J., Held, S., Paul, E. et al. (2015). Social buffering in a bird. *Animal Behaviour* 105: 11–19.

Ekstrand, C., Algers, B., and Svedberg, J. (1997). Rearing conditions and foot-pad dermatitis in Swedish broiler chickens. *Preventive Veterinary Medicine* 31: 167–174.

Erasmus, M.A., Turner, P.V., and Widowski, T.M. (2010). Measures of insensibility used to determine effective stunning and killing of poultry. *Journal of Applied Poultry Research* 19: 288–298.

Evans, C.S. and Evans, L. (1999). Chicken calls are functionally referential. *Animal Behaviour* 58: 307–319.

Evans, C., Evans, L., and Marler, P. (1993). On the meaning of alarm calls: functional reference in an avian vocal system. *Animal Behaviour* 46: 23–38.

Fritz, J. and Kotrschal, K. (1999). Social learning in common ravens, *Corvus corax*. *Animal Behaviour* 57: 785–793.

Gentle, M.J. (1992). Pain in birds. *Animal Welfare* 1: 235–247.

Gentle, M.J. (2011). Pain issues in poultry. *Applied Animal Behaviour Science* 135: 252–258.

Gil, D. and Gahr, M. (2002). The honesty of bird song: multiple constraints for multiple traits. *Trends in Ecology & Evolution* 3: 133–141.

Gill, E.L. (1994). Environmental enrichment for captive starlings. *Animal Technology* 45: 89–93.

Greenwood, V.J., Smith, E.L., Cuthill, L.C. et al. (2002). Do European starlings prefer light environments containing UV? *Animal Behaviour* 64: 923–928.

Gregory, N.G. and Wotton, S.B. (1990). Comparison of neck dislocation and percussion of the head on visual evoked responses in the chicken's brain. *Veterinary Record* 126: 570–572.

Griffin, A.S., Savani, R.S., Hausmanis, K., and Lefebvre, L. (2005). Mixed-species aggregations in birds: Zenaida doves, *Zenaida aurita*, respond to the alarm calls of carib grackles, *Quiscalus lugubris*. *Animal Behaviour* 70 (3): 507–515.

Gunnarsson, S., Yngvesson, J., Keeling, L.J., and Forkman, B. (2000). Rearing with early access to perches impairs spatial skills of laying hens. *Applied Animal Behaviour Science* 67: 217–228.

Harper, J. and Skinner, N.D. (1998). Clinical nutrition of small psittacines and passerines. *Journal of Exotic Pet Medicine* 7 (3): 116–127.

Hawkins, P. (2010). The welfare implications of housing captive wild and domesticated birds. In: *The Welfare of Domestic Fowl and Other Captive Birds* (ed. D. IJH and P. Hawkins), 53–102. New York, USA: Springer.

Hegelund, L., Sørensen, J.T., Kjær, J.B., and Kristensen, I.S. (2005). Use of the range area in organic egg production systems: effect of climatic factors, flock size, age and artificial cover. *British Poultry Science* 46 (1): 1–8.

Heidenreich, B. (2007). An introduction to positive reinforcement training and its benefits. *Journal of Exotic Pet Medicine* 16: 19–23.

Hestermann, H., Gregory, N.G., and Boardman, W.S.J. (2001). Deflighting procedures and their welfare implications in captive birds. *Animal Welfare* 10: 405–419.

Heyers, D., Manns, M., Luksch, H. et al. (2007). A visual pathway links brain structures active during magnetic compass orientation in migratory birds. *PLoS One* 2: e937.

Hill, G.E. (1991). Plumage coloration is a sexually selected indicator of male quality. *Nature* 350: 337–339.

Horsted, K. and Hermansen, J.E. (2007). Whole wheat versus mixed layer diet as supplementary feed to layers foraging a sequence of different forage crops. *Animal* 1 (4): 575–585.

Horsted, K., Hammershøj, M., and Hermansen, J.E. (2006). Short-term effects on productivity and egg quality in nutrient-restricted versus nonrestricted organic layers with access to different forage crops. *Acta Agriculturae Scandinavica Section A: Animal Science* 256: 42–54.

Huber-Eicher, B. and Sebö, F. (2001). Reducing feather pecking when raising laying hen chicks in aviary systems. *Applied Animal Behaviour Science* 73: 59–68.

Hudson, A., Inglis, I., Jones, A. et al. (2001). Laboratory birds: refinements in husbandry and procedures. *Laboratory Animals* 35 (S): 1–163.

Inglis, I.R. and Ferguson, N.J.K. (1986). Starlings search for food rather than eat readily available food. *Animal Behaviour* 34: 614–616.

Inglis, I.R. and Hudson, A. (1999). European wild birds. In: *The UFAW Handbook on the Care and Management of Laboratory Animals* (ed. T. Poole and P. English), 670–676. Oxford, UK: UFAW/Blackwell.

Jennings, J. (1996). The collared Aracani. *AFA Watchbird* 23 (2): 56–57.

Jones, R.B. and Faure, J.M. (1981). The effects of regular handling on fear responses in the domestic chick. *Behavioural Processes* 6: 135–143.

Jones, R.B., Carmichael, N.L., and Rayner, E. (2000). Pecking preferences and predispositions in domestic chicks: implications for the development of environmental enrichment devices. *Applied Animal Behaviour Science* 69: 291–312.

Jones, T., Feber, R., Hemery, G. et al. (2007). Welfare and environmental benefits of integrating commercially viable free-range broiler chickens into newly planted woodland: a UK case study. *Agricultural Systems* 94: 177–188.

Keeling, L.J. and Duncan, I.J.H. (1989). Interindividual distances and orientation in laying hens housed in groups of three in two differently sized enclosures. *Applied Animal Behaviour Science* 24: 325–342.

Keels, S.J. (2009). Polly can make you sick: pet bird-associated diseases. *Cleveland Clinic Journal of Medicine* 76 (4): 235–243.

Keiper, R.R. (1970). Studies of stereotypy function in the canary, Serina canarius. *Animal Behaviour* 18: 353–357.

Kirkwood, J. (1999). Introduction to birds. In: *The UFAW Handbook on the Care and Management of Laboratory Animals* (ed. T. Poole and P. English), 661–669. Oxford, UK: UFAW/Blackwell.

Kjaer, J.B., Sørensen, P., and Su, G. (2001). Divergent selection on feather pecking behaviour in laying hens (Gallus gallus domesticus). *Applied Animal Behaviour Science* 71 (3): 229–239.

Knierim, U. (2006). Animal welfare aspects of outdoor runs for laying hens: a review. *NJAS Wageningen Journal of Life Sciences* 54 (2): 133–145.

Koutsos, E.A., Matson, K.D., and Klasing, K.C. (2001). Nutrition of birds in the order Psittaciformes: a review. *Journal of Avian Medicine and Surgery* 15: 257–275.

Landys, M.M., Wingfield, J.C., and Ramenofsky, M. (2004). Plasma corticosterone increases during migratory restlessness in the captive white-crowned sparrow *Zonotrichia leucophrys gambelli*. *Hormones and Behavior* 46: 574–581.

Lauber, J.K. and Kinnear, A. (1979). Eye enlargement in birds induced by dim light. *Canadian Journal of Ophthalmology* 14: 265–269.

Lazarus, J. and Symonds, M. (1992). Contrasting effects of protective and obstructive cover on avian vigilance. *Animal Behaviour* 43 (3): 519–521.

Lenouvel, P., Gomez, D., Théry, M., and Kreutzer, M. (2009). Do grooming behaviours affect visual properties of feathers in male domestic canaries, *Serinus canaria*? *Animal Behaviour* 77: 1253–1260.

Li, T., Troilo, D., Glasser, A., and Howland, H.C. (1995). Constant light produces severe corneal flattening and hyperopia in chickens. *Vision Research* 35: 1203–1209.

Li, T., Howland, H.C., and Troilo, D. (2000). Diurnal illumination patterns affect the development of the chick eye. *Vision Research* 40: 2387–2393.

Lightfoot, T.L. and Yeager, J.M. (2008). Pet bird toxicity and related environmental concerns. *Vet Clin North Am Exot Anim Pract* 11 (2): 229–259.

Machin, K.L. (2005). Avian pain: physiology and evaluation. *Compendium on Continuing Education for the Practicing Veterinarian* 27: 98–108.

Maddocks, A.A., Goldsmith, A.R., and Cuthilll, J.C. (2002). Behavioural and physiological effects of absence of ultraviolet wavelengths on European starlings *Sturnus vulgaris*. *Journal of Avian Biology* 33: 103–106.

McAdie, T. and Keeling, L. (2002). Effects of manipulating feathers of laying hens on the incidence of feather pecking and cannibalism. *Applied Animal Behaviour Science* 68: 215–229.

Mendoza, A. (1996). A 'Flintstone wheel' for enrichment. *Shape of Enrichment* 5: 9–10.

Mete, A., Dorrestein, G.M., Marx, J.J. et al. (2001). A comparative study of iron retention in mynahs, doves and rats. *Avian Pathology* 30: 479–486.

Mirabito, L. and Lubac, S. (2001). Descriptive study of outdoor run occupation by 'red label' type chickens. *British Poultry Science* 42: S16–S17.

Moberley, R.L., White, P.C.L., and Harris, S. (2004). Mortality due to fox predation in free-range poultry flocks in Britain. *Veterinary Record* 155: 48–52.

Mourtizen, H. and Ritz, T. (2005). Magnetoreception and its use in bird navigation. *Current Opinion in Neurobiology* 15: 406–414.

Müller, W., Vergauwen, J., and Eens, M. (2010). Testing the developmental stress hypothesis in canaries: consequences of nutritional stress on adult song phenotype and mate attractiveness. *Behavioral Ecology and Sociobiology* 64: 1767–1777.

Murphy, L.B. and Duncan, I.J.H. (1978). Attempts to modify the responses of domestic fowl towards human beings. II. The effect of early experience. *Applied Animal Ethology* 4: 5–12.

Mwalusanya, N.A., Katule, A.M., Mutayoba, S.K. et al. (2002). Nutrient status of crop contents of rural scavenging local chickens in Tanzania. *British Poultry Science* 43: 64–69.

Newberry, R.C. and Shackleton, D.C. (1992). Use of visual cover by domestic fowl: a venetian blind effect. *Animal Behaviour* 54: 387–395.

Newberry, R.C. and Shackleton, D.M. (1997). Use of visual cover by domestic fowl: a venetian blind effect? *Animal Behaviour* 54: 387–395.

Nicol, C.J. and Pope, S.J. (1999). The effects of demonstrator social status and prior foraging success on social learning in laying hens. *Animal Behaviour* 57: 163–171.

Nicol, C.J., Lindberg, A.C., Phillips, A.J. et al. (2001). Influence of prior exposure to wood shavings on feather pecking, dust bathing and foraging in adult laying hens. *Applied Animal Behaviour Science* 73: 141–155.

Nowicki, S., Searcy, W.A., and Peters, S. (2002). Brain development, song learning and mate choice in birds: a review and experimental test of the "nutritional stress hypothesis". *Journal of Comparative Physiology A* 188: 1003–1014.

Owen, A., Wilkinson, R., and Sözer, R. (2014). In situ conservation breeding and the role of zoological institutions and private breeders in the recovery of highly endangered Indonesian passerine birds. *International Zoo Yearbook* 48 (1): 199–211.

Pasteau, M., Nagle, L., and Kreutzer, M. (2004 May 1). Preferences and predispositions for intra-syllabic diversity in female canaries (Serinus canaria). *Behaviour* 141 (5): 571–583.

Pasteau, M., Nagle, L., and Kreutzer, M. (2009 Apr 1). Preferences and predispositions of female canaries (Serinus canaria) for loud intensity of male sexy phrases. *Biological Journal of the Linnean Society* 96 (4): 808–814.

Pet Food Manufacturers' Association (PFMA) 2014 Bird Size-O-Meter. Available at www.pfma.org.uk/bird-size-o-meter. Accessed 2 December 2014

Preuss, S.E., Bartels, T., Schmidt, V., and Krautwald-Junghanns, M.-E. (2007). Vitamin a requirements of alipochromatic ('recessive-white') and coloured canaries (Serinus canaria) during the breeding season. *Veterinary Record* 160: 14–19.

Pryke, S.R. and Griffin, S.C. (2006). Red dominates black Signalling among head morphs in colour polymorphic Gouldian finches. *Proceedings of the Royal Society B: Biological Sciences* 273 (1589): 949–957.

Pryke, S.R., Astheimer, L.B., Buttemer, W.A., and Griffith, S.C. (2007). Frequency-dependent physiological trade-offs between competing colour morphs. *Biology Letters* 3 (5): 494–497.

Remage-Healey, L. and Romero, L.M. (2000). Daily and seasonal variation in response to stress in captive starlings (*Sturnus vulgaris*): glucose. *General and Comparative Endocrinology* 119: 60–68.

Riedstra, B. and Groothuis, T.G.G. (2002). Early feather pecking as a form of social exploration: the effect of group stability on feather pecking and tonic immobility in domestic chicks. *Applied Animal Behaviour Science* 77: 127–138.

Savory, C.J. and Duncan, I.J.H. (1982). Voluntary regulation of lighting by domestic fowls in skinner boxes. *Applied Animal Ethology* 9: 73–81.

Smith, E.L., Greenwood, V.J., Goldsmith, A.R., and Cuthill, I.C. (2005a). Effect of repetitive visual stimuli on behaviour and plasma corticosterone of European starlings. *Animal Biology* 55: 245–258.

Smith, E.L., Evans, J.E., and Parraga, C.A. (2005b). Myoclonus induced by cathode ray tube screens and low-frequency lighting in the European starling (*Sturnus vulgaris*). *The Veterinary Record* 157: 148–150.

Sodhi, N.S., Şekercioğlu, C.H., Barlow, J., and Robinson, S.K. (2011). Harvesting of tropical birds. In: *Conservation of Tropical Birds* (ed. N.S. Sodhi, C.H. Şekercioğlu, J. Barlow and S.K. Robinson), 152–172. Oxford, UK: Blackwell.

Soma, M., Takahasi, M., Ikebuchi, M. et al. (2006). Early rearing conditions affect the development of body size and song in Bengalese finches. *Ethology* 112: 1071–1078.

Spencer, K.A., Buchanan, K.L., Leitner, S. et al. (2005). Parasites affect song complexity and neural development in a songbird. *Proceedings of the Royal Society of London B: Biological Sciences* 272: 2037–2043.

Struelens, E., Tuyttens, F.A.M., Janssen, A. et al. (2005). Design of laying nests in furnished cages: influence of nesting material, nest box position and seclusion. *British Poultry Science* 46: 9–15.

Styrsky, J.D., Berthold, P., and Robinson, W.D. (2004). Endogenous control of migration and calendar effects in an intratropical migrant, the yellow-green vireo. *Animal Behaviour* 67: 1141–1149.

Sung, W. (2010). Passerines. In: *Behaviour of Exotic Pets* (ed. V.V. Tynes), 12–20. Oxford, UK: Wiley-Blackwell.

Tauson, R. (1998). Health and production in improved cage designs. *Poultry Science* 77: 1820–1827.

Van de Weerd, H.A., Keatinge, R., and Roderick, S. (2009). A review of key health-related welfare issues in organic poultry production. *World's Poultry Science Journal* 65: 649–684.

Vasquez, R.A. and Kacelnik, A. (2000). Foraging rate versus sociality in the starling, *Sturnus vulgaris. Proceedings of the Royal Society B: Biological Sciences* 267: 157–164.

Vestergaard, K.S., Damm, B.I., Abbott, U.K., and Bidsøe, M. (1999). Regulation of dustbathing in feathered and featherless domestic chicks: the Lorenzian model revisted. *Animal Behaviour* 58: 1017–1025.

Webster, A.B., Fletcher, D.L., and Savage, S.I. (1996). Humane on-farm killing of spent hens. *Journal of Applied Poultry Research* 5: 191–200.

Widowski, T.M. and Duncan, I.J.H. (1996). Laying hens do not have a preference for high-frequency versus low-frequency compact fluorescent light sources. *Canadian Journal of Animal Science* 76: 177–181.

Widowski, Y.M. and Duncan, I.J.H. (2000). Working for a dustbath: are hens increasing pleasure rather than reducing suffering? *Applied Animal Behaviour Science* 68: 39–53.

Wolf, P., Bartels, T., Sallmann, H.-P. et al. (2000). Recessive-white canaries. *Animal Welfare* 9: 153–165.

Wright, T.F., Brittan–Powell, E.F., Dooling, R.J., and Mundinger, P.C. (2004). Sex–linked inheritance of hearing and song in the Belgian Waterslager canary. *Proceedings of the Royal Society of London B: Biological Sciences* 271 (Suppl 6): S409–S412.

Zhang, S.L., Yang, S.H., Li, B. et al. (2011). An alternate and reversible method for flight restraint of cranes. *Zoo Biology* 30: 342–348.

Zebra Finches (*Taeniopygia guttata*)

15

Graham Law, Rudolf Nager, and Michael Wilkinson

15.1 History and Context

15.1.1 Natural History

Zebra finches are weaver finch members of the class Avia, order Passeriformes, and family Estrildidae, within its own genus *Taeniopygia* (Christidis 1987). Zebra finches are widespread and abundant in their native Australasia. One subspecies, *Taeniopygia guttata castanotis*, are found in most of the continental arid and semi-arid zones, only avoiding the cool, moist south, and the tropical far north. Another subspecies, *T. g. guttata*, are found on the Lesser Sundas and neighbouring islands north of Australia. The Lesser Sundas zebra finches are slightly smaller, and the males have a less ornate plumage than Australian zebra finches. *T. guttata* is classified as being of Least Concern (IUCN 2016).

In the wild, zebra finches live in arid open steppes with scattered bushes and trees that provide nesting and roosting opportunities usually close to water sources. Outside of the breeding time, brood nests are constructed for sleeping in. They are adaptable and varied in their nesting habits, with nests being found in cavities, scrub, low trees, bushes, on the ground, in termite hills, rabbit burrows, nests of other birds, and in

Companion Animal Care and Welfare: The UFAW Companion Animal Handbook,
First Edition. Edited by James Yeates.
© 2019 Universities Federation for Animal Welfare. Published 2019 by John Wiley & Sons Ltd.

crevices and ledges of human structures. In their native habitat, they are usually active in the mornings and late evenings when temperatures are cooler.

Like all finches, they have strong and stubby beaks, one of several adaptations to their diet of hard grass seeds. They do not have teeth but instead they have a muscular gizzard that functions as a gastric mill to break down the seed. The mechanical breakdown of food is aided by the birds hulling the seed before swallowing, abrasion by a tough keratin-like layer of koilin lining the gizzard, and the birds' deliberate ingestion of small stones and grit. Wild birds forage on the ground, perch on grass stalks to pick seeds from the seed heads, and also eat the occasional insect. They usually feed on greener diets after substantial rains. These can occur at any time of the year, and zebra finches opportunistically travel to follow the best food sources as precipitation patterns change. As a consequence they are a highly gregarious species, gathering in large flocks of a hundred or more birds when conditions are favourable.

15.1.2 Domestic History

Finches have been kept in captivity for the last millennium, for example in China. The zebra finch is often recommended to bird-keeping beginners and novice fanciers because of its brightly coloured plumage, low cost, high adaptability, and ease of reproduction (Aschenborn 1990; Kelvey 1994). They are also exhibited at many cage bird shows held in most parts of the world. In mixed collections, they are used as foster parents because of their readiness to incubate eggs of other species (Fisher 1997). Zebra finches are also one of the most commonly used laboratory birds (Bateson and Feenders 2010).

In the nineteenth century, large numbers of wild-caught zebra finches were exported from Australia as cage birds, and by the late 1800s, they were also frequently bred in captivity. From World War I onwards, imports from Australia, which were then mainly birds bred in captivity there, were much reduced, and in 1960 the Australian government banned exports of all native wildlife. The zebra finches used today as companion animals are therefore all captive bred and have been for at least half a century. As a result, domestic zebra finches are genetically distinct from the wild stock (Forstmeier et al. 2007).

This process has altered a number of behavioural and other traits. Female domestic zebra finches take longer to reach adult size and sexual maturity is delayed. Domestic zebra finches in Europe, but not North America, are larger in body size presumably because of selection by aviculturists. The structure of distance calls and duration of song phrases have also changed (Zann 1996). In addition, captive breeding has given rise to about 30 different main colour morphs. The most frequently found colour mutant is fawn, which was discovered in wild birds in 1927 and formed the breeding stock from which many of the other colour morphs were developed. Most colour mutations are recessive, so unexpected colour morphs may appear in later generations, and some are sex-linked (e.g. fawn, Kilner 1998). However, the physical and behavioural needs of birds bred in captivity remain unchanged.

15.2 Principles of Zebra Finch Care

15.2.1 Diet

Zebra finches are obligate omnivores, with nutritional needs as described in Table 15.1. Feeding the right diet to zebra finches is particularly challenging, not least because

Table 15.1   Nutritional requirements of adult, nonbreeding zebra finches.

Nutrient	Amount required per day for adult
Protein	0.5 g of protein; 12–14% protein content of feed, hence 4 g of seed
Carbohydrate	48–117 kcal
Lipid	4% lipid content
Calcium	0.5%
Phosphorus	0.25% available phosphorus
Calcium-to-phosphorus ratio	around 2 : 1
Vitamin D	16 IU (biological equivalent of 4 μg cholecalciferol/ ergocalciferol)
Water	Ad libitum

All figures assume animals are of normal physiology, healthy, and non-breeding.
Source: Robbins (1993), Stockdale (2008), Tully et al. (2009).

nutritional needs are not static and the actual nutrient requirements for specific species are poorly defined. Like many other finches, they can do well on a mixed diet of seeds and greens. Proprietary brands for specific species are available from most pet suppliers. They usually consist of mixes of millet that can be provided either on the floor or in feeders attached to the wall.

Feeding seeds soaked until they just begin to sprout can make several nutrients more readily available to the finches than would be available from the dry seed mix. This can be particularly useful when coming into the breeding season – a time when wild birds feed on a greener diet at a seasonally wetter time of the year. It is also useful during chick rearing as developing chicks thrive better on the more readily available nutrients in soaked seeds. Such soaked food should not be left till next day because it becomes a growing medium for microorganisms. Additional soft diet conditioning foods, or alternatively minced boiled egg, can also be fed once a week.

However, exclusively seed-based diets can lead to nutritional deficiencies (Stockdale 2008). In particular, the seeds commonly provided to zebra finches are either rich in carbohydrate (canary seed, millets) or oils (sunflower, rape, hemp, linseed) but are generally low in fibre, protein (especially essential amino acids), minerals, and the majority of vitamins. Zebra finches also tend to be rather selective in which seeds they eat and which they leave out. Feeding only commercially available seeds may therefore lead to nutritional imbalances which can manifest themselves in clinical (e.g. poor feather quality, delayed moults, scaly feet and legs, egg binding, and obesity), behavioural (e.g. poor parenting, failure to sing or court), or other signs (Stockdale 2008).

Other plant matter can provide additional fibre that grains lack and be offered to the birds for them to investigate and feed. Suitable plants include freshly cut grass stalks with their seed heads, dandelions, and tree whips with the leaves in place (e.g. lime trees, sycamore, and fruit tree branches). Spinach, lettuce or cucumber can also be offered once a week. In all cases, it is important to make sure that plants have not been sprayed with insecticides and are washed thoroughly because these chemicals can have sublethal effects on zebra finches (LaBonde 1996; Albert et al. 2008; Kitulagodage et al. 2008; Fildes et al. 2009).

Insoluble grit, flint, or quartz chips are said to assist seed digestion, but providing such grit is no longer considered to be essential for seed-eating passerine birds (Taylor 1996). Provision of some soluble grit, however, may serve another purpose: the provision of calcium. Such grit may be given in the form of cuttlefish bone or soluble grit (e.g. powdered oyster shell or a proprietary water-soluble supplement) or as pulverised plaster of Paris (Martin 1984). The amount of calcium needed depends, among other things, on the amount of dietary calcium and the presence of ultraviolet (UV) light. Insoluble grit can cause digestive disturbances if it is consumed as a substitute for soluble calcium.

Zebra finches are active and constantly forage on the ground and from seed heads if provided. Millet sprays with seed still on the stalk can also simulate the natural feeding behaviour from intact seed heads (Figure 15.1). Suspending sprays from the roof of the enclosure, rather than placing them next to the perches, can encourage more exercise from the bird against the calorific reward it receives (Law et al. 2010).

Zebra finches should have constant access to water, although they can survive without water for several days if necessary. When drinking, they suck water into their bills instead of scooping it like most birds, and therefore an appropriately designed water source (e.g. a water font) needs to be provided and kept clean.

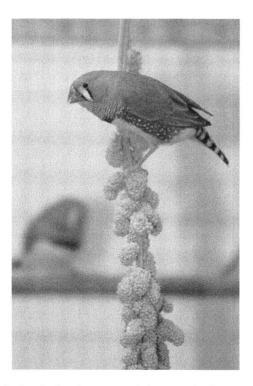

Figure 15.1 Zebra finches feeding from suspended sprays of millet.

15.2.2 Environment

Zebra finches should be given the largest enclosure that can be afforded and accommodated. Horizontal flight is more important than vertical flight and therefore longer rather than taller enclosures are preferable (Hawkins et al. 2001).

Careful consideration should also be paid to the placement of the enclosure. Draughts, for example, should be avoided in indoor accommodation because this can quickly debilitate birds and lead to illness and death. Another consideration is that most birds do not like to be viewed from all sides because this can make them feel insecure and vulnerable. Situating the enclosure with its back to a wall or, better still, constructing it in such a way that it can only be viewed from the front is generally preferable. Despite their tropical and subtropical distribution, overnight temperature in arid steppes can fall below freezing, and zebra finches tolerate such low temperatures perfectly well. Thus, depending on geographical location, many finches can survive outdoors all year round if given suitable flights and warm, dry, frost-free shelters. The outdoor aviary should be constructed in such a way that it does not encourage sunbathing cats or local raptors to perch above the enclosures' occupants. Roofs should allow light but prevent wild bird faeces from entering the enclosure. The bars of any finch enclosure should not be more than 1 cm apart.

Where birds are being kept indoors, enclosures should be placed in rooms with ample daylight cover (e.g. south-facing rooms with large windows in the northern hemisphere). Rooms with little or no daylight should be lit by high-frequency, fluorescent tubes, which are always safe (Nager and Law 2010). Low-frequency tubes should be avoided because they have a flicker rate that the birds can perceive and this may cause stress. If the birds are near a window they should have sufficient areas of shade to escape the full glare of the sun and choose their preferred thermal zone. For birds held indoors without natural light or for breeding purposes, it is a good idea to provide them with a source of UV light (usually on a 12-hours on, 12-hours off cycle) to prevent problems with calcium metabolism. UV-emitting bulbs can be installed, no more than 60 cm away from the bird (Figure 15.2) and replaced regularly as per the manufacturer's recommendations. Birds can see in the UV range and can use this to assess the suitability of a potential mate. Birds may also use this range of vision to find food and perhaps to avoid predators (Stoddard and Prum 2011).

Perches should be given careful consideration taking into account different sizes, textures, and shapes. Perches, such as twist perches that are only attached at one end, have much more potential for movement than perches secured at both ends and provide for a more natural range of movements (Law et al. 2010). Flexible perches can also help exercise the birds' muscles each time another bird lands or leaves the perch (Figure 15.3). Perches are best placed at different heights without cluttering the enclosure in a way that would restrict flight opportunities. The highest perches should be located at the rear of the enclosure, where the birds feel secure, and these are often the ones the birds select for roosting. Perches should not be located directly above food or water bowls to reduce faecal contamination. The base of the enclosure can be protected using paper tray liners and substrates such as sand, wood chippings or hemp core can be scattered over this allowing the birds an opportunity to forage for spilled seed on a more natural substrate.

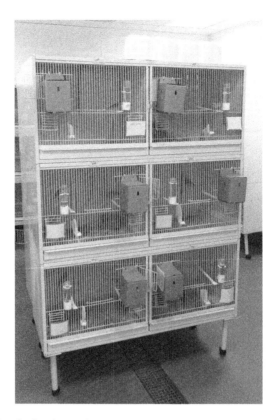

Figure 15.2 Zebra finches kept indoors provided with visible and ultraviolet light sources.

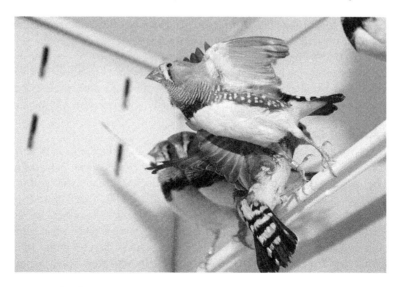

Figure 15.3 Zebra finches on a flexible perch that exercises their muscle each time another bird lands or leaves the perch.

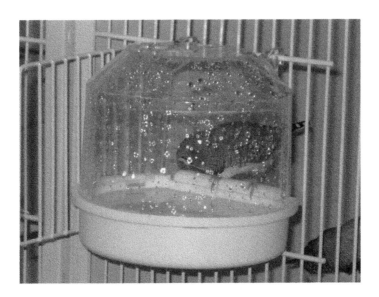

Figure 15.4 Suitable water bath that minimises water spillage.

Zebra finches should be given water baths (Figure 15.4) or showers to maintain good feather condition. These should minimise water spillage that would wet the cage and surroundings. Zebra finches in captivity are ready to breed year-round and use nests to sleep in. Therefore, it is a good idea to provide them with nesting opportunities in captivity (e.g. nest boxes, nest baskets, half coconut shells) and nesting material (e.g. long stalks of hay, coconut fibres) year round. The deprivation of natural behaviours can lead to the development of various maladaptive behaviours (Coulon et al. 2014). Therefore, aiming to simulate relevant features of the zebra finch natural habitat in the captive situation generally allows the animals to display a broader range of natural behaviours and avoids the development of abnormal ones. When introducing novel enrichment to the birds' enclosures it is important to monitor the effect that they have to ensure that it is beneficial because some proposed enrichments, such as providing cover, have been found to make the birds more fearful (Collins et al. 2008).

15.2.3 Animal Company
Zebra finches are a social species that should be kept in groups and may be stressed, anxious, and susceptible to illness if kept alone (Martin 1984). Social play has not been described in finches (Diamond and Bond 2003), but finches interact with and preen one another, and in preparation for the night, they typically huddle together and spend the night in close proximity. Social interactions therefore appear to be critical for the birds' normal, healthy life. Zebra finches also stay in contact with each other acoustically through calls and songs. When a male zebra finch produces directed songs to attract a female, special 'reward' areas of its brain are strongly activated, resulting in similar changes in brain reward function to those caused by positive rewards in humans thus stimulating a positive emotional state in the animal. Conversely, 'undirected song' produced by males kept alone, possibly for practice or to communicate with birds they

cannot see, did not induce a similar reward function in the birds' brains (Huang and Hessler 2008).

Nevertheless, the right group composition is usually one of same-sex groups, unless the intention is to produce offspring. Having mixed-sex groups as the norm risks generating large numbers of birds and quickly exhausting resources and housing capacity. Males and females differ in their appearance, with males having a more ornate plumage and a redder bill than females (Figure 15.5). Male–female pairs usually breed quite readily; if they do, both the female and the male incubate the eggs and feed the young and so the pair should be left together. Sexual imprinting is a learned behaviour that depends on the way the animals are raised, and altering birds' context during their 'learning' phase by, for example, cross-fostering or early weaning, can profoundly affect their behavioural development. The ideal group size depends on the space and resources available. The larger the group the larger the enclosure needs to be. Some finches, when perching for the night, compete with one another to be at the centre of the perching group because this is one of the safest and warmest positions to be in. They achieve this by hopping over one another and pushing in to secure the desired position (Morris 2006). Birds who are incompatible or given insufficient resources may also peck at one another (Figure 15.6).

Because there are many species available in the pet trade that have similar husbandry requirements, it is tempting to keep a variety of them in the same enclosure. However, care has to be taken with such mixes because one species can interfere with the other's breeding arrangements. In addition, although many of the finch species kept in captivity live in sociable flocks, dominance hierarchy and related bullying can occur and needs to be carefully monitored. If other companion animals such as cats and dogs are around, the birds should be kept inside their enclosure and the enclosure should be placed well out of reach of these potential predators so that the birds feel as secure as possible.

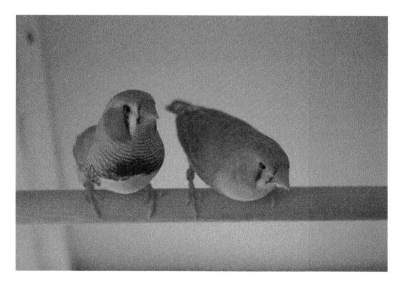

Figure 15.5 Pair of zebra finches with the male (on the left) having a more ornamented plumage compared to the female (on the right).

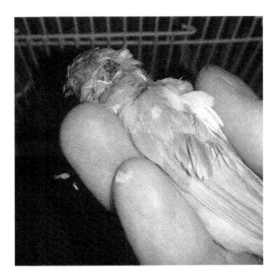

Figure 15.6 Female zebra finch with pecking injuries (feather loss, ulceration, crusting) at the back of the neck.

15.2.4 Human Interaction

Although zebra finches are a highly gregarious species, they do not bond strongly to people. However, they can become quite tame, especially if hand-reared, and may readily respond to talking or whistling or greet their owners with songs and beeps – especially at feeding time. They are thus good for watching and listening to, but not so much for handling. Rewarding zebra finches with a preferred food (e.g. lettuce, carrot, or mealworm) immediately after a handling event can help to settle the birds more quickly and allow them to return to normal behaviours faster (Collins et al. 2008). Rewarding birds after a disturbance, therefore, appears to be an effective and simple way to improve habituation to human presence.

15.2.5 Health

Zebra finches can be affected by a variety of health problems (Table 15.2; Figure 15.7). In fairly stable environments in indoor enclosures health problems are unlikely to be caused by infectious agents. Exceptions to this general rule can occur because of the introduction of new birds, the presence of a pre-existing, chronic infectious agent (e.g. gastric *Macrorhabdus ornithogaster*), or in birds kept outdoors at least some of the time coming into contact with infectious agents carried by wild animals or by the elements. Outdoor aviaries and group housing are common with fanciers, creating an increased risk of introducing novel infections. Some of these (e.g. atoxoplasmosis, avian pox, and pseudotuberculosis) can have devastating effects when introduced into a naïve population, causing high mortality rates.

A chronic gastric condition can be caused by the yeast *M. ornithogaster*. This organism can grow in large numbers in the gizzard, resulting in the destruction of the koilin layer and the subsequent inability to digest food. As a consequence, affected birds may become 'light', fluffed up, may regurgitate, and pass voluminous droppings containing

Table 15.2 Selected health problems in zebra finches.

Condition			Welfare effects
Infectious or Parasitic	Bacterial	Salmonella[a]	Regurgitation, dysphagia, difficulty breathing, conjunctivitis, peracute deaths
		Yersinia[a]	Regurgitation, dysphagia, difficulty breathing, conjunctivitis, peracute deaths
		Chlamydophila[a]	Apathy, diarrhoea, nasal and ocular discharge, difficulty breathing
		Campylobacter[a]	Pale voluminous droppings, apathy, deaths among nestlings
		Mycoplasma	Conjunctivitis, upper respiratory disease
		Mycobacteria[a]	Fluffed up, weight loss, deaths
		Escherichia coli	Conjunctivitis, metritis, diarrhoea, septicaemia
	Viral	Paramyxovirus	Diarrhoea, respiratory disease, loss of appetite, torticollis, deaths
		Polyomavirus (V)	Fluffed up, poor feathers, abdominal haemorrhage, deaths in nestlings
		Papillomavirus	Wartlike masses in skin of feet and legs
		Cytomegalovirus	Apathy, difficulty breathing, loss of appetite, swollen eyelids, deaths
	Fungal	Macrorhabdosis	Fluffed up, apathy, weight loss but always hungry, anaemia
		Aspergillosis[a]	Difficulty breathing, respiratory distress, acute deaths
		Candidiasis[a]	Loss of appetite, crop stasis, regurgitation, diarrhoea
		Dermatomycoses[a]	Feather loss, hyperkeratosis
	Internal Parasitic	Atoxoplasmosis	Ruffled feathers, diarrhoea, swollen coelom, neurological signs, death
		Coccidiosis (Isospora)	Ruffled feathers, diarrhoea, swollen coelom, neurological signs, death
		Cochlosomosis	Yellow diarrhoea in young birds, whole seeds in droppings, deaths
		Cryptosporidiosis[a]	Weight loss, depression, pale, or bulky droppings, difficulty breathing
		Toxoplasmosis[a]	Respiratory disease, blindness, neurological signs
		Trichomoniasis	Regurgitation, sinusitis, difficulty breathing and eating, weight loss
		Gapeworm	Respiratory distress, gasping, coughing, sneezing
		Capillariasis	Diarrhoea, weight loss
		Sternostoma	Wheezing, gasping, head shaking, loss of voice, respiratory distress
	External Parasitic	Cnemidocoptes	Scaly beak, eyes and feet, itchiness
		Dermanyssus[a]	Depression, anaemia, itchiness, respiratory distress

(Continued)

Table 15.2 (Continued)

Condition		Welfare effects
Metabolic or Nutritional problems	Obesity/fatty liver	Loss of appetite, depression, swollen abdomen, diarrhoea, sudden death
	Gout	Shuffling gait, swollen joints, loss of appetite, polyuria/polydipsia, death
	Vitamin A deficiency	Lethargy, nasal discharge, sneezing, conjunctivitis, rinoliths
	Calcium or Vitamin D deficiency	Fractures, misshapen bones, tremors, egg retention
	Calcium or Vitamin D excess	Increased drinking or urination, difficulty breathing, neurological signs, sudden deaths
	Amyloidosis	Diarrhoea, weight loss, lethargy, lameness, polyuria or polydipsia
Neoplastic	Renal or gonadal adenocarcinoma	Emaciation, abdominal distension, dyspnoea, lameness
	Lymphosarcoma	Emaciation, abdominal distension, dyspnoea
	Thymoma	Dyspnoea, emaciation
	Fibromas, Lipomas	Localised growths
Degenerative	Joint disease	Enlarged joints, lameness
Toxic	Inhalant	Carbon monoxide, Teflon cookware, hair spray, glues, paints, smoke, formaldehyde Dyspnoea, sudden death
	Plants	Avocado, yew, oleander, lupine Diarrhoea, regurgitation
	Pesticides	Organophosphates Diarrhoea, ataxia, tremors, seizures
Traumatic	Concussion, fractures	Depression, seizures, blindness, immobility, abnormal wing position
	Air sac rupture	Dyspnoea, abnormal swelling
	Limb constriction	Necrosis, loss of function
	Pecking	Feather loss, wounds, bleeding, eye injuries

[a] Denotes zoonotic diseases.
(V) denotes that a vaccine is available in some countries.

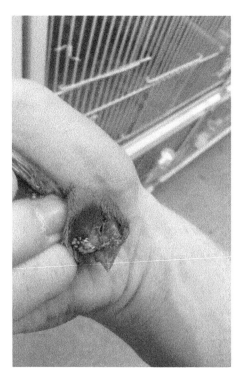

Figure 15.7 Male zebra finch with swelling around the eye.

undigested seeds but also appear dull and may display 'fearless' sham-eating behaviour (i.e. they go about picking up seeds without actually swallowing them even in the near presence of human strangers). Important zoonotic agents that may affect finches include *Campylobacter* spp., *Salmonella* spp., *Mycobacterium avium, Yersinia pseudotuberculosis, Pasteurella multocida, Toxoplasma* spp., and red mites (*Dermanyssus gallinae*). *Chlamydophila psittaci* (the cause of psittacosis or ornithosis) is quite rare in passerines, although it remains a potential risk.

Being small animals with a high metabolic rate, serious diseases can take a rapid course, allowing little time for intervention and limiting the range of diagnostic and treatment options. In addition, finches tend not to reveal signs of their ill health, making disease identification and diagnosis difficult even for the skilful observer. For these reasons, an emphasis on prevention of potential health problems is particularly important when it comes to small pet birds. However, few vaccines have been developed for use in pet birds, and the few available (e.g. against canary pox, polyomavirus) are only licensed in some countries. Nevertheless, diseases can be somewhat prevented by simple measures such as regular and thorough cleaning of enclosures and their furniture; quarantining for a sufficient time of any newcomers; providing a balanced diet and suitable environment; and avoiding overcrowding and sources of stress such as bullying, the presence of predators, sudden unfamiliar noises, or extremes of temperature.

When ailments appear, owners should not provide 'home-made' remedies or initiate proprietary treatments before taking the sick animal to an experienced veterinarian because these treatments may interfere with tests and possibly delay reaching a diagnosis. Taking the animal to the veterinarian in its own enclosure is generally less stressful for the bird and allows assessment of the animal's normal environment and collection of faecal or other samples. Isolating sick individuals from other birds can help limit the spread of the problem if it is infectious and facilitate the monitoring, treating, and nursing of the affected animals. In all cases, keeping good records of what was noticed and when, helps build an accurate clinical history and hopefully reach a diagnosis. Minor health issues such as overgrown claws or beaks can often be corrected by experienced owners or veterinary professionals. Because zebra finches are totally reliant on flight to properly move about the enclosure, wing clipping is generally discouraged (Table 15.3). Owners should prevent possible indoor injuries by other means.

15.2.6 Euthanasia

Acceptable methods of euthanasia of zebra finches are listed in Table 15.4. Because of their small size, the best method is usually an overdose of inhaled anaesthetics such as halogenated ethers (Eatwell 2008). Where this is not an available option, neck dislocation is a rapid and humane method of euthanasia when carried out competently.

Table 15.3 Nontherapeutic elective surgical procedures performed on zebra finches.

Mutilation	Reasons and benefits for the animal	Reasons and benefits for owners (or other humans)	Perioperative welfare risks	Welfare risks due to the behaviours prevented
Wing pinioning	Can be kept outdoors	To avoid losing animals	Pain, distress	Inability to fly prevents primary means of locomotion

Table 15.4 Methods of euthanasia for zebra finches kept as companion animals.

Method	Restraint required	Welfare benefits	Welfare risks
Inhalation of anaesthetic overdose	Free or in small cotton bag and then inside small sealed chamber	Rapid loss of consciousness Little restraint required No pain	Confinement
Cervical dislocation	Secure handling	Immediate loss of consciousness	Momentary pain, distress Poor technique can lead to severe pain

Source: Hawkins et al. (2001), Rae (2006), Eatwell (2008), and AVMA (2013).

15.3 Signs of Zebra Finch Welfare

15.3.1 Pathophysiological Signs

A number of pathophysiological signs can indicate poor welfare in finches (Table 15.5; Figure 15.8). Other measures that may be used as adjuncts in a welfare assessment include alterations in stress hormones such as catecholamines and corticosterone (Palme et al. 2005; Wada et al. 2008; Banerjee and Adkins-Regan 2011; Norris and Carr 2013), glucose (Marsh et al. 1984; Remage-Healey and Romero 2000), leukocyte profiles (Davis et al. 2008; Cirule et al. 2012), markers of oxidative stress (Costantini 2008; Romero and Alonso 2014), and telomere length (Heidinger et al. 2012). However, these are unlikely to be of much use to the general practitioner or pet owner and are usually restricted to research laboratories. Few, if any, pathophysiological signs are

Table 15.5 Pathophysiological signs of poor welfare in zebra finches.

Sign	What to look for
Loss of weight or body condition	Loss of pectoral muscle mass, 'going light'
Regurgitation	Dried semi-digested seed on commissure of beak or in the enclosure, matted feathers around face, salivation
Nasal or ocular discharge or swelling	Inflammation or irritation of eyes, blocked sinuses, presence of pus, 'wet eye'
Abnormal respiration (dyspnoea)	Rapid and shallow respiratory movements, abnormal extension of neck, 'tail bobbing', respiratory noises, head shaking, open-mouth breathing
Damage to, or loss of, feathers, skin changes	Bald patches, feather cysts, colour breaks, fret marks, bleeding, scaly crusts, skin nodules
Fluffed appearance	Feathers ruffled up all or most of the time when ambient temperature is not cold, possibly shivering
Semi-closed, dull eyes	Eyes not fully open or not showing their normal brightness
Abdominal swelling	Abnormal convexity of abdominal wall, unusual protrusions
Changes in consistency, colour, regularity or quantity of dropping; vent staining	Watery, yellow, pale, blood-stained, presence of whole seeds or grit, fewer, bulkier, straining, redness around vent, stained feathers around vent
Abnormal masses or growths	Soft or hard lumps protruding over or under the skin or bulging from inside a body cavity
Lameness, drooping wing(s), abnormal perching	Holding up a limb, inability to perch or walk properly, abnormal wing position, instability
Neurological signs	Tremors, ataxia, paralysis, abnormal or absent flight, lack of balance, head tilt, head shaking

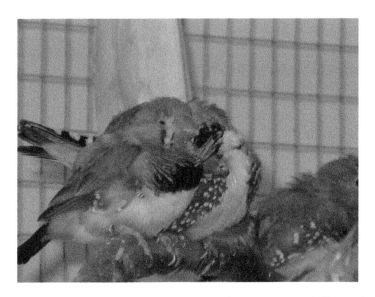

Figure 15.8 Male zebra finch showing general signs of ill health such as fluffed-up feathers and semi-closed, dull eyes.

Table 15.6 Basic measures and clinical standards of zebra finches (*Taeniopygia guttata*).

Parameter	Normal measures	
Life expectancy	4–7 years	
Mean weight (adult)	11–15 g	
Cloacal temperature (diurnal)	38–44 °C	
Pubescence	90 days	
Incubation	11–14 days	
Clutch size	4–6	
Food intake	20–30 °C: 3–4 g day^{-1}	>30 °C: 1–2 g day^{-1}
Water intake (at 23 °C)	3–5 mL day^{-1}	
Blood volume	0.75–1.0 mL (approx. 69 mL kg^{-1})	
Haematocrit	Males and nonbreeding females: 44–62%	Breeding females: 31–55%

Sources: Zann (1996), Wolfensohn and Lloyd (2003), Nager and Law (2010), Williams et al. (2012), and Miksys et al. (2013).

specific to a particular disease or pathological condition. More often than not, signs are non-specific and tend to manifest themselves in variable combinations such that they do not lend themselves to being rigidly classified into categories. It is often more useful to approach them in a holistic manner and consider that what affects the physiology of the animal also tends to affect its behaviour. Careful attention to detail and thorough knowledge of the birds, their environment, and of species-specific characteristics (Table 15.6) go a long way in helping detect the presence of such signs. The approach to welfare assessment should vary depending on whether it involves one pet animal, a small group, or a large number of birds. In the latter situation, it is harder to assess some signs such as the type of stools passed by one individual, and therefore it is important to spend time observing and whenever necessary, to isolate birds whose welfare raises concerns. Similarly, when groups of birds are kept as pets, it is useful to thoroughly investigate any unexpected death because the information gleaned by an experienced avian practitioner from such investigations (e.g. a necropsy) can result in important benefits to the rest of the group.

15.3.2 Behavioural Signs

Many of the pathophysiological signs listed are likely to be accompanied by one or more behavioural changes indicative of poor welfare (Table 15.7). In general, abnormal behaviour is less well-described in finches than those of other bird species. Self-directed feather-plucking appears to be relatively uncommon in captive passerines, where it is more likely to be a normal behaviour associated with reproduction (Sung 2010). More often than not, feather loss in captive finches is related to bullying and pecking by other zebra finches, a problem that requires more attention than it has been given so far.

Table 15.7 Behavioural signs of poor welfare in zebra finches.

Behavioural sign	Possible accompanying pathophysiological signs
Reduced food or water consumption	Loss of body condition, 'going light'
Increased food or water consumption	Changed droppings
Increased bullying or pecking behaviour	Feather loss, feather damage
Away from others, lack of interest in surroundings, apathy	Fluffed-up appearance, dull eyes
Increased or reduced performance of 'comfort' behaviours such as preening or dust bathing	Changed quality of plumage
Hiding head in plumage	Fluffed-up appearance, dull eyes, 'going light', shivering
Abnormal nesting behaviours, neglect of young, cannibalism	Loss of body condition, neurological signs, changed droppings, dyspnoea
Excessive attention to some part of the body	Abnormal masses or growths, damaged or loss feathers, skin changes
Stereotypic behaviour (see text)	Loss of condition, changed plumage
Loss of shyness or fear towards humans	Fluffed up, regurgitation, dull eyes
Immobility, lethargy	Neurological signs, fluffed up, dull eyes
Unusual perching height or position in enclosure	Swellings, lameness, dyspnoea
Changed singing patterns	Loss of condition, changed droppings, dyspnoea

Apart from the obvious establishment of social hierarchies, it is likely that other factors play an important role in this aberrant behaviour that can have such a negative welfare impact in the bullied individuals. Situations of overcrowding, lack of social stability, and lack of appropriate environmental stimulation (e.g. foraging opportunities) are likely to contribute to its inception or maintenance (Sung 2010).

Two stereotypic behaviours described in domestic songbirds kept in cages are the so-called 'route-tracing' and 'spot picking' (van Hoek and Ten Cate 1998; Garner et al. 2003). Route-tracing consists in a bird repeatedly following a precise and invariable route within its cage whilst spot picking is a stereotypy in which a bird repeatedly touches a specific spot in its body or in the cage environment with the tip or side of the bill. If present, these and other stereotypic behaviours are an indication of poor welfare and should prompt a thorough revision of the animal's captive environment (including enrichment and social interactions) and its opportunities for performing species-specific behaviours.

Finally, singing is not, per se, a reliable sign of good welfare (Huang and Hessler 2008). It is a learned behaviour that depends on the way the animals are raised, but changes in song may indicate an altered welfare state.

15.4 Worldwide Action Plan for Improving Zebra Finch Welfare

Nutritional health problems and those related to an inadequate captive environment are of particular concern in pet passerines. Lack of appropriate information, misguided affection, or a general lack of knowledge of the species, can lead even well-intentioned owners to provide inadequate conditions to their pets (Young 2003). Typical problems encountered in captive environments are insufficient space, poor enclosure design and location, lack of enrichment, incompatible social groups, and inappropriate handling and care. Novice owners are strongly recommended to seek advice from their veterinary surgeon and from more experienced owners before acquiring zebra finches as pets.

Guidelines for keeping zebra finches are mostly based on 'best practice' advice by bird breeders and researchers who have kept this species for many years. Their use in research laboratories means there is increasing knowledge from fundamental research on zebra finches, which has the potential to address some of the welfare problems arising from keeping them as companion animals. However, even for laboratory birds, our understanding of how to best address their welfare problems is far from complete (Nager and Law 2010). One of the most important action points is therefore increased research to understand their nutritional, husbandry, and behavioural needs (including social context, human interaction), and disease control, as well as more effective assessment of welfare (including pain).

Any insights gained by such studies need proper dissemination and education at all levels if it is to result in real improvements to the welfare of so many zebra finches kept in captivity. Owners and potential owners, as well as suppliers and manufactures of bird food, caging, and enclosure furniture must be made aware of the legal and moral responsibilities towards their companion animals, including associated costs such as veterinary care. For example, although there are clear guidelines for suitable dimensions for enclosures (e.g. Hawkins et al. 2001), many cages seen in pet shops and used at homes have entirely unsuitable dimensions for zebra finches.

Bibliography

Albert, C.A., Williams, T.D., Morrissey, C.A. et al. (2008). Dose-dependent uptake, elimination, and toxicity of monosodium methanearsonate in adult zebra finches (*Taeniopygia guttata*). *Environmental Toxicology and Chemistry* 27: 605–611.

Aschenborn, C. (1990). *Finches and Their Care*. Neptune City, NJ: TFH Publications Inc.

AVMA (American Veterinary Medical Association). (2013). AVMA Guidelines for the Euthanasia of Animals: 2013 Edition. Available at https://www.avma.org/KB/Policies/Pages/Euthanasia-Guidelines.aspx. Accessed 7 October 2015.

Banerjee, S.B. and Adkins-Regan, E. (2011). Effect of isolation and conspecific presence in a novel environment on corticosterone concentrations in a social avian species, the zebra finch (*Taeniopygia guttata*). *Hormones and Behavior* 60: 233–238.

Bateson, M. and Feenders, G. (2010). The use of passerine bird species in laboratory research: implications of basic biology for husbandry and welfare. *ILAR Journal* 51: 394–408.

Chitty, J. and Lierz, M. (eds.) (2008). *BSAVA Manual of Raptors, Pigeons and Passerine Birds*. Gloucester UK: BSAVA.

Christidis, L. (1987). Phylogeny and systematics of estrildine finches and their relationships to other seed-eating passerines. *Emu* 87: 119–123.

Cirule, D., Krama, T., Vrublevska, J. et al. (2012). A rapid effect of handling on counts of white blood cells in a wintering passerine bird: a more practical measure of stress? *Journal für Ornithologie* 153: 161–166.

Collins, S.A., Archer, J.A., and Barnard, C.J. (2008). Welfare and mate choice in zebra finches: effect of handling regime and presence of cover. *Animal Welfare* 17: 11–17.

Costantini, D. (2008). Oxidative stress in ecology and evolution: lessons from avian studies. *Ecology Letters* 11: 1238–1251.

Coulon, M., Henry, L., Perret, A. et al. (2014). Assessing video presentations as environmental enrichment for laboratory birds. *PLoS One* 9 (5): e96949.

Davis, A.K., Maney, D.L., and Maerz, J.C. (2008). The use of leukocyte profiles to measure stress in vertebrates: a review for ecologists. *Functional Ecology* 22: 760–772.

Diamond, J. and Bond, A.B. (2003). A comparative analysis of social play in birds. *Behaviour* 140: 1091–1115.

Eatwell, K. (2008). Passerine birds: investigation of flock mortality/morbidity. In: *BSAVA Manual of Raptors, Pigeons and Passerine Birds* (ed. J. Chitty and M. Lierz), 370–376. Gloucester UK: BSAVA.

Fildes, K., Astheimer, L.B., and Buttemer, W.A. (2009). The effect of acute fenitrothion exposure on a variety of physiological indices, including avian aerobic metabolism during exercise and cold exposure. *Environmental Toxicology and Chemistry* 28: 388–394.

Fisher, R. (1997). *Guide to Owning a Finch*. Neptune City, NJ: TFH Publications Inc.

Forstmeier, W., Segelbacher, G., Mueller, J.C. et al. (2007). Gemetic variation and differentiation in captive and wild zebra finches (*Taeniopygia guttata*). *Molecular Ecology* 16: 4039–4050.

Garner, J.P., Mason, G.J., and Smith, R. (2003). Stereotypic route-tracing in experimentally caged songbirds correlates with general behavioural disinhibition. *Animal Behaviour* 66: 711–727.

Hawkins, P., Morton, D.B., Cameron, D. et al. (2001). Laboratory birds: refinement in husbandry and procedures. Fifth report of BVAAWF/FRAME/RSPCA/UFAW Joint Working Group on Refinement. *Laboratory Animals* 35: 1–163.

Heidinger, B.J., Blount, J.D., Boner, W. et al. (2012). Telomere length in early life predicts lifespan. *Proceedings of the National Academy of Sciences of the United States of America* 109: 1743–1748.

van Hoek, C.S. and Ten Cate, C. (1998). Abnormal behaviour in caged birds kept as pets. *Journal of Applied Animal Welfare Science* 1: 51–64.

Huang, Y.-C. and Hessler, N.A. (2008). Social modulation during songbird courtship potentiates midbrain dopaminergic neurons. *PLoS One* 3 (10): e3281. doi: 10.1371/journal.pone.0003281.

IUCN (International Union for the Conservation of Nature). (2016). The IUCN Red List of Threatened Species. Available at https://www.iucn.org/theme/species/our-work/iucn-red-list-threatened-species. Accessed 22 August 2016.

Kelvey, M. (1994). *Finches as a New Pet*. Neptune City, NJ: TFH Publications Inc.

Kilner, R. (1998). Primary and secondary sex ratio manipulation by zebra finches. *Animal Behaviour* 56: 155–164.

Kitulagodage, M., Astheimer, L.H., and Buttemer, W.A. (2008). Diacetone alcohol, a dispersant solvent, contributes to acute toxicity of a fipronil-based insecticide in a passerine bird. *Ecotoxicology and Environmental Safety* 71: 597–600.

LaBonde, J. (1996). Toxic disorders. In: *Diseases of Cage and Aviary Birds*, 3, Chapter 39e (ed. W. Rosskopf and R. Woerpel), 511–522. Baltimore: William & Wilkins.

Law, G., Nager, R., Laurie, J. et al. (2010). Aspects of the design of a new birdhouse at the University of Glasgow's Faculty of Biomedical and Life Sciences. *Animal Technology and Welfare* 9: 25–30.

Marsh, R.L., Carey, C., and Dawson, W.R. (1984). Substrate concentrations and turnover of plasma glucose during cold exposure in seasonally acclimatized house finches, Carpodacus mexicanus. *Journal of Comparative Physiology. B* 154: 469–476.

Martin, H. (1984). *Zebra Finches. A Complete Pet Owners Manual*. Barron's Educational Inc.

Miksys, S., Cappendijk, S.L.T., Perry, W.M. et al. (2013). Nicotine kinetics in zebra finches *in vivo* and *in vitro*. *Drug Metabolism and Disposition* 41: 1240–1246.

Morris, D. (2006). *Watching: Encounters with Humans and Other Animals*. London: MAX.

Nager, R.G. and Law, G. (2010). The zebra finch. In: *The UFAW Handbook on the Care and Management of Laboratory and Other Research Animals*, 8e (ed. J. Kirkwood and R. Hubrecht), 674–685. Oxford: Wiley-Blackwell.

Norris, D.O. and Carr, J.A. (2013). *Vertebrate Endocrinology*, 5e. San Diego, CA: Academic Press, Elsevier.

Palme, R., Rettenbacher, S., Touma, C. et al. (2005). Stress hormones in mammals and birds. Comparative aspects regarding metabolism, excretion and noninvasive measurement in fecal samples. *Annales New York Academy of Sciences* 1040: 162–171.

Rae, M.A. (2006). Diagnostic value of necropsy. In: *Clinical Avian Medicine*, vol. II (ed. G.J. Harrison and T.L. Lightfoot), 661–678. Palm Beach, Florida: Spix Publishing Inc.

Remage-Healey, L. and Romero, L.M. (2000). Daily and seasonal variation in response to stress in captive starlings (*Sturnus vulgaris*): glucose. *General and Comparative Endocrinology* 119: 60–68.

Robbins, C.T. (1993). *Wildlife Feeding and Nutrition*, 2e. San Diego: Academic Press.

Romero, A.A. and Alonso, C. (2014). Covariation in oxidative stress markers in the blood of nestling and adult birds. *Physiological and Biochemical Zoology* 87: 353–362.

Stockdale, B. (2008). Passerine birds: nutrition and nutritional diseases. In: *BSAVA Manual of Raptors, Pigeons and Passerine Birds* (ed. J. Chitty and M. Lierz), 347–355. Gloucester UK: BSAVA.

Stoddard, M.C. and Prum, R.O. (2011). How colorful are birds? Evolution of the avian plumage color gamut. *Behavioral Ecology* 22: 1042–1042.

Sung, W. (2010). Passerines. In: *Behavior of Exotic Pets*, 1e (ed. V.V. Tynes), 12–20. Chichester, England: Wiley.

Taylor, E.J. (1996). An evaluation of the importance of insoluble versus soluble grit in the diet of canaries. *Journal of Avian Medicine and Surgery* 10: 248–251.

Tully, T.N. Jr., Dorrestein, G.M., and Jones, A.K. (2009). *Handbook of Avian Medicine*, 2e. Edinburgh: Saunders Ltd Publishing.

Wada, H., Salvante, K.G., Stables, C. et al. (2008). Adrenocortical responses in zebra finches (*Taeniopygia guttata*): individual variation, repeatability, and relationship to phenotypic quality. *Hormones and Behavior* 53: 472–480.

Williams, T.D., Fronstin, R.B., Otomo, A., and Wagner, E. (2012). Validation of the use of phenylhydrazine hydrochloride (PHZ) for experimental manipulation of haematocrit and plasma haemoglobin in birds. *Ibis* 154: 21–29.

Wolfensohn, S. and Lloyd, M. (2003). *Handbook of Laboratory Animal Management and Welfare*, 3e, 378. Oxford, UK: Blackwell Publishing Ltd.

Young, R.J. (2003). *Environmental Enrichment in Captive Animals*, UFAW Series. Oxford: Blackwell Publishing.

Zann, R.A. (1996). *The Zebra Finch*. Oxford: Oxford University Press.

True Parrots (*Psittacoidea*)

16

Joy Mench, Joanne Paul-Murphy, Kirk Klasing, and Victoria Cussen

16.1 History and Context

16.1.1 Natural History

Parrots are members of the class Aves, order Psittaciformes, and superfamily Psittacoidea, which has more than 330 recognised species including parrots, lories, macaws, parakeets, and budgerigars, widely distributed across the Americas, Australia, Africa, and Asia. Parrots are the most endangered group of birds in the world, and the parrot trade is a major contributor to the decline in wild parrot populations (Tella and Hiraldo 2014). Of the 300 known parrot species, 52 are considered endangered, and almost all remaining species are considered threatened (CITES n.d.), except peach-faced lovebirds, cockatiels, budgerigars, and rose-ringed parakeets (Parrot Travel n.d.).

Diet composition is poorly documented for many psittacine species but varies between species and seasonally within species (Table 16.1; Matuzak et al. 2008). The majority of daily activity is spent engaged in foraging, feeding, and preening behaviours. Foraging and feeding has been reported to account for 67% of the daily activity of some species in the wild (Rozek et al. 2010). Psittacines are highly social, gregarious birds that typically form lifelong pair bonds and engage in bi-parental care of their

Companion Animal Care and Welfare: The UFAW Companion Animal Handbook,
First Edition. Edited by James Yeates.

Table 16.1 Dominant food items consumed by some wild parrots.

Species	Food types
Blue and Gold macaw *(Ara ararauna)*	Seeds, fruits, nuts
Budgerigar (*Melopsittacus undulatus*)	Seeds
Hooded parrot (*Psephotellus dissimilis*)	Seeds, flowers, invertebrates
Hyacinth macaw (*Anodorhynchus hyacinthinus*)	Palm nuts (50% lipid content)
Orange-winged amazon *(Amazona amazonica)*	Fruits (85% from palm fruit)
Red-fronted macaw *(Ara rubrogenys)*	Fruits, seeds
Scaly-headed parrot *(Pionus maximiliani)*	Seeds (70%), flowers (20%)
Scarlet macaw *(Ara macao)*	Fruits, nuts, bark, leaves
Spix's macaw *(Cyanopsitta spixii)*	Palm nuts

Source: Koutsos et al. (2001) and Matson and Koutsos (2006).

altricial young. Pairs live within larger colonies or flocks, the size of which may change seasonally. Flocks may also aggregate at clay licks or water resources in mixed-species groups that can number several thousand individuals.

The behaviour and ecology of avian species are critical selection pressures that have affected brain evolution (Ricklefs 2004; Iwaniuk and Hurd 2005; Lefebvre and Sol 2008). The brain regions associated with information integration, learning, and innovation are particularly large in parrots in comparison to other birds and many mammals (Iwaniuk and Hurd 2005). It is thought that this allows parrots to be flexible in their behaviour (e.g. Emery 2006), employing innovative foraging strategies and successfully colonising new environments (Sol et al. 2005). Indeed, psittacines are considered by many to possess sophisticated cognitive abilities comparable to those of primates (Cussen and Mench 2013).

16.1.2 Domestic History

Many different species of parrots are kept as companions. The budgerigar *(Melopsittacus undulates)* is the most common pet bird species in North America and western Canada and is the second-most common pet bird species in northern Europe. Other common species in the United Kingdom, for example, are African grey parrots *(Psittacus erithacus)*, Senegal parrots *(Poicephalus senegalus)*, Meyer's parrots *(Poicephalus meyeri)*, Amazon parrots *(Amazonas* spp.), pionus parrots *(Pionus* spp.), caiques *(Pionites* spp.), macaws, conures, loriesor lorkikeets, budgerigars, parakeets, and lovebirds *(Agapornis)*, as well as cockatoos and cockatiels (Parrot Society 2014). Parrots are also used for research, mainly studying their behaviour and cognitive abilities (Mench and Blatchford 2013).

Although parrots have been kept in captivity for more than 2500 years, they are generally not considered to be domesticated. Companion cockatiels, lovebirds, small conures, and budgerigars are commonly captive-bred (Engbretson 2006), and captive-bred parrots may be hand-reared to increase their tameness and desirability as companions. Nevertheless, many pet parrot species are still wild-caught (van Hoek and ten Cate 1998) and should be thought of as wild animals in terms of meeting their physiological, nutritional, and behavioural needs. Indeed, most of the tropical birds that are captured as part of either the legal or illegal wildlife trade are destined for the pet markets, with the European Union the major importing region (Sodhi et al. 2011). Parrots make up a substantial portion of this trade. For example, it is estimated that about 1.2 million wild-caught Neotropical parrots were traded between 1991 and 1996 (Beissinger 2001), and this figure does not include the numbers traded illegally or domestically. In the United States, the Wild Bird Conservation Act, which was passed in 1992, does limit the importation of wild birds, including parrots (http://www.fws.gov/international/pdf/ factsheet-wild-bird-conservation-act-summary-of-effects-2013.pdf).

16.2 Inputs

16.2.1 Suitable Diet

The natural diets of different psittacines are diverse, but most of the species that are typically kept in captivity consume a varied diet in the wild that consists of sugary fruits, high fat fruits, nuts, seeds, leaves, nectars, pollens, flower parts, and often invertebrates and small vertebrates (e.g. Table 16.2). Food preferences may change throughout life. For example, females increase their consumption of higher nutrient food items when they begin to form eggs, and they also feed their chicks food items that have a higher nutrient density than those that they consume themselves.

Captive birds are fed several different diets that match the nutrient content of the food to their changing nutrient needs. Typically a diet containing high levels of energy, protein, and other nutrients is hand-fed to growing chicks or provided to the female so that she may feed it to the chicks. After fledging, a maintenance type diet is fed, which has lower levels of energy, protein, and other nutrients. In addition to being less expensive, a maintenance diet prevents obesity and metabolic diseases that may be caused by high levels of dietary nutrients. Finally, breeding birds need to have a diet introduced at the time of reproduction that has higher levels of protein, calcium, and trace nutrients.

Table 16.2 Nutritional requirements of adult, nonbreeding budgerigars (*Melopsittacus undulates*).

Nutrient	Key sources	Amount required, adult
Daily food intake	Mixture of seeds or pelleted grains	25% of body weight per day of hulled seeds
Metabolizable energy	Carbohydrates, lipids and protein in seeds	20 kcal per day for adults housed in aviaries at thermoneutral temperatures
Protein	Sunflowers, soybeans, canary seeds, egg	12% of the diet as high quality protein, increasing to 13.2% for egg production
Calcium	Calciferous grit	≈0.8% of the diet for egg production
Water	High moisture foods or supplemental	2.4% of body weight per day at thermoneutral temperatures

All figures assume animals are of normal physiology, healthy, and non-breeding.
Source: Koutsos et al. (2001).

It is difficult to provide a blend of domestic seeds and fruits that will provide sufficient nutrients for successful breeding and chick rearing. Domestic seeds and fruits have a nutrient composition that is different from that consumed by free-living psittacines. In particular, domestic seeds, and fruits are higher in energy and lower in protein and trace nutrients. Furthermore, parrots may select seeds with the highest levels of fat and lower levels of several required nutrients, which leads to obesity and malnutrition (Kalmar et al. 2010).

For these reasons, parrots should be fed pelleted or extruded diets that contain grains and legumes, supplemented with vitamins and minerals. Scientifically formulated pelleted diets are nutritionally superior to mixtures of seeds and fruits, especially for egg production and chick rearing (Ullrey et al. 1991; Harrison 1998; Klasing 1998). The disadvantage of feeding pelleted diets is that they provide less behavioural enrichment. For this reason, pelleted diets are often complemented with small amounts (less than 25% of the dry matter) of fruits and vegetables. Vegetables are considerably more nutritious than fruits and should dominate the enrichment foods provided to breeding birds.

The method used to provide food to parrots is also important (Pèron and Grosset 2014). Wild parrots spend a considerable proportion of their day foraging, and the lack of opportunity to forage may contribute to the development of behavioural pathologies in pet parrots. Foraging time can be extended in orange-winged Amazon parrots by giving them oversized food pellets that require them to use both their beaks and feet to manipulate them. The parrots prefer these to small pellets and are also more active when provided with them (Rozek et al. 2010; Rozek and Millam 2011). Foraging enrichments like mixing food with inedible items, providing raw foods that require manipulation, and providing food via puzzle-feeders that require the parrots to work for their food (Figure 16.1) can also be used to increase foraging time (van Zeeland et al. 2013; Pèron and Grosset 2014).

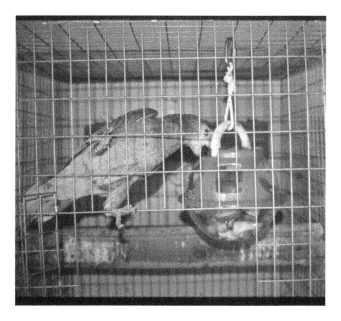

Figure 16.1   Puzzle-feeder that requires the parrot to work for the food.

Parrots should be provided with fresh water at all times. Supplementing vitamins and minerals in the water to control for deficiencies in seeds in not recommended. First, the bitter taste of some of these trace nutrients decreases water intake. Second, supplying an adequate yet non-toxic amount of nutrients is extremely difficult because water intake is extremely variable and unpredictable between individual birds. Compounding the problem, some vitamins are unstable in water and are quickly destroyed (Koutsos et al. 2001).

16.2.2 Suitable Environment

Because so many different parrot species are kept as companions, it is impossible to provide detailed information in this chapter about suitable environments for each species. Enclosures can vary in size and shape depending on parrot size and whether the birds are being housed individually, in pairs, or in groups. At a minimum, any enclosure should allow the parrots to spread their wings and turn around while perched without touching the cage floor or sides (Kalmar et al. 2010). It is important for parrots to get exercise, so enclosures that are sufficiently high and wide to allow flight are considered most desirable (Hawkins et al. 2001). However, a 2005 survey of parrot owners in the United States found that nearly 65% of owners of larger parrots housed them in cages that were too small to allow flight. Parrots that are kept in enclosures that do not allow flight should be let out daily for exercise.

Enclosures should be designed such that they are safe, easily cleaned and disinfected, and with doors that are wide enough for easy access. The sides of parrot enclosures should be made of a material that allows the parrots to climb (e.g. wire mesh, horizontal bars). Galvanised steel should be avoided because zinc is toxic to birds that lick or bite at the caging (Howard 1992). Additionally, rough welds at joints provide an opportunity for birds to ingest toxic minerals, especially when cages are new. Other important factors to consider in the parrot's living environment are temperature, humidity, lighting, and noise (Hawkins et al. 2001; Hawkins 2010; Kalmar et al. 2010; Mench and Blatchford 2013).

Parrots need adequate perches in their enclosure, which should be flexible, non-slippery, non-toxic, and non-abrasive and of a size that allows the birds to wrap their toes most of the way around them (Luescher and Wilson 2006). Providing several perch types of various diameters that provide opportunities for the bird to move around the cage can help prevent nail overgrowth and pododermatitis. Sand-covered perches are not advised because they are abrasive to the skin on the bottom of the foot. Chewable perches can also provide environmental enrichment (Kalmar et al. 2010). Perches should be arranged such that the birds do not foul the food and water when they are perching and be placed at approximately human shoulder height to minimise fear reactions by the birds (Luescher and Wilson 2006). If parrots are being bred, they will also require adequate provisions for incubating their eggs and raising the young to fledging (Martin and Romagnano 2006; Spoon 2006). Many parrot species are motivated to use properly designed nest boxes in captivity (Martin and Romagnano 2006).

16.2.3 Animal Company

The parrots typically kept as companions are all social animals, and should be housed in compatible social pairs or groups when possible. Despite their social nature, it appears that companion parrots are often housed alone. In a 2005 survey of parrot owners in the United States, 56% of parrot owners housed their birds alone (Leonard 2005). African Grey parrots who have been singly housed long term have shorter telomeres than pair-housed birds, which is an indicator that they are experiencing chronic stress (Aydinonat et al. 2014). Parrots housed alone may be more likely than those housed in pairs or groups to show feather picking, incompatibility with other parrots, noisiness, mating displays towards humans, and aggression towards humans and other animals (Leonard 2005). Having direct social contact with other parrots may be important to reduce some of these problems because singly caged orange-winged Amazon parrots spent twice as much time screaming as those caged in pairs even when they were able to see other parrots in the room (Meehan et al. 2003). Parrot owners may be concerned that socially housed parrots will bond to other birds rather than humans, but the reverse may be true. For example, pair-housed Amazons respond less fearfully than individually housed birds to humans with whom they are not familiar (Meehan et al. 2003).

16.2.4 Human Interactions

Adequate human companionship can potentially meet some of the social needs of companion parrots. However, many parrots may experience relatively limited human contact on a daily basis. For example, parrot owners in a 2005 U.S. survey reported that they only interacted with their parrot for an average of about 15 minutes per day, although the larger, more-expensive species received more attention than the smaller, less-expensive species (Leonard 2005). One concern is that some parrots may bond so closely to their owner that they experience separation anxiety (Bergman and Reinisch 2006).

Human company can also be stressful to parrots, insofar as they are effectively wild prey animals kept in captivity. Handling of parrots early in life is critical to reduce this problem (Figure 16.2). Captive breeding should ideally allow human interaction alongside parent rearing (Aengus and Millam 1999). Parent rearing improves reproductive success (Myers et al. 1988) and decreases abnormal behaviours and aggression associated with sexual bonding to human handlers (Schmid et al. 2006), whereas

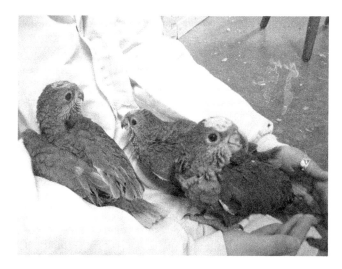

Figure 16.2 Handling of parrot chicks early in life.

periodic handling of parent-reared parrot chicks increases tameness and decreases physiological indicators of stress (Collette et al. 2000). If parrots are hand-reared, this should be done using syringes or spoons because parrots who are instead fed using gastric tubes can show additional signs of stress such as increased aggression to humans (Schmid et al. 2006). Handler attitudes are particularly important for taming parrots, and parrot chicks have been found to be less fearful when handled by individuals who express empathetic attitudes towards pets in general (Cramton 2006).

Parrots' cognitive abilities and behavioural flexibility also allow them to be trained. Veterinarians and keepers should work with parrots to train them to participate in necessary procedures to reduce stress during handling, which can increase the birds' overall health and allow more frequent and less stressful applications of preventive medicine (Daugette et al. 2012).

16.2.5 Health

Parrots can be affected by a variety of health problems, and medical and behavioural disorders will vary by species as well as by regional location. As an example for budgerigars as a common pet bird species, a table of common health disorders of the budgerigar is provided in Table 16.3. Many of the medical conditions seen in companion birds around the world have direct or indirect origins in nutrition, husbandry, and lack of owner knowledge (Speer et al. 2016).

There are a few diseases that can be transmitted from parrots to humans or from humans to parrots (Table 16.4). The risks of zoonotic diseases can be reduced by simple precautions such as keeping the birds indoors to reduce exposure to wild birds and mosquitos, not feeding wild birds nearby, regular veterinary examinations, good hygiene in and around the birds, while handling any birds, while preparing food, and not handling dead or sick wild birds. As with most species, the elderly, young, or immuno-compromised individual may be at particular risk of infection.

All parrots should receive regular health checks from specialist avian veterinary surgeons, especially as the birds get older. Routine procedures during an annual wellness examination for a companion bird may include physical examination, obtaining a small blood sample for diagnostic tests including a complete blood count and a biochemistry panel to assess organ health, and radiographs to evaluate body systems such as lungs, air sacs, kidneys, or heart size that are difficult to evaluate by physical examination.

Parrots may have overgrown nails when their captive environment does not provide adequate substrate for natural wearing of the keratin or as a result of poor diet, liver disease, or arthritis, which can lead to uneven weight bearing. When a nail becomes 'overgrown', the keratin sheath is elongated and sharp and leads to abnormal perching as well as possible entanglement. Trimming overgrown nails requires careful restraint of the bird while using a nail clipper, Emery board, or rotary sanding tool to blunt the tips. Using positive reinforcement training, parrots can be trained to perch and allow owners to gently file the nail tips with an Emery board, thereby avoiding the need for restraint (Heidenreich 2007). If the nail is clipped inappropriately, haemorrhage will occur, caused by damaging the blood vessels around the bone or cutting the bone itself – a painful condition for the bird (Figure 16.3). Such an experience may generate distrust and damage the nature of the owner-bird relationship (Speer 2001). Hence it is advised to seek the assistance of veterinary staff with avian experience to restrain and trim overgrown nails.

Table 16.3 Selected health problems in budgerigars.

Condition			Welfare effects
Infectious or parasitic diseases	Viral	Avian polyomavirus (budgie fledging disease)	Depression; diarrhoea; paralysis; abnormal feathers
		Psittacine beak and feather disease	Depression; damage to beak and feathers; secondary infections
	Bacterial	Bacterial enteritis	Depression; diarrhoea; respiratory difficulty; sinus inflammation
		Mycoplasma	Difficulty breathing; respiratory inflammation
	Fungal	*Candida* (Candidiasis)	Crop infection
		Macrorhabdus ornithogaster (megabacteria; going light)	Vomiting; weight loss
	Internal parasites	Trichomoniasis	Weight loss; vomiting; diarrhoea; depression; difficulty breathing
		Giardiasis	
		Coccidiosis	
	External parasites	Knemidokoptes	Beak and cere deformities
Hormonal or metabolic disorders		Chronic egg laying and egg binding	Exhaustion, weakness, painful straining
		Goitre – iodide deficiency, thyroid hyperplasia	Weight loss, crop enlargement, regurgitation
Neoplastic		Lipoma	May be benign; discomfort; skin ulceration
		Renal adenocarcinoma	Lameness, increased water intake and urine production
		Pituitary gland adenoma	Malcoordination; seizures; blindness Increased thirst
Degenerative or geriatric conditions		Arthritis	Pain; difficulty moving; nail overgrowth
Toxic		Heavy metals	Regurgitation
Trauma		Head leg and wing injuries	Pain associated with area of injury

Source: Adapted from Speer et al. (2016).

Table 16.4 Example zoonoses of parrots.

Condition			Transmission	Disease in humans
Infectious	Bacterial	Psittacosis (*Chlamydia psittaci*)	Via respiratory and oral secretions, feather dander and faeces	Symptoms often mild, nonspecific flulike symptoms but severe infection includes pneumonia
		Salmonellosis (*Salmonella* spp.)	Via faeces and feather material	Diarrhoea, vomiting, fever, abdominal cramps
		Collibacilosis (*Escherichia coli*)	Shed in faeces	Diarrhoea, abdominal cramps, malaise, fever, dysentery
		Mycobacteriosis (*Mycobacterium avium* complex)	This bacteria is in soil and water and can become established in carrier birds or humans and shed through oral and faecal material. Infections from same environmental source as parrots	Pulmonary involvement: similar to tuberculosis Gastrointestinal involvement: diarrhoea and abdominal cramps
	Viral	Newcastle Disease (Paramyxovirus-1)	Shed through faecal material and respiratory and oral secretions	Mild conjunctivitis and flulike symptoms
		West Nile Disease	Parrots and humans both susceptible to virus transmitted by bite of infected mosquito, but no known case of human getting infection from parrot	Most symptoms mild, fever, headache however severe cases include meningoencephalitis

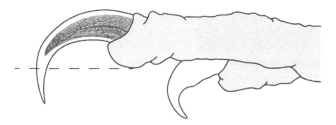

Figure 16.3 An imaginary line from the bottom of the toe pad across the nail approximates where an overgrown nail can be trimmed.

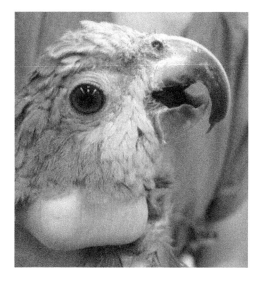

Figure 16.4 Adult Amazon parrot with overgrowth of the upper and lower beak linked to chronic malnutrition.

Beak trimming should not be needed if the bird eats an appropriate diet and uses the beak for normal behaviours. If keratin builds up along the lateral aspects of the beak, this can be smoothed using a rotary sanding tool. An excessively long beak is often associated with malnutrition or liver disease, and a thorough veterinary examination is indicated. In budgerigars, the presence of a small mite called *Knemidokoptes* can also cause the beak to be overly soft and overgrown, but it responds well to prescribed treatment (not over-the-counter therapies). Malformation and malocclusion of the upper and lower beak is a serious problem, which can be congenital or caused by damage to the beak during improper hand feeding or trimming (Figure 16.4). Trauma to the tip of the beak or the rictus of the maxillary beak (the soft and highly innervated tissue at the commissures) is often painful, causing the bird to grasp its food abnormally, leading to permanent malocclusions (Lucas and Stettenheim 1972; Abramson and Speer 1995). These may require surgical repair or regular trimming by a specialised veterinarian to keep the beak functional and less painful.

Wing trimming is not a routine recommendation because flight and exercise improve the overall well-being of pet birds. Wing feathers can be temporarily trimmed to improve safety in the home if free flight endangers the bird (as a result of the presence of other pets, ceiling fans, open windows, etc.). The number and type of feathers to be trimmed will depend on the species of parrot and the desired outcome of the trim. Feathers that are still growing are vascular and should not be trimmed.

16.2.6 Euthanasia

Acceptable methods of euthanasia of parrots are listed in Table 16.5. The best method is usually sedation or anaesthesia, followed by the injection of an overdose of pentobarbitone into a vein. Sedation or anaesthesia may be particularly beneficial when the pentobarbitone injection would be distressful, dangerous, or difficult. High concentrations of inhaled anaesthetics may be used as a sole method of euthanasia for large numbers of parrots, such as in flock or aviary situations, to minimise handling.

16.3 Signs of Welfare Problems

16.3.1 Pathophysiological Signs

The outward behaviour of a companion bird acclimated to handling may not accurately reflect the physiologic changes occurring in stress-related hormone levels, respiratory rate, or body temperature (Le Maho et al. 1992; Heatley et al. 2000). When healthy birds are transported, restrained, or stressed, their outward appearance can be unchanged from their daily resting appearance. Stress can, however, lead to an increased white blood cell count, altered types of white blood cells in circulation, elevated glucose levels, and effects on several enzymes (Scope et al. 2002). Underlying disease will further alter blood parameters, which can therefore be extremely useful to differentiate infectious from noninfectious causes of disease. Stress may also be indicated by elevated respiratory rate or body temperature (Le Maho et al. 1992; Heatley et al. 2000). Other general signs include weight loss and feather loss, which may indicate feather picking generally, or feather loss or damage on a specific body area which may indicate localised pain.

Table 16.5 Methods of euthanasia for parrots kept as companion animals.

Method	Restraint required	Welfare benefits	Welfare risks
Injection of anaesthetic into a vein (pentobarbitone)	Secure handling (or anaesthesia)	Rapid loss of consciousness	Pain from injection
Inhalation of anaes-thetic overdose[a]	Free or in small cotton bag and then inside small sealed chamber	No pain	Confinement

[a] May be suitable for large numbers of birds or for birds difficult to handle.
Source: AVMA (2013).

16.3.2 Behavioural Signs

Behavioural changes can be cryptic and subtle but are often the earliest signs of welfare problems detected by animal caretakers or owners. In the wild, showing overt signs of illness or pain could attract unwanted attention from predators and can lower the parrot's status in the social order of the flock (Graham 1998). To notice subtle changes, owners of companion parrots should ensure they are sufficiently familiar with the full range of normal behaviours for the species and with each individual bird's normal behaviour.

The classic description of a 'sick bird' includes being less active than usual and perching in a corner or on the cage floor in a huddled, fluffed-up position with eyes closed. Such signs usually indicate that birds are very ill. Previous indicators in some parrots are increased restlessness, slight changes in vocalising, or increased aggression (Le Maho et al. 1992). Pain may cause guarding behaviour that leads to the bird showing decreased interest in its surroundings and less social interaction with the owner or other parrots. Mobility may be impaired and abnormal. Other classic indicators of pain, especially chronic pain, include loss of appetite and lack of grooming or, conversely, overgrooming of a painful site or other compulsive behaviour.

Even when not ill or in pain, parrots may engage in a variety of abnormal behaviours (Meehan and Mench 2006), including stereotypic locomotor or oral behaviours (e.g. repetitive pacing, flipping, or cage bar biting) and feather picking (also called feather pecking, feather plucking, feather pulling, feather-damaging behaviour, or feather-destructive behaviour). These abnormal behaviours often arise because the birds are kept in unstimulating environments (Luescher and Wilson 2006; Meehan and Mench 2006) and may be extremely difficult to stop once started. It is therefore important to provide conditions that prevent them from developing in the first place or to intervene effectively once they are observed.

Feather-picking behaviour may be particularly distressing to parrot owners because parrots are often prized for their beautiful plumage but may make themselves almost completely bald (Figure 16.5) and even inflict injuries on themselves. Feather-picking behaviour is more commonly reported in some parrot species than others (van Zeeland et al. 2009; Jayson et al. 2014), but the overall incidence of the problem is unknown. It may be widespread because a recent survey of the owners of more than 700 African grey parrots and cockatoos registered with veterinary practices in the United Kingdom found that approximately 40% of their birds feather picked (Jayson et al. 2014). Feather picking may be caused by nutritional deficiencies, exposure to toxins or environmental irritants, parasites, diseases, dermatitis, allergies, or endocrine imbalances (Seibert 2006) and may be socially copied from other birds when parrots are housed together or can see one another (Garner et al. 2006). Although medical causes should first be ruled out if parrots start feather picking, a common cause is a lack of environmental complexity, in particular a lack of foraging opportunities (Meehan and Mench 2006; van Zeeland et al. 2009).

Other behaviours that are not abnormal per se may nevertheless indicate that the parrot's environment is inadequate in some way. One of these is incessant screaming, which may be associated with insufficient social stimulation or distress or having been hand-reared (Leonard 2005; Bergman and Reinisch 2006). Excessive fearfulness and aggression towards either humans or other animals are also common problems and can

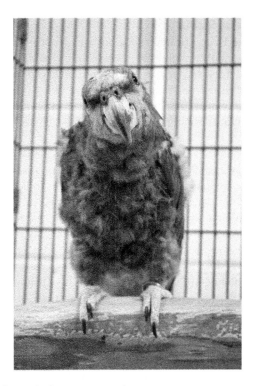

Figure 16.5   A feather picked orange winged Amazon parrot.

be affected by many factors including being wild-caught, lack of sufficient social or physical enrichment, hand-rearing, lack of handling when young, and other factors that either cause inappropriate bonding or failure to bond to humans (Meehan and Mench 2006; Welle and Luescher 2006; Wilson and Luescher 2006).

16.4 Action Plan for Improving Parrot Welfare Worldwide

The capture of wild parrots involves high rates of nest poaching of fledglings and often poor housing, nutritional, and transport conditions for the captured birds (Weston and Memon 2009; Sodhi et al. 2011). This can lead to high mortality – for example, it has been estimated that approximately 30% of the parrots caught in Mexico die in transit (Weston and Memon 2009). There is disagreement about whether parrot species can be sustainably harvested for the pet trade and whether the parrot trade can be adequately regulated or instead should be stopped entirely (Cooney and Jepson 2006; Engbretson 2006; Gilardi 2006; Sodhi et al. 2011). In 2000, the International Union for the Conservation of Nature (Snyder et al. 2000) published an action plan for parrot conservation that advocated raising public awareness about parrots and the threats that face them, and preventing illegal trapping and trade.

One of the major challenges for the welfare of wild parrots is their popularity as companions. The popularity of parrots can make them attractive to owners who lack the ability to care for them properly. Caring for parrots poses significant financial, time, and logistical challenges, especially because parrots have complex cognitive abilities and can live for several decades.

It appears that an increasing number of parrots are relinquished by their owners to shelters or sanctuaries or to other individuals or organisations. In the United States, various organisations and individuals involved with parrot relinquishment indicated that they had nearly 5400 parrots relinquished to them within a 12-month period (Meehan n.d). Although many of these relinquished parrots were rehomed, about 2000 remained in need of a permanent home at the end of the year. One survey of more than 1200 parrot owners in the United States found that about 6% of owners had relinquished a parrot during the preceding year (Leonard 2005). A large proportion of relinquished parrots are cockatiels or parakeets (Meehan n.d.), which also appear to be the species that are easier to rehome, whereas Conures and Amazons are more difficult to rehome. Common reasons for owner relinquishment include: compatibility factors such as inability of owners to dedicate adequate time to the birds, inadequate space, failure to get along with family members or other parrots in the household and cost; personal factors such as owners' lifestyle changes, illness, death, divorce, moving, and allergies; lack of bonding; and behavioural problems such as feather picking, aggression, messiness, noisiness, and difficulty of training (Leonard 2005).

Leonard's survey (2005) also found that owners who received instruction when they obtained their parrot were more likely to be satisfied with their relationship with that parrot. Given that there are broad differences between parrot species in terms of life expectancy, behaviour, husbandry, and space requirements, this emphasises the critical need for better education of potential owners about selecting the appropriate species of parrot and the challenges associated with keeping parrots to reduce the number of birds relinquished to sanctuaries or euthanised.

Bibliography

Abramson, J. and Speer, B.L. (1995). Anatomy and physiology. In: *The Large Macaws* (ed. J. Abramson, B.L. Speer and J.B. Thomsen), 39–71. Raintree Publications: Fort Bragg, USA.

Aengus, W.L. and Millam, J.R. (1999). Taming parent-reared Orange-winged Amazon parrots by neonatal handling. *Zoo Biology* 18: 177–187.

AVMA (American Veterinary Medical Association). (2013). AVMA Guidelines for the Euthanasia of Animals: 2013 Edition. Available at https://www.avma.org/KB/Policies/Pages/Euthanasia-Guidelines.aspx. Accessed 7 October 2015.

Aydinonat, D., Penn, D.J., Smith, S. et al. (2014). Social isolation shortens telomeres in African Grey parrots (*Psittacus erithacus erithacus*). *PLOS One* 9: e93839.

Beissinger, S.R. (2001). Trade of live wild birds: potentials, principles and practices of sustainable use. In: *Conservation of Endangered Species* (ed. J.D. Reynolds, G.M. Mace, K.H. Redford and J.G. Robinson), 182–202. Cambridge: Cambridge University Press.

Bergman, L. and Reinisch, U.S. (2006). Parrot vocalization. In: *Manual of Parrot Behavior* (ed. A.U. Luescher), 219–224. Ames, IA, USA: Blackwell.

CITES n.d. The CITES Species. Available at https://www.cites.org/eng/disc/species.php. Accessed 11 July 2018.

Collette, J.C., Millam, J.R., Klasing, K.C., and Wakenell, P.S. (2000). Neonatal handling of Amazon parrots alters the stress response and immune function. *Applied Animal Behaviour Science* 66: 335–349.

Cooney, R. and Jepson, P. (2006). The international wild bird trade: what's wrong with blanket bans? *Oryx* 40: 18–23.

Cramton, B. (2006). Handler attitude and chick development. In: *Manual of Parrot Behavior* (ed. A.U. Luescher), 113–131. Ames, IA, USA: Blackwell.

Cussen, V.A. and Mench, J.A. (2013). Performance on the Hamilton search task, and the influence of lateralization, in captive orange-winged Amazon parrots (*Amazona amazonica*). *Animal Cognition* 17: 901–909.

Daugette, K.F., Hoppes, S., Tizard, I., and Brightsmith, D. (2012). Positive reinforcement training facilitates the voluntary participation of laboratory macaws with veterinary procedures. *Journal of Avian Medicine and Surgery* 26: 248–254.

Emery, N.J. (2006). Cognitive ethology: the evolution of avian intelligence. *Proceedings of the Royal Society B* 361: 23–43.

Engbretson, M. (2006). The welfare and sustainability of parrots as companion animals: a review. *Animal Welfare* 15: 263–276.

Garner, J.P., Meehan, C.L., Famula, T.R., and Mench, J.A. (2006). Genetic, environmental, and neighbor effects on the severity of stereotypies and feather picking in Orange-winged Amazon parrots (*Amazona amazonica*): an epidemiological study. *Applied Animal Behaviour Science* 96: 153–168.

Gilardi, J.D. (2006). Captured for conservation: will cages save wild birds? A respone to Cooney & Jepson. *Oryx* 40: 24–26.

Graham, D.L. (1998). Pet birds: historical and modern perspectives on the keeper and the kept. *Journal of the American Veterinary Medical Association* 212: 1216–1219.

Harrison, G.J. (1998). Twenty years of progress in pet bird nutrition. *Journal of the American Veterinary Medical Association* 212: 1226–1230.

Hawkins, P. (2010). The welfare implications of housing captive wild and domesticated birds. In: *The Welfare of Domestic Fowl and Other Captive Birds* (ed. I.J.H. Duncan and P. Hawkins), 53–10. New York, NY: Springer.

Hawkins, P., Morton, D.B., Cameron, D. et al. (2001). Laboratory birds: refinements in husbandry and procedures. *Laboratory Animals* 35 (Suppl. 1): 1–163.

Heatley, J.J., Oliver, J.W., Hosgood, G. et al. (2000). Serum corticosterone concentrations in response to restraint, anesthesia, and skin testing in Hispaniolan Amazon parrots (*Amazona ventralis*). *Journal of Avian Medicine and Surgery* 14: 172–176.

Heidenreich, B. (2007). An introduction to positive reinforcement training and its benefits. *Journal of Exotic Pet Medicine* 16: 19–23.

van Hoek, C.S. and ten Cate, C. (1998). Abnormal behavior in caged birds kept as pets. *Journal of Applied Animal Welfare Science* 1: 51–64.

Howard, B.R. (1992). Health risks of housing small psittacines in galvanized wire mesh cages. *Journal of the American Veterinary Medical Association* 200: 1667–1674.

Iwaniuk, A.N. and Hurd, P.L. (2005). The evolution of cerebrotypes in birds. *Brain Behavior and Evolution* 65: 215–230.

Jayson, S.A., Williams, D.L., and Wood, J.L.N. (2014). Prevalence and risk factors of feather plucking in African Grey parrots (*Psittacus erithacus erithacus* and *Psittaus eritahcus timneh*) and cockatoos (*Cacatua spp.*). *Journal of Exotic Pet Medicine* 23: 250–257.

Kalmar, I.D., Janssesns, G.P.J., and Moons, C.P.H. (2010). Guidelines and ethical considerations housing and management of psittacine birds used in research. *ILAR Journal* 51: 409–423.

Klasing, K. (1998). *Comparative Avian Nutrition*. Wallingford, UK: CABI.

Koutsos, E.A., Matson, K.D., and Klasing, K.C. (2001). Nutrition of birds in the order Psittaciformes: a review. *Journal of Avian Medicine and Surgery* 15: 257–275.

Lefebvre, L. and Sol, D. (2008). Brains, lifestyles and cognition: are there general trends? *Brain Behavior and Evolution* 72: 135–144.

Le Maho, Y., Karmann, H., Briot, D. et al. (1992). Stress in birds due to routine handling and a technique to avoid it. *American Journal of Physiology* 263: R775–R775.

Leonard, A.L. (2005). Companion parrots and their owners: a survey of United States households. M.S. Thesis, University of California, Davis, California.

Luescher, A.U. and Wilson, L. (2006). Housing and management considerations for problem prevention. In: *Manual of Parrot Behavior* (ed. A.U. Luescher), 291–300. Ames, IA, USA: Blackwell.

Lucas, A.M. and Stettenheim, P.R. (1972). *Avian Anatomy: Integument*. Publication No. 362. Washington: US Government Printing Office.

Martin, S.G. and Romagnano, A. (2006). Nest box preferences. In: *Manual of Parrot Behavior* (ed. A.U. Luescher), 79–82. Ames, IA, USA: Blackwell.

Matson, K.D. and Koutsos, E.A. (2006). Captive parrot nutrition: interactions with anatomy, physiology, and behavior. In: *Mannual of Parrot Behavior* (ed. A.U. Luescher), 49–58. Ames, IA, USA: Blackwell.

Matuzak, G.D., Bezy, M.B., and Brightsmith, D.J. (2008). Foraging ecology of parrots in a modified landscape: seasonal trends and introduced species. *The Wilson Journal of Ornithology* 120: 353–365.

Meehan, C.L. (2004). National Parrot Relinquishment Research Project: Report to PETsMART Charities. Available at http://www.thegabrielfoundation.org/documents/NPRRPReport.pdf. Accessed 24 May 2018.

Meehan, C.L. and Mench, J.A. (2006). Captive parrot welfare. In: *Manual of Parrot Behavior* (ed. A.U. Luescher), 301–318. Ames, IA, USA: Blackwell.

Meehan, C.L., Garner, J.P., and Mench, J.A. (2003). Isosexual pair housing improves the welfare of young Amazon parrots. *Applied Animal Behaviour Science* 81: 73–88.

Mench, J.A. and Blatchford, R.A. (2013). Birds as laboratory animals. In: *Laboratory Animal Welfare* (ed. K. Bayne and P.V. Turner), 279–300. New York, USA: Academic Press.

Myers, S.A., Millam, J.R., Roudybush, T.E., and Grau, C.R. (1988). Reproductive success of hand-reared vs. parent-reared cockatiels *Nymphicus hollandicus*. *Auk* 105: 536–542.

Parrot Society, UK. (2014). Pet Parrots. A Complete Beginner's Guide. Available at http://www.theparrotsocietyuk.org/pet-parrots/a-complete-beginners-guide. Accessed 11 July 2018.

Parrot Travel. n.d. CITES. Available at http://www.parrottravel.org/cites. Accessed 11 July 2018.

Péron, F. and Grosset, C. (2014). The diet of adult ositticides: veterinarian and ethological approaches. *Journal of Animal Physiology and Animal Nutrition* 98: 403–416.

Ricklefs, R.E. (2004). The cognitive face of avian life histories. *The Wilson Bulletin* 116: 119–133.

Rozek, J.C. and Millam, J.R. (2011). Preference and motivation for different diet forms and their effect on motivation for a foraging enrichment in captive Orange-winged Amazon parrots (*Amazona amazonica*). *Applied Animal Behaviour Science* 129: 153–161.

Rozek, J.C., Danner, L.M., Stucky, P.A., and Millam, J.R. (2010). Over-sized pellets naturalize foraging time of captive Orange-winged Amazon parrots (*Amazona amazonica*). *Applied Animal Behaviour Science* 125: 80–87.

Scope, A., Filip, T., Gabler, C., and Resch, F. (2002). The influence of stress from transport and handling on hematologic and clinical chemistry blood parameters of racing pigeons (*Columba livia domestica*). *Avian Diseases* 46: 224–229.

Schmid, R., Doherr, M.G., and Steiger, A. (2006). The influence of breeding method on the behaviour of adult African grey parrots (*Psittacus erithacus*). *Applied Animal Behaviour Science* 98: 293–307.

Seibert, L. (2006). Feather-picking disorder in pet birds. In: *Manual of Parrot Behavior* (ed. A.U. Luescher), 255–266. Ames, IA, USA: Blackwell.

Snyder, N., McGowan, P., Gilardi, J., and Grajal, A. (eds.) (2000). *Parrots: Status Survey and Conservation Action Plan 2000–2004*. Cambridge, UK: International Union for the Conservation of Nature.

Sodhi, N.S., Şekercioğlu, C.H., Barlow, J., and Robinson, S.K. (2011). Harvesting of tropical birds. In: *Conservation of Tropical Birds* (ed. N.S. Sodhi, C.H. Şekercioğlu, J. Barlow and S.K. Robinson), 152–172. Oxford, UK: Blackwell.

Sol, D., Duncan, R.P., Blackburn, T.M. et al. (2005). Big brains, enhanced cognition, and response of birds to novel environments. *Proceedings of the National Academy of Sciences United States of America* 102: 5460–5465. doi: 10.1073/pnas.0408145102.

Speer, BL. (2001). The clinical consequences of routine grooming. *Proceedings of the Association of Avian Veterinarians*, pp. 109–115.

Speer, B.L., Olsen, G.P., Doneley, R. et al. (2016). Common conditions of commonly held companion birds in multiple parts of the world. In: *Current Therapy in Avian Medicine and Surgery*, 777–781. St Louis, MO, USA: Elsevier.

Spoon, T. (2006). Parrot reproductive behavior, or who associates, who mates, and who cares? In: *Manual of Parrot Behavior* (ed. A.U. Luescher), 63–78. Ames, IA, USA: Blackwell.

Tella, J.L. and Hiraldo, F. (2014). Illegal and legal parrot trade shows a long-term, cross-cultural preference for the most attractive species, increasing their risk of extinction. *PLOS One* 9: e107546.

Ullrey, D.E., Allen, M.A., and Baer, D.J. (1991). Formulated diets versus seed mixtures for psittacines. *Journal of Nutrition* 121: S193–S205.

van Zeeland, Y.R.A., Spruit, B.M., Rodenburg, T.B. et al. (2009). Feather damaging behaviour in parrots: a review with consideration of comparative aspects. *Applied Animal Behaviour Science* 121: 75–95.

van Zeeland, Y.R.A., Schoemaker, N.J., Ravenstein, M.M. et al. (2013). Efficiency of foraging enrichments to increase foraging time in Grey parrots (*Psittacuc erithacus eritahcus*). *Applied Animal Behaviour Science* 149: 87–102.

Welle, K.R. and Luescher, A.U. (2006). Aggressive behavior in pet birds. In: *Manual of Parrot Behavior* (ed. A.U. Luescher), 211–218. Ames, IA, USA: Blackwell.

Weston, M.K. and Memon, M.A. (2009). The illegal parrot trade in Latin America and its consequences to parrot nutrition, health and conservation. *Bird Populations* 9: 76–83.

Wilson, L. and Luescher, A.U. (2006). Parrots and fear. In: *Manual of Parrot Behavior* (ed. A.U. Luescher), 225–232. Ames, IA, USA: Blackwell.

Pigeons (*Columba livia*)

17

John Chitty

17.1 History and Context

17.1.1 Natural History

Pigeons and doves are members of the class Avia, order Columbiformes, and family Columbidae, which consists of 309 species in 42 genera (del Hoyo et al. 1997). Within this family, all forms of domestic pigeons are descended from the Rock dove, *Columba livia*. There are possibly 13 *C. livia* subspecies, although the differences in classification are essentially of academic interest only. It is, in fact, difficult to determine which wild populations are 'natural Rock doves' and which are 'feral pigeons'. The species as a whole is extremely common worldwide with the exception of areas of climate extremes (Arctic, Antarctic, rainforest, and desert). Because of their widespread colonisation, rock pigeons are classified as being of Least Concern (IUCN 2016).

Indeed, pigeons are found almost everywhere that man has colonised because of their ability to adapt to the urban environment (del Hoyo et al. 1997). In particular, pigeons' natural nesting and perching positions are on rock ledges, which are effectively replicated by many buildings. Birds typically nest in pairs within colonies, producing well-formed nests from plant material and feathers. In the wild, birds do not form lasting

Companion Animal Care and Welfare: The UFAW Companion Animal Handbook,
First Edition. Edited by James Yeates.
© 2019 Universities Federation for Animal Welfare. Published 2019 by John Wiley & Sons Ltd.

pair bonds although they do stay together during rearing. Young pigeons ('squabs') are altricial but can fly by 5 weeks old. Parents feed them a crop milk, produced from the thickened lining of the crop that it is shed, regurgitated, and given to young. Wild adult pigeons predominantly eat grain, although they may also eat some invertebrates (del Hoyo et al. 1997). They follow diurnal patterns of activity.

17.1.2 Domestic History

Pigeons were first kept several thousand years ago in the Middle East, presumably assisted by the natural affinity between the species and man-made buildings. Typically, they have been used for a number of purposes. In ancient times, birds were prized for their guano for fertiliser, and message carrying (including in wartime) has been used for at least 2000 years. Meat production is of minor significance other than in the United States, and there is some use of pigeons in scientific research. Other pigeons are kept for exhibition or showing.

Racing is comparatively modern as a competition, with the main increase in interest occurring in the nineteenth century, although it is now widespread and of high economic value. Pigeon racing can involve hundreds or thousands of birds released in each race. The European racing season runs from April to September with the length of races increasing as the season progresses (typically 100–700 km, although some longer races do occur). It is largely males that race. A racing ring is applied to the leg, which is read when birds return at the end of the race and winners are decided on average speed (Hooimeijer 2006; Becker 2008a). Other forms of performance flying are also now widespread and of high economic value in many countries. Some competitions involve scoring the extent to which multiple pigeons 'tumble' or 'roll' (i.e. somersault backwards). Some judge the unity of multiple birds' tumbles during flight; others judge birds' high-speed vertical spiralling down from high altitudes to near the ground or how far birds tumble backwards without flying.

Selective breeding has produced a wide variety in colour, feathering, and body shape. It has also selected for exaggerated body features amongst 'fancy' or show pigeons. One example is the greatly enhanced ceres (skin around the nares) of some males that totally preclude them seeing where they are flying. 'Tumbler' and 'roller' pigeons have been selected to somersault backwards during flight and fall. Some (e.g. Parlour tumblers) can no longer fly but only tumble as soon as they intend to take wing (Godfrey and Godfrey 2011). Individual prize exhibition, racing, and tumbling pigeons can attract high values of more than €10 000.

17.2 Principles of Pigeon Care

17.2.1 Diet

Pigeons are herbivorous and their diet should be grain based. This can be a mixture of cereals or cereal-based pellets. Grains should be supplemented with both soluble grit for calcium (e.g. oyster shell) because birds can use up calcium in egg production (Figure 17.1), and insoluble stones for grinding food in the ventriculus. Vegetables or forage are rarely needed. Precise dietary needs depend on the individual and the time of year (Table 17.1).

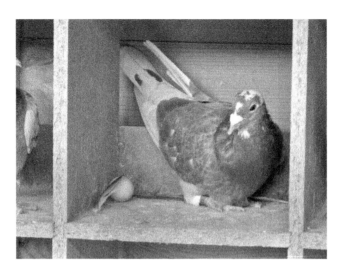

Figure 17.1 Pigeon with laid egg.

Table 17.1 Nutritional requirements of normal racing pigeons during the 'Racing Year'.

Period	Requirements
Racing season	Higher fibre rations between races, except for high-energy fatty foods immediately before and after races
	Additional electrolytes after races may aid recovery
	Additives containing high-digestibility amino acids, vitamins, and minerals may be beneficial
Moult	Specific moulting mixtures made up of diverse grains and legumes and containing high quantities of extruded corn
	Essential amino acid supplements may also be beneficial
Breeding	Increased dietary protein from pairing to the end of the rearing period
	High levels of soluble grit and fat-soluble vitamins
Weaning	Balanced energy and protein
	Easily digestible diet
	Reduced (or no) maize content
Resting	Comparatively low-fat, protein and fibre levels to avoid excessive weight gain Maize may be added if the environmental temperature is low

Measured feeding twice daily is generally preferred to ad libitum feeding. Feeding enrichment is typically not used other than in young birds, for whom feed may be scattered on wide 'tables' rather than long troughs to encourage flocking behaviours. Such scatter-feeding may provide some enrichment (BVAAWF/FRAME/RSPCA/UFAW Joint Working Group on Refinement 2001), although additional hygiene measures should be employed to reduce faecal contamination of the food. For older racing birds, such enrichments should be balanced with the need to provide adequate calorific intake because increasing the time needed to feed may ultimately result in insufficient energy intake. However, feeding enrichments should be considered when intake is restricted during the resting phase and also if birds are kept singly (Turner 2010).

Water is generally given in troughs or round 'hoppers'. Drinking is achieved by means of immersion of the beak into water and then creation of a negative pressure inside the oral cavity. This method allows some water to pass back from the oral cavity into the water bowl which can facilitate the spread of pathogens. Drinking devices should be designed for groups of four or less to minimise spread of disease between birds (Hooimeijer 2006; Becker 2008b). Both feed and water troughs should be provided such that there is sufficient space for all birds to reduce competition between birds and ensure all receive adequate provision.

17.2.2 Environment

Traditional dovecotes are used for small groups of ornamental birds (Hooimeijer 2006; Becker 2008a). In comparison, racing birds are generally kept in 'lofts' of around 60–70 birds, with some lofts housing more than a thousand birds. Lofts range from attic-type rooms over garages, through bird aviaries attached to sheds (Figure 17.2), up to large, complex buildings with indoor breeding compartments, outside flights, and openings to

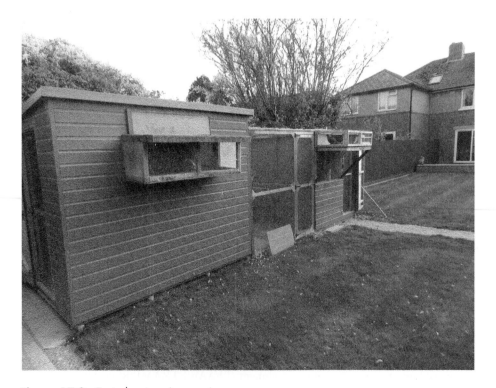

Figure 17.2 Typical racing pigeon aviary.

allow birds to enter and exit (Figure 17.3). All pigeons should have space to exercise adequately; if birds are housed in smaller cages, they should be given access to flight rooms at least once a day (Figure 17.4). Lofts should be also situated in sheltered and quiet locations because loud noises also provoke panic responses.

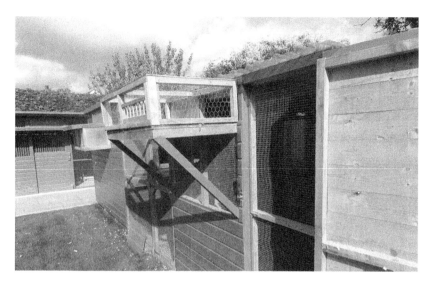

Figure 17.3 Aviary opening to allow entry/exit of birds.

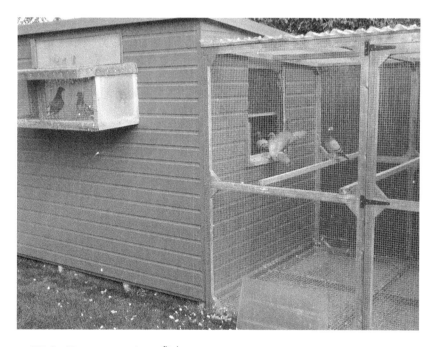

Figure 17.4 Pigeons accessing a flight area.

Ventilation and cleaning must be adequate to disperse irritants such as ammonia, remove feathers and feather dust, and limit humidity (Nepote 1999). Air should flow from young stock to old and preferably not between groups to minimise spread of potential pathogens to immunologically naive stock. Construction materials should be easy to clean and disinfect and without cavities or crevices that allow organic material to build-up. Surfaces and troughs should be easily accessible for cleaning, especially in indoor breeding areas, and a regular cleaning routine should be implemented. Ease of access is also important to allow regular cleaning and for food and water to be provided in a hygienic manner. Poor environmental conditions are major causes of disease in racing pigeons, particularly respiratory disease.

The welfare impact of racing is unclear. Losses during races are poorly studied, and most are ascribed to outside influences. However, these losses can be on a large scale, especially in young birds being trained and in particular races. For example, some sources have quoted very low return numbers from races across the English Channel. Because not all returning birds are always clocked in, it is not known how well this reflects actual loss rates. Nonetheless, the scale of these losses must represent a serious welfare concern.

17.2.3 Animal Company

Pigeons are not solitary birds and should not be kept alone. They should be kept either in pairs (with or without young) or as small flocks (Figure 17.5). These flocks can include males and females or can be single-sex flocks, although aggression may be more frequent in the latter (McGregor and Haselgrove 2010). Differentiating sex in immature birds is

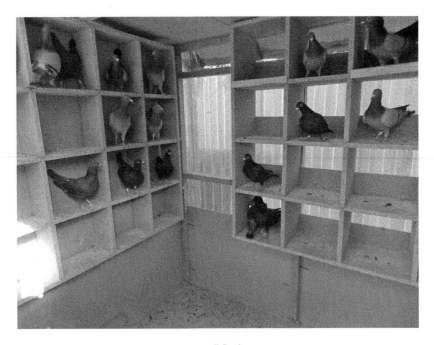

Figure 17.5 Pigeons living together as a small flock.

difficult, with traditional techniques such as head shape, vent shape, or length of digit 3 being unreliable. In mature birds, some males develop a cere hypertrophy, but otherwise sex differentiation is made on the basis of courtship behaviours and whether the bird lays eggs. DNA sexing using feathers or blood may also be performed.

Aggression may occur between individual pigeons. It is usually related to territory, especially roosting sites, and may also be elicited by food. Aggression normally begins with visual threat displays, such as erection of the plumage, spreading of tails, and raising of wings. This can progress to pecking, in particular at the eyes and head. However, if sufficient space, roosting sites and food are provided, aggressive interactions between birds are rarely seen, although problems may be more frequent when birds from different sources are mixed (Nepote 1999). Although the majority of birds are parent reared, hand rearing birds does not appear to affect their later social and sexual interactions with other pigeons or cause them to suffer when mixed with other pigeons if sufficient resources are provided.

Overcrowding can be a major problem and can predispose pigeons to disease through reduced hygiene, competition at feeding or drinking sites, and general stress (Hooimeijer 2006; Becker 2008a). As a general rule, there should be an absolute maximum stocking rate of one adult male, two adult females, and two young birds per cubic metre. Ideally levels should be half of these. Higher rates may be acceptable for short periods when young newly fledged birds are being encouraged to flock. There is a frequent temptation for owners to increase flock sizes to increase production. Where this is done, accommodation must be enlarged accordingly.

Birds spontaneously pair within groups. Males perform elaborate display flights, bowing (often accompanied by vocalisation), drive the female away from the main flock, and then feed her as if she is a juvenile. The speed of pairing and the length and complexity of these stages are dictated by whether or not the birds are in breeding season, and pairing can occur in just a few minutes when both male and female are at their most receptive. Immature juvenile birds may also show such behaviours to each other although they rarely progress through all stages (Goodwin 1983). A common method of motivating older male birds to race is the 'widower' system. Following pairing, males and females are separated for a week for daily training before being briefly reunited before the race. The pair is normally reunited for a long period on return. Hormonal influences on this technique appear important (Schmidt-Koenig 1963). The separation of the established pair seems likely to induce significant stress in both birds, and some hypthosise that this underlies the male's motivation the return to the loft.

Pigeons should be kept away from the sight and sounds of possible predators. Avian predators in particular may induce panic responses and self-injury. However, pigeons may be mixed with other nonpredatory bird species because they are typically not aggressive.

17.2.4 Human Interactions

Humans are naturally perceived as potential predators. Aggression toward humans is extremely unusual, which reflects their lack of mobbing behaviour toward predators (Goodwin 1983) and should not be taken as a lack of fear. Pigeons do show 'freeze' or 'panic' fear responses in the presence of unknown or threatening humans, for example when captured by strangers or during veterinary treatment. Sudden changes in routine or in keeping staff may also cause alterations in flock behaviour or feeding, which may lead to physical disease and decreased reproductive or race performance.

Handling and other interactions should therefore be done by familiar caregivers wherever possible, and within a maintained routine. If the birds are used to the particular caregiver, it may be best to move birds out of areas during cleaning or maintenance if another caregiver is performing these tasks. Approaches to birds should be made in a quiet calm manner and capture should be done by regular handlers in a calm manner. Pigeons can usually be captured and restrained with bare hands. Nervous birds may be captured using a net. Tractable birds can be restrained with one hand, with the bird 'sat' on the upward-facing palm, the legs extended caudally together, and held along with the tail between first and second fingers and the thumb (Wildpro 2015).

Frequent human proximity and handling birds from an early age should induce a tolerance of human company, and well-handled birds appear calm and confident when held. Well-handled birds will react socially to humans as well other birds, whether they were PARENT-REARED or hand-reared. Furthermore, hand-reared birds may imprint on humans and then react both socially and sexually to humans as well as to other pigeons (Goodwin 1983), whereas parent-reared birds may react socially but not sexually to humans. In either case, birds do not appear to suffer if deprived of human company if they are mixed with other pigeons, beyond learned associations with food. Various forms of learning and conditioning have also been demonstrated in pigeons (Delius 1983; Bonardi et al. 1993), which explains their high degree of trainability and the importance of daily routine in reducing stress and disease in racing flocks. It also means that appropriate training techniques may be used to reduce stress. For example, the stress of being caught up by hand may be reduced by training birds to walk into transport boxes.

17.2.5 Health

Pigeons can suffer from many diseases, particularly within flocks (Table 17.2), including zoonoses such as chlamydiosis, salmonellosis, and campylobacteriosis (Chitty and Lierz 2008). Infectious diseases may be spread via drinking systems or when birds are mixed with other flocks or feral birds, for example at races or shows. Poor husbandry can also exacerbate disease and facilitate entry and spread of infectious disease within the flock. Preventative measures should therefore include the use of quarantine facilities for birds entering or re-entering the flock; suitable treatment facilities so sick birds can be temporarily removed from the flock; regular examination and clinical sampling within the flock; and regular review and maintenance of the loft and hygiene procedures.

Medical problems may be suffered by single individuals or as part of an overall flock problem. Investigation of disease should therefore always involve clinical assessments of the affected individuals, other individuals, and the flock as a whole; examination of the loft; evaluation of husbandry methods (Hooimeijer 2006; Becker 2008a); appropriate sampling (e.g. faecal testing for parasites); and postmortem examination of dead or culled individuals and unhatched eggs. In some cases (e.g. parasitism), it is easy to determine that there are welfare issues throughout the flock. In other cases (e.g. noninfectious disease or trauma), there is a temptation to regard issues as being related to individuals only and not to assess the flock adequately. Investigations should be led by a veterinary surgeon because even experienced keepers may misdiagnose problems, use inappropriate

Table 17.2 Selected health problems in domestic pigeons.

		Condition	Welfare effects
Infections or infestations	Viral	Paramyxovirus-1 (V) aka. Newcastle Disease	Altered posture; malcoordination; tremors; disorientation; tremors; increased thirst
		Aviopoxvirus columbae (V)	Skin damage; eyelid swelling
		Pigeon herpesvirus	Acute: sneezing; eye inflammation; ulcers; vomiting; diarrhoea; lethargy Chronic: difficulty breathing; (secondary infections)
	Bacterial	*Salmonella* spp. (V)	Altered posture; poor balance; abscesses; reduced vision; joint inflammation, dropped wing; paralysis; reduced appetite; weight loss; diarrhoea
		Chlamydia psittaci	Often no effects; Difficulty breathing; sneezing; eye inflammation; weight loss; reduced appetite; diarrhoea
		Mycoplasmosis	Respiratory disease; sinusitis. Lifetime carriage or subclinical infection possible even with treatment
		Staphylococcal or streptococcal infections	These may cause a variety of clinical signs including generalised illness and death. Usually seen as opportunist infections; *Staphylococcus intermuedius* has been isolated as a commensal in pigeons
	Fungal	*Trichophyton megnini*	Skin damage
		Aspergillius spp.	Lower respiratory disease causing granuloma or abscess formation. Clinical signs include respiratory disease a more generalised weight loss or lethargy
	Internal Parasites	*Trichomonas gallinae* (canker)	Upper respiratory inflammation or plaques; poor exercise tolerance; weight loss; diarrhoea
		Ascaridia spp. *Capillaria* spp.	Weight loss; reduced exercise tolerance
		Eimeria spp. *Hexamita* spp.	Weight loss; diarrhoea
	External Parasites	Various mites	Itchiness; feather damage; anaemia
Toxic		Dimetridazole	Malcoordination; tremors
Traumatic		Flight injuries	Pain; difficulty in movement
		Shooting	Pain; internal organ damage

(V) means vaccine available.

diagnostic tests, or delay too long so that disease outbreaks are far progressed by the time veterinary assistance is sought. Pigeons should be given pre-emptive analgesia before or after an event that is likely to be painful, such as trauma or crop repair surgery, even if the bird appears normal.

Breeding has led to some genetic abnormalities. In addition, selection for tumbling and rolling may effectively select for abnormal serotonin brain function (Smith et al. 1987) or for epilepsy-like convulsions (Entrikin and Erway 1972), with anti-convulsant drugs reducing its performance (Kabir 2012). Such birds may also have a reduced ability to fly, with Parlour tumblers being effectively unable to fly, which may cause frustration and an inability to escape threats (Godfrey and Godfrey 2011). The behaviour itself may also cause exhaustion or injuries from impact.

17.2.6 Euthanasia

Acceptable methods of euthanasia of pigeons are listed in Table 17.3. The best method is usually sedation or anaesthesia, if needed, followed by the injection of an overdose of pentobarbitone into the ulnar or basilic vein because pigeons do not have an easily identifiable jugular vein (Chitty 2008). Intramuscular pentobarbital injections are highly irritant and painful. Neck dislocation may be humane if performed efficiently by an experienced operator.

17.3 Signs of Pigeon Welfare

17.3.1 Pathophysiological Signs

Physical signs of welfare problems may be seen in either the flock as a whole or in individuals. Problems in individuals may indicate welfare concerns in the flock and vice versa. In many cases, it is easier to assess welfare problems in the flock because there are a number of parameters that may indicate a failure to perform or thrive and thus the presence of underlying stressors. In particular, the presence of disease signs in a number of birds or increased mortality rates should stimulate suspicion of the presence of infectious disease agents and of underlying husbandry or dietary defects.

Disease in an individual may reflect stress or other welfare compromises. In essence, any departure from the norm for a particular bird may be an indication of disease or

Table 17.3 Methods of euthanasia for pigeons kept as companion animals.

Method	Restraint required	Welfare benefits	Welfare risks
Injection of anaesthetic into a vein (pentobarbitone)	Secure handling (or anaesthesia)	Rapid loss of consciousness	Pain from injection
Cervical dislocation	Secure handling	Rapid loss of consciousness	Momentary pain, distress Poor technique

Source: AVMA (2013).

Table 17.4   Key pathophysiological signs of welfare compromises in pigeons.

Body area	Specific symptoms
General	Loss of weight or body condition
Head or face	Nasal or ocular discharge
	Ocular or sinus swelling
Plumage and skin	Damage or loss of plumage
	Increased presence of ectoparasites
	Fluffed appearance
	Injuries (e.g. pecking)
Abdomen	Abdominal swelling
Excretion	Vent staining
	Changes in consistency, colour, regularity, or quantity of dropping
Decreased reproductive rates	Reduced pairing
	Reduced egg laying or infertile eggs
	Reduced hatching
	Poor chick survival

stress (Table 17.4). A proper diagnostic investigation of disease issues is therefore required when presented with a sick bird, rather than owners relying on 'traditional' methods. For example, faecal samples are extremely useful when assessing loss of condition or poor performance (i.e. where intestinal parasites may be important). However, they can be less useful – and even misleading – in other cases, such as respiratory disease. Physiological measures of stress include alterations of body temperature and alterations in stress hormones (especially catecholamines and corticosterone [Jeronen et al. 1976]), glucose and white cell parameters (Jeronen et al. 1976; Scope et al. 2002).

Poor performance can be assessed at the individual level, for example, in poor race performance, training performance or growth rate, and can indicate welfare problems for each individual (Tables 17.5 and 17.6). Performance can also be assessed at the flock level, for example, poor return of birds post release. This may be a sign of overall flock issues such as underlying subclinical disease, inadequate diet, or poor husbandry. Similarly, poor exercise management, training methods, and pair bonding may also contribute to poor performance. It is tempting to blame external factors (e.g. threats of predation from raptors) when the real problems may be poor flight performance, sites, or pair-bonding (Chitty and Lierz 2008). Similarly a reduced breeding success, such as pigeons producing fewer than around five broods of two eggs each year, may suggest a number of problems (Table 17.5). Records should be kept and reviewed to establish whether reduced chick numbers stem from certain pairs or from reduced performance of the whole flock.

17.3.2 Behavioural Signs
Behavioural signs are often subtle and are frequently overlooked, especially if the keeper is not familiar with the normal behaviour of the flock as a whole and of individual birds within the flock. Changes in behaviour may not be recognised as disease signs until the

Table 17.5 Differential diagnoses for decreased reproductive rates.

Indicator	Likely implications
Reduced pairing	Environmental problems or poor matching
Reduced egg laying or infertile eggs	Non-mating
	Parental dietary problems or disease
Reduced hatch	Poor diet
	Parental illness reducing chick viability
	Environmental factors
	Disturbance affecting egg incubation
Poor chick survival	Disease, especially subclinical disease in parents
	Disturbance
	Poor diet

Table 17.6 Basic measures and clinical standards of pigeons.

Parameter	Normal measures	
Life expectancy	20–30 years	
Mean weight	Males: 400–550 g	Females: 400–550 g
Body temperature	37–39 °C	
Respiratory frequency	25–30 breaths/min(resting)	
Heart rate	260–450 beats/min	
Pubescence	Males: 6–8 months	Females: 6–8 months
Blood volume	40–50 mL (approx. 10% bodyweight)	
Haematocrit	45–55	

Source: Chitty and Lierz (2008).

development of physical signs. Nevertheless, behavioural signs can be important indicators and may be seen in association with physical disease or often as a precursor to physical disease (Table 17.7). As with physical signs, behavioural indicators may be assessed at the level of the flock and the individual. Behavioural signs of welfare issues are more likely to be identified in individual birds. Nonetheless, flock alterations may be seen, especially where disturbances or issues in husbandry have affected a large number of individuals. In particular, alteration in site use can indicate current or previous disturbances; for example, the presence of potential predators can lead to the avoidance of particular feeders, drinkers, or nest sites. Poor relationships can also be seen at the flock level, such as rates of aggression between individuals, poor pair bonding, and failure to incubate eggs or rear chicks.

Although the pigeon has been well-studied with respect to pain physiology and analgesia (Hawkins and Machin 2004; Hawkins and Paul-Murphy 2011; Desmarchelier et al. 2012), the actual assessment of pain in individuals is extremely difficult, reflecting

Table 17.7 Key behavioural signs of welfare compromises in pigeons.

Aspect of behaviour	Specific responses
Altered activity or responsiveness	Reduced flying ability; poor flight performance
	Immobility or lethargy
Avoidance	Not interacting with other birds or humans
	Not using certain perches or nest sites. Escape attempts
	Failure to return from flights
Altered posture or expression	Closed eyes
	Reduced ability to perch
Altered metabolic processes and maintenance or other common behaviour	Dyspnoea or tachypnoea and tail bobbing
	Reduced appetite; anorexia
	Increased or reduced preening behaviour
Attack or preattack behaviours	Aggressive displays
	Aggression to other birds or handlers
Abnormal behaviours	Head bobbing
	Adjunctive pecking
Specific local signs of local pain	Lameness
	Wing drooping
	'Guarding' of limbs

their stoical nature and status as a prey species where overt displays of pain or illness may stimulate predator attack. However, some signs have been linked to pain in pigeons (Table 17.5). Other signs may additionally be regarded as indicators of potential underlying stressors or disease. Birds may show avoidance behaviours, such as not interacting with other birds or humans or not using certain perches or nest sites. Birds may also show escape attempts, which can manifest as failure to return from training or race flights. Changes in vocalisations may also indicate a compromise in pigeons' welfare, such as a lack of voice, altered voice, or excessive vocalisation.

Aggressive behaviours may indicate a lack of space, roosting sites, food quantity, or feeding space. Redirected aggression has been reported in response to 'frustration' (Campagnoni et al. 1986) in pigeons, and so the investigation of aggression in birds must not only look for causes of pain and so on but also assess whether or not they are restricted in their ability to perform normal behaviours. Displacement behaviours, such as altered preening, may also indicate an underlying anxiety disorder. Longer-term development of abnormal behaviours has been recorded in pigeons, including stereotypical behaviours such as head bobbing and adjunctive pecking (Palya and Zacny 1980). The identification of stereotypical behaviour in a bird should stimulate investigation of likely stressors and removal or correction of all possible causes. Pigeon navigation also shows aspects of stereotypical behaviour (Meade et al. 2005), even if this reduces route efficiency. Whether or not this is a sign of active ongoing welfare problems is debatable but may suggest that behavioural problems can be linked to poor individual performance.

17.4 Worldwide Action Plan to Improve Pigeon Welfare

Pigeons have been kept for centuries and some pigeon-keeping methods are rooted in the past. This tradition and experience brings significant value and experienced keepers have a great deal of knowledge of their birds both individually and collectively. However, it also means that there is often a resistance to adopt new methods, as reflected, for example, in the overreliance on faecal samples in investigating any clinical illness whether or not related to the gastrointestinal system. New ideas, underpinned by developments in animal welfare and veterinary science, should be better communicated and accepted. A greater recognition of the welfare needs of all pigeons as individuals is needed to promote better care. This includes recognition and promotion of the husbandry requirements of fancy and tumbling doves and the review of particular practices within the showing, fancying, and racing communities.

There is significant potential for welfare problems in the keeping, training, and competing of pigeons. Some racing flights have large-scale financial and staff investment and appropriately treat racing pigeons as athletes. However, this is not always seen throughout the pigeon racing or fancying communities, especially where young or non-winning birds have low financial value. The extremes of performance mean that even minor discrepancies in training or feeding can cause serious welfare problems, and wider recognition of the need to treat racing and performance pigeons as athletes should increase the level of their care.

Particular priorities for research include assessment of the welfare impact of breeding changes and the development and implementation of breeding recommendations. Studies tracking training and racing birds, the recovery of bodies for postmortem examination, and simple measures such as compulsory 'clocking in' of all birds would help establish true loss rates and shed further light on the causes and means of prevention of underlying welfare problems and racing losses. Further work in evaluating fitness, especially physiological measurements, are also needed to prevent the release of unfit birds and reduce race losses. Once such parameters are established and causes of race losses accurately determined, then more definite recommendations for training can be established. The difficulties in assessing pain in birds also means there is a need to develop pain scales to assist with this. For example, the subtlety of signs of pain and disease has led to many believing analgesia or anaesthesia to be unnecessary. Therefore better methods of pain assessment and 'scoring' are necessary to determine genuine levels of pain and needs for pain relief.

Pigeon keepers also need to be encouraged to seek veterinary intervention, rather than relying on their own diagnoses or consulting other peers. The reasons given for not doing so include the cost of veterinary fees, the lack of interest or knowledge of some veterinary surgeons (in their experience), and in many countries, the easy availability of prescription-only drugs on the Internet or from other pigeon keepers. However, avian veterinary medicine is growing worldwide and veterinary surgeons can add significant value. The veterinary profession needs to convey this to the pigeon owners and to demonstrate its abilities. In addition, regulations on veterinary medicines need tightening and to be consistently enforced especially in the light of current concerns on drug resistance.

Bibliography

AVMA (American Veterinary Medical Association). (2013). AVMA Guidelines for the Euthanasia of Animals: 2013 Edition. Available at https://www.avma.org/KB/Policies/Pages/Euthanasia-Guidelines.aspx. Accessed 7 October 2015.

Becker, R. (2008a). Pigeon husbandry and racing management. In: *BSAVA Manual of Raptors, Pigeons and Passerine Birds* (ed. J. Chitty and M. Lierz), 14–18. Gloucester, UK: BSAVA.

Becker, R. (2008b). Pigeons: nutrition. In: *BSAVA Manual of Raptors, Pigeons and Passerine Birds* (ed. J. Chitty and M. Lierz), 299–304. Gloucester, UK: BSAVA.

Bonardi, C., Rey, V., Richmond, M., and Hall, G. (1993). Acquired equivalence of cues in pigeon autoshaping: effects of training with common consequences and with common antecedents. *Animal Learning and Behavior* 21: 369–376.

BVAAWF/FRAME/RSPCA/UFAW Joint Working Group on Refinement (2001). Laboratory birds: refinements in husbandry and procedures. Fifth report of BVAAWF/FRAME/SPCA/UFAW Joint Working Group on Refinement. *Laboratory Animals* 35 (supp 1): 1–163.

Chitty, J. (2008). Basic techniques. In: *BSAVA Manual of Raptors, Pigeons and Passerine Birds* (ed. J. Chitty and M. Lierz). Gloucester, UK: BSAVA.

Chitty, J. and Lierz, M. (2008). *BSAVA Manual of Raptors, Pigeons and Passerine Birds*. Gloucester, UK: BSAVA.

Campagnoni, F.R., Lawler, C.P., and Cohen, P.S. (1986). Temporal patterns of reinforcer-induced general activity and attack in pigeons. *Physiology and Behavior* 37: 577–582.

Delius, J. (1983). Learning. In: *Physiology and Behaviour of the Pigeon* (ed. M. Abs). Academic Press.

Desmarchelier, M., Troncy, E., Fitzgerald, G., and Lair, S. (2012). Analgesic effects of meloxicam administration on postoperative orthopedic pain in domestic pigeons (*Columba livia*). *American Journal of Veterinary Research* 73 (3): 361–367.

Entrikin, R.K. and Erway, L.C. (1972). A genetic investigation of roller and tumbler pigeons. *Journal of Heredity* 63: 351–354.

Godfrey R, Godfrey D (2011). Rolling and Tumbling. Available at www.ufaw.org.uk/birds/pigeons-rolling-and-tumbling. Last accessed 13 June 2015

Goodwin, D. (1983). Behaviour. In: *Physiology and Behaviour of the Pigeon* (ed. M. Abs). Academic Press.

Hawkins, M.G. and Machin, K.L. (2004). Avian pain and analgesia. *Proceedings of the Association of Avian Veterinarians* 165–174.

Hawkins, M.G. and Paul-Murphy, J. (2011). Avian Analgesia. *Veterinary Clinics of North America Exotic Animal Practice* 14: 61–80.

Heatley, J.J., Oliver, J.W., Hosgood, G. et al. (2000). Serum corticosterone concentrations in response to restraint, anaesthesia, and skin testing in Hispaniolan Amazon parrots (*Amazona ventralis*). *Journal of Avian Medicine and Surgery* 14: 172–176.

Hooimeijer, J. (2006). Management of racing pigeons. In: *Clinical Avian Medicine* (ed. G.J. Harrison and T.L. Lightfoot), 849–860. Palm Beach, FL: Spix Publishing.

del Hoyo, J., Elliott, A., and Sargatal, J. (1997). *Handbook of the Birds of the World Volume 4: Sandgrouse to Cuckoos*. Barcelona: Lynx Edicions.

IUCN (2016). The IUCN Red List of Threatened Species. Available at https://www.iucn.org/theme/species/our-work/iucn-red-list-threatened-species. Accessed 22 August 2016.

Jeronen, E., Isometsa, P., Hissa, R., and Pyornila, A. (1976). Effect of acute temperature stress on the plasma catecholamine, corticosterone and metabolite levels in the pigeon. *Comparative Biochemistry and Physiology part C; Comparative Pharmacology* 55: 17–22.

Kabir, M.A. (2012). Tumbling behaviour of pigeons. *Global Journal of Science Frontier Research Biological Sciences* 12 (6): 17–19.

Le Maho, Y., Karmann, H., Briot, D. et al. (1992). Stress in birds due to routine handling and a technique to avoid it. *American Journal of Physiology-Regulatory, Integrative and Comparative Physiology* 263: 775–781.

McGregor, A. and Haselgrove, M. (2010). Doves and pigeons. In: *The UFAW Handbook on the Care and Management of Laboratory Animals*, 8e (ed. R.C. Hubrecht and J. Kirkwood), 686–696. Oxford: Wiley-Blackwell.

Meade, J., Biro, D., and Guilford, T. (2005). Homing pigeons develop local route stereotypy. *Proceedings of the Royal Society B: Biological Sciences* 272 (1558): 17–23.

Nepote, K. (1999). Pigeon housing: practical considerations and welfare implications. *Laboratory Animals* 28 (2): 34–37.

Palya, W.L. and Zacny, J.P. (1980). Stereotyped adjunctive pecking by caged pigeons. *Animal Learning and Behavior* 8: 293–302.

Rooney N et al (2012). RSPCA Welfare Guidelines for Performing Animals- Pigeons & Doves. Available at https://www.rspca.org.uk/adviceandwelfare/performinganimals/guidelines. Accessed 1 October 2018.

Schmidt-Koenig, K. (1963). Hormones and homing in pigeons. *Physiological Zoology* 36: 264–272.

Scope, A., Filip, T., Gabler, C., and Resch, F. (2002). The influence of stress from transport and handling on hematologic and clinical chemistry blood parameters of racing pigeons (*Columba livia domestica*). *Avian Diseases* 46: 224–229.

Smith, G.N., Hingtgen, J., and William DeMyer, W. (1987). Serotonergic involvement in the backward tumbling response of the parlor tumbler pigeon. *Brain Research* 400: 399–402.

Turner, T. (2010). Enrichment for Carneaux pigeons used in behavioral learning research. *Laboratory Animals (New York)* 39 (2): 40–41.

Wildpro (2015). Catching and Handling of Pigeons & Doves (Wildlife Casualty Management). Available at http://wildpro.twycrosszoo.org/S/00Man/AvianHusbandryTechniques/UKBHusbIndTech/handle_av_doves_pigeons.htm. Accessed 13 June 2015.

Reptiles (*Reptilia*)

18

Joanna Hedley, Robert Johnson, and James Yeates

18.1 History and Context

18.1.1 Common Natural History

Reptiles include more than 10 000 species, including turtles, tortoises, snakes, lizards, and crocodilians (Table 18.1). Reptiles are found on every continent except Antarctica and in a wide range of environments, including on land, in trees, in freshwater, and in seas, with some spending almost all their time in the water. Wild reptiles are still caught for trade in many countries, in particular turtles and green iguanas (Praud and Moutou 2010), but the conservation status of many species is under threat (IUCN 2016).

Most reptiles depend almost entirely on their environment for warmth, and control their body temperature through their behaviour. They can lose heat via respiration, urination, and behaviours such as moving into the shade or water. They can maintain their temperature by burrowing or postural changes such as coiling up. They can gain heat from the sun and warm surfaces via radiation, conduction, and convection by altering their location, position, skin-colour, and body posture and from digesting food in some species (e.g. South American rattlesnakes [*Crotalus durissus terrificus*], Tattersall et al. 2004). A few reptiles (not usually kept as pets) can tolerate subzero

Companion Animal Care and Welfare: The UFAW Companion Animal Handbook,
First Edition. Edited by James Yeates.

Table 18.1 Examples of reptile species kept as companion animals.

Crocodilians (Crocodilia)	Snakes and lizards (Squamata)	Tortoises, turtles and terrapins (Testudines)
African dwarf crocodile(*Osteolaemus tetraspis*)	Ball or Royal python (*Python regius*)	Red-eared sliders (*Trachemys scripta elegans*)
Cuvier's dwarf caiman (*Paleosuchus palpebrosus*)	*Boa constrictor* (*Boa constrictor*)	Mediterranean tortoises (*Testudo* spp.)
	Cornsnakes (*Pantherophis guttatus*)	
	Bearded dragons (*Pogona vitticeps*)	
	Green Iguanas (*Iguana iguana*)	
	Leopard gecko (*Eublepharis macularius*)	
	Yemen or veiled chameleon (*Chamaeleo calyptratus*)	

temperatures through specific adaptations that either prevent or allow their body to cope with water freezing in their bodies (e.g. European common lizards [*Lacerta vivipara*]). Several species enter a period of dormancy or 'brumation', triggered by low temperatures and shortening day lengths, in which they are less active, less responsive and eat less (e.g. Box turtles [*Terrapene* spp.]), but others do not (e.g. Fijian crested iguanas [*Brachylophus vitiensis*]), or may 'aestivate' during hot or dry periods. A period of brumation often precedes and stimulates subsequent reproductive activity.

Nearly all reptiles have a thickened and hardened outer skin, which is shed regularly, covered in overlapping scales, and some also possess thicker protective shells. Reptiles engage in a wide range of activities, from swimming (including several snakes) to climbing (including some terrapins). Some reptiles are often relatively inactive, for example green iguanas (*Iguana iguana*) may spend 90% of their time immobile (Van Marken Lichtenbelt et al. 1993). Some hunt either actively or by ambush, and crocodiles have even been seen to use tools as lures for prey (Dinets et al. 2015). Many reptiles are able to sense ultraviolet (UV), infrared, ground, or water vibrations or various chemicals to detect food, mates, and predators and to identify other individuals. The importance of each sense varies between orders and species; for example, snakes generally rely less on vision and more on 'smell' than turtles, tortoises, and lizards. Some reptiles may also vocalise, including underwater (e.g. long-necked freshwater turtles [*Chelodina oblonga*], Giles et al. 2009).

Many reptiles are largely solitary, coming together almost solely for reproduction. However, some species naturally form groups with family members or others, for reasons such as defence (e.g. Australian black rock skinks [*Egernia saxatilis*], O'Connor and Shine 2003) or cooperative hunting (e.g. crocodilians, Dinets 2015). Even some seemingly asocial animals may come together, for example as juveniles or reproducing females (e.g. timber rattlesnakes, *Crotalus horridus*: Clark et al. 2012). A few species exhibit a limited period of maternal care (e.g. Eastern Diamondback rattlesnakes [*Crotalus adamanteus*], Butler and others 1995). Most reptiles lay eggs, with some exceptions such as many skinks (*Scincomorpha*) and most boas (*Boidae*) who are live bearing. Some female reptiles can produce offspring without sexual interaction; sometimes with the females engaging in 'male' courtship behaviour (e.g. *Cnemidophorus* spp., Moore et al. 1985).

18.1.2 Common Domestic History

Reptile keeping seems more prominent in 'Western' countries, perhaps because reptiles may be considered dangerous and unappealing wild animals in their native countries. For example, it has been estimated that there are around 2 million pet reptiles kept in the United Kingdom (PFMA 2014), where native reptile species are sparse and generally small and benign. Reptiles are kept by a variety of owners, ranging from specialist 'hobby' enthusiasts and amateur private 'pet' keepers, to reptiles kept as interior decoration (e.g. chameleons) or even souvenirs for tourists (e.g. small turtles). A wide variety of species are kept as pets. Some species may be considered particularly 'exotic' (e.g. rare species), dangerous (e.g. venomous species such as rattlesnakes [*Crotalus* spp.] and mambas [*Dendroaspis* spp.]), unsuitable to be handled (e.g. chameleons), or difficult to breed in captivity. A small number of species appear to be becoming more popular, at least in some countries, for example, bearded dragons and cornsnakes because these are marketed as generally easy to keep and a suitable 'beginner' species.

In many countries, the most common reptile species are at least partly captive-bred. Some strains have been selected for particular colour 'morphs' and shapes (e.g. in Royal or ball pythons [*Python regius*]). Nevertheless, reptiles have undergone limited, if any, genuine domestication. Reptile breeding and trade occurs on large scales, with estimates of annual live reptile imports (including many on CITES Appendix II) reaching 2.2 million into the European Union and around 2 million into and 9 million from the United States (Laidlaw 2005; UNEP/WCMC 2009; ENDCAP 2012).

18.2 Principles of Reptile Care

18.2.1 Diets

Most snakes and crocodilian reptiles are carnivorous, whereas many tortoises and turtles are herbivorous or omnivorous. Each reptiles' specific requirements and preferences depend on their species, age, activity, environment, reproduction status (e.g. some reptiles may stop eating when about to lay eggs), and season (e.g. before brumation). Commercial diets may not reflect these differences, and owners need to adapt their pet's diet to meet any changes in their nutritional needs. There is a danger of owners overfeeding their reptiles, perhaps because they enjoy watching food being eaten and because reptiles' metabolic rates are approximately 25% of equivalent mammals' (Donoghue 1998), with some species having particularly low metabolic rates (e.g. larger boids in comparison to colubrids). Overfeeding can lead to obesity or hyperlipidosis, with excessive fat deposited in the coelom, under the skin and within organ tissues. Owners should

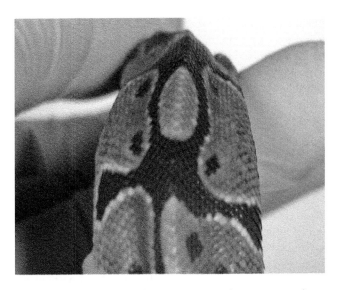

Figure 18.1 Ball python with triangular cross-sectional appearance because of marked body-condition loss. (*Source:* Courtesy Kevin Eatwell).

regularly monitor their reptiles' weight and body condition (e.g. using silhouette and tail base width; Figure 18.1) and keep feeding records to monitor intake and feeding behaviours.

Reptiles' requirements for micronutrients, such as calcium, phosphorus, and vitamins A, D, and E, depend on environmental conditions (e.g. temperature and UV-light levels) and reproductive status, and inadequate nutrition can lead to problems such as skin conditions and metabolic bone disease. Nutrition can often be improved by ensuring prey (whether invertebrate or vertebrate) are adequately housed and fed before being fed out to reptiles to ensure they are adequately nutritious. Depending on the quality of the diet, many pet reptiles may require vitamin and mineral supplementation, particularly for calcium, for example, through dusting their food or giving them cuttlefish. However, not all need this; for example, many snakes on appropriate diets may consume enough calcium and vitamin D to avoid metabolic bone conditions. Furthermore, there is a danger of overdosing reptiles, especially small lizards. Some reptiles (e.g. some tortoises) can be selective feeders, making it hard to ensure a balanced diet.

Feeding frequency needs to be appropriate to the species and the individual. Smaller and herbivorous reptiles usually need feeding at least daily but more frequent small feeds, or continuous access to foraging or grazing, may provide enrichment. In contrast, feeds may be separated by several weeks for other reptiles such as some larger snakes – although this can be fatal for already undernourished or ill animals. Many reptiles are motivated to browse or hunt, and opportunities to replicate such behaviour should be provided. Some may be reluctant to eat in captivity, especially if provided with nonwhole, nonmoving, or dead prey.

Provision of live animals as prey, however, raises serious welfare concerns (Cooper and Williams 2014). The vertebrate prey animals suffer from fear, stress and injury before death, and may have been kept in unsuitable environments before being fed.

(The welfare effects on invertebrate prey animals are less clear). Live invertebrate and vertebrate prey can also cause injuries or spread diseases (in addition to those spread by prekilled prey); for example, rats may attack reptiles in self-defence, and crickets may damage eyes or skin, causing damage. Wherever possible, live feeding should be avoided and prey scents and behaviour should be simulated, for example, by owners moving prey with tongs or using automatic 'shakers'. If live feeding is adopted, feeding must be observed and any uneaten prey should be removed from the enclosure when reptiles are less active.

Although many lizards and snakes obtain water from food, fresh water should be provided. A rule of thumb is at least 20–30 mL/kg a day (Calvert 2004), but species needs vary. Depending on reptile species' natural drinking behaviour, the best water provision may be misting, drip systems, or bowls shallow enough to prevent drowning. Although reptiles cannot absorb their water requirements through the skin, bathing may encourage reptiles to drink, and some chelonians can take water in through their cloaca. Water should not be withdrawn to encourage eating because this risks kidney damage from raised serum levels of uric acid; indeed, anorexic animals should always be hydrated before feeding. Dehydration can be associated with heart, kidney, and bone problems (especially in herbivores with higher potassium intake) or gout (especially in terrestrial reptiles who secrete uric acid more than ammonia).

18.2.2 Environments

Pet reptiles may be housed in an indoor, enclosed, climate-controlled area, or 'vivarium', although some might be kept in more open outdoor environments. All environments need to provide a certain amount of three-dimensional space and refuges so that every reptile can move around freely and have a choice of different microenvironments within the enclosure. Even reptiles who naturally spend much of their time within smaller hides or burrows should be able to access a larger space. Environments should allow adequate space for exercise, especially because many small reptiles are highly active. Enough space is also needed for animals kept in larger groups or who need space to avoid one another. Lastly, enough space is needed for essential resources – in particular adequate height for reptiles that climb and sufficient access to a body of water for aquatic and semi-aquatic species.

Reptiles need the right interactions of environmental temperature, humidity, air, and water flow to maintain adequate comfort, behaviour patterns, digestion, and immune responses (Table 18.2). Inappropriate temperatures or humidity can lead to problems such as skin conditions, poor shedding, and deformities (e.g. African spurred tortoises, [*Geochelone sulcata*], Weisner and Iben 2003) or aggression (e.g. leopard geckos [*Eublepharus macularis*], Flores et al. 1994). Relative humidity should not be too high, although many reptiles (e.g. tropical species) need a higher humidity than that often found in centrally heated homes, and even many desert species can benefit from humid areas. Humidity can be increased by spraying objects in the environment and providing compartments packed with damp sphagnum moss, vermiculite, or peat kept moistened. Ventilation and water flow should avoid excessive drying or cooling while preventing a build-up of harmful microorganisms. All reptiles need a background temperature in their preferred optimum temperature zone (e.g. nocturnal tropical geckos) and need a temperature *gradient* so they can choose to warm up, cool off, or maintain their

Table 18.2 General requirements for reptile "climates".

Aspects	Requirements
Temperature and light	A suitable thermostatically controlled background temperature, varying by day and night
	An appropriate temperature gradient across all usable areas of the enclosure, including a basking area if appropriate for the species
	Sufficient safe places to obtain direct light and heat
	Fire-alarms and back-up heat sources (e.g. power generators or microwavable heat bags)
Humidity	A safe water bath (for some species)
	Drier areas (for some species)
Temperature and humidity	Monitoring of temperature and humidity (in addition to the thermostat)
	Humid areas at different temperatures
Temperature, ventilation, hygiene and water quality	Adequate air and water filtration and changes, without drafts, water-currents or excessive cooling

temperature at any given time. Heat sources should be protected or located to avoid overheating (e.g. from floor heating) or burns from the reptile being in direct contact or unable to move away from them (e.g. lamps).

Light should cover the appropriate range of infrared, visual, and UV wavelengths, to allow vision, thermal regulation, and vitamin D production. UV-A may be important for natural interactions between individuals and reproduction. Many reptiles rely on UV-B for production of vitamin D (e.g. green iguanas, Allen and Oftedal 1994), and insufficient UV light can result in metabolic bone disease. Some reptiles can also obtain vitamin D from their diet (e.g. panther chameleons [*Chameleo pardalis*], Ferguson et al. 2003), but may benefit from both sources. Natural light can provide appropriate lighting in native countries, although vivaria should not be placed entirely in direct sunlight from which animals cannot escape, and reptiles may need supplementary light in other climates. Artificial UV light sources should be designed for the particular species, used according to manufacturers' instructions, tailored to the individual (e.g. placed where animals enjoy basking and at an appropriate distance to be effective), and replaced when required. Owners should also monitor UV output with a UV meter to ensure appropriate light reaches the animals and that bulbs are not wearing out. All UV and visible wavelengths should be provided in naturalistic light–dark cycles, and some reptiles are more active at night or during dawn and dusk.

Environments should be secure to prevent both escape and any injuries from escape attempts. In particular, reptiles may not perceive clear glass or plastic as barriers, risking accidental facial damage unless the glass is made visible (e.g., using tape at nose-height). Glass walls may also create reflections that are perceived as another, possibly threatening, reptile.

In addition, all reptiles should be given opportunities to hide, such as tunnels, boxes, or substrates for burrowing. There should be sufficient and well-located hides so that each animal can hide separately, escape from each other, and control their body temperatures at the same time. Aquatic reptiles also need underwater hides and burrowing substrates. Camouflaging or mimicking species such as chameleons may benefit from naturalistic contents (e.g. leaves) and colours with which they can blend in and may decrease their stress levels. Alarming noise and physical vibrations should be avoided because these may be interpreted as predators. Resources such as food and heat sources should be placed in quiet and sheltered areas, so that animals do not have to choose between security and other resources.

Reptiles should be provided with appropriate substrates (Figure 18.2) and water for swimming or bathing. Substrates should be safe if they are ingested, for example, when feeding or tongue-flicking to explore their environment. Burrowing reptiles should have deep enough substrate to make a genuine burrow. Aquatic and semi-aquatic reptiles should have access to an area of water of sufficient width, length, and depth for simultaneous full immersion and swimming of all reptiles in the group. This should be kept clean to avoid conditions such as dermatitis (Figure 18.3), while minimising disturbance. Most reptiles therefore benefit from regular spot cleaning as required rather than frequently having their substrate replaced completely, although occasional deep cleaning may help to remove persistent pathogens such as snake mites (*Ophionyssus natricis*). However, the right approach varies between different reptiles; for example, leaving small quantities of faeces may benefit some snakes (e.g. reducing investigatory tongue flicks and defaecation responses in rattlesnakes, Chiszar et al. 1980) but be unpleasant for some geckos (e.g. Brown et al. 1998).

Environments should have sufficient resources to allow motivated behaviour. Enrichment can increase reptiles' behavioural repertoires and increase activity (e.g.

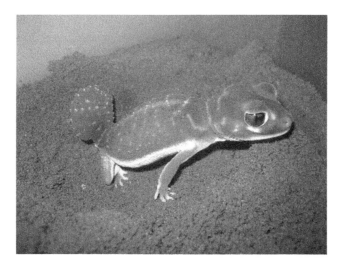

Figure 18.2 Knob-tailed gecko (*Nephrurus levis*) on sand-based substrate. (*Source:* Courtesy of C Johnson).

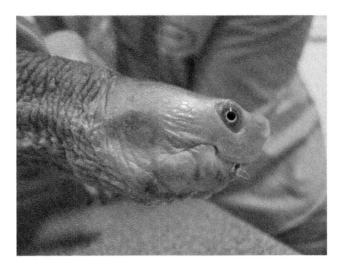

Figure 18.3 Short necked turtle (*Emydura macquarrii*) with dermatitis resulting from poor water quality. (*Source:* Courtesy R Johnson).

Eastern Box Turtles [*Terrapene carolina carolina*], Case et al. 2005; loggerhead turtles [*Caretta caretta*], Therrien et al. 2007; ratsnakes [*Elaphe obsolete*], Almli and Burghardt 2006) and may reduce some problems such as self-mutilation (e.g. African soft shell turtle [*Trionyx triunguis*], Burghardt et al. 1996). Some reptiles also prefer more complex environments (e.g. Eastern Box Turtles: Case 2003), and minor modifications can stimulate exploration. Reptiles need specific enrichments to perform particular behaviours such as climbing and basking, and they need to have three-dimensional frameworks, branches and platforms to do so (Figure 18.4). Many reptiles sit, bathe, or defaecate in water, and need water baths that are large enough for them to become submerged, as well as fresh water sources for drinking. If not, they may otherwise defaecate in their drinking water. Other reptiles, such as leopard geckos, can drown in very small depths of water, so any water provided for such reptiles should be in a small, shallow dish to prevent drowning.

18.2.3 Animal Company
Reptiles are generally not sociable and many reptiles may suffer when housed in groups. Competition can deprive reptiles of accessing food, basking, or shelter, especially when there are significant size differences (Figure 18.5). Aggression can cause injuries, infections, and fatalities. In the wild, reptiles may avoid physical aggression by a variety of postural and other threatening behaviours, depending on the species (some of which can also represent courtship behaviours). One reptile may then safely retreat in response. In contrast, captive animals lack the ability to retreat. For example, the pheromones and sight of adult green iguanas may also cause stress and decreased health in juveniles (Alberts et al. 1994). Most reptiles should therefore be kept out of sight and smell of each other.

However, some reptiles can have complex social interactions, varying with age, sex, and seasonality, and such sociable animals may benefit from compatible company. Some reptiles can form stable social groups (e.g. Australian skinks [*Egernia* spp.],

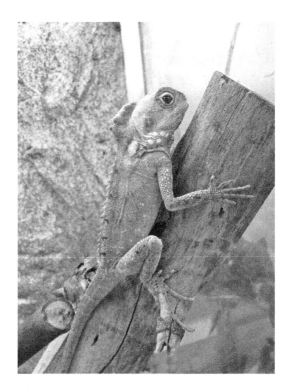

Figure 18.4 Boyd's forest dragon (*Hypsilurus boydii*) resting on a bare branch. (*Source:* Courtesy R Johnson).

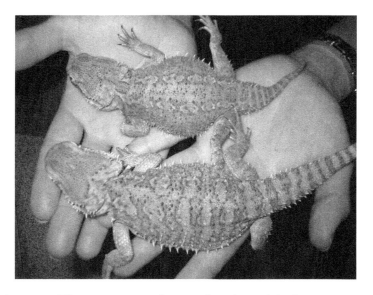

Figure 18.5 Size difference in Lawson's dragon (*P. henrylawsoni*) clutch mates. (*Source:* Courtesy Robert Johnson).

Gardner et al. 2001; Chapple 2003; desert night lizards [*Xantusia vigilis*], Davis 2011). Reptiles may also engage in social play (e.g. emidyd turtles, Kramer and Burghardt 1998) and cooperative behaviour including tunnelling (e.g. great desert skinks [*Liopholis kintorei*], McAlpin et al. 2011); nesting (e.g. some Australian lizards, Doody et al. 2009); huddling (e.g. desert night lizards, Rabosky et al. 2012); and group vigilance (e.g. green iguanas, Burghardt 1977; Burghardt et al. 1977; gidgee skink [*Egernia stokesii*], Lanham and Bull 2004). Reptiles may also be able to follow others' gaze (e.g. red-footed tortoises [*Geochelone carbonaria*], Wilkinson et al. 2010a) and learn from one another (e.g. Florida redbelly turtles [*Pseudemys nelson*, Davis and Burghardt 2011; red-footed tortoises, Wilkinson et al. 2010b).

Both social and unsocial reptiles can suffer from being in overly large groups, having insufficient space, size discrepancies, and insufficient resources. Any groups should be carefully managed to ensure animals are compatible, provide adequate resources, allow escape, and prevent overcrowding in terms of both space and access to resources. The signs of social stress can be subtle, and groups need to be carefully monitored. In some species, parental behaviours may also include protection and incubation of the eggs or young (e.g. many crocodilians), although the welfare impacts of depriving parents or young of such interactions in captivity are not well known. However, courtship and copulation can also be traumatic, and females may be injured if they are unable to escape. In some cases, parental behaviours may include predatory cannibalisation if young are left with adults.

Mixed-species groupings are generally stressful for reptiles and should be avoided. Some species can carry pathogens, without any symptoms, that can cause a disease in another species (e.g. boas can carry an inclusion body disease virus that can cause serious disease in pythons, Keeble 2004). Other species may be seen as predators or prey and reptiles may attack other pets.

18.2.4 Human Interactions

Human company is not a need for reptiles, and there is no convincing evidence that reptiles enjoy human presence or contact. Some well-handled reptiles may tolerate human presence or approach humans for rewards such as food or warmth. However, many reptiles appear to perceive humans as predators and find interactions stressful. Handling can also damage the fragile skin of lizards such as chameleons and geckos or any reptile during shedding. Handling reptiles outside their vivarium can also remove them from UV sources and reduce their body temperature, which can cause an immunosuppressive response (e.g. desert iguanas [*Dipsosaurus dorsalis*], Evans and Cowles 1959). Generally, pet reptiles should be handled minimally and only when necessary for health checks, management, or getting them used to humans.

When reptiles are handled, they should be gently supported. For large snakes this may involve use of the handler's body or even two people. For safety reasons, it may be necessary to control the head, legs, or tail, but reptiles should not be held by these alone. Some reptiles may also prefer to have something underfoot (e.g. tortoises), to walk or wriggle from one hand to another or rest on a hand, or to wrap around the handler. Handlers should ensure their bodies do not smell of or move like prey (e.g. rapidly or partially hidden). Other reptiles may show more passive reactions to handling, such as 'playing dead' (e.g. many chameleons), coiling up into a 'ball' (e.g. ball pythons;

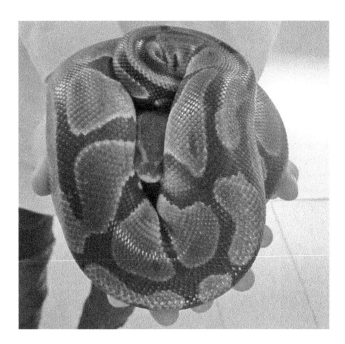

Figure 18.6   Ball python curling into a ball. (*Source:* Courtesy Kevin Eatwell).

Figure 18.6) or retracting into their shell (e.g. chelonians). Owners therefore cannot use ease of handling as a trustworthy indicator of stress. Some reptiles may perform bluff or sham bites with a closed mouth.

Fearful reptiles may attempt to escape by rolling or thrash around, trying to climb higher (e.g. onto the handler's head), dropping to the ground, wrapping more tightly (e.g. many snakes), or shedding part of their tail. Some reptiles may threaten using sham strikes or by making themselves look bigger (e.g. frilled lizards; Figure 18.7). As a last resort, reptiles may show aggression such as tail strikes, biting, or defensively spraying urine, faeces, or musk. Some reptiles can cause serious injuries (e.g. marine turtles and crocodilians), envenomation (e.g. venomous snakes or Komodo dragon saliva; Fry et al. 2006, 2009), or infections (e.g. monitor lizards and iguana). Human-directed aggression may also be the result of pain, seasonal hormonal changes, or poor environments (Varga 2004). Aggression may be reduced by decreasing sunlight or temperatures, but these methods fail to address the underlying fear or pain and, arguably, a need to routinely down-regulate animals' metabolism to allow handling suggests they are not suitable as pets.

Gentle handling, especially of young animals, can be used to habituate animals to handling and to particular procedures. Reptiles may be trained to go to particular places, enter tubes or other apparatus for handling, to follow a target or scent, or to approach a person on command (e.g. green sea turtle, [*Chelonia mydas*], Streeter and Floyd 1998) and clicker-trained (e.g. Aldabra tortoises [*Geochelone gigantean*], Weiss and Wilson 2003; Caiman lizards [*Dracaena guianensis*], Hellmuth et al. 2012). Reptiles may learn to associate certain events or actions with food rewards (e.g. elapids, Loaring

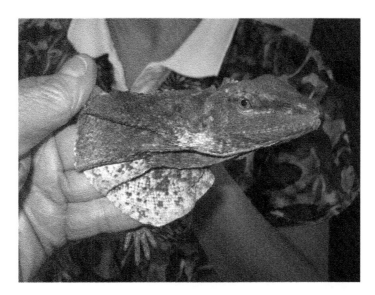

Figure 18.7 Frilled lizard (*Chlamydosaurus kingie*). (*Source:* Courtesy R Johnson).

and Trim 2012), although predators may learn to associate humans with food. They may also associate other provisions as rewards, including water for bathing (e.g. indigo snakes [*Drymarchon couperi*], Kleinginna 1970).

18.2.5 Health

Some diseases are common to many reptile species, including those caused by viruses (e.g. herpesviruses, iridoviruses, paramyxoviruses, and poxviruses); bacteria (e.g. abscesses, blister disease, septic arthritis, and stomatitis); fungi (especially in aquatic species); protozoa (e.g. *Entamoeba*, flagellates, ciliates, and coccidia); worms (e.g. nematodes, hookworms, tapeworms, and tongueworms) and mites (Figure 18.8) such as *O. natricis*. Several infections are zoonotic, including *Escherichia coli*, *Pseudomonas*, several tick-borne ricketsiall diseases, and pentastomid parasites. Salmonella is normally present in many healthy reptiles and may be found on their bodies and in their environments and presents a specific risk for humans with insufficient immunity (Barten 1993).

Retained skin from incomplete shedding ('dysecdysis') may result in restricted blood supply to the limb, leading to necrosis or infection. Posthibernation anorexia may be a result of poor management or disease. Reptiles may also suffer from reproductive problems such as egg retention, and some species should be neutered to avoid welfare problems during reproduction. There is limited evidence of widespread inherited disorders resulting from breeding, although there is an increasing suspicion of some neurological problems associated with a 'spider' colouring pattern in ball pythons (Rose and Williams 2014).

There are effectively no vaccinations available for pet reptiles. Nevertheless, disease risks can be reduced by selecting uninfected breeding animals and by housing animals singly or in small, closed, single-species groups. Owners should avoid accumulating large numbers of animals, especially mixed-species groups. If an owner keeps multiple

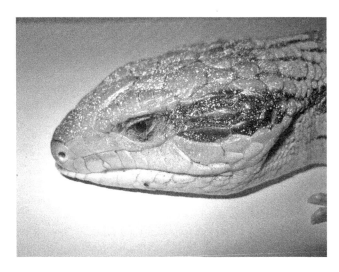

Figure 18.8   Eastern blue tongued skink (*Tiliqua scincoides*) with heavy *Ophionyssus natricis* mite infestation. (*Source:* Courtesy R Johnson).

Table 18.3   Examples of veterinary specialisations specifically relevant for reptiles kept as companion animals (see also Chapter 1).

Recognising organisation	Example veterinary specialties
American Veterinary Medical Association	American Board of Veterinary Practitioners in Reptile and Amphibian Practice
European Board of Veterinary Specialisation	European College of Zoological Medicine (Herpetology)
Australian and New Zealand College of Veterinary Scientists	Australian and New Zealand College of Veterinary Scientists: Zoo and Wildlife Medicine Chapter
Royal College of Veterinary Surgeons	RCVS Specialists in Zoological Medicine (Reptilan)

animals, then each species, and where appropriate, individuals, should be kept sufficiently isolated to avoid disease transmission. Owners should employ adequate quarantine and barrier hygiene methods. New animals should be routinely screened (e.g. viral and parasite screening of faeces; polymerase chain reaction (PCR) screening of blood or oesophagus; serology for paramyxoviruses) and quarantined.

The critical determinant for good health is avoiding bad husbandry. In particular, immune function can be reduced by malnutrition and overly low temperatures (Guillette et al. 1995). All reptiles should be checked by a veterinary surgeon, from specialist veterinary surgeons where possible and available (Table 18.3) and undergo species-appropriate sampling for both testing and to establish basal values for the animal, at least annually. Reptiles should be presented before diseases become chronic, so owners need to monitor for subtle signs of disease and slowly progressing conditions. Owners also should follow sensible hygiene precautions regarding even healthy animals, although this cannot eliminate human health risks, and young children, pregnant women, elderly, or frail adults and other immunosuppressed people should avoid or minimise all contact with reptiles.

18.2.6 Euthanasia

The euthanasia of reptiles can be challenging and should involve two stages (Table 18.4). The first stage is to cause unconsciousness. The best method for this is often sedation if necessary, followed by an injection of an overdose of pentobarbitone (or, in some cases, tricaine methanesulfonate) into a vein or head trauma in some reptiles (e.g. shooting in large crocodilians). Particular issues for reptiles include access for injections, especially in reptiles with a shell and reptiles' slow metabolic rates and high tolerance of hypoxia (e.g. in aquatic species). Many are able to survive on only anaerobic metabolism, holding their breath and slowing their heart to virtually undetectable rates. These factors make inhaled anaesthesics, hypothermia (e.g. freezing large reptiles or species that can tolerate subzero temperatures), and decapitation unacceptably slow. These factors can also make it challenging to confirm death in reptiles without specialist equipment such as Doppler probes. Consequently, the second stage of euthanasia is to ensure death by destroying the brain by crushing or 'pithing'. Fertilised eggs should also be destroyed completely and instantaneously or injected with an anaesthetic overdose.

18.3 Signs of Reptile Welfare

18.3.1 Pathophysiological Signs

Signs of disease, poor growth, or reproduction can be general indicators of extremely bad welfare. Stress may reduce immune function or affect healing (e.g. tree lizards [*Urosaurus ornatus*], French et al. 2006), and many health problems are the result of management. For example, poor shedding may suggest inappropriate husbandry, malnutrition, dehydration, pathology, or hormonal imbalances (Avery 1994), and stress may reduce mating behaviour in garter snakes (Moore and Mason 2001). However, the absence of such changes is not an indicator of acceptable welfare. In some species, colour changes can also indicate stress or other physiological processes (e.g. green anoles [*Anole carolensis*], Plavicki et al. 2004). Elevated cardiac activity may also indicate

Table 18.4 Methods of euthanasia for (some) reptiles kept as companion animals.

Method	Restraint required	Welfare benefits	Welfare risks
Injection of anaesthetic into a vein, followed by brain destruction	Secure handling (or anaesthesia)	Rapid loss of consciousness	Pain from injection
Instantaneous destruction of brain tissue	Secure handling (or anaesthesia)	Immediate loss of consciousness	Severe pain if done inaccurately

Source: AVMA (2013).

distress (e.g. turtles, Cabanac and Bernieri 2000). Changes in levels of catecholamines or reproductive hormone might also suggest stress but may vary seasonally (Mahmoud et al. 1989; Hamann et al. 2003). Corticosteroid levels may indicate 'stress' in chelonians, squamatans, and crocodilians (Table 18.5), although levels may not change during stress (Warwick et al. 2013).

18.3.2 Behavioural Signs

Identifying signs of suffering can be difficult because many are quite subtle and owners may be quite poor at perceiving them. Owners are also unable to pick up most subtle chemical cues (as opposed to visible cues) that reptiles use for communication. Nevertheless, useful information about reptiles' welfare can be gained from observing how they share their time between eating, thermoregulatory behaviour, UV-B basking, energy-conserving behaviours, and energy-expending activities such as reproduction and exploration. For example, a reduced appetite can suggest disease, low ambient temperatures, unsuitable food content or presentation, skin shedding, inappropriate substrate, social stress, overhandling or poorly managed hibernation; or also normal responses (e.g. of many male snakes during the breeding season). Inactivity may represent disease, low ambient temperatures, insufficient food intake, stress, or dormancy. Owners may inaccurately attribute inactivity as contentment, in particular some may interpret a posture of eyes closed and head and limbs extended as 'contentment'.

Particular behaviours may indicate particular problems such as fear or pain (Table 18.6), although many can occur in a range of other contexts (e.g. food regurgitation during diseases and apparent aggressive behaviours during courtship). Behavioural stereotypies have been recorded in reptiles (e.g. Burghardt et al. 1996; Case et al. 2005), although there is limited understanding of their causes and significance. While reptiles do not regulate their body temperature as mammals and birds do (as a physiological measure), their thermoregulatory behaviour can indicate welfare problems. Seeking out

Table 18.5 Examples of corticosteroid assessment in reptiles.

Example Species		References
Snakes and lizards	Brown treesnakes (*Boiga irregularis*)	Mathies et al. (2001)
	Tree lizards (*Urosaurus ornatus*)	Moore et al. (1991)
	Skinks (*Egernia whitii*)	Jones and Bell (2004)
	Western fence lizards (*Sceloporus occidentalis*)	Dunlap and Wingfield (1995)
Chelonians	Loggerhead sea turtles (*Caretta caretta*)	Gregory et al. (1996)
	Hawksbill turtles (*Eretmochelys imbricate*)	Jessop et al. (2004)
	Red-eared slider turtles (*Trachemys scripta elegans*)	Cash et al. (1997)
Crocodilians	American alligators (*Alligator mississipiensis*)	Lance and Lauren (1984)
	Caimans, *Caiman crocodiles*	Gist and Kaplan (1976)

Table 18.6 Key behavioural signs of possible welfare compromises in reptiles.

Aspect of behaviour	Specific Responses
Increased activity or responsiveness	Agitation
	General hypersensitivity
	Increased vigilance
	Elevated stance
	Attention to particular threats
	Reaction on palpation
	Withdrawal of body part from contact
Avoidance	Hiding
	Immobility
	Coiling, shell retraction
	Playing dead
Looking bigger or threats	Turning side on
	Dewlap extension
	Colour changes
	Displaying throat colours
	Head bobbing
	Doing push-ups
	Waving
	Open-mouthed threats
	Tongue flicking
	Tail whipping
Alarm or distress signals	Barking (e.g. some geckos)
Escape	Wriggling, writhing, or rolling during handling
	Flight (jumping, running, slithering)
	Tail 'drop'
Passive defence	U-shaped posture with abdomen protected between head and tail presented as weapons
Preattack behaviours	Hissing (e.g. snakes)
	'Sighing' (e.g. iguanas)
	'Symbolic' bites
	Elevated head, ready to strike
Attack	Food regurgitation (e.g. some snakes)
	Musk spraying
	Spraying urine or faeces
	Tail strikes
	Biting
Altered metabolic processes	Reduced appetite
	Increased drinking or urination
	Immobility, lethargy
	Closed or partly closed eyes
	Increased respiratory rate

Table 18.6   (Continued)

Aspect of behaviour	Specific Responses
Specific signs of local pain	Hunched posture
	Tucked up abdomen
	Raised, extended head
	Biting a specific area
	Scratching a specific area
	Flicking a foot at specific area
	Lameness
	Holding part of length uncoiled
Other signs of pain	Darkening colour
	Excessive swallowing

Source: Bennett (1998), Bradley Bays et al. (2006), Chiszar et al. (1980, 1995), Girling and Raiti (2004), Hernandex-Divers (2001), Kreger and Mench (1993), Lance (1990, 1992), Moore and Mason (2001), Mooreet al. (2000), Mosley (2009), (2011), Read (2004), Rossi (2006), Varga (2004), Warwick (1990a, 1990b), Warwick et al. (1995/2004), (2013).

higher temperatures may indicate overly low ambient temperatures, infections (e.g. *Agama agama*, Ramos et al. 1993) or more general distress (e.g. *Clemmys insculpta*, Cabanac and Bernieri 2000), and seeking out low temperature areas may also be a general indicator of welfare problems (Warwick 1990b). Spending time in a water bowl may be usual or indicate high ambient temperatures, low humidity, or parasite infections (Mayer and Bradley Bays 2006).

18.4 Action Plan for Improving Reptile Welfare Worldwide

Priorities for reptile care include nutrition, lighting, and space. Many reptiles are kept indoors and in climates different from those of their native countries, particularly in terms of UV-B, temperature and relative humidity. Keeping reptiles in vivaria allows owners to control these environments, while limiting the reptiles' abilities to do so. Owners, therefore, have both the opportunity to ensure environments are correct and the responsibility to do so. There remains a perception amongst some owners that reptiles need minimal space and environmental enrichment. These attitudes need to change, and scientific research can help this. However, in the absence of scientific research, reptiles should be given the benefit of the doubt; for example, it is a reasonable assumption that all animals should be able to extend to their full length, even if they spend a lot of time curled up. The burden of proof should be on showing that they do not suffer when their environments are restricted or impoverished. Similarly, care is needed to reduce to a minimum the practice of live feeding of vertebrates or other animals thought to be sentient and any consequent suffering, either through generic welfare laws or through specific codes of practice.

Keepers and sellers should also ensure that reptiles are kept only by competent owners and only for the right reasons. Governments and vendors should limit the importation, trade, and ownership by the public to those reptile species that are able and likely to be kept safely and according to good practice. Owners should avoid deliberately choosing 'exotic', less common, or challenging species. Some of these may be dangerous or difficult to keep in a state of good welfare, and there is likely to be limited knowledge and experience within the public or reptile keeping community at large about them. Reptiles of such species may be more likely to come from wild-caught stock or be inbred (because there are not sufficient numbers for large-scale captive-breeding programmes). Hobby breeders who deliberately breed less-common or easy species should take extra care to ensure that all the offspring are taken by owners who can care for them. For any species, it is important to prevent deliberate or accidental release into the environment as escapees can be invasive non-native species or may pose a risk of spreading disease into existing wild populations.

Finally, research on reptiles is limited, compared to that on mammals and birds (Bonnet et al. 2002). There is a need for more high-quality research on reptile welfare and for the findings to be disseminated to owners and policy makers. Research is needed to identify species' capabilities, needs, and how to assess their welfare. Any barriers to such research, such as funding constraints or priorities, need to be addressed to keep pace with increases in the popularity of keeping particular species and reptiles in general. This should ensure that policies and ownership practices are based on robust scientific findings wherever possible.

Bibliography

Alberts, A.C., Jackintell, L.A., and Phillips, J.A. (1994). Effects of chemical and visual exposure to adults on growth hormones and behavior of juvenile green iguanas. *Physiology and Behaviour* 55: 987–992.

Allen, M.E. and Oftedal, O.T. (1994). The nutrition of carnivorous reptiles. In: *Captive Management and Conservation of Amphibians and Reptiles* (ed. J.B. Murphy, K. Adler, J.T. Collins and J.B. Murphy), 71–82. Ithaca, USA: Society for the Study of Reptiles and Amphibians.

Almli, L.M. and Burghardt, G.M. (2006). Environmental enrichment alters the behavioral profile of ratsnakes (Elaphe). *Journal of Applied Animal Welfare Science* 9: 85–109.

Avery, R.A. (1994). The effects of termperature on captive amphibians and reptiles. In: *Captive Management and Conservation of Amphibians and Reptiles* (ed. J.B. Murphy, K. Adler and J.T. Collins), 47–51. Ithaca, NY, USA: Society for the Study of Amphibians and Reptiles.

AVMA (American Veterinary Medical Association). (2013). AVMA Guidelines for the Euthanasia of Animals: 2013 Edition. Available at https://www.avma.org/KB/Policies/Pages/Euthanasia-Guidelines.aspx. Accessed 7 October 2015.

Barten, S. (1993). The medical care of iguanas and other common pet lizards. *Veterinary Clinics of North America: Small Animal Practice* 23: 1213–1249.

Bennett, R.A. (1998). Pain and analgesia in reptiles and amphibians. Proc. Assoc. Rept. Amphib. Vet., Kansas City, pp. 1–5

Bonnet, X., Shine, R., and Lourdais, O. (2002). Taxonomic chauvinism. *Trends in Ecology & Evolution* 17 (1): 1–3.

Bradley Bays, T., Lightfoot, T., and Mayer, J. (2006). *Exotic Pet Behaviour*. UK: Saunders.

Burghardt, G.M. (1977). Of iguanas and dinosaurs: social behavior and communication in neonate reptiles. *American Zoologist* 17: 177–190.

Burghardt, G.M. (1998). The evolutionary origins of play revisited. Lessons from turtles. In: *Animal Play: Evolutionary, Comparative and Ecological Perspectives* (ed. M. Bekoff and J.A. Byers), 1–26. New York, NY: Cambridge University Press.

Burghardt, G.M. (2013). Environmental enrichment and cognitive complexity in reptiles and amphibians: concepts, review, and implications for captive populations. *Applied Animal Behaviour Science* 147 (2013): 286–298.

Burghardt, G.M., Greene, H.W., and Rand, A.S. (1977). Social behavior in hatchling green iguanas: life at a reptile rookery. *Science* 195: 689–691.

Burghardt, G.M., Ward, B., and Rosscoe, R. (1996). 1996 Problem of reptile play: environmental enrichment and play behavior in a captive Nile soft-shelled turtle, Trionyx triunguis. *Zoo Biology* 15: 223–238.

Butler, J.A., Hull, T.W., and Franz, R. (1995). Neonate aggregations and maternal attendance of young in the eastern diamondback rattlesnake, *Crotalus adamanteus*. *Copeia* 1: 196–198.

BVZS (2003). *Guidelines for Acceptable Methods of Euthanasia for Zoo, Exotic, Pet and Wildlife Species 1: Reptiles*. London, UK: BVZS.

Cabanac, M. and Bernieri, C. (2000). Behavioral rise in body temperature and tachycardia by handling of a turtle (Clemmys insculpta). *Behavioural Processes* 49 (2): 61–68.

Calvert, I. (2004). Nutrition. In: *BSAVA Manual of Reptiles* (ed. S.J. Girling and P. Raiti), 18–39. Gloucester, UK: BSAVA.

Carmel, B. and Johnson, R. (2014). *A Guide to Health and Disease in Reptiles and Amphibians*. Burleigh, Qld: Reptile Publications.

Case, B. C. (2003) Environmental Enrichment for Captive Eastern Box Turtles (Terrapene carolina carolina). A thesis submitted to the Graduate Faculty of North Carolina State University in partial fulfillment of the requirements for the Degree of Master of Science

Case, B.C., Lewbart, G.A., and Doerr, P.D. (2005). The physiological and behavioural impacts of and preference for an enriched environment in the eastern box turtle (Terrapene carolina carolina). *Applied Animal Behaviour Science* 92: 353–365.

Cash, W.B., Holberton, R.L., and Knight, S.S. (1997). Corticosterone secretion in response to capture and handling in free-living red-eared slider turtles. *General and Comparative Endocrinology* 108: 427–433.

Chapple, D.G. (2003). Ecology, life-history and behavior in the Australian scincid genus Egernia, with comments on the evolution of complex sociality in lizards. *Herpetological Monographs* 17: 145–180.

Chiszar, D., Wellborn, S., Wand, M.A. et al. (1980). Investigatory behaviour in snakes II. Cage cleaning and the induction of defecation in snakes. *Animal Learning and Behaviour* 8: 505–510.

Chiszar, D., Murphy, J.B., and Radcliffe, C.W. (1995). Behavioural consequences of husbandry manipulations: indicators of arousal, quiescence and environmental awareness. In: *Health and Welfare of Captive Reptiles* (ed. C. Warwick, F.L. Frye, J.B. Murphy, et al.), 186–204. London, UK: Chapman and Hall.

Clark, R.W., Brown, W.S., Stechert, R., and Greene, H.W. (2012). Cryptic sociality in rattlesnakes (*Crotalus horridus*) detected by kinship analysis. *Biology Letters* 8: 523–525.

Cooper, J.E. and Williams, D.L. (2014). The feeding of live food to exotic pets: issues of welfare and ethics. *Journal of Exotic Pet Medicine* 23: 244–249.

Cooper, J.E., Ewbank, R., Platt, C., and Warwick, C. (1989). Euthanasia of amphibians and reptiles, Universities Federation for Animal Welfare/World Society for the Protection of AnimalsCooper, J. E. & Williams, D. L. 2014 the feeding of live food to exotic pets: issues of welfare and ethics. *Journal of Exotic Pet Medicine* 23: 244–249.

Davis, A.R. (2011). Kin presence drives philopatry and social aggregation in juvenile Desert Night Lizards (*Xantusia vigilis*). *Behavioral Ecology* 23 (1): 18–24.

Davis, K.M. and Burghardt, G.M. (2011). Turtles (Pseudemys nelsoni) learn about visual cues indicating food from experienced turtles. *Journal of Comparative Psychology* 125: 404–410.

De Vosjoli, P. (1999). Designing environments for captive amphibians and reptiles. *The Veterinary Clinics of North America. Exotic Animal Practice* 2: 43–68.

Dinets, V. (2015). Apparent coordination and collaboration in cooperatively hunting crocodilians. *Ethology Ecology and Evolution* 27 (2): 244–250.

Dinets, V., Brueggen, J.C., and Brueggen, J.D. (2015 Jan 2). Crocodilians use tools for hunting. *Ethology Ecology and Evolution* 27 (1): 74–78.

Divers, S.J. (1996). Basic reptile husbandry, history taking and clinical examination. *In Practice* 18: 51–65.

Donoghue, S. (1996). Veterinary nutritional management of amphibians and reptiles. *Journal of the American Veterinary Medical Association* 208 (11): 1816–1820.

Donoghue, S. (1998). Nutrition of pet amphibians and reptiles. *Seminars in Avian and Exotic Pet Medicine* 7 (3): 148–153.

Doody, J.S., Freedberg, S., and Keogh, J.S. (2009). Communal egg-laying in reptiles and amphibians: evolutionary patterns and hypotheses. *The Quarterly Review of Biology* 84: 229–252.

Doody, J.S., Burghardt, G.M., and Dinets, V. (2013 Feb 1). Breaking the social–non-social dichotomy: a role for reptiles in vertebrate social behavior research? *Ethology* 119 (2): 95–103.

Dunlap, K.D. and Wingfield, J.C. (1995). External and internal influences on indices of physiological stress: seasonal and population variation in adrenocortical secretion of free-living lizards, *Sceloporus occidentalis*. *Journal of Experimental Zoology* 271: 36–46.

Eatwell, K. (2010). Options for analgesia and anaesthesia in reptiles. *In Practice* 32: 306–311.

ENDCAP (2012). *Wild Pets in the European Union*. Available at: http://endcap.eu/wp-content/uploads/2013/02/Report-Wild-Pets-in-the-European-Union.pdf. Accessed 6 June 2018.

Evans, E.E. and Cowles, R.B. (1959). Effect of temperature on antibody synthesis in the reptile, *Dipsosaurus dorsalis*. *Proceedings of the Society for Experimental Biology and Medicine* 101 (3): 482–483.

Ferguson, G.W., Gehrmann, W.H., Karsten, K.B. et al. (2003). Do panther chameleons bask to regulate endogenous vitamin D_3 production? *Physiological and Biochemical Zoology* 76 (1): 52–59.

Flores, D., Tousignant, A., and Crews, D. (1994). Incubation temperature affects the behaviour of adult leopard geckos (*Eublepharus macularis*). *Physiology and Behaviour* 55 (6): 1067–1072.

French, S.S., Matt, K.S., and Moore, M.C. (2006). The effects of stress on wound healing in male tree lizards (*Urosaurus ornatus*). *General and Comparative Endocrinology* 145: 128–132.

Fry, B.G., Vidal, N., Norman, J.A. et al. (2006). Early evolution of the venom system in lizards and snakes. *Nature* 439: 584–588.

Fry, B.G., Wroe, S., Teeuwisse, W. (2009). A central role for venom in predation by Varanus komodoensis (Komodo Dragon) and the extinct giant Varanus (Megalania) priscus. *Proceedings of the National Academy of Sciences* 106(22): 8969–8974. doi: 10.1073/pnas.0810883106.

Gardner, M.G., Bull, C.M., Cooper, S.J.B., and Duffield, G.A. (2001). Genetic evidence for a family structure in stable social aggregations of the Australian lizard *Egernia stokesii*. *Molecular Ecology* 10: 175–183.

Giles, J.C., Davis, J.A., McCauley, R.D., and Kuchling, G. (2009). Voice of the turtle: the underwater acoustic repertoire of the long-necked freshwater turtle, *Chelodina oblonga*. *Journal of the Acoustical Society of America* 126: 434–443.

Girling, S.J. and Raiti, P. (eds.) (2004). *BSAVA Manual of Reptiles*. Gloucester, UK: BSAVA.

Gist, D.H. and Kaplan, M.L. (1976). Effects of stress and ACTH on plasma corticosterone levels in the caiman *Caiman crocodilus*. *General and Comparative Endocrinology* 28: 413–419.

Gregory, L.F., Gross, T.S., Bolten, A.B. et al. (1996). Plasma corticosterone concentrations associated with acute captivity stress in wild loggerhead sea turtles (*Caretta caretta*). *General and Comparative Endocrinology* 104: 312–320.

Guillette, L.J., Cree, A., and Rooney, A.A. (1995). Biology of stress: interactions with reproduction, immunology and intermediary etabolism. In: *Health and Welfare of Captive Reptiles* (ed. C. Warwick, F.L. Frye and J.B. Murphy), 32–81. London, UK: Chapman and Halls.

Hamann, M., Limpus, C.J., and Whittier, J.M. (2003). Seasonal variation in plasma catecholamines and adipose tissue lipolysis in adult female green sea turtles (*Cheloniamydas*). *General and Comparative Endocrinology* 130: 308–316.

Hellmuth, H., Augustine, L., Watkins, B., and Hope, K. (2012). Using operant conditioning and desensitization to facilitate veterinary care with captive reptiles. *Veterinary Clinics of North America: Exotic Animals* 15: 425–443.

Hernandex-Divers, S.J. (2001). Clinical aspects of reptile behavior. *Veterinry Clinics of North America: Exotic Animal Practice* 4: 599–612.

Hyndman, T.H., Shilton, C.M., and Marschang, R.E. (2013). Paramyxoviruses in reptiles: a review. *Veterinary Microbiology* 165: 200–213.

IUCN. (2016). *The IUCN Red List of Threatened Species*. Available at https://www.iucn.org/theme/species/our-work/iucn-red-list-threatened-species. Accessed 22 August 2016.

Jacobson, E.R., Morris, P., Norton, T.M., and Wright, K. (2001). Quarantine. *Journal of Herpetological Medicine and Surgery* 11: 24–30.

Jessop, T.S., Sumner, J.M., Limpus, C.J., and Whittier, J.M. (2004). Interplay between plasma hormone profiles, sex and body condition in immature hawksbill turtles (*Eretmochelys imbricata*) subjected to a capture stress protocol. *Comparative Biochemistry and Physiology. Part A* 137: 197–204.

Jones, S.M. and Bell, K. (2004). Plasma corticosterone concentrations in males of the skink Egernia whitii during acute and chronic confinement, and over a diel period. *Comparative Biochemistry and Physiology* 137: 105–113.

Keeble, E. (2004). Neurology. In: *BSAVA Manual of Reptiles* (ed. S.J. Girling and P. Raiti), 273–289. Gloucester, UK: BSAVA.

Kleinginna, P. (1970). Operant conditioning of the indigo snake. *Psychonomic Science* 18: 53–55.

Kramer, M. and Burghardt, G.M. (1998). Precocious courtship and play in emydid turtles. *Ethology* 104: 38–56.

Kreger, M.D. and Mench, J.A. (1993). Physiological and behavioural effects of handling in the ball python (*Python regius*) and the blue-tongues skink (*Tiliqua scincoides*). *Applied Animal Behaviour Science* 38: 323–336.

Laidlaw, R. (2005). *Scales and tails. The welfare and trade of reptiles kept as pets in Canada*. New York, NY: World Society for the Protection of Animals.

Lance, V.A. (1990). Stress in reptiles. In: Progress in comparative endocrinology. Proceedings of the eleventh international symposium on comparative endocrinology. A. Epple, C.G. Scanes and M.H. Stetson, editors. New York, NY. Pp. 461–466

Lance, V.A. (1992). Evaluating pain and stress in reptiles. In: *The Care and Use of Amphibians, Reptiles and Fish in Research* (ed. D.O. Schaeffer, K.M. Klienow and L. Krulisch), 101–106. Bethesda MD: Scientists Center for Animal Welfare.

Lance, V.A. and Lauren, D. (1984). Circadian variation in plasma corticosterone in the American alligator, *Alligator mississippiensis*, and the effects of ACTH injections. *General and Comparative Endocrinology* 54: 1–7.

Lanham, E.J. and Bull, C.M. (2004). Enhanced vigilance in groups in Egernia stokesii, a lizard with stable social aggregations. *Journal of Zoology* 263: 95–99.

Loaring, C. and Trim, S. (2012). Refining laboratory husbandry of venomous snakes of the family Elapidae. *Animal Technology and Welfare* 11 (3): 157–164.

Locke, B. (2008). Venomous snake restraint and handling. *Journal of Exotic Pet Medicine* 17: 273–284.

Mader, D.R. (2006). *Reptile Medicine and Surgery*. St Louis, MS: Saunders Elsevier.

Mahmoud, I.Y., Guillette, L.J. Jr., McAsey, M.E., and Cady, C. (1989). Stress-induced changes in serum testosterone, estradiol-17B and progesterone in the turtle *Chelydra serpentina*. *Comparative Biochemistry and Physiology* 93: 423–427.

Mason, R.T. and Rockwell Parker, M. (2010). Social behavior and pheromonal communication in reptiles. *Journal of Comparative Physiology. A* 196: 729–749.

Mathies, T., Felix, T.A., and Lance, V.A. (2001). Effects of trapping and subsequent short-term confinement stress on plasma corticosterone in the brown treesnake (Boiga irregularis) on Guam. *General and Comparative Endocrinology* 124: 106–114.

Mayer, J. and Bays, T.B. (2006). Reptile behavior. In: *Exotic Pet Behavior: Birds, Reptiles, and Small Mammals* (ed. T.B. Bays, T. Lightfoot and J. Mayer), 103–162. St. Louis, MO: Elsevier.

McAlpin, S., Duckett, P., and Stow, A. (2011). Lizards cooperatively tunnel to construct a long-term home for family members. *PLoS One* 6 (5): e19041.

Moore, I.T. and Jessop, T.S. (2003). Stress, reproduction, and adrenocortical modulation in amphibians and reptiles. *Hormones and Behavior* 43: 39–47.

Moore, I.R. and Mason, R.T. (2001). Behavioral and hormonal responses to corticosterone in the male red slider garter snake. Thamnophis sirtalis parietalis. *Physiology and Behavior* 72 (5): 669–674.

Moore, M.C., Whittier, J.M., and Crews, D. (1985). Sex steroid hormones during the ovarian cycle of an all-female, parthenogenetic lizard and their correlation with pseudosexual behavior. *General and Comparative Endocrinology* 60 (2): 144–153.

Moore, M.C., Thompson, C.W., and Marler, C.A. (1991). Reciprocal changes in corticosterone and testosterone levels following acute and chronic handling stress in the tree lizard, *Urosaurus ornatus*. *General and Comparative Endocrinology* 81: 217–226.

Moore, I.T., LeMaster, M.P., and Mason, R.T. (2000). Behavioral and hormonal responses to capture stress in the male red-sided garter snake, *Thamnophis sirtalis parietalis*. *Animal Behaviour* 59: 529–534.

Mosley, C. (2009). Clinical approaches to analgesia in reptiles. In: *Handbook of Veterinary Pain Management*, 2e (ed. J.S. Gaynor and W.W. Muir), 481–493. Missouri: Mosby, Elsevier.

Mosley, C. (2011). Pain and nociception in reptiles. *The Veterinary Clinics of North America. Exotic Animal Practice* 14 (1): 45–60.

O'Connor, D. and Shine, R. (2003). Lizards in "nuclear families": a novel reptilian social system in *Egernia saxatilis* (Scincidae). *Molecular Ecology* 12 (3): 743–752.

Pasmans, F., Blahak, S., Martel, A., and Pantchev, N. (2008). Introducing reptiles into a captive collection: the role of the veterinarian. *The Veterinary Journal* 175: 53–68.

PFMA (Pet Food Manufacturers Association). (2014). Pet Population Statistics. Available from http://www.pfma.org.uk/pet-population-2014/. Accessed 27 November 2014.

Plavicki, J., Yang, E.J., and Wilczynski, W. (2004). Dominance status predicts response to non-social forced movement stress in green anole lizard (*Anole carolinensis*). *Physiology and Behavior* 80: 547–555.

Praud, A. and Moutou, F. (2010). *Health Risks from New Companion Animals*. Brussels, Belgium: Eurogroup for Animals.

Rabosky, A.R., Corl, A., Liwanag, H.E. et al. (2012). Direct fitness correlates and thermal consequences of facultative aggregation in a desert lizard. *PLoS One* 7 (7): e40866.

Ramos, A.B., Don, M.T., and Muchlinski, A.W. (1993). The effect of bacteria ingestion on mean selected body temperature in the common agama, *Agama agama*: a dose-dependent study. *Comparative Biochemistry and Physiology. A* 105: 479–484.

Read, M.R. (2004). Evaluation of the use of anaesthesia and analgesia in reptiles. *Journal of the American Veterinary Medical Association* 224 (4): 547–552.

Rose, M.P. and Williams, D.L. (2014). Neurological dysfunction in a ball python (*Python regius*) colour morph and implications for welfare. *Journal of Exotic Pet Medicine* 23: 234–239.

Rossi, J.V. (2006). General husbandry and management. In: *BSAVA Manual of Reptiles* (ed. S.J. Girling and P. Raiti), 25–41. Gloucester: BSAVA.

Streeter, K. and Floyd, S. (1999). Exploring operant conditioning in a green sea turtle. In: Kalb, H., Wibbels, T. (eds) *Proceedings of the 19th annual symposium on sea turtle conservation and biology*. NOAA Tech Memo NMFS-SEFSC-443, Pp. 8–10.

Tattersall, G.J., Milsom, W.K., Abe, A.S. et al. (2004). The thermogenesis of digestion in rattlesnakes. *Journal of Experimental Biology* 207 (4): 579–585.

Therrien, C.L., Gaster, L., Cunningham-Smith, P., and Manire, C.A. (2007). Experimental evaluation of environmental enrichment of sea turtles. *Zoo Biology* 26: 407–416.

UNEP/WCMC. (2009). Wildlife Trade 2009. Available at http://ec.europa.eu/environment/cites/pdf/2009_yearbook.pdf. Accessed 7 June 2018.

Van Marken Lichtenbelt, W.D., Wesselingh, R.A., Vogel, J.T., and Albers, K.B. (1993). Energy budgets in free-living green iguanas in a seasonal environment. *Ecology* 74: 1157–1172.

Varga, M. (2004). Captive maintenance and welfare. In: *BSAVA Manual of Reptiles* (ed. S.J. Girling and P. Raiti), 6–17. Gloucester, UK: BSAVA.

Warwick, C. (1990a). Important ethological and other considerations of the study and maintenance of reptiles in captivity. *Applied Animal Behaviour Science* 27: 363–366.

Warwick, C. (1990b). Reptilian ethology in captivity: observations of some problems and an evaluation of their aetiology. *Applied Animal Behaviour Science* 26: 1–13.

Warwick, C., Frye, F.L., and Murphy, J.B. (eds.) (1995/2004). *Health and Welfare of Captive Reptiles*. London and New York: Chapman & Hall/Kluwer.

Warwick, C., Arena, P.C., Steedman, C., and Jessop, M. (2012). A review of captive exotic animal-linked zoonoses. *Journal of Environmental Health Research* 12: 9–24. http://www.cieh.org/jehr/default.aspx?id=41594.

Warwick, C., Arena, P., Lindley, S. et al. (2013). Assessing reptile welfare using behavioural criteria. *In Practice* 35: 123–131.

Wiesner, C.S. and Iben, C. (2003). Influence of environmental humidity and dietary protein on pyramidal growth of carapaces in African spurred tortoises (*Geochelone sulcata*). *Journal of Animal Physiology and Animal Nutrition* 87 (1–2): 66–74.

Weiss, E. and Wilson, S. (2003). The use of classical and operant conditioning in training Aldabra tortoises (Geochelone gigantea) for venipuncture and other husbandry issues. *Journal of Applied Animal Welfare Science* 6 (1): 33–38.

Wildlife, P. (2001). *Morbidity and Mortality in Private Husbandry of Reptiles*. RSPCA: Horsham, UK.

Wilkinson, A., Mandl, I., Bugnyar, T., and Huber, L. (2010a). Gaze following in the red-footed tortoise (Geochelone carbonaria). *Animal Cognition* 13: 765–769.

Wilkinson, A., Kuenstner, K., Mueller, J., and Huber, L. (2010b). Social learning in a non-social reptile (Geochelone carbonaria). *Biology Letters* 6: 614–616.

Central Bearded Dragons (*Pogona vitticeps*)

19

Robert Johnson and Sophie Adwick

19.1 History and Context

19.1.1 Natural History

Central or inland bearded dragons (*Pogona vitticeps*) are agamid members of the class Reptilia, order Squamata, and family *Agamidae*. There are currently thought to be seven or eight existing *Pogona* species (Grenard 2001; Cannon 2003), including the Rankin's or Lawson's dragon (*Pogona henrylawsoni*). This chapter is limited to *P. vitticeps*; other species, even within the same genus, may have different needs. These reptiles are native to Australia, where their conservation status has not been assessed (International Union for the Conservation of Nature [IUCN] 2015).

Their natural habitat is semi-desert and dry, open woodland. These environments are relatively hot and rich in ultraviolet (UV) light by day and cool at night. Central bearded dragons are mostly terrestrial, although they spend considerable time off the ground, often perching upright on rock piles, fence posts, bushes, and trees during the heat of the day (Figure 19.1). This allows dragons to monitor neighbours and watch for predators and food, and bearded dragons are among the most visually oriented of all Australian lizards (Greer 1989). They are naturally territorial and largely solitary.

Companion Animal Care and Welfare: The UFAW Companion Animal Handbook,
First Edition. Edited by James Yeates.
© 2019 Universities Federation for Animal Welfare. Published 2019 by John Wiley & Sons Ltd.

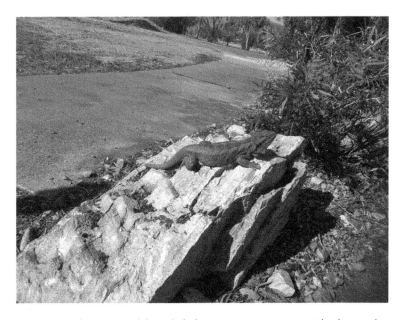

Figure 19.1 Free living central bearded dragon (*Pogona vitticeps*) basking, Alice Springs (*Source:* courtesy Robert Johnson).

Elevation also helps dragons to gain heat from the sun, escape the hot desert floor, and take advantage of passing breezes. They maintain body temperatures by changing their location; panting; excreting faeces and urates; and colour change, for example, beginning each day dark grey and becoming increasingly pale as they reach their optimum temperature (Wilson 2012).

Once a sufficient body temperature is achieved, dragons engage in other activities such as seeking food. They eat a variety of soft vegetation, flowers, invertebrates, frogs, small lizards, and birds (Greer 1997; Jepson 2011; Brown 2012). As their internal temperature drops, heat-seeking behaviour is triggered once again. At night, dragons rest in protected refuges, and their body temperatures drop to match that of the surrounding environment (Jepson 2011). A period of dormancy known as 'brumation' can be triggered by falling temperatures and shorter day lengths, and brumating lizards are less active, less responsive, and take food only opportunistically. Breeding typically follows brumation.

19.1.2 Domestic History

Central bearded dragons were not commonly kept as pets until the 1990s in the United States. Since then, they have become one of the most commonly kept pet lizards across Australia, North America, and Europe (Cannon 2003; Wright 2008). Bearded dragons are not legally exported from Australia for the pet trade. Captive breeding essentially sustains the pet population there and elsewhere in the world. This has led to artificial selection for aesthetic traits such as colour, size, and scaliness, resulting in numerous 'morphs' being available and new types continuously being created. The extent to which artificial selection results in negative welfare consequences for individual animals is not yet clear.

19.2 Principles of Bearded Dragon Care

19.2.1 Diet

Bearded dragons are obligate omnivores with nutritional requirements as described in Table 19.1. Vegetables and leafy greens should be provided to all ages of lizards every day in a form suitable to the size of dragon. Fruits should only be offered occasionally, and high-carbohydrate fruits such as bananas can cause gastric disturbance (Jepson 2011). All dragons also need animal-based protein, with juveniles needing approximately 50% invertebrate matter compared with 10–40% for adults (Macmillan et al. 1989; Brown 2012). Guidance regarding the frequency of giving animal protein varies, for example, from once per week (Jepson 2011) to two to four times per week (Brown 2012) for adults.

Excess calorie intake may lead to overly rapid growth in juveniles and obesity in adults (Donoghue 2006), particularly if combined with a lack of activity, especially activities related to food acquisition. Energy calorie intake can be reduced by limiting the number of invertebrate prey items offered, combined with increasing activity by habitat enlargement, enclosure enrichment, and improved feeding strategies. Colonic impactions, often accompanied by loss of appetite, can also be caused by overfeeding, particularly of chitin within prey exoskeletons or by insufficient water or roughage from leafy greens (Wright 2008). Conversely, malnutrition can compromise a dragon's immune system and invite infections.

Dragons, particularly juveniles and egg-laying females (Jepson 2011; Brown 2012), usually need supplementary minerals and vitamins, especially calcium and vitamin D_3 (Table 19.2). Low dietary calcium, an improper calcium-to-phosphorus ratio, excessive dietary protein, or excessive dietary vitamin D may cause metabolic bone diseases. These can cause disorientation, tremors, twitching of the digits, abnormal movement, prolapse of the cloaca (Figure 19.2), constipation, weakness, paralysis, seizures, spinal and bony deformities such as scoliosis, fractures, and soft pliable bones such as mandibles. Powdered calcium or cuttlefish should always be available for all animals of all

Table 19.1 Nutritional requirements of nonbreeding central bearded dragons.

Nutrient	Amount required (% dry matter)
(Invertebrate) Protein	Adults: 10–40%
	Juveniles: 50%
Fibre	15–10%
Calcium	1–1.5%
Phosphorus	0.5–0.9%
Calcium-to-phosphorus ratio	2 : 1
Water	Ad libitum

All figures assume animals are of normal physiology, healthy, and non-breeding.
Source: Macmillan et al. (1989), de Vosjoli et al. (2001), Jepson (2011), and Brown (2012).

Table 19.2 Suggested calcium provision for central bearded dragons.

Life stage	Suggested provision
Hatchlings and juveniles	Food dusted every day with a calcium and D_3 supplement
Subadults and reproductively active females	Food dusted with a calcium supplement and a combined calcium and vitamin D_3 supplement continuously on alternate days
Nonbreeding adults	Food dusted with a calcium and D_3 supplement three to four times each week
All ages	Ad lib from bowl of powdered calcium or cuttlefish in addition to food dusting

ages. Invertebrate prey can also be pre-fed additional calcium (Meredith and Redrobe 2002), or prey and vegetation can be dusted with calcium powder (Donoghue 2006; Rossi 2006). Dandelion and watercress are high in calcium, whereas rhubarb leaves, spinach, daffodils, peas, and beans contain oxalic or phytic acid, which render calcium unusable to dragons and can cause bladder stones or gastrointestinal irritation (Jepson 2011). Hatchlings should also be given supplementary vitamins A and C daily, and adults every 7–14 days.

Commercial foods can be relatively nutritious, although many have been evaluated as having overly low crude fibre, high calcium, or high iron content (Kik and Beynen 2003). Dragons may be less interested in eating commercial foods because of their appearance, texture, and lack of natural movement, and such diets can lead to dental problems (Jepson 2011). In comparison, feeding live animals provides environmental enrichment and encourages activity, but the welfare of the prey should be considered. No live prey should remain in the vivarium overnight because they may injure and feed on the lizards. Any uneaten vegetation should also be removed and bowls cleaned after feeding (RSPCA personal communication).

Some dragons suffer gut impactions from eating substrates such as wood or bark chips, coco coir, grass pellets, walnut shells, ground corn cob (Meredith and Redrobe 2002; Wright 2008; Jepson 2011; Brown 2012), and sand for juvenile dragons. Dragons may eat such substrates accidentally during feeding or deliberately if they are understimulated (Frye 1995), so the risks of ingestion can be reduced by careful observation, feeding animals in separate containers, offering food on solid material such as a shallow bowl or large leaf or enriching their enclosures.

Captive individuals should be given direct access to water at all times. Lack of water can lead to chronic subclinical dehydration (Wright 2008), which can decrease nutrient utilisation, as well as risk metabolic bone disease and colonic impactions. Bearded dragons can obtain water through their diet, and vegetables such as cucumbers, courgettes, and lettuces are useful sources of water (Jepson 2011). Dragons also naturally drink water droplets collected in plants, and pet dragons may benefit from spraying plants daily (for juveniles) or twice weekly (for adults) or a drip system (Grenard 2001; Jepson 2011). A shallow dish of fresh water should be provided to adults (in addition to water for bathing), but not to young juveniles who may drown.

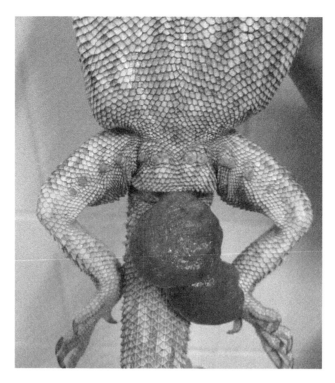

Figure 19.2   Prolapse of the cloaca and large intestine (*Source:* courtesy Robert Johnson).

19.2.2 Environment

Captive environments should resemble dragons' natural habitats as closely as possible (Cannon 2003; Figure 19.3). Bearded dragons are regularly active lizards across horizontal and vertical dimensions, and therefore need a large three-dimensional space. Enclosure dimensions also need to have enough space to ensure that certain fundamental environmental conditions can be achieved, such as an appropriate temperature gradient and space for sufficient climbing, shelter, feeding, and watering sites for each animal to perform motivated behaviours. Enclosure dimensions of at least 100 × 40 × 40 cm (L × W × H) for a single adult to 150 × 60 × 100 cm for two to three adults have been suggested (Cannon 2003; Jepson 2011; RSPCA personal communication).

Full-spectrum light is important in providing a 'daytime' photoperiod as well as facilitating vision. Lighting regimes should be connected to a timer to ensure a 12:12 or 14:10 day-to-night pattern is maintained year round, unless brumation is being induced through the shortening of day lengths, in which case a 14:10 pattern can be gradually inversed (Meredith and Redrobe 2002; Jepson 2011; Brown 2012). Vivarium day-to-night temperature should cycle with the light and brightness should be raised and lowered gradually to match natural conditions more closely.

UV light is also important. UVA is necessary for normal vision and in triggering behaviour such as feeding. UVB is essential for the synthesis of vitamin D_3 by the skin and the health consequences of incorrect UVB levels can be severe, permanent, and even

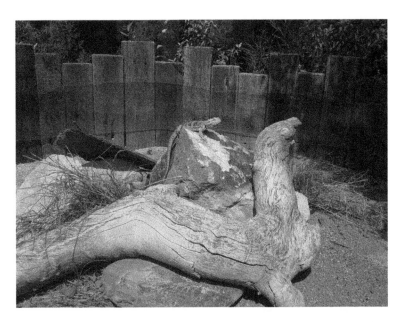

Figure 19.3 Outdoor sunning enclosure providing security and natural ultraviolet exposure (*Source:* courtesy Robert Johnson).

fatal. UV sources should be those specifically developed for use in reptile husbandry, with a UV rating of 10.0 or 12.0 (Jepson 2011), and used in accordance with manufacturer instructions. Dragons have ridges above their eyes to protect them from overhead light; serious eye problems can result from exposure to UVB rays from the side (Jepson 2011). Because light intensity decreases with distance from the bulb, the UV source should be placed above their basking area, 15 cm (Cannon 2003) to 45 cm (Jepson 2011) above the animal's highest reach point. Bulbs should usually be replaced every 6–12 months because UV output decreases over time (Cannon 2003).

Dragons' biological processes work optimally at body temperatures around 35–36 °C (Greer 1989; Cannon 2003). Background daytime enclosure temperatures have been recommended of 27–35 °C, 22–28 °C (Jepson 2011), or 28–30 °C (Brown 2012), and reduced temperatures at night of 15–20 °C (Jepson 2011) or 20–25 °C (Brown 2012). More importantly, dragons should be allowed to regulate their own temperatures within a thermal gradient, so environments should provide a range from cooler areas as low as 15 °C at night up to daytime basking areas as high as 35 °C or even 40 °C (Jepson 2011; Brown 2012). Providing the correct thermal conditions requires multiple thermometers to monitor each 'extreme' of the temperature gradient and at least two thermostatically controlled heat sources: one for ambient heat and one for a basking spot. Some owners reduce overnight temperatures further to stimulate brumation and thus reproduction. However, bearded dragons do not appear to suffer negative welfare effects from not brumating in captivity, and overly low temperatures can lead to suboptimal physiological condition, poor digestion, compromised immune function, and increased risk of diseases such as stomatitis and receding gums, especially if combined with poor hygiene.

Humidity should be no greater than 30% (Brown 2012). High humidity can lead to blister disease; low humidity can lead to abnormal skin shedding (Meredith and Redrobe 2002). As well as drinking water, dragons need additional water containers large enough for bathing. These should be placed at the cooler end of the vivarium to reduce evaporation, and a consequent rise in humidity. Dragons should also be given free access to a humid hide, especially during shedding. Excessive humidity can be avoided by minimising water spillage and subsequent evaporation, removing damp substrate, avoiding broad-leafed vegetation, and regular monitoring using a hygrometer. Ventilation should also be adequate to limit bacterial and fungal growth and avoid draughts, which can otherwise lead to respiratory disease (Meredith and Redrobe 2002; Jepson 2011).

Although a variety of substrate materials are available and marketed for bearded dragons, not all are appropriate (Table 19.3). A mixture of silver or play sand and chemical-free soil offers a substrate that retains heat, enables digging behaviour, and does not encourage bacterial growth. Sharp or building sand should be avoided because these are abrasive and may cause eye or skin irritation. Reptile carpet and moisture-retaining products such as coir and bark can harbour high levels of bacteria and fungi (Jepson 2011). When using substrates that do not allow burrowing behaviour, opportunities to dig should be provided, for example through a container of moistened fine-grained sand (Brown 2012).

Table 19.3 Suitability of various substrates for bearded dragon enclosures.

Substrate	Advantages	Disadvantages
Silver or play sand + chemical-free soil	Attractive	Risk of gut impaction if swallowed in large amounts
Fine-grained sand	Enables dragons to dig	Avoid for juveniles because of impaction risk, unless fed outside enclosure
Wood or bark chips		Fumes from pine may cause respiratory distress
		Risk of impaction
Grass pellets	Relatively digestible if consumed accidentally	Become mouldy and decompose quickly
Coco coir	Absorbent	Risk of gut impaction
Walnut shells		Wet substrate will harbour bacteria and other microorganisms
Ground corn cob		
Reptile carpet	Absorbent	Wet substrate will harbour bacteria and other microorganisms
		Need to supplement with a container of dirt or sand so dragons can have the opportunity to dig
Newspaper or paper towel	Clean, cheap, and absorbent	Need to supplement with a container of dirt or sand so dragons can have the opportunity to dig

Bearded dragons produce considerable waste, so frequent cleaning is needed. Spot cleaning should be performed to remove faecal matter as it is produced. Dragons may also defaecate in their water bowl, resulting in bacterial overgrowth that could lead to infection (Meredith and Redrobe 2002). Water bowls should therefore be cleaned daily, using reptile-safe cleaning products, before being rinsed and refilled with fresh water. The inside of the enclosure should be wiped down weekly, and the entire contents thoroughly cleaned, rinsed, dried, and reset monthly (RSPCA personal communication). Items collected from outside (e.g. the garden) should not be introduced into the vivarium because they may harbour insects, parasites, and pathogens. Leaving small amounts of faecal matter in enclosures can provide familiar chemical cues, which may have a calming effect on captive individuals (Chiszar 1995).

Dragons should be given ample opportunities to climb and perch off the ground, including at least one sturdy, secure branch per individual. The inability to perform such behaviour can result in stress, poor muscle tone, and weakness. Abrasive materials such as rocks and branches also provide surfaces on which dragons can rub their skin during shedding, and which wear down their claws, thereby helping to avoid overgrown nails, feet deformities, skin infections, and loss of digits. Rostral trauma from rubbing on cage sides as a result of escape attempts or interaction with lizards in neighbouring enclosures is seen in dragons housed both in indoor vivaria and outdoors in wire enclosures; visual barriers at ground level can reduce the chances of this behaviour.

Hides should be provided throughout the thermal gradient and in sufficient numbers to allow all dragons to secrete themselves at the same temperature and at the same time. Such hides can take the form of cork logs, bark pieces, well-supported rocks, empty plant pots, wooden constructions, real or artificial plants, and some commercially produced shelters. Water containers of sufficient size to enable bathing should be provided for adult dragons, placed at the cooler end of the vivarium to reduce evaporation and a consequent rise in humidity.

Transportation should be minimised to avoid stress. When it is necessary, dragons should be transported at a suitable temperature, in secure but well-ventilated and well-insulated containers that protect them from crushing injuries (Table 19.3). Each dragon can be placed individually in a large cloth bag or pillowcase, the opening of which is then tied up, and placed within an appropriate wooden or plastic container. Bags should be packed, but not stacked, securely in a container to limit movement during transit but still provide adequate ventilation. Polystyrene or crumpled or shredded paper should be added to provide insulation while allowing sufficient ventilation. Keeping the animal in a dark and secure environment during transport helps to reduce stress, and containers should not be placed in direct sunlight or draughts. During transportation, dragons should be maintained at a temperature within their natural range, around 25 °C and never above 30 °C to keep them comfortable and healthy. Reptiles may cool during transportation and therefore digest food more slowly, so smaller dragons should be fed no less than 6 hours and larger dragons no less than 12 hours before transport (Brown 2012).

19.2.3 Animal Company

Central bearded dragons are not social animals and as a rule, should not be kept together in captivity. Any lizard of any size can become injured or out-competed by co-occupants, and small animals are especially vulnerable to severe or fatal injury. Males are often aggressive to each other and tend to harass females, particularly in the breeding season. Females are also territorial but can form more tolerant hierarchies. Sex identification becomes easier as dragons mature. Male bearded dragons have symmetrical hemipenis swellings just caudal to the cloaca, a thicker tail base, and more prominent femoral pores inside the hindlimbs (Figure 19.4).

Dragons may respond to social and other threats, such as newly arriving dragons, by rapid head bobbing; substrate licking; expanding and darkening their beard; showing the yellow lining of the mouth; raising the body with the sides compressed; raising the tail; flattening the body and tilting towards the aggressor to look bigger; or rapidly rotating a forelimb, which gives the impression that the lizard is waving (Wilson 2012). The other dragon may then either flee or stand and show reciprocal head bobbing and beard extension. A fight usually occurs if neither individual flees.

(a)

(b)

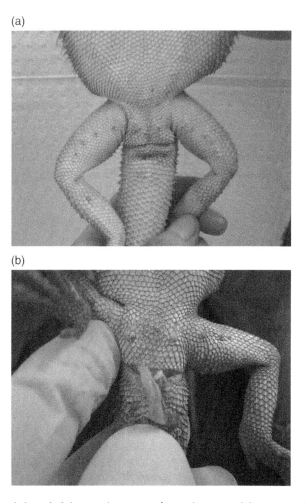

Figure 19.4 Male bearded dragon showing (a) femoral pores and (b) a seminal plug protruding from the hemipenis pouch (*Source:* courtesy Robert Johnson).

The use of a hormone implant, deslorelin, may reduce male bearded dragons' aggression (Rowland 2011). Presently this is not a widely recognised practice, no research has been performed into potential negative impacts, and the drug used is not licensed for use in reptiles. Aggressive behaviour has evolved for biological reasons, and it is unclear whether chemical treatment reduces the welfare impact of stress on animals or simply masks the outward signs of aggression – for example, studies on the use of deslorelin to manage aggression in iguanas have revealed equivocal results (Z. Knotek, personal communication). Dragons should not be housed with other species because of risks of aggression and disease transmission.

19.2.4 Human Interaction

Dragons have a reputation for being easy to handle, but non-reactivity does not necessarily represent a lack of distress. In fact, humans may be seen as predators (Kreger and Mench 1993). Dragons should therefore be approached and handled calmly, and extra care should be taken with young and apparently 'flighty' animals. Dragons should be fully supported under their forelimbs and hindlimbs, without restricting their breathing. They should never be picked up by their tails, which do not regenerate if injured. Frequent handling outside the vivarium can also lead to excessive time away from UV light and heat sources, and clinical experience suggests there is a correlation between handling time and manifestation of metabolic bone diseases in bearded dragons. Fear of perceived predators may be shown by freezing, 'flashing' their beard with their mouths open and flight. Bearded dragons generally try to escape by making themselves as spiky as possible, struggling, and attempting to jump or run. Uncommonly, grasped dragons may bite or lash with the tail as a last resort (Greer 1989). Although gentle handling may decrease such responses, some individuals may never get used to, or tolerate, close human contact.

19.2.5 Health

Bearded dragons can be affected by a variety of health problems (Table 19.4). For example, juvenile lizards are susceptible to contracting adenovirus by ingesting food contaminated with faeces, often from clinically normal carriers (Doneley and Buckle 2012). There is no specific treatment for adenovirus infection beyond supportive care, such as fluids, warmth, nutritional support, and treatment for any concurrent intestinal parasites. Such parasites include intestinal and hepatic coccidiosis, cryptosporidiosis, and isosporiasis. *Coccidia*, oxyurids, and flagellate parasites may normally be commensal organisms or of no pathogenic significance, but 'superinfested' lizards may be visibly ill and require treatment (Stahl 2003). One survey of captive reptiles reported that 43.5% of agamids were infested with *Isospora* sp. and 61.6% with oxyurids (Pasmans et al. 2008). Ticks can also become common on dragons housed outdoors during the warmer parts of the year. Some infections can infect humans, sometimes without the animal showing any signs, including *Salmonella, Mycobacteria, Campylobacter,* and *Chlamydia* (Kramer 2006; Johnson-Delaney 2006; Mitchell 2010; Weiss et al. 2011).

A key prevention method is ensuring all dragons receive adequate care because most problems are related to poor husbandry practices (Stahl 2003). New introductions and breeding animals should be routinely screened for adenovirus. Any affected or in contact animals should then be quarantined. Indeed, any bearded dragon introduced into a household with other reptiles should be routinely quarantined for at least 2 months in

Table 19.4 Selected health problems in central bearded dragons.

Condition			Welfare effects
Infectious or parasitic	Viral	Adenovirus	Reduced appetite, weight loss; weakness; neurological disorders
		Iridovirus or ranavirus	Difficulty eating; drooling; difficulty breathing; rostral damage; dental disease; weight loss; skin inflammation; bone infections
	Bacterial	*Mycobacterium*	Weight loss; lethargy; abscesses
		Dermatophilus congolensis	Skin swelling, irritation, ulcers, damage; pain
		Bacterial conjunctivitis	Eyelid swelling; irritation
		Salmonella	Diarrhoea; weight loss; decreased appetite
	Fungal	Fungal skin infections (various)	Skin damage; granulomas
		Nannizziopsis spp.	Skin and deep tissue damage
	Internal Parasites	*Cryptosporidium serpentis*	Middle-ear infections
		Coccidiosis (*Isospora amphiboluri*)	Gastrointestinal pain; malabsorption; pain; loss of appetite;
		Pinworms (Oxyurids)	weight loss; malnutrition;
		Flagellate protozoans	diarrhoea; secondary infections
		Microsporidia	Loss of appetite; depression; lethargy; neurological disturbances
		Lungworm (*Entomelas* spp.)	Respiratory distress
	External Parasites	Snake mites (*Ophionyssus natricis*)	Skin swelling and irritation; infections; abscesses; shedding problems
		Ticks (e.g. *Ixodes pacificus*)	
Hormonal disorders		Metabolic bone disease (nutritional secondary hyperparathyroidism)	Gut stasis; bloating; impaction Tremors; paralysis Reduced growth; deformed or soft bones; bone fractures
		Fatty liver (Hepatic lipidosis)	Reduced appetite; inactivity; weight loss; infections
Neoplastic		Leukaemia	Weight loss; lethargy
Degenerative or geriatric conditions		Gout	Joint pain; difficulty walking and climbing

(*Continued*)

Table 19.4 (Continued)

Condition		Welfare effects
Malfunction	Gut impaction	Reduced appetite; weight loss; pain; lack of faeces; lack of energy
		Severe cases: deformed spine; full or partial hind leg paralysis
	Abnormal skin shedding	Discomfort; constriction or loss of extremities; skin infection
	Egg binding	Restlessness; persistent straining
Toxic	Firefly toxicity (cardenolides)	Gasping; difficulty breathing; head shaking
	Pyrethrins	Diarrhoea; malcoordination; tremors; seizures
Traumatic	Rostral trauma	Pain; infection
	Thermal burns	Pain; infection

a separate room. During this period the activity and feeding behaviour of the bearded dragon should be observed and faecal samples should be taken (at least one at the start of quarantine and another at the end) and tested for parasites. Dragons should not leave quarantine until the final faecal test and examination are complete. Owners should also take sufficient hygiene precautions to reduce the risks of being infected, especially by *Salmonella*. Annual veterinary checks are also recommended for all pet dragons or more frequently if their behaviour or appearance change.

The shedding process is dependent upon a reptile's health, ambient temperature, humidity, and other environmental factors (Maderson 1965; Maderson et al. 1970, 1998). Healthy adult dragons shed approximately every 2 to 3 months, and younger lizards more often, shedding the skin in patches rather than as one entire piece. The underlying new skin should be soft and free of blemishes: crusts, ulcers, and retained skin fragments should be investigated. Poor environmental conditions, such as suboptimal temperature, low humidity, and poor enclosure hygiene, can cause problems with shedding such as skin retention around the digits and tail, ischaemic necrosis (a type of 'gangrene'), and respiratory noise. 'Soaking' the lizard in warm water or misting the lizard with tepid water may help to loosen adhered skin that has failed to separate.

19.2.6 Euthanasia

Acceptable methods of euthanasia of bearded dragons are listed in Table 19.5. The best method is usually sedation or anaesthesia, followed by the injection of an overdose of pentobarbitone (140 mg/kg) into the ventral caudal venous sinus. This should cause death within 3–30 minutes (RSPCA personal communication). Other chemicals can cause pain on injection or other undesirable effects; for example, volatile anaesthetic agents may lead to breath holding. Manually applied blunt force trauma to the head is acceptable, when other options are unavailable, if performed by well-trained and skilled personnel and promptly followed by a further procedure, such as decapitation or pithing, to ensure death.

Table 19.5 Methods of euthanasia for central bearded dragons kept as companion animals.

Method	Restraint required	Welfare benefits	Welfare risks
Injection of anaesthetic (pentobarbitone), followed by overdose injection of pentobarbitone into ventral caudal venous sinus	Secure handling and deep sedation or anaesthesia	Rapid loss of consciousness	Pain from injection
Injection of anaesthetic into a vein, followed by brain destruction	Secure handling and deep sedation or anaesthesia	Rapid loss of consciousness	Pain from injection
Head trauma	Secure handling or deep sedation or anaesthesia	Rapid loss of consciousness	Severe pain if inaccurate or not followed by prompt secondary method

Source: RSPCA (personal communication), AVMA (2013).

19.3 Signs of Bearded Dragon Welfare

19.3.1 Pathophysiological Signs

Many signs of poor welfare are general and do not indicate a specific disease. In particular, loss of body condition, including poor muscle tone and skin changes, can be early signs of serious problems. Weight loss may present as generalised muscle wastage of the pelvic region and tail base. The ribs may also become more prominent. Such signs could indicate a number of problems, including malnourishment; dehydration; parasites; cachexia (body weakness and wasting); or other illnesses. Size disparity may be the result of gastrointestinal parasites or bullying over food and basking sites. Skin tenting, sunken eyes, and prominent skin folds may indicate dehydration. Generalised weakness or lethargy can occur as a result of dehydration but may also be present in conditions such as metabolic bone diseases, parasitism, or infection.

Traumatic wounds, such as missing toes or tail tips, may indicate fighting, aggression related to mating, or poor skin shedding. Skin burns point to inappropriate heat sources or their location. An inability to swallow or manipulate food within the mouth may be the result of a primary oral problem or generalised weakness. Similarly, vomiting, regurgitation, or rejection of food may indicate an upper gastrointestinal issue or an underlying condition. Colonic impaction, often accompanied by loss of appetite, can indicate dietary problems and metabolic diseases but also inappropriate substrate (e.g. leading to ingestion and impaction), vitellogenesis (yolk deposition), poor hygiene, recent acquisition, or recent changes in housing, overhandling, old age, or trauma. Diarrhoea can indicate poor environmental conditions including low environmental temperatures, inappropriate diets, sudden dietary changes, or infection (Barten 2006).

Infections can also often be attributed to a compromised immune system as a consequence of inappropriate husbandry and related stress (Meredith and Redrobe 2002).

19.3.2 Behavioural Signs

A healthy bearded dragon should be bright-eyed and alert, regularly active, showing an interest in the environment and food items, and should move 'decisively' and, if disturbed, quickly. A lizard placed in a new environment should actively explore the enclosure and seek elevated vantage points to view the surroundings. Poor welfare is therefore suggested where a dragon is regularly seen staying on the ground, not climbing or basking, or not eating. Dragons should readily stand erect when stimulated, pushing their chests off the ground and their bodies upwards as their front limbs are extended, which may be described as a 'proud' stance or that they appear 'able to do push-ups'. Unhealthy animals may be unable or reluctant to raise the head or body.

Rapid colour changes (within minutes) may indicate thermoregulatory, social, or predator avoidance behaviours. Dragons may change their skin colour according to the ambient temperature, colour of substrate. or as a stress response. In general, colour change is most often associated with temperature regulation, whereas pattern change is generally associated with social interactions (Greer 1989). Seeking areas of higher or cooler temperatures, inactivity, or increased aggression towards other dragons are signs of inappropriate enclosure environment. Repetitive opening and closing of the mouth and 'popping' or 'crackling' noises are usually signs of respiratory disease. Open-mouthed breathing when at rest can be a behavioural thermoregulatory response; a yawn; a defensive display; or a sign of serious respiratory disease. Panting may suggest distress, overheating, or conversely, near optimal temperature. Healthy lizards may hold their mouths agape when basking without this indicating a problem.

19.4 Worldwide Action Plan for Improving Bearded Dragon Welfare

All bearded dragon owners should have adequate competence, information, expertise, and facilities to provide a captive environment and diet that meets their animal's needs and allows their pets to experience the widest possible range of safe natural behaviours. This is a responsibility of individual owners, but pet shops are well placed to provide best practice guidance to owners. Those selling or otherwise providing animals have a responsibility to ensure that the animals they provide will be looked after as well as possible. Information should also be available on the management of breeding, focusing on the number of individuals in need of rehoming because of over breeding, and wider welfare issues associated with selective breeding.

Research is needed to determine the physical and behavioural needs of captive dragons. Baseline data obtained from field-based ecological studies of wild dragons would help to determine best practice for captive husbandry. Pathophysiological research should determine normal faecal cortisol levels, health issues, life span, and microflora (e.g. Cushing et al. 2011). Behavioural observations should determine normal natural behaviour and their contexts, degree of sociability, and home range size. Clinic-based studies of captive dragons are also required to identify and record pathophysiological baselines, captive survival rates, health problem incidences, normal behaviours, and the extent to which owners are meeting their pet bearded dragons' needs.

Reptile medicine is developing as a discipline, although a great deal remains to be learned with respect to the health and veterinary care of these animals. As bearded dragons become more popular pets, many owners may expect a high level of veterinary care (Whitehead 2011), and the veterinary profession must adapt accordingly. Veterinarians must develop a good understanding of bearded dragon husbandry, the conditions that frequently affect them, and diagnostic techniques and advice appropriate to the species. Veterinary training on particular species like the central bearded dragon should be aimed at vets in general practice as well as more specialist clinicians within international and national specialist veterinary associations. International, national, regional, and local groups should be established and developed to facilitate the transfer of knowledge and share best practice, not only among veterinary surgeons but also owners and breeders.

Bibliography

Alworth, L.C., Hernandez, S.M., and Divers, S.J. (2011). Laboratory reptile surgery: principles and techniques. *Journal of the American Association for Laboratory Animal Science* 50 (1): 11–26.

Anon (2014a). Multistate *outbreak of Human Salmonella Cotham and Salmonella Kisarawe* infections linked to contact with pet bearded dragons (Final Update). Available at http://www.cdc.gov/salmonella/cotham-04-14/index.html?s_cid=cs_002. Accessed 11 July 2018.

Anon (2014b). Salmonella *outbreak that infected 132 people linked to bearded dragons bought* at pet stores. Available at http://www.dailymail.co.uk/news/article-2613154/Salmonella-outbreak-infected-132-people-linked-bearded-dragons-bought-pet-stores.html. Accessed 10 October 2013.

Arena, P.C. and Warwick, C. (1995). Miscellaneous considerations. In: *Health and Welfare of Captive Reptiles* (ed. C. Warwick, F.L. Frye and Murphy), 263–283. London and New York: Chapman & Hall/Kluwer.

Avery, R.A. (1999). Terrestrial reptiles: lizards, snakes and tortoises. In: *The UFAW Handbook on the Care and Management of Laboratory Animals. Volume 1: Terrestrial Vertebrates*, 7e (ed. T. Poole), 733–746. Blackwell Science Ltd.

AVMA (American Veterinary Medical Association). (2013). AVMA Guidelines for the Euthanasia of Animals: 2013 Edition. Available at https://www.avma.org/KB/Policies/Pages/Euthanasia-Guidelines.aspx. Accessed 7 October 2015.

Barten, S.L. (2006). Lizards. In: *Reptile medicine and surgery*, 2e (ed. D.R. Mader), 683–695. Philadelphia (PA): WB Saunders.

Brown, D. (2012). *A Guide to Australian Dragons in Captivity*. Burleigh, Qld: Reptile Publications.

Cannon, M.J. (2003). Husbandry and veterinary aspects of the bearded dragon (*Pogona spp.*) in Australia. *Seminars in Avian & Exotic Pet Medicine* 12 (4): 205–214.

Chiszar, D.C. (1995). Behavioural consequences of husbandry manipulations: indicators of arousal, quiescence and comfort awareness. In: *Health and Welfare of Captive Reptiles* (ed. C. Warwick, F.L. Frye and J.B. Murphy), 186–204. London and New York: Chapman & Hall/Kluwer.

Close, B., Bannister, K., Baumans, V. et al. (1996a). Recommendations for euthanasia of experimental animals. Part 2. *Laboratory Animals* 31: 1–32.

Close, B., Bannister, K., Baumans, V. et al. (1996b). Recommendations for euthanasia of experimental animals. Part 1. *Laboratory Animals* 30: 293–316.

Cooper, J.E. (2010). Terrestrial reptiles: lizards, snakes & tortoises. In: *The UFAW Handbook on the Care and Management of Laboratory and Other Research Animals*, 8e (ed. R. Hubrecht and J. Kirkwood), 707–730. Wiley-Blackwell: Chichester.

Cooper, J.E., Ewbank, R., Platt, C., and Warwick, C. (1989). *Euthanasia of Amphibians and Reptiles*, 35. Universities Federation for Animal Welfare/World Society for the Protection of Animals.

Cushing, A., Pinborough, M., and Stanford, M. (2011). Review of bacterial and fungal culture and sensitivity results from reptilian samples submitted to a UK laboratory. *Veterinary Record* 169: 390.

Doneley, R.J., Buckle, K.N. and Hulse, L. (2012). Adenoviral infection in a collection of juvenile inland bearded dragons (Pogona vitticeps). *Australian Veterinary Journal* 92(1–2):41–45. doi: 10.1111/avj.12136.

Donoghue, S. (2006). Nutrition. In: *Reptile Medicine and Surgery*, 2e (ed. D.R. Mader), 251–298. Philadelphia (PA): WB Saunders.

Frye, F.L. (1993). *A Practical Guide for Feeding Captive Reptiles*. Malabar, Florida: Krieger.

Frye, F.L. (1995). Nutritional considerations. In: *Health and Welfare of Captive Reptiles* (ed. C. Warwick, F.L. Frye and Murphy), 82–97. London and New York: Chapman & Hall/Kluwer.

Greer, A.E. (1989). Agamidae – Dragon lizards. In: *The Biology and Evolution of Australian Lizards* (ed. A.E. Greer), 9–50. Chipping Norton, NSW: Surrey, Beatty and Sons.

Greer, A.E. (1997). Agamidae—Dragon lizards. In: *The Biology and Evolution of Australian Lizards* (ed. A.E. Greer), 9–50. Chipping Norton, NSW: Surrey, Beatty and Sons.

Grenard, S. (2001). *The Bearded Dragon*. New York: Wiley Publishing.

International Union for the Conservation of Nature (IUCN) Red List of Threatened Species Version 2015.1. www.iucnredlist.org. Downloaded 7 June 2015.

Jepson, L. (2011). *Bearded Dragons: Understanding and Caring for your Pet*. Indonesia: Magnet & Steel Ltd.

Johnson-Delaney, C.A. (2006). Reptile zoonoses and threats to public health. In: *Reptile Medicine and Surgery* (ed. D.R. Mader), 1017–1030. Philadelphia, PA: Saunders.

Kik, M.J. and Beynen, A.C. (2003). Evaluation of a number of commercial diets for iguana (*Iguana iguana*), bearded dragons (*Pogona vitticeps*), and land and marsh tortoises. *Tijdschrift voor Diergeneeskunde* 128 (18): 550–554.

Kramer, M.H. (2006). Granulomatous osteomyelitis associated with atypical mycobacteriosis in a bearded dragon (*Pogona vitticeps*). *The Veterinary Clinics of North America. Exotic Animal Practice* 9 (3): 563–568.

Kreger, M.D. and Mench, J.A. (1993). Physiological and behavioural effects of handling and restraint in the ball python (*Python regius*) and the blue-tongued skink (*Tiliqua scincoides*). *Applied Animal Behaviour Science* 38: 323–336.

Macmillan, R.E., Augee, M.L., and Ellis, B.A. (1989). Thermal ecology and diet of some xerophilous lizards from western New South Wales. *Journal of Arid Environments* 16: 193–201.

Maderson, P.F.A. (1965). Histological changes in the epidermis of snakes during the sloughing cycle. *Journal of Zoology* 146: 98–113.

Maderson, P.F.A., Chiu, K.W., and Phillips, J.G. (1970). Changes in the epidermal histology during the sloughing cycle in the Rat snake *Ptyas korros* Schlegel, with correlated observations on the thyroid gland. *Biological Bulletin* 139 (2): 304–312.

Maderson, P.F.A., Rabinowitz, T., Tandler, B., and Alibardi, L. (1998). Ultrastructural contributions to an understanding of the cellular mechanisms involved in lizard skin shedding with comments on the function and evolution of a unique Lepidosaurian phenomenon. *Journal of Morphology* 236: 1–24.

Meredith, A. and Redrobe, S. (eds.) (2002). *BSAVA Manual of Exotic Pets*, 4e. Gloucester: BSAVA.

Mitchell, M.A. (2010). Managing the reptile patient in the veterinary hospital: Establishing a standards of care model for nontraditional species. *Journal of Exotic Pet Medicine* 19 (1): 56–72.

Pasmans, F., Blahak, S., Martel, A., and Pantchev, N. (2008). Introducing reptiles into a captive collection: the role of the veterinarian. *The Veterinary Journal* 175: 53–68.

Rossi, J.V. (2006). General husbandry and management. In: *Reptile Medicine and Surgery*, 2e (ed. D.R. Mader), 25–41. Philadelphia (PA): WB Saunders.

Rowland, M. (2011). Use of a deslorelin implant to control aggression in a male bearded dragon (*Pogona vitticeps*). *Veterinary Record* 169: 127.

Stahl, S. (2003). Pet lizard conditions and syndromes. *Seminars in Avian & Exotic Pet Medicine* 12 (3): 162–182.

Taddei, S., Dodi, P.L., Di Ianni, F. et al. (2010). Conjunctival flora of clinically normal captive green iguanas (*Iguana iguana*). *Veterinary Record* 167: 29–30.

de Vosjoli, P., Mailloux, R., Donoghue, S. et al. (2001). *The Bearded Dragon Manual*. Singapore: Advanced Vivarium Systems (AVS) Books.

Warwick, C. (1990). Reptilian ethology in captivity: observations of some problems and an evaluation of their aetiology. *Applied Animal Behaviour Science* 26: 1–13.

Warwick, C., Arena, P.C., Steedman, C., and Jessop, M. (2012). A review of captive exotic animal-linked zoonoses. *Journal of Environmental Health Research* 12: 9–24.

Warwick, C., Arena, P.C., Lindley, S. et al. (2013). *Assessing reptile welfare using behavioural criteria. In Practice* 35 (3): 123–131. doi: 10.1136/inp.f1197.

Weiss, B., Rabsch, W., Prager, R. et al. (2011). Babies and bearded dragons: sudden increase in reptile-associated Salmonella enterica serovar Tennessee infections, Germany 2008. *Vector Borne and Zoonotic Diseases* 11 (9): 1299–1301.

Whitehead, M. (2011). Enter the dragon. *The Veterinary Record* 169 (12): 318.

Wilson, S.K. (2012). *Australian Lizards: A Natural History*. Collingwood: CSIRO Publishing.

Wright, K. (2008). Two common disorders of captive bearded dragons (*Pogona vitticeps*): nutritional secondary hyperparathyroidism and constipation. *Journal of Exotic Pet Medicine* 17 (4): 267–272.

Nonvenomous Colubrid Snakes (*Colubridae*)

20

Joanna Hedley and Kevin Eatwell

20.1 History and Context

20.1.1 Natural History

Colubrid snakes are members of the class Reptilia, order Squamata, and family Colubridae. There are more than 3400 species of snakes found throughout the world on every continent with the exception of Antarctica (Reptile Database 2013), most of which are included in the Colubrid family. A small number of colubrid species are endangered or critically endangered (IUCN 2016). Although species may vary widely in terms of their biology and ecology, they share a number of characteristics which are important to understand to address their welfare needs.

Energy requirements are 2–6% of those of a similarly sized mammal and unnecessary energy is rarely expended (Galvao et al. 1965). This influences their dietary and thermal behaviour. Snakes maintain their optimum body temperatures by moving towards or away from sources of radiation and conduction, for example, cooling down by moving into shade, burying into substrate, or bathing. All snakes are carnivorous, eating small mammals, birds, amphibians, fish, insects, and even other reptiles. Some snakes hunt actively, but many employ a 'sit-and-wait ambush method of hunting. Prey

Companion Animal Care and Welfare: The UFAW Companion Animal Handbook,
First Edition. Edited by James Yeates.
© 2019 Universities Federation for Animal Welfare. Published 2019 by John Wiley & Sons Ltd.

may be killed or incapacitated by constriction or venom before being swallowed whole and alive to die from suffocation. Digestion takes several days to weeks. In temperate regions, food scarcity and temperatures can limit activity in winter periods, and certain species such as garter snakes naturally hibernate during this time. As a general rule, snakes are solitary except at times of mating. Garter snakes come together to share a space for hibernation, and snakes may be being found in the same vicinity to benefit from resources such as a heat source or shelter.

20.1.2 Domestic History

Snakes have been kept in captivity for thousands of years, as status symbols, for religious reasons, as a food source, and for their skins. In recent years, the number of snakes kept as household pets has increased dramatically. For example in the United Kingdom in 2013, there were an estimated 300 000 pet snakes (Pet Food Manufacturers' Association [PFMA] 2013). These include both wild-caught and captive-bred individuals, although the proportions for each source are unknown. Commonly kept species such as corn snakes (*Pantherophis guttatus*) are often captive-bred, and captive-breeding of snakes in general does appear to be increasing, although wild-caught individuals are also falsely offered as captive-bred. Captive breeding can be successful for several species and various colour and pattern morphs have been developed that are not naturally seen in the wild. Despite this, snakes cannot be considered as domestic animals and still appear to retain the same instincts as their wild counterparts. Snakes may become accustomed over time to regular handling, showing less aggressive and defensive behaviour, but this is not equivalent to this animal becoming domesticated.

20.2 Principles of Snake Welfare

20.2.1 Diet

All snakes are carnivores, although they inevitably also ingest plant matter via the stomachs of some of their prey (Frye 1995), which may have some potential nutritional value. Most commonly kept species can be fed on whole mammalian prey such as mice, rats, guinea pigs, or rabbits.

Snakes can become obese, particularly if overfeeding is combined with insufficient opportunities for exercise. There are also no validated condition scoring methods for snakes, but generally, reduced epaxial muscle mass is used as an indication of starvation, anorexia, or cachexia, with poor condition making snakes appear more triangular in cross section. Obesity is usually judged by the lack of clear muscle definition and increased rounding of the coelomic cavity because of the storage of excess fat along the coelomic cavity. Fat is stored in the caudal third and soft-tissue swellings can be clearly evident on some snakes, such as corn snakes. Obese snakes find it difficult to coil effectively.

The feeding of live vertebrate prey is generally not recommended (see previous chapter) because it results in a highly stressful death for the prey species and also puts the snake at risk of injuries from rodent attack. If prey are bred by the owner for feeding, they should be killed humanely immediately before feeding. To simulate live prey and increase exploratory or hunting behaviours, dead prey can be dragged around the enclosure to create a scent trail for the snake to follow simulating prey pursuit (Frye 1995). Alternatively prey can be fed from feeding tongs and moved from side to side to provoke a feed response. Carcases can also be opened to make them smell stronger. These techniques can increase the rate of tongue flicking (used for scent detection) and trailing behaviour in some species (Chiszar et al. 1981).

Feeding frequency depends on the snake's size, age, season, activity levels, and other factors but usually varies from weekly to monthly. Overfeeding is a significant problem in captivity and can lead to obesity, especially if the snake is allowed insufficient opportunity to exercise. However, colubrid snakes' higher metabolic rates mean obesity is less likely than for larger boid snakes. Certain snakes have specific dietary requirements (e.g. garter snakes), and diets should be appropriate for the particular species.

Many snakes receive a large amount of their water requirements in their food, but fresh water should always be offered and most snakes will drink water. Overheating or low environmental humidity for snakes may also increase water requirements. Insufficient water, overly high temperatures, low humidity, or cachexia can be associated with dehydration. Dehydration can lead to the formation of cloacal stones, weight loss, and rectal prolapses in some arboreal snakes requiring high humidity levels.

20.2.2 Environment

All snakes should be given the opportunity to stretch out to their full length with room to move around if desired (Arena and Warwick 1995, and Warwick et al. 2013) and a daily opportunity for brief exercise outside of their enclosure. Many snakes move over large distances; for example, indigo snakes have an average home range of 76 ha for females and 202 ha for males (Breininger et al. 2011). Even more sedentary species which ambush their prey would naturally move between feeds. Insufficient opportunity for exercise may predispose snakes to health problems such as obesity (Laidlaw 2005). Exercise should however be supervised at all times and care should be taken to prevent injury or escape.

An appropriate environmental temperature range and gradient requires both a primary background heat source and a secondary local heat source to produce a thermal gradient that allows the snake to select its preferred temperature. Care should be taken to protect snakes from direct contact with heat sources (e.g. by fitting a guard over heat lamps) because thermal burns are common especially if background temperatures are low, and snakes appear unable to adequately perceive focal areas of burning until damage is severe (Arena and Warwick 1995).

The range of humidity required varies between species, taking into account the natural habitat and temperature. Incorrect humidity can lead to dehydration, problems shedding, respiratory tract diseases, and kidney disease. Species from more tropical climates require extra spraying, misting, or water drippers to provide an adequate level of humidity, and water should be given in a container large enough for the snake to submerge its whole body at once if so desired; some snakes may also use water baths for the purposes of defaecation.

Lighting should be provided for an appropriate photoperiod (12 hours for tropical snakes and 10–14 hours depending on the season for temperate snakes). Ideally this lighting would provide a full spectrum of visible and ultraviolet (UV)light. Corn snakes can increase their vitamin D levels when exposed to UVB light (Acierno et al. 2008), but the true health and behavioural benefits are unknown for most species. Enclosures should also be positioned away from direct sunlight, draughts, and televisions, which can be a source of both noise and vibrations that may disturb the snake.

For tree-dwelling snakes, branches should be provided to allow them to stretch out and move in a vertical direction. All enclosures should contain appropriate hide areas to ensure that the snake may feel secure (Figure 20.1). Transparent boundaries may not always be perceived by snakes, resulting in self-trauma (Figure 20.2), and lack of

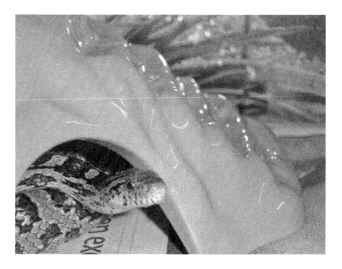

Figure 20.1 Rat snake using a commercial hide.

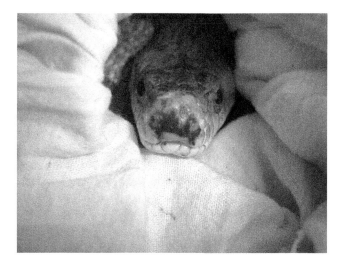

Figure 20.2 Corn snake with rostral ulceration as a result of rubbing on the glass of the enclosure.

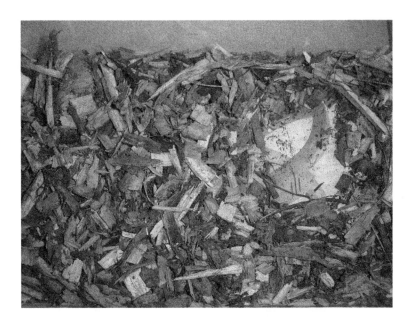

Figure 20.3 Corn snake hiding in substrate.

opportunities to hide may result in chronic stress (Warwick 1990). Substrates should also be chosen that allow snakes to bury themselves, such as commercially available aspen bedding (Figure 20.3). The enclosure should be spot cleaned whenever urates or faeces are passed, and the substrate completely changed and enclosure disinfected on at least a monthly basis. Enclosures should be accessible and easy to clean to minimise stress for the snake.

20.2.3 Animal Company

In general, company does not appear to be important for snakes. Snakes may be put together for breeding, although this is for human benefits rather than the snakes' welfare because there is no evidence that company (or breeding) is necessary from a welfare viewpoint. Indeed, although snakes are rarely territorial, they may perceive others of their own species as prey (e.g. king snakes [*Lampropeltis* spp.]). These snakes should always be kept in isolation. Furthermore, overcrowding is a significant concern in many commercial enclosures and some collections. Owners are best advised to keep single snakes in individual enclosures.

Once snakes are mature, their sex can be determined by gently inserting a small probe into the corner of the cloaca and directing it caudally towards the tail tip. In the male, the probe can usually be easily passed without resistance to a distance of greater than six scales. In the female, resistance is generally met at a distance of less than six scales. This should only be performed by a veterinary surgeon or other experienced and competent person.

Snakes similarly derive no positive benefit from the company of other animal species. They are more likely to regard them as either potential predators or prey. Mixing of species is therefore not advised both from a social viewpoint and also in terms of cross-species disease transmission.

20.2.4 Human Interaction

Although snakes may become accustomed to human company, there is no evidence that they derive pleasure from handling interactions unlike some other pet animal species. Indeed, handling can be a source of stress. Handling should not be performed when snakes are in the process of shedding, when they may feel more vulnerable, and their skin may be easily damaged. Handling is also not advised at or immediately after feeding because of the risks of 'aggression' and regurgitation. Docile snakes may be handled by gently lifting from their container whilst supporting their body, whereas potentially aggressive snakes are likely to need their head firmly restrained to prevent bites. Snakes should not be held only by the head or neck because of the risk of vertebral damage if allowed to thrash about unsupported.

However, regular brief periods of gentle handling may help the snake get used to human contact and to decrease aggressive and defensive behaviour (Kreger and Mench 1993). Cornsnakes are capable of learning simple tasks (Holtzman et al. 1999) and getting snakes to allow safe feeding, weighing, and health checks is generally advisable especially for large or potentially dangerous animals.

20.2.5 Health

Snakes can be affected by a variety of health problems, many of which are linked to environmental and general husbandry deficiencies (Table 20.1). All snakes may potentially carry *Salmonella* bacteria. These bacteria typically cause no clinical problems for snakes but are of potential concern to the keeper and any other in-contact animals especially if they are young, old, or immune suppressed. Both direct and indirect contact with snakes involve risk factors; thus, intermediate surfaces and items may also harbour *Salmonella*. Good hygiene principles are always advised when dealing with any reptiles. However, even conscientious hand washing alone does not always offer reliable protection from infection (Warwick et al. 2012). Any new snakes in a collection should be quarantined for 90–180 days to prevent introduction of disease, and informed observations should be made of their general health and behaviour. Faecal screens are advisable to check for internal parasites, especially in the case of wild-caught animals. In certain situations, particular disease screening may be advised, such as for Inclusion Body disease or Paramyxovirus.

20.2.6 Euthanasia

Acceptable methods of euthanasia of colubrid snakes are listed in Table 20.2. The best method is usually deep sedation or anaesthesia, followed by the injection of an overdose of pentobarbitone (60–100 mg/kg, although higher doses may sometimes be required) into the ventral tail vein. In small snakes, the tail vein may not be easily accessible, and pentobarbitone may need to be injected into the heart following anaesthesia. Because of their slow metabolism, cardiac arrest may take several minutes. The heart should be checked by means of a Doppler probe and once heartbeat has ceased, the animal should be pithed in order to establish brain death.

Table 20.1 Selected health problems in corn snakes.

Condition			Welfare effects
Infectious or parasitic	Viral	Adenovirus	Diarrhoea; regurgitation; neurological problems
		Ophidian Paramyxovirus	Difficulty breathing; reduced eating; regurgitation; head tremors; stargazing; loss of balance; weakness; abnormal behaviour
	Bacterial	*Mycobacterium*	Difficulty breathing; weight loss; lethargy; abscesses
	Fungal	Various	Skin damage; granulomas
	Internal Parasites	Amoebiasis (e.g. *Entamoeba invadens*)	Loss of appetite; weight loss; dehydration
		Cryptosporidium serpentis	Acute: Regurgitation; lethargy; abdominal discomfort; infections Chronic: Reduced eating; Weight loss
		Lungworm *(Rhabdias spp.)*	Respiratory distress
		Strongyloid nematodes	Lethargy; gastrointestinal disturbance; loss of appetite; regurgitation; diarrhoea; respiratory disease; skin blistering
	External Parasites	Snake mites (*Ophionyssus natricis*)	Skin swelling and irritation; infections; shedding problems; anaemia
Hormonal or metabolic disorders		Gout	Lethargy; reduced eating
		Fatty liver (Hepatic lipidosis)	Reduced appetite; reduced activity; weakness; weight loss or gain
Neoplastic		Adenocarcinoma Chondrosarcoma Liposarcoma	Pain; discomfort; malaise
Toxic		Organoposphate	Loss of balance; malcoordination; muscle tremors; increased salivation
Traumatic		Burns	Pain

Table 20.2 Methods of euthanasia for colubrid snakes kept as companion animals.

Method	Restraint required	Welfare benefits	Welfare risks
Injection of anaesthetic into a vein (pentobarbitone), followed by brain destruction	Secure handling (or anaesthesia)	Rapid loss of consciousness	Pain from injection

Source: AVMA (2013).

20.3 Signs of Snake Welfare

20.3.1 Pathophysiological Signs

Signs of welfare problems may be subtle even to the experienced keeper or veterinarian. Emaciation, oral discharge, egg binding, and dyspnoea (Figure 20.4) are common to a wide range of health problems. In turn, disease is often a sign of chronic stress, such as those resulting from poor husbandry conditions. For example, blister disease may suggest high humidity, parasitism, or stress. Detailed records should be kept of a snake's body weight and condition, reproductive activity, shedding, and behaviour to detect changes. There are no species-specific weight ranges as all snakes grow throughout their life, so generally body weight is evaluated relative to each snake's previous weight. Shedding should occur regularly, and failure to shed normally may suggest underlying husbandry or welfare problems (Figure 20.5). Shedding can also indicate the snake's growth rate. Failure to mature as expected for the species – including both poor growth and overly rapid growth and obesity – may indicate long-term welfare problems.

Weight change can also indicate water intake because some snakes may take a lot of water on board, which may not be appreciated by the observer. Dehydrated snakes may have weight loss without reduced body condition and increased body weight after water is offered (as well as show signs such as decreased amounts of urine, hardened uric acid concretions, or tacky, and pale mucous membranes). Blood measures such as electrolytes, haematology, proteins, and uric acid can also indicate the hydration status of the snake.

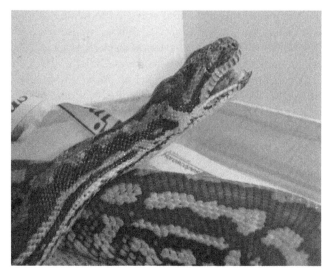

Figure 20.4 Carpet python showing a positional change associated with severe dyspnoea resulting from a bacterial pneumonia.

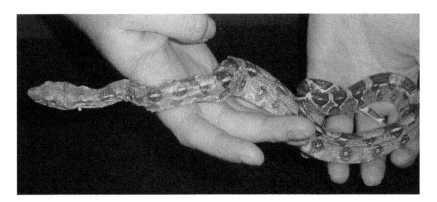

Figure 20.5 Juvenile red-tailed boa with retained exuvium present, which can reflect underlying illness or poor husbandry.

20.3.2 Behavioural Signs

Changes in feeding can also indicate problems. A snake's appetite may be assessed by evaluating the feed response. Anorexia may suggest pain or disease, hypothermia from suboptimal conditions, or debilitation. A diminished feed response may suggest a well satiated snake, making them more tractable. Hungry snakes often demonstrate a feeding response whenever their enclosure is approached, including striking the enclosure in response to movement outside or appearing aggressive when the enclosure is opened. A feed response, followed by regurgitation may indicate illness. Feeding frequencies are an important guide to the snake's overall long-term welfare, and owners should keep accurate feeding records. Most snakes also normally drink voluntarily if offered, but generally a dehydrated but otherwise well snake can be seen to actively drink a large volume when water is made available, unless they are too weakened to drink.

Chronic fear or distress can induce anorexia, immobility, or increased hiding. Acute fear or distress typically evoke subtle behavioural signs (Eatwell 2010). Nevertheless, owners may notice a number of defensive behaviours. Initially, increased tongue flicking as the snake gathers information on the novel situation can often be interpreted as an indicator of stress (or during exploration after their enclosure has been cleaned or the snake moved to a novel environment). 'Bluff displays' can include inflating their air sacs fully to distend the snake followed by quick release of the air to create a loud hiss. 'S' coiling of the neck, in readiness to strike, and fake strikes with a closed or open mouth are also often employed (Figure 20.6). Other bluff displays include tail vibration and mimicry of more dangerous species. Violent writhing, defaecation, and or regurgitation may also indicate stress, for example during handling.

Other defensive behaviours from snakes include a variety of adaptive behaviours such as catalepsy, death feigning and tonic immobility (e.g. hog-nosed snakes [*Heterodon* spp.]). These involve continued unresponsiveness to external stimuli and are often evoked after an elaborate bluff display. The snake's mouth may hang open limply, with the tongue out and all movement ceased. Haemorrhage from the mouth, nostrils, and cloaca and hemipenile eversion may also occur. Such snakes typically lie on their backs, and then assume a normal posture and move away once the threat has diminished.

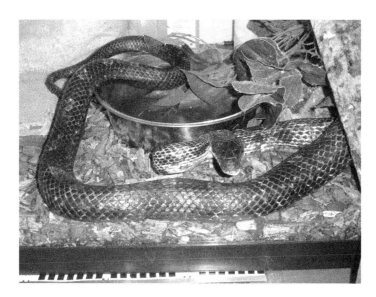

Figure 20.6 Juvenile corn snake sitting in a striking position with flattened head to appear more triangular and ready to strike if approached.

This response is evoked naturally in response to attacks from potential predators; it is thought the lack of movement diminishes the kill response of predators, and the smeared bowel contents makes the snake taste unpleasant.

Tail display or tail vibrating occurs in a number of species including cornsnakes (*Elaphe* spp.). This is believed to be a display to divert a predator's attention to the tail. It also mimics more aggressive species such as rattlesnakes (*Crotalus* spp.) discouraging predation as an audible buzz can be created when performed in a dry substrate. Tail displays can also coincide with hiding the head (Figure 20.7), or tail movements may mimic head movements encouraging a potential predator to bite the tail instead. A final defence can include flattening of the skull by moving the quadrate bones laterally giving the head a triangular appearance mimicking the head shape of vipers.

Snakes may show behavioural responses to pain modulation (Oleson et al. 2008; Sladky et al. 2008). Some can be best identified by extended remote observation. Acute local pain can lead to immobility or guarding of the affected area (e.g. reluctance to coil a section) or abnormal resting postures may be used to alleviate pressure. Altered respiration may occur as a result of discomfort from muscles and ribs (or indicate genuine respiratory pathology). Snakes may also rub the area on the substrate or rocks. Chronic pain is likely to reduce exploratory behaviour and lead to immobility, but more overt displays are unlikely to be seen.

Pain-related or fear-related responses can be induced by handing or close proximity of the owner to the snake in pain as a result of the protective response being heightened by pain. For example, a snake in pain may show an initial flight response to avoid handling followed by increased aggressiveness once restrained. The significance of such behaviour also depends on the species (e.g. predator species versus prey species); the tameness of the snake considered; the competence of the handler; and the time of day,

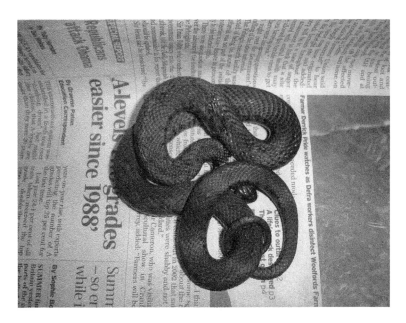

Figure 20.7   Grass snake with head hidden under other body loops for protection.

lighting, temperature, and the timing of feeds and sheds. As examples: disturbing a snake at an unusual time of day may provoke an aggressive response; snakes exposed to UV lighting may show increased activity; a cold snake may have a reduced or delayed aggressive response; a hungry snake may well strike as it is anticipating food; and snakes who have just eaten or are due to shed are usually more defensive or aggressive.

20.4 Worldwide Action Plan for Improving Pet Snake Welfare

The largest area for improvement in pets snake welfare worldwide is in improving our evidence base of appropriate captive care. This involves finding out more about how the captive environment influences chronic stress and which aspects of husbandry can be modified to reduce the effects of this. Knowledge then needs to be transferred to veterinarians, the pet trade, owners, and zoological collections, so that they can improve current husbandry practices and provide better, prompt veterinary treatment. Particularly important areas for education include incorrect social groupings, presence of potential predators, exposure through lack of hides, and the need for appropriate analgesia. Information should also be used to develop minimum welfare standards and welfare assessment guidelines. Some may be simpler to create, such as guidelines on diet, enclosure design, and climatic requirements. It may be more difficult to create outcome-based approaches, for example, to reduce abnormal behaviours or improve biological performance, which may result from a wide variety of changes. Input-based guidelines should therefore be currently used as a baseline for captive colubrids.

Bibliography

Acierno, M.J., Mitchell, M.A., Zachariah, T.T. et al. (2008). Effects of ultraviolet radiation on plasma 25-hydroxyvitamin D3 concentrations in corn snakes (*Elaphe guttata*). *American Journal of Veterinary Research* 69: 294–297.

Arena, P.C. and Warwick, C. (1995). Miscellaneous factors affecting health and welfare. In: *Health and Welfare of Captive Reptiles* (ed. C. Warwick, F.L. Frye and Murphy), 263–283. London, UK: Chapman & Hall/Kluwer.

AVMA (American Veterinary Medical Association). (2013). AVMA Guidelines for the Euthanasia of Animals: 2013 Edition. Available at https://www.avma.org/KB/Policies/Pages/Euthanasia-Guidelines.aspx. Accessed 7 October 2015.

Breininger, D.R., Bolt, R., Legare, M.L. et al. (2011). Factors influencing home-range sizes of eastern indigo snakes in Central Florida. *Journal of Herpetology* 45 (4): 484–490.

Chiszar, D.C., Taylor, S.V., Radcliffe, C.W. et al. (1981). Effects of chemical and visual stimuli upon chemosensory searching by garter snakes and rattlesnakes. *Journal of Herpetology* 15 (4): 415–423.

Eatwell, K. (2010). Options for analgesia and anaesthesia in reptiles. *In Practice* 32: 306–311.

Frye, F.L. (1995). Nutritional considerations. In: *Health and Welfare of Captive Reptiles* (ed. C. Warrick, F.L. Frye and J.B. Murphy), 83–97. London: Chapman and Hall.

Galvao, P.E., Tarasantchi, J., and Guertzenstein, P. (1965). Heat production of tropical snakes in relation to body weight and body surface. *American Journal of Physiology* 209 (3): 501–506.

Holtzman, D.A., Harris, T.W., Aranguren, G., and Bostock, E. (1999). Spatial learning of an escape task by young corn snakes, *Elaphe guttata guttata*. *Animal Behaviour* 57: 51–60.

IUCN (International Union for the Conservation of Nature). (2016). *The IUCN Red List of Threatened Species*. Available at https://www.iucn.org/theme/species/our-work/iucn-red-list-threatened-species. Accessed 22 August 2016.

Kreger, M.D. and Mench, J.A. (1993). Physiological and behavioral effects of handling and restraint in the ball python (Python regius) and the blue-tongued skink (Tiliqua scincoides). *Applied Animal Behaviour Science* 38: 323–336.

Laidlaw, R. (2005). *Scales and tails. The welfare and trade of reptiles kept as pets in Canada.* New York, NY: World Society for the Protection of Animals.

Liang, Y.F. and Terashima, S. (1993). Physiological properties and morphological characteristics of cutaneous and mucosal mechanical nociceptive neurons with A- delta peripheral axons in the trigeminal ganglia of crotaline snakes. *Journal of Comparative Neurology* 328: 88–102.

Mosley, C. (2009). Clinical approaches to analgesia in reptiles. In: *Handbook of Veterinary Pain Management*, 2e (ed. J.S. Gaynor and W.W. Muir), 481–493. Missouri: Mosby, Elsevier.

Oleson, M.G., Bertelsen, M.F., Perry, S.F., and Wang, T. (2008). Effects of preoperative administration of butorphanol or meloxicam on physiologic responses to surgery in ball pythons. *Journal of the American Medical Association* 233: 1833–1888.

Pet Food Manufacturers' Association (PFMA) (2013). Available at https://www.pfma.org.uk/pet-population. Accessed 18 December 2013.

Reptile Database (2013). Species Numbers. Available at http://www.reptile-database.org/db-info/SpeciesStat.html. Accessed 29 September 2013.

Sladky, K.K., Kinnet, M.E., and Johnson, S.M. (2008). Analgesic efficacy of butorphanol and morphine in bearded dragons and corn snakes. *Journal of the American Veterinary Medical Association* 233 (2): 267–273.

Warwick, C. (1990). Reptilian ethology in captivity: observations of some problems and an evaluation of their aetiology. *Applied Animal Behaviour Science* 26: 1–13.

Warwick, C., Arena, P.C., Steedman, C., and Jessop, M. (2012). A review of captive exotic animal-linked zoonoses. *Journal of Environmental Health Research* 12: 9–24.

Warwick, C., Arena, P., Lindley, S. et al. (2013). Assessing reptile welfare using behavioural criteria. *In Practice* 35: 123–131.

Mediterranean Tortoises (*Testudo* spp.)

21

Andrew C. Highfield

21.1 History and Context

21.1.1 Natural History

Mediterranean tortoises (*Testudo* spp.) are members of the class Reptilia, order Testudines, and family Testudinae. There are four widely acknowledged species of terrestrial tortoise found in the Mediterranean region. Members of the Spur-thighed tortoises(*Testudo graeca* complex), Hermann's tortoise (*T. hermanni*), Marginated tortoise (*T. marginata*), and Egyptian tortoise (*T. kleinmanni*). Taxonomic status of these reptiles and the ability to differentiate them in practice, therefore, also has important welfare implications because biological habits and needs vary. That said, in general terms their broad environmental and dietary requirements are somewhat similar. *T. marginata* are classified as 'Least Concern'; *T. graeca* as Vulnerable; *T. hermanni* as Near Threatened; and *T. kleinmanni* are Critically Endangered.

The taxonomy of the *T. graeca* complex is particularly confused with numerous species and subspecies proposed (Bonin et al. 2006). There is rarely much agreement on validity. It is clear that there are a large number of different geographical forms, each with unique morphological and sometimes behavioral features. There are two primary

Companion Animal Care and Welfare: The UFAW Companion Animal Handbook,
First Edition. Edited by James Yeates.

geographical groups within the *T. graeca* complex: those occurring in North Africa and Southern Spain, and those occurring in Turkey, the Caucasus, and the Middle East. The North African group contains the prototypical *T. graeca* L. 1758. The Caucasian group is dominated by *Testudo (graeca) ibera*. Many commentators consider this to be a separate species entirely. A detailed review of this confused and controversial taxonomic situation is beyond the scope of the present text. However, it should be noted that these different forms do have significantly differing patterns of behaviour, different structural features, different responses to common pathogens. and can prove to be mutually incompatible.

T. g. graeca occur in semi-arid to arid environments, typified by hot, dry summers, and by relatively mild, short winters (Figure 21.1). *T. hermanni*, *T. g. ibera*, and *T. marginata* tend to occur in similar, though somewhat less arid and more densely vegetated habitats, often including the edges of forests. *T. kleinmanni* occurs in a narrow band of coastal dune habitats in Libya, Egypt, and Israel. Winter temperatures experienced in the Mediterranean are strongly correlated with altitude, where populations at higher, inland sites tend to experience lower temperatures and for longer periods than those inhabiting more moderate coastal zones.

Tortoises respond to extended periods of cold weather by burying underground and entering a state of torpor (hibernation). This may not be continuous, but periodic, with

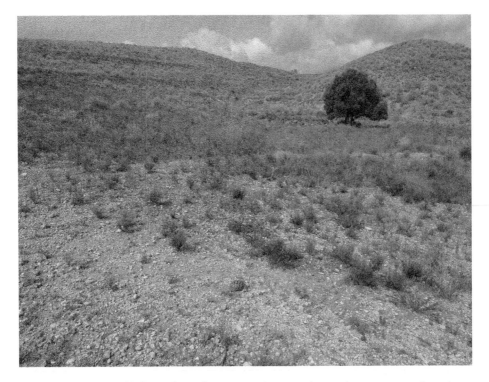

Figure 21.1 Natural habitat of *Testudo graeca*, rich in varied microclimates across a large home range.

occasional emergences in warmer periods. It is not unusual to find the same species in the same general location remaining active at low altitudes, whereas those at higher, colder altitudes remain buried and inactive. In summer, a similar, but reversed pattern may be observed with regard to aestivation. In Spain, for example, where daytime temperatures can exceed 35 °C, *T. graeca* aestivate underground from late June until mid-September at lower altitudes. Periodic emergences can occur, usually coinciding with precipitation. A substantial part of the year is spent buried, or semi-buried, to escape conditions that are either too cold, too hot, or too dry.

Juveniles have the same dietary and environmental requirements as adults and follow the same activity cycles. Nocturnal activity may also occur during this period. Diurnal activity tends to occur in three distinct periods: early morning basking, feeding, or mating, followed by retreat into a burrow or scrape, and a secondary period of activity in late afternoon or early evening. The precise times vary as the seasons advance and as a result of local climatic variables. Peak activity for all Mediterranean zone tortoises occurs in spring, with a secondary activity peak in early autumn. Eggs are normally laid in May–June, and hatchlings emerge following the first rains of autumn which typically occur in early September. Activity and feeding is strongly cyclic and coincides with vegetation peaks and more moderate temperatures. Tortoises are behavioral thermoregulators and are adept at using body posture, natural shade, and varying degrees of contact or isolation from the surrounding environment to adjust their body temperatures.

Mediterranean tortoises consume a wide variety of plant species. One population of *T. g. graeca* living in the Donana Park in southern Spain consumed at least 88 different plant species (Andreu 1987), and a population living in an overgrazed area in the Atlas Mountains in Morocco during the spring season consumed a range of 34 different plant species (Mouden et al. 2006). Some species (particularly *T. hermanni*) also opportunistically consume small insects, snails, or slugs, but this remains an extremely small proportion of their overall intake. The availability of fresh forage varies seasonally, with a sharp peak in early spring and a steep decline in the heat of summer when only dried and desiccated material may be available. At such times tortoises are normally aestivating but may emerge to feed on this during episodes of rain, before returning to aestivation. The natural diet of all Mediterranean tortoises is extremely high in fibre content, typically ranging from 30 to 49%, rich in calcium, and low in phosphorus (a mean ratio of 14 : 1 was recorded in a dietary analysis of plants consumed by free ranging *T. kleinmanni*), and with protein levels in the range of 17% (dry matter basis) and 4–6% (as-fed basis).

Mediterranean tortoises are typically solitary animals in the wild. Brief contact for male–male combat and mating occurs mainly in spring, and often again, depending on climate and location, in early autumn. Other contacts occur infrequently, by chance. There is no maternal care. Hatchlings emerge from the nest and are solitary and self-sufficient immediately. Mediterranean tortoises typically use a large home range of several hectares, with females frequently ranging further (to 7.4 ha) than males (to 4.6 ha) in the case of *T. hermanni* (Mazzotti et al. 2002). This has important implications for space requirements in captivity. *T. graeca* can reach very high ages, sometimes exceeding a century.

Tortoises can feel pain but may not demonstrate it in the same way as mammals (MacArthur et al. 2004). They, possess very developed network of nerve endings throughout their bodies, including directly beneath the scutes of the carapace and plastron (Bonin et al. 2006), which appear sensitive to physical stimulation and to temperature variations. Chelonian skin is also rich in two distinct classes of mechanoreceptors with a similarity to mammalian pressure and touch receptors (Kenton et al. 1971).

21.1.2 Domestic History

In the eighteenth and nineteenth centuries, tortoises were prized as rare and valuable curiosities. One of the most famous animals acquired in this way was the tortoise of the naturalist Gilbert White of Selborne. The earliest documented accounts of commercial importation began to appear in 1886 when Sir Peter Eade recorded purchasing some tortoises from a street trader in Norwich (Loveridge and Williams 1957). By the turn of the twentieth century, the trade was numbered in thousands annually; by the mid-twentieth century, numbers had risen to hundreds of thousands annually. Lambert (1969) quotes figures of more than 300 000 tortoises being exported from Morocco alone to Britain each year in the 1950s. Now, Spur-thighed, Hermann's, and Marginated tortoises are all relatively common in captivity.

Because of the adoption of legislation in exporting countries, the trade in wild-caught tortoises from North Africa declined sharply from 1976 onwards. Traders responded by increasing imports from other areas such as Turkey. In 1984 CITES restrictions came into effect, further reducing the wild-caught trade. Bulk imports of farmed or 'ranched' Hermann's tortoises (*T. hermanni*), typically exported as juveniles, have also become a significant factor in continuing trade. Concerns persist that many of the tortoises which are sold as captive-bred have wild-caught origins (TRAFFIC 2012) Domestically produced captive-bred Mediterranean tortoises are typically offered for sale by enthusiasts operating on a small scale but relatively few of these enter the commercial pet trade. Within the European Union, trade in all *Testudo* spp. requires A10 paperwork under Wildlife Trade Regulation 338/97. The Egyptian tortoise, *T. kleinmanni*, however, is a CITES Appendix I listed species and trade is strictly controlled.

21.2 Principles of Mediterranean Tortoise Care

21.2.1 Diet

All Mediterranean tortoises are primarily herbivorous and need a wide variety of plant species. In captivity a mix of fresh, green, high-fibre vegetation based on flowers and herbs combined with dried, coarse vegetation of also high (more than 35%) fibre, supplied on a cyclic basis, closely approximates the natural diet of Mediterranean tortoises (Highfield 2010b). This makes it extremely difficult, if not impossible, to provide perfect nutrition in captivity. Captive diets often are too high in available protein, too low in fibre, contain excessive quantities of highly digestible carbohydrates and phosphorus (e.g. fruits), include a limited range of plant species, and offer inadequate levels of calcium.

Overfeeding combined with a lack of natural inactivity periods also contribute to artificially accelerated rates of growth in captivity compared to growth in the wild.

Provision of completely unsuitable foodstuffs can also cause malnutrition. For example, eggs, dog food, peas, beans, canned tomatoes, and tofu are unsuitable. Excess fruits can severely disrupt their digestive processes which are geared to a very high fibre, low sugar intake (Highfield 2000). These imbalances may lead to lactate-induced diarrhoea and consequent dehydration (Donoghue and Langenberg 1996). These problems are avoidable with careful dietary (and environmental) management.

Tortoises require access to fresh drinking water, especially if maintained indoors for any period. Dehydration (which may present as inelastic skin and sunken eyes) is a common finding and is associated with the formation of bladder 'stones' formed from insoluble urates.

21.2.2 Environment

Tortoise species from Mediterranean habitats require correspondingly appropriate macro- and microclimates. Such environments are challenging to create outside of the natural habitat, especially in a limited space.

Mediterranean tortoises are ill-suited to confinement in vivaria or similarly restricted indoor enclosures which almost invariably fail to offer suitable thermal environments such as gradient and convection effects and frequently subject inhabitants to extremes of relative humidity (Highfield 2009). The best captive environments provide a combination of extensive outdoor accommodation, with well-drained substrates in a sunny location, shade for retreat in hot weather, and (in cooler climates) provision of additional means of achieving adequate body temperatures, such as access to greenhouses, cold-frame terraria, or poly tunnel systems (Highfield 2014b). Provision of artificial light and heat may also be required. Tortoises should not, on both welfare and physiological grounds, be maintained in small glass or wooden enclosures indoors, except on a very temporary basis. Long-term housing in glass tanks and small vivaria should be regarded as inhumane (Highfield 2010a, Animal Protection Agency 2012).

Tortoises rely almost exclusively upon the environment that they are kept in to meet their physiological and metabolic needs. They employ complex behaviours and make use of microclimates to regulate their body temperatures. They must be able to attain adequate temperatures to permit normal activity patterns and must be able to self-regulate their body temperature using the environment provided (Heatwole and Taylor 1987). Whilst broad optimum thermal ranges are reasonably well understood, subtle variations may be essential to well-being. Such refined regulation may only be self-determined by tortoises at a given time and in a given situation, for example as a behavioural strategy in the mediation of disease (Warwick et al. 2013). Mediterranean tortoises are typically most active between ambient temperatures of approximately 22–34 °C. At night, temperatures can safely fall to between 5 and 10 °C. These species require a minimum basking zone temperature of 30 °C, and this must be large enough to cover the entire body evenly. Large tortoises require large basking zones. A suitable basking zone temperature would be in the 34–38 °C range.

Basking zone tortoises also require access to a cooler or shaded and cooler retreat area so that they can voluntarily reduce their body temperature on demand. An optimum gradient or differential from the basking zone is in the 10–15 °C range. If an adequate thermal gradient is not available, animals may overheat and become unable to self-regulate their body temperature with potentially lethal consequences.

Temperatures in excess of 40 °C can be rapidly lethal to tortoises as they cause general-ised overheating beyond the animal's critical thermal maximum (the point at which first collapse and immobility, and then death occurs). The critical thermal maximum of most tortoises is in the range 39–41 °C (Hutchison et al. 1966.) Excessively high surface tem-peratures can also produce thermal contact burns in tortoises. These injuries can also be common where base mounted heat pads are employed (MacArthur et al. 2004). Uneven heating can occur from reptile basking lamps as a result of proximity and to differences between the infrared spectrum produced by artificial lamps compared to natu-ral infrared (Figure 21.2). Basking lamps can also lead to altered light patterns and severe reductions in local relative humidity (Figure 21.3).

Mediterranean tortoises also have specific requirements with regard to relative humid-ity and lighting. Very low (<30% relative humidity) levels for extended periods can result in chronic dehydration with consequential renal stress and extended exposure to high levels (>70% relative humidity) increases the risk of cutaneous disorders and respiratory disease. Optimum levels of ambient humidity would be in the 40–55% range for most Mediterranean species but can vary. Lighting when indoors or under glass must include sufficient levels of ultraviolet (UV) B to permit vitamin D_3 synthesis. Heat sources must, therefore, be carefully designed to permit normal photoregulatory, hydroregulatory, and thermoregulatory behaviours, which can be difficult to achieve (Highfield 2014a).

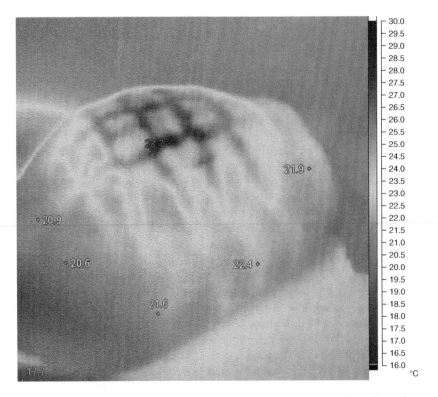

Figure 21.2 Uneven heating from a typical reptile basking lamp as recorded by a thermal imaging camera.

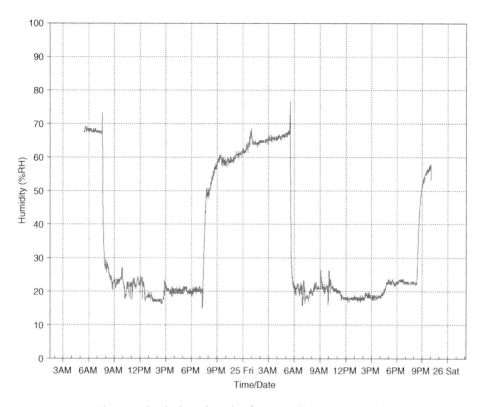

Figure 21.3 Reduction in local relative humidity, from 70 to below 20%, recorded under a basking lamp during lamp 'on' cycles.

Tortoises receive little or no vitamin D_3 from dietary sources, and rely almost exclusively upon UVB from unfiltered sunlight to synthesize D_3 internally. Insufficient vitamin D_3 availability can lead to reduced bone density (Figure 21.4) and other serious metabolic problems. Signs of metabolic bone disease include swellings, lethargy, general weakness, tremors, and bones becoming thicker, soft, and pliable. Metabolic bone disease is a primary, and perhaps the most common, cause of premature death among captive tortoises. Rapidly growing animals such as hatchlings are most at risk because their bones are generally softer and their requirements for minerals make them particularly susceptible to malnutrition. Egg laying females are also at particular risk because of the extra demands that egg production places on their calcium metabolism. However, all adults can be affected if maintained in a state of deficiency for long enough.

Metabolic bone disease can be associated with the carapace deformity observed in many captive-reared tortoises. As the external skeletal bones of the carapace can get less dense, they become thicker and softer and more easily deformed by external forces such as the pull of the tortoise's limb and respiratory muscles. The bone can also grow to conform to the keratin scutes, which can thicken, build-up, and dry out during periods of low humidity or dehydration. These combined factors can then deform the soft skeleton, forming it into a pyramid shape (Figure 21.5). Soaking the tortoise may soften

(a)   (b)

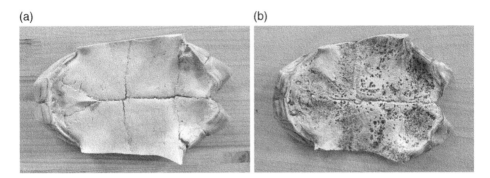

Figure 21.4 Bone densities of *Testudo graeca*: (a) Typical plastron from a wild tortoise; (b) Plastron with lesions from a tortoise raised on an inappropriate captive diet.

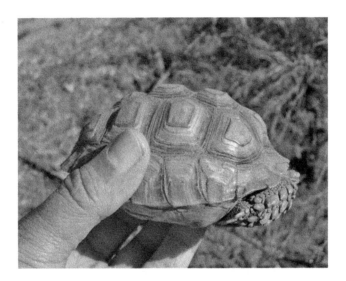

Figure 21.5 Carapace deformity resulting from incorrect husbandry.

the keratin, thereby reducing the symptom of pyramiding but does not address the metabolic bone disease itself. To prevent metabolic bone disease, as well as adequate levels of calcium in the diet, tortoises need adequate (but not excessive) quantities of D_3. This may be provided by means of dietary supplementation or by exposure to adequate levels of UVB lighting and sufficient basking temperatures for them to be exposed to the UV light.

21.2.3 Animal Company

Mediterranean tortoises do not maintain sustained social groupings of any kind in nature, except briefly during mating or other purely random encounters. For the most part, they live a solitary existence in low-density populations. Male and female Mediterranean tortoises may be highly territorial as they enter their breeding cycle. Overcrowding because of lack of space, inadequate retreats in which to conceal themselves, or a greater than 1:1 ratio of males to females, amplify such behaviours and greatly increase the risk of stress and traumatic injury.

The different species (and some geographical variants) of Mediterranean tortoise demonstrate different patterns of behaviour, to such a degree that keeping mixed groups is extremely inadvisable and is likely to lead to heightened levels of stress and also potentially to serious injuries. The best known example of this mismatching of species is the tendency of *T. graeca* and *Testudo ibera* to violently ram each other as a precursor to mating or to maintain social hierarchies, a behaviour virtually unknown in *T. hermanni*. If *T. hermanni* and *T. graeca* are mixed, the former may therefore typically sustain severe shell injuries as a result. Conversely, *T. hermanni* engage in mutual biting behaviour, whereas North African *T. graeca* do not, and in this case the latter may sustain serious soft-tissue injuries. *T. marginata* also bite and ram and are capable of inflicting serious trauma injuries on other species (and occasionally, on each other). There are also anatomical differences between these species that preclude safe mixing. For example, male *T. hermanni* possess a tail 'spur' that is compatible with the female's clocal configuration but which is capable of causing severe internal injuries if they attempt to mate with other species.

Tortoises should not be kept with other reptiles because lizards, snakes, and chelonia carry many mutually antagonistic pathogens. Keeping them in areas with high concentrations of avian faeces should also be avoided because this is associated with a number of parasitic diseases and bacterial infections and infections in chelonia, including the formation of aural abscesses and shell infections. Tortoises should never be kept where dogs or rodents have access to them because both are routinely linked to often fatal attacks.

21.2.4 Human Interactions

Mediterranean tortoises display no affinity or need for human company. In the wild, being picked up or moved is likely to be associated with predators. They may also have experienced being dropped by a human. Fearful healthy tortoises may attempt to escape, to bite, to retract into the shell, or to become flaccid. Tortoises should therefore be picked up as little as possible, except for necessary interactions and for getting them used to being picked up. When necessary, tortoises should be restrained by supporting the shell, while allowing the feet to touch a solid surface. Larger tortoises may need to be held using two hands, and an additional person may be needed, for example, to administer medicines. Tortoises are unlikely to be coaxed out of their shell; they are more likely to come out when relaxed or when they need (e.g. for easier respiration). However, tortoises may be trained to approach humans by associating human interactions or particular cues with food.

21.2.5 Health

Mediterranean tortoises can suffer from several diseases (Table 21.1). Some of these are zoonotic and can pose particular risks to humans with immature or compromised immune systems. *Salmonella* is of particular concern, although many other potentially pathogenic agents also pose a threat including clostridium and campylobacter. Anyone who handles tortoises should follow a strict hand-washing protocol and take care to reduce any possibility of transmission on clothes or food utensils.

Table 21.1 Selected health problems in Mediterranean tortoises.

Condition			Welfare effects
Infectious or Parasitic	Viral	Paramyxovirus	Skin inflammation
		Poxvirus	Papules on the eyelids; reduced appetite; weight loss
		Herpesvirus Iridovirus or ranavirus Picornavirus	Upper respiratory tract, mouth and tongue inflammation; nasal discharge; abscesses; respiratory distress; malaise; difficulty eating; drooling;
	Bacteria	*Mycoplasa agassizii*	reduced appetite; eye irritation; skin irritation; neck oedema; depression; neurological disorders
		Dermatophilus congolensis	Skin swelling, irritation, ulcers, damage; pain
	Fungal	Fungal skin infections (various)	Skin damage; granulomas; 'shell-rot'
	Internal Parasites	Flagellate protozoans	Gastrointestinal pain; malabsorption; loss of appetite; weight loss; malnutrition; secondary infections
		Cryptosporidium serpentis	Reduced appetite; lethargy; regurgitation; dehydration; infections
		Plasmodium	Anemia; lethargy; neurological or cardiac problems
		Pinworms (*Oxyuris* spp.)	Gastrointestinal blockage
	External Parasites	Ticks (e.g. *Ixodes pacificus*)	Skin swelling and irritation; infections; abscesses; shedding problems
		Flystrike (e.g. *Phormia* spp.; *Sacrophaga* spp.)	Skin damage; loss of appetite; irritation; pain; septicaemia
Hormonal disorders		Metabolic Bone Disease (nutritional secondary hyperparathyroidism)	Gut stasis; bloating Tremors; paralysis Reduced growth; deformed or soft bones; bone fractures
		Fatty liver (Hepatic lipidosis)	Reduced appetite; inactivity; weight loss; infections
Toxic		Ivermectin	Neurological signs
Traumatic		Dog attacks	Skin damage; pain

Mediterranean tortoises are highly susceptible to a number of highly lethal viral pathogens (Jacobson 2007), including chelonian herpes virus. Mortality rates can exceed 90% of affected animals within 3 months of infection. Outbreaks have been recorded from Europe, the United States, and South Africa. The mixing of different

Table 21.2 Methods of euthanasia for Mediterranean tortoises.

Method	Restraint required	Welfare benefits	Welfare risks
Injection of anaesthetic (pentobarbitone) into the heart, followed by brain destruction	Anaesthesia	Rapid loss of consciousness	Pain from injection

Source: AVMA (2013).

species, even on a fleeting basis, appears to considerably amplify the infection risk. It is advised that tortoises should be maintained in same-species groups based on geographical origin, and all new arrivals are subjected to extended periods of quarantine. In northern climates, poor hibernation techniques by keepers result in many cases of injury and premature death associated with exposure to subzero temperatures. Frost-blinded tortoises are particularly common after a harsh winter.

By far the greatest proportion of health problems reported in tortoises can be attributed to poor dietary and environmental management and to inappropriate contact with other species. Dietary-related conditions of both deficiency and excess are common. Thermal burns from artificial heat sources and dehydration from inappropriate use of basking lamps and unsuitable accommodation are also frequently encountered. Failure to provide adequate temperatures, adequate gradients to permit natural thermoregulation, and inadequate lighting further contribute to the high rates of ill-health observed in captive tortoises that are maintained outside of their natural bioclimatic zone (Highfield 2013). Respiratory diseases (including persistent nasal discharges) are also common in animals maintained in suboptimum temperature ranges and that have been exposed to other affected tortoises.

21.2.6 Euthanasia
Acceptable methods of euthanasia of tortoises are listed in Table 21.2. The best method is usually anaesthesia followed (once non-responsiveness is evident) by the injection of an overdose of pentobarbitone (200 mg/kg) into the heart, followed by pithing (see Chapter 18). Chelonia have an extremely high tolerance to anoxia (Milton 2008), with some demonstrating an ability to survive for up to 27 hours in a 100% nitrogen environment (Johlin and Moreland 1933). Methods such as decapitation, freezing, and inhaled anaesthesia are therefore inappropriate.

21.3 Signs of Mediterranean Tortoise Welfare

21.3.1 Pathophysiological Signs
General measures of overall welfare include survival, health, growth, and breeding (Griffiths et al. 2012). Poor body condition or low body mass compared to carapace length may suggest recent health, nutritional, or other problems. Poor quality of deformed carapaces may suggest current or previous nutritional or environmental problems, not least vitamin D deficiency.

Haematological and biochemical parameters can be used (Christopher 1999; López-Olvera et al. 2003). Red blood cell levels can indicate hydration (Peterson 2002). Corticosterone and cortisol can be measured in tortoises, and the latter becomes significantly higher 30 minutes after handling and release, and remains high for 4 weeks after handling, confinement, and transportation (Fazio et al. 2014), although handling and transportation may not lead to increases in other tortoise species (e.g. *Gopherus polyphemus*, Kahn et al. 2007; *Gopherus agassizii*, Drake et al. 2012). There may be differences between individuals, for example in other species, male tortoises may have higher corticosteroid levels and females may show seasonal variations (e.g. Ott et al. 2000; Lance et al. 2001; Drake et al. 2012).

21.3.2 Behavioural Signs

Tortoises do not readily display obvious and highly specific signs of distress. Distressed tortoises may not issue any vocal sounds, even under conditions of severe pain, with the possible exception of a squeak or hiss. The absence of vocalisation, therefore, should not be interpreted as the absence of pain or distress. Tortoises may instead demonstrate distress through increased or decreased activity or by trying to move away from sources of discomfort or to sharply retract their affected limbs. Other indicators include sudden, sharp, withdrawal of the head as far back as possible into the shell and silent gaping with the lower jaw. It is important not confuse this latter sign with one of the signs also associated with respiratory disease, however. Trembling and grating of the jaws is an additional indicator of pain and distress in chelonia (Warwick et al. 2013). These indicators are normally present in cases of acute pain and distress only. In cases of chronic or lower level stress and anxiety, few such obvious behavioural indicators may be present. Instead, otherwise 'normal' behaviours may be extended for unusual periods of time, or manifest in unusual circumstances.

Many different behaviours are associated with specific types of stress and distress. For example, confinement in small enclosures, especially those with transparent walls, frequently results in apparent hyperactivity and patrolling of the perimeter (often resulting in rostral abrasions), whereas exposure to excess temperatures may produce either attempts to burrow beneath the substrate and inactivity or hyperactivity accompanied by salivation, depending on the temperatures involved. Confinement in inadequately sized accommodation can also result in loss of muscle tone, lethargy, and unhealthy weight gain. Similarly, exposure to suboptimum temperatures results in inactivity, inappetence, and over time, weight loss.

21.4 Worldwide Action Plan for Improving Tortoise Welfare

In captivity, priorities for improvement are preventing poor housing conditions, incorrect and inadequate environments, excessive and inappropriate handling, excess intraspecific competition as a result of overcrowding, behavioural incompatibilities as a consequence of inappropriate mixing of species, and lack of environmental enrichment (Ackerman 1997; Jepson 2009). This last factor is frequently overlooked when considering chelonia but nevertheless warrants greater attention. In the largest-ever survey of purchasers of pet tortoises conducted by the Tortoise Trust over 4 years from 2009 to 2013, the provision of completely inadequate housing systems and poor dietary

advice were comprehensively identified as key problem areas (Tortoise Trust 2014). There has been, in the United Kingdom, a move away from leaving tortoises in gardens to manage as best they could in an unsuitable climate, which led to high levels of mortality. However, the more recent trend towards indoor accommodation produces an entirely different set of problems that needs resolution.

The single-largest contributor to welfare problems with these species is probably poor and misleading information on husbandry, both at the point of sale and in outdated or inaccurate information published in books and on the Internet. In the study by the Tortoise Trust, more than 85% of purchasers felt that the advice they received initially on these subjects was both inadequate and misleading. More than 50% of purchasers reported health problems and mortalities that could be attributed to following such advice (Tortoise Trust 2014). Many owners commented that if they had fully understood the housing, environmental, and dietary requirements of tortoises, then they would not have purchased them in the first place. Public education on pet ownership, particularly regarding the requirements of tortoises, is often inadequate, which can generate major welfare (and subsequent rehoming) problems. A related major area of concern is the level of care and advice provided by retailers. Improved training of authorities responsible for pet shops, so that they are better able to assess provision of care for exotic animals, would represent an important step forward.

Bibliography

Ackerman, L. (1997). *The Biology, Husbandry and Health Care of Reptiles*. Neptune City: TFH Publications.

Andreu, A. C (1987). Ecologia dinamica poblacional de la tortuga mora, Testudo graeca, en Donana. Thesis doctoral, University of Seville.

Animal Protection Agency (2012). Environment Audit Committee, House of Commons. Written evidence submitted by the Animal Protection Agency.

AVMA (American Veterinary Medical Association). (2013). AVMA Guidelines for the Euthanasia of Animals: 2013 Edition. Available at https://www.avma.org/KB/Policies/Pages/Euthanasia-Guidelines.aspx. Accessed 7 October 2015.

Bonin, F., Devaux, B., and Dupre, A. (2006). *Turtles of the World*. London: A. C. Black.

Christopher, M.M. (1999). Physical and biochemical abnormalities associated with prolonged entrapment in a desert tortoise. *Journal of Wildlife Diseases* 35: 361–366.

Donoghue, S. and Langenberg, L. (1996). Nutrition. In: *Reptile Medicine and Surgery* (ed. D. Mader), 148–174. Philadelphia: W. B Saunders.

Drake, K.K., Nussear, K.E., Esque, T.C. et al. (2012). Does translocation influence physiological stress in the desert tortoise? *Animal Conservation* doi: 10.1111/j.1469-1795.2012.00549.x.

Fazio, E., Medica, P., Bruschetta, G., and Ferlazzo, A. (2014). Do handling and transport stress influence adrenocortical response in the tortoises (*Testudo hermanni*)? *ISRN Veterinary Science* doi: 10.1155/2014/798273.

Griffiths, C.J., Zuel, N., Tatayah, V. et al. (2012). The welfare implications of using exotic tortoises as ecological replacements. *PLoS One* 7 (6): e39395.

Heatwole, H.F. and Taylor, J. (1987). *Ecology of Reptiles*. New South Wales: Surrey Beatty & Sons, Pty.

Highfield, A.C. (2000). *The Tortoise & Turtle Feeding Manual*. London: Carapace Press.

Highfield, A. C. (2009). A comparative analysis of indoor housing systems for terrestrial tortoises. Tortoise Trust, London. Tortoise Trust Website.

Highfield, A.C. (2010a). *Evaluating Indoor Tortoise Housing for Compliance with the Animal Welfare Act (2006) – Practical Guidelines for Retailers, Trading Standards Officers, Keepers and Animal Welfare Officers*. London: Tortoise Trust & Jill Martin Fund for Tortoise Welfare & Conservation Tortoise Trust Website.

Highfield, A. C. (2010b). Dietary Fibre in the diet of the Herbivorous Tortoise Testudo graeca graeca in Spain: Some implications for captive husbandry. Tortoise Trust Website

Highfield, A. C. (2013). The Tortoise Trust Guide to Tortoises and Turtles. Kindle Edition.

Highfield, A. C. (2014a). The Effect of Basking Lamps on the Health of Captive Tortoises and other Reptiles.

Highfield, A. C. (2014b). The Climate Frame: An innovative outdoor housing system for arid and tropical habitat tortoises. Tortoise Trust Website.

Hutchison, V., Vinegar, A., and Kosh, R. (1966). Critical thermal maxima in turtles. *Herpetologica* 22 (1): 32–41.

Jacobson, E. (2007). *Infectious Diseases and Pathology of Reptiles*. London: CRC Press.

Jepson, L. (2009). *Exotic Animal Medicine*. Saunders Elsevier.

Johlin, J.M. and Moreland, F.B. (1933). Studies of the blood picture of the turtle after complete anoxia. *Journal of Biological Chemistry* 103 (1): 107–114.

Kahn, P.F., Guyer, C., and Mendonca, M.T. (2007). Handling, blood sampling, and temporary captivity do not affect plasma corticosterone or movement patterns of gopher tortoises (*Gopherus polyphemus*). Copeia 3: 614–621.

Kenton, B., Kruger, L., and Woo, M. (1971). Two classes of slowly adapting mechanoreceptor fibres in reptile cutaneous nerve. *Journal of Physiology (London)* 212: 21–44.

Lambert, M.R.K. (1969). Tortoise drain in Morocco. *Oryx* 10: 161–172.

Lance, V.A., Grumbles, J.S., and Rostal, D.C. (2001). Sex differences in plasma corticosterone in desert tortoises, *Gopherus agassizii*, during the reproductive cycle. *The Journal of Experimental Zoology* 289: 285–289.

López-Olvera, J.R., Montane, J., Marco, I. et al. (2003). Effect of venipuncture site on hematologic and serum biochemical parameters in marginated tortoise (*Testudo marginata*). *Journal of Wildlife Diseases* 39: 830–836.

Loveridge, A. and Williams, E.E. (1957). *Revision of the African Tortoises and Turtles of the Suborder Cryptodira*. Cambridge.

MacArthur, S., Wilkinson, R., and Meyer, J. (2004). *Medicine and Surgery of Tortoises and Turtles*, 579. Blackwell Publishing.

MacArthur, S. (2006). Chelonian Anaesthesia and Surgery. Testudo (6): 3.

Mazzotti, S., Pisapia, A., and Fasola, M. (2002). Activity and home range of *Testudo hermanni* in northern Italy. *Amphibia-Reptilia* 23 (3): 305–312.

Milton, S.K. (2008). The physiology and anatomy of anoxia tolerance in the freshwater turtle brain. In: *Biology of Turtles: From Structures to Strategies of Life* (ed. J. Wyneken, M.H. Godfrey and V. Bels), 301–344. CRC Press. Taylor & Francis Group.

Mouden, E., Slimani, E.H., Kaddour, T. et al. (2006). *Testudo graeca graeca* feeding ecology in an arid and overgrazed zone in Morocco. *Journal of Arid Environments* 64 (2006): 422–435.

Ott, J.A., Mendonc, M.T., Guyer, A.C., and Michener, W.K. (2000). Seasonal changes in sex and adrenal steroid hormones of gopher tortoises (*Gopherus polyphemus*). *General and Comparative Endocrinolog* 117: 299–312.

Peterson, C.C. (2002). Temporal, population, and sexual variation in hematocrit of free-living desert tortoises: correlational tests of causal hypotheses. *Canadian Journal of Zoology* 80: 461–470.

Tortoise Trust (2014). *A Report on Pet Tortoise Purchases over a Four Year Period: Health and Welfare Aspects*. London: Tortoise Trust.

TRAFFIC (2012). *Captive-Bred or Wild-Taken? Examples of Possible Illegal Trade in Wild Animals Through Fraudulent Claims of Captive-Breeding*. Cambridge, UK: TRAFFIC International.

Warwick, C., Arena, P., Lindley, S. et al. (2013). Assessing reptile welfare using behavioural criteria. *In Practice* 35: 123–131.

Ornamental Fish (*Actinopterygii*)

22

Lynne Sneddon and David Wolfenden

22.1 History and Context

22.1.1 Natural History

Fish include more than 32 700 discovered species, broadly categorised into three main groups: the jawless hagfish and lampreys; the cartilaginous fish (elasmobranchs including sharks, skates, and rays); and the bony fishes (including the lungfishes, bichirs, sturgeons, gars, and teleosts). The vast majority of pet fish are teleosts (Table 22.1).

Fish have adapted to inhabit a range of freshwater and marine habitats (Andrews et al. 2011; Fishbase 2014), with approximately half of all fish species found within marine habitats, slightly less than half inhabiting freshwater and around 1% of species able to move between the two environments. Most species kept as pets are tropical fish (e.g. coral reef fishes and South American and African freshwater species), with two notable exceptions of goldfish and koi, which are temperate to subtropical fish. Some species can tolerate extreme conditions including very low oxygen levels in stagnant pools (e.g. gouramis and bettas), oxygen supersaturation (e.g. 115% in rock carp, temperatures of −1.8 or 43 °C, hard water (e.g. Rift Valley cichlids), soft, acidic water (e.g. Amazon species), acidic conditions of a pH below 7 (e.g. Amazonian Discus fishes), a

Companion Animal Care and Welfare: The UFAW Companion Animal Handbook,
First Edition. Edited by James Yeates.

Table 22.1 Examples of pet teleost fish families and species.

Family	Example species
Cyprinids or Barbs (Cyprinidae)	Goldfish (*Carassius auratus*)
	Koi carp (*Cyprinus carpio*)
	Zebrafish (*Danio rerio*)
	Tiger barb (*Puntius tetrazona*)
	Ruby barb (*Pethia nigrofasciata*)
	White Cloud Mountain minnow (*Tanichthys albonubes*)
Gouramis (Osphronemidae)	Siamese fighting fish (*Betta splendens*)
	Three spot gourami (*Trichopodus trichopterus*)
	Dwarf gourami (*Trichogaster lalius*)
Cichlids (Cichlidae)	Oscar (*Astronotus ocellatus*)
	Freshwater angelfish (*Pterophyllum* spp.)
	Discus (*Symphysodon* spp.)
Characidae	Neon tetra (*Paracheirodon innesi*)
	Cardinal tetra (*Paracheirodon axelrodi*)
Poeciliidae	Guppy (*Poecilia reticulata*)
	Molly (*Poecilia sphenops*)
Loricariids (Loricariidae)	Common Plecostomus or Suckermouth catfish (*Hypostomus plecostomus*)
Pomacentridae	Common clownfish (*Amphiprion ocellaris*)
	Yellow-tailed damselfish (*Microspathodon chrysurus*)
Gobiidae	Catalina goby (*Lythrypnus dalli*)
Bleniidae	Midas blenny (*Ecsenius midas*)

basic pH above 7 (e.g. Rift Valley cichlids), and high water pressure in deep oceanic trenches (Moyle and Cech 2004).

The behaviour of fish is as equally diverse with some species defending a territory (e.g. freshwater cichlids and marine damselfish), and others existing in large, highly organised groups or shoals (e.g. minnows and other cyprinid fish). Some social groups have a single 'alpha' male in a harem of females (e.g. Mexican mollies [*Poecilia sphenops*]). Many fish are hermaphroditic, with the dominant fish in a pair or group becoming the breeding female and the next highest status fish the breeding male (e.g. clownfish [*Amphiprion* spp.]). Some species form symbiotic relationships with other species, such as with an anemone host (e.g. clownfish) or shrimp that maintain their burrow (e.g. sand gobies), and many marine fish visit cleaner wrasse.

In general, the energy requirements of fish are lower than those of similar sized mammals or birds and most fish have to obtain their vitamin C from their diet. Different species have various feeding strategies. Natural foods include fish (e.g. for marine lionfish), invertebrates such as rotifers and copepods or other zooplankton (e.g. for clownfish), algae, or vegetation (e.g. for tangs or surgeonfish [*Acanthuridae*]) to wood (e.g. for panaques). Some fish feed almost constantly in the wild (e.g. clownfish or tangs), whereas others feed infrequently (e.g. lionfish), often depending on their diet. Some fish are nocturnal hunters or foragers (e.g. some types of catfish). Some are anatomically adapted for surface feeding (e.g. position of the mouth), whereas others forage on or within the substrate. Ammonia and other by-products of digested food are excreted across the gills and in faeces, directly into the water.

22.1.2 Domestic History

Ornamental fish are kept or reared for their visual appeal rather than for any edible or angling qualities. The keeping and breeding of ornamental fish began more than 1000 years ago, and nowadays many fish species are prized for their beauty and distinct markings (e.g. koi carp). Around 1 in 10 households possess pet fish in the United Kingdom (*The Telegraph* 2012) and in the United States (Davenport 1996), and the numbers of individual fish held as companion animals are estimated at up to 20–25 million in aquaria and 20 million in ponds in the United Kingdom alone (PFMA 2014) with some 4000 freshwater and marine species kept as pets or held in public exhibits. Overall, the global trade in ornamental fish is estimated to be worth around GBP£3–4 billion (OATA). The retail values of individual pet fish range from around €1 (e.g. for a guppy) to more than €10 000 (e.g. for a top-quality koi).

Many freshwater species and several marine fish are bred in captivity (Figure 22.1). On average, 90% of freshwater fish species are farmed and 10% collected in the wild; whereas almost 95% of marine species are collected in the wild and just 5% are reared (Oliver 2001, 2003; Sea Shepherd 2012). As a result of captive breeding, various extreme morphologies have been developed by ornamental fish breeders, some of which

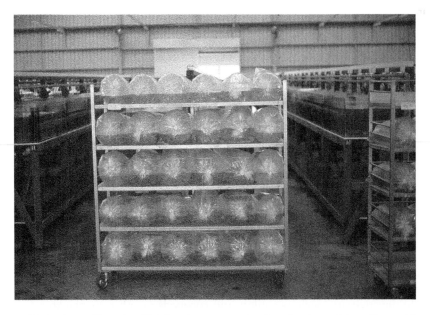

Figure 22.1   Bags of farm-bred fish for air transportation from Southeast Asia to Europe (*Source: courtesy Peter Burgess*).

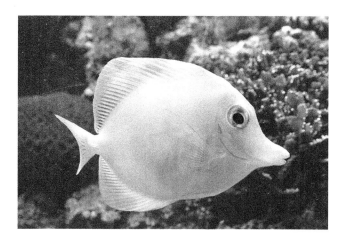

Figure 22.2 Yellow Tang harvested from coral reefs to supply the pet fish market (*Source: courtesy Peter Burgess*).

may compromise welfare, such as fancy 'bubble eye goldfish' (UFAW 2013) and 'balloon' mollies (mollies with stunted body shape and distended abdomens), plus a number of hybridised species have been produced (e.g. the parrot cichlid) for their ornamental appeal.

However, many fish are wild caught and transported from areas such as the Amazon and coral reefs (Walster 2008). Between 40 and 50 million fish annually are imported into the United Kingdom, mainly from South America, Africa, and Indo-Pacific and Caribbean coral reef regions (Sea Shepherd 2012). As one example, thousands of yellow tangs are harvested from coral reefs to supply the pet fish market annually, and an estimated 150 000 yellow tangs (*Zebrasoma flavescens*) were harvested in a single year from Hawaiian coral reefs (Figure 22.2). Mortality rates can be from 1 to 30% in shipments of wild-caught fish (Ploeg 2007), due in part to the often poor conditions under which the fish are held and to the impact of transportation and acclimation stress as the animals pass through various stages in the live-fish chain. Capture of marine fishes can threaten habitat integrity through damage to the environment during capture and reduce the biodiversity of tropical marine ecosystems by reducing the sustainability of native fish populations and reducing the genetic diversity of those populations.

22.2 Principles of Fish Welfare

22.2.1 Suitable Diets

The nutritional requirements of pet fish vary considerably between species (Lewbart 1998). Herbivorous and many omnivorous fish need sufficient plant material in their diet, whereas live foods are essential for many carnivorous fish, and in particular, for rearing marine and freshwater fish fry. Plant material can be provided either as specialist commercially available feeds, including 'plec pellets' (e.g. for freshwater herbivores), or as sushi 'nori' seaweed sheets (e.g. for tangs). Flake formulations can form the main

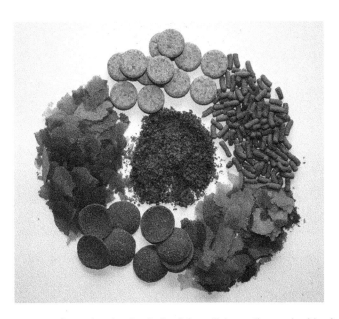

Figure 22.3 Range of popular dry foods for fish in flake, pellet, and tablet forms (*Source:* courtesy Peter Burgess).

diet for many species (Figure 22.3), although supplementary feeds are recommended to add nutritional variety and feeding enrichment. Frozen feeds range from 'staple' diets (e.g. Mysis shrimps) to specialised foods (e.g. containing sponges for marine angelfish) and are generally highly palatable. Some carnivorous fish may be fed whole invertebrate prey, such as rotifers, copepods, and brine shrimp.

The correct quantity of food provision varies between species. Overfeeding can lead to uneaten food decomposing and damaging water quality and the health of the fish. Starvation can occur from owners' failure to provide food, or due to a lack of suitable food; for example, many marine dragonets die in captivity because of lack of appropriate animate foods (Wood and Dakin 2003). Manufacturer's directions are usually set as a rate of percentage body weight (e.g. 1–3% body weight/day) and should be followed, although many owners do not weigh their fish while trying to reproduce the natural diet of the species.

Some commercial diets do not meet the nutritional requirements of many ornamental fish without adequate supplementation; as examples, flakes can lose their water-soluble vitamins rapidly upon introduction to the water and chronic vitamin C deficiency can cause spinal deformities, internal and external haemorrhaging, anaemia, poor growth rate, and increased mortalities (Tacon 1992). Frozen foods can decompose rapidly in air and frozen food should never be used past the expiry date because the free radicals formed during prolonged freezing may be harmful. Incorrect food choices such as feeding fatty red meat are unsuitable and can cause liver damage.

The frequency and manner of provision is also important, and owners should try to replicate the feeding behaviour of the species. In terms of frequency, some fish may benefit from feeding every other day (e.g. lionfish), whereas others usually need regular, small feeds (e.g. planktivorous species and fry). Feeding methods also vary, and multiple feeding methods (e.g. floating and sinking) may be required to suit all the fish kept in a multispecies community tank. Some fish forage, for example in picking algae of rocks or sifting substrate such as sand. Others catch live prey, and some fish and fry respond only to 'animate' food items and can be difficult to wean onto inanimate foods (e.g. marine dragonets [*Synchiropus* spp]). Live brine shrimp can be cultured from dried cysts that hatch in saltwater. Rotifers and copepods can be more difficult to culture, requiring strict cleanliness and precise feeding. However, live foods may lack important nutrients (e.g. fatty acids, Yanong 2001) and wild-harvested live foods risk spreading bacteria (e.g. *Streptococcus*), external parasites (e.g. *Icthyophthirius* and *Epistylis*), or internal parasites (e.g. *Eustronglyides*; microsporidia; *Capillaria*; Yanong 2001). Feeding live 'feeder fish' (e.g. goldfish) to predators (e.g. piranha) is unethical and may additionally cause nutritional deficiencies since commercial diets are supplemented with essential vitamins and minerals.

22.2.2 Suitable Environment

All fish need appropriate space for exercise to maintain adequate stocking densities and to express their full normal behavioural repertoire. For example, sufficient space should be provided to allow nest-guarding species, such as cichlids, to establish a territory. Tanks should also be large enough to accommodate the fish when adult. Smaller tanks can also make it harder to maintain optimal, stable conditions, and water conditions are far more prone to suddenly deteriorate in a small bowl than in a large aquarium. Small goldfish tanks, 'Betta bowls', or novelty enclosures are therefore unsuitable. Some fish can become too large for the average home aquarium (e.g. pacu, iridescent sharks, giant gourami, red tailed catfish, shovel-nosed catfish, common pleco, arowana, high fin banded loach, bala shark, tin foil barb, and sturgeons).

Because of the intimate relationship between fish and their aquatic environment, maintaining optimal water quality is paramount to fish health and welfare. Water quality should be monitored daily in newly set-up tanks and ponds and at least once a week in established systems, and filtration, aeration, and temperature-control equipment should be regularly checked. Effective filtration or regular part-water changes are essential to delivering optimal water conditions for captive fish. Owners should keep a stock of spare equipment and water-treatment products, in case they urgently need to improve water parameters (e.g. pH) or to reduce levels of toxic by-products such as ammonia and nitrite. There are three main methods of filtration: mechanical, biological, and chemical. These respectively facilitate the removal of particulate waste from the water; the conversion of toxic metabolites into less toxic compounds; and the binding or neutralisation of toxins and other undesirable chemicals.

The aim of mechanical filtration is to remove solid waste such as fish faeces and uneaten food. Otherwise, this is broken down by microorganisms, producing toxic products and using up oxygen, potentially leading to suffocation of fish or compromising the biofilter. Solid waste can also allow parasites and pathogenic harmful bacteria to reach dangerous population levels, and organic compounds dissolved in the water can be difficult to remove in recirculating systems (Wheaton 2002). Solid waste can be removed by trapping or settling them, and the resulting waste regularly removed, for example, through rinsing, pressure-washing, backwashing, or siphoning. In marine aquaria (and some large freshwater systems), protein skimming can be employed to attract waste products to air bubbles, forming a foam that is pushed up into a collection cup and removed from the water. Combining the air with ozone (O_3) also helps to breakdown long-chain dissolved organic compounds and (to a certain extent) control pathogen levels. However, O_3 can be extremely dangerous and requires adequate redox (reduction–oxidation) potential control and 'scrubbing' of the air exiting the skimmer to remove residual free ozone.

Biological filtration uses microorganisms to convert toxic chemicals in the water to less toxic forms, and in this sense, biological filters can be thought of as 'biological reactors'. Ammonia from fish and uneaten food can be toxic at below 1 ppm in its unionised form (NH_3), causing damage to the gills and skin, disruption of the fish's haemoglobin, neurological damage, and, indirectly, secondary diseases such as 'fin rot'. The water should be tested regularly and ammonia concentrations kept below 0.1 mg/L. The first step of biological filtration is for ammonia-oxidising bacteria (AOBs) to convert ammonia to nitrite (NO_2^-). This is still toxic at levels under 1 ppm for some fish, leading to 'brown blood disease' or suffocation. Owners should ensure the biofilter is able to maintain nitrite levels below 0.1 ppm or undetectable. In emergency situations, as a last resort, the effects of nitrite poisoning in freshwater fish can usually be alleviated through the addition of salt (sodium chloride) at a concentration of 0.1 g/L while the cause of nitrite in the water is investigated and dealt with.

Nitrite-oxidising bacteria (NOBs) can then convert nitrite to nitrate (NO_3^-). This is less toxic to fish, although sensitivity varies; juvenile stages can be particularly sensitive (Camargo et al. 2005) and prolonged sublethal concentrations may be a chronic stressor. Whilst some fish can develop a tolerance to nitrate, allowing some individuals to survive in concentrations of several hundred parts per million NO_3^-, over 50 ppm NO_3^- should be considered unacceptable, with marine systems housing delicate fish and invertebrates often requiring less than 10 ppm NO_3^-. Nitrate levels can be reduced by limiting nutrient input (i.e. through not overfeeding or overstocking); assimilation into plants in freshwater aquaria and macroalgae (such as *Caulerpa* spp. or *Chaetomorpha* spp.); microbial denitrification or utilising 'live rock' (chunks of coral rubble harbouring various macro- and microorganisms) in marine systems; or water changes. Any water changes should avoid changing more than a third of the total volume to allow fish to slowly become accustomed to the alteration in water quality.

Adding fish to a newly established aquarium or pond can expose them to potentially lethal levels of ammonia because the biological filter needs time to be colonised by microbes. Introducing small numbers of fish gradually can allow sufficient populations of bacteria until ammonia and nitrite are at <0.1 ppm, when more fish may be added, and so on until full stocking density is reached. However, this approach is difficult to manage, requiring regular testing of parameters and water changes, and can risk lethal spikes of ammonia and nitrite. A better means of biofilter establishment is to add inorganic ammonia (e.g. ammonium chloride) until the biofilter can maintain both ammonia and nitrite at <0.1 ppm, even when ammonia is added. At this point, the aquarium or pond is safe for its first small stock of fish. Owners can speed up biofilter development by using commercially available preparations of microorganisms or 'cloning' an established, disease-free filter, but these should not be relied on to instantly mature an aquarium.

Chemical filtration uses specialised media, such as granular activated carbon (GAC), to chemically bind (adsorb) pollutants such as heavy metals and medications. GAC can last up to several weeks depending on the levels of pollutants within the aquarium and the quantity of carbon used and should be discarded and replaced after use. GAC may adsorb free chlorine in the mains water; chlorine in mains tap water can damage fish health and reduce microbial activity. Levels lower than 0.003 ppm should be achieved to prevent long-term chronic effects on the aquarium or pond's inhabitants. Free chlorine gas can also be driven off by aerating the water before use, but chloramine needs to be neutralised using specific water conditioners.

Water should be maintained at the correct 'hardness', with the right levels of metallic ions, for the particular species. For example, breeding discus may need very soft water of around 2°general hardness (GH) and 1°carbonate hardness (CH), whereas Lake Tanganyika cichlids may be kept in hard water of approximately 20°GH and 10°KH. Regional variations in the chemical properties of mains water can be dramatic, and owners may need to alter its hardness. Water can be softened by using resins designed specifically for aquarium use (domestic water softening resins are unsuitable because they introduce sodium into the water) or by adding the water or specific salts to clean, filtered rainwater or reverse-osmosis water by carefully calculating the relative amounts, for example, using 'Pearson's Square' (Figure 22.4). Reverse-osmosis water is virtually devoid of minerals and must never be used by itself for keeping fish because the lack of minerals makes it unable to sustain them. Water can be hardened by adding specific salts, and the use of calcareous media such as coral gravel in the filter, or as a substrate, can help to maintain the hardness at required levels.

Salinity is a measure of the total dissolved salts in water, sometimes expressed as specific gravity. The correct salinity depends on the species, but in general, marine aquaria should be maintained at a stable salinity of around 35‰ and brackish fish such

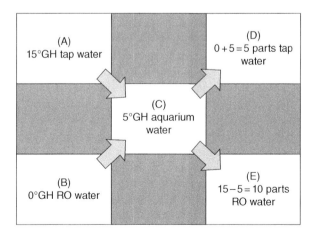

Figure 22.4 Pearson's square to calculate correct mix of (A) Mains and (B) Reverse osmosis (RO) water hardness by calculating (C) the desired GH of the aquarium water; (D) Calculate the proportion of tap water to use (=B+C); (E) the proportion of RO water to use (=A−C), with an example ratio of 1 : 2 tap water to RO.

as scats and mudskippers between 1 and 10‰. Evaporation of freshwater can increase the salinity of marine aquaria to stressful levels by increasing the work needed by the fish to maintain water and salt balance. Salinity or specific gravity may be measured using a refractometer, electronically, or using a hydrometer. Salinity can be decreased by adding freshwater (not saltwater), and stabilised by using automatic freshwater top-up systems or 'osmolators'.

Water should also be kept at the correct pH for the species. Whilst some freshwater community species can adapt well to a range of pH conditions, oceans vary little in their pH, and most off-shore marine fish have a narrow pH tolerance, between pH 7.8 and 8.4. If the pH is significantly outside ideal levels, fish may suffer from acidosis or alkalosis, often affecting their respiratory system and causing skin damage. Because the pH scale is logarithmic, a seemingly small change in pH can have significant physiological effects on fish, so sudden changes should be avoided.

Fish rely on their environment to regulate their body temperature so water temperature has a profound influence on their growth, physiology, immunocompetence, and breeding cycles. In particular, excessively high or low temperatures may cause respiratory distress, osmoregulatory problems, immunosuppression, and a breakdown of the central nervous system. Some temperate freshwater pond fish are able to tolerate temperatures from 4 to 35 °C (e.g. carp and goldfish); whereas tropical marine and freshwater fish are unable to withstand such extremes of temperature, and most commonly kept aquarium fish have a relatively narrow temperature tolerance range. Owners should maintain a stable water temperature, using heaters or chiller units if necessary.

Sufficient dissolved oxygen is crucial for the fish, the biofilter bacteria, and other aerobic organisms within the aquarium or pond. Water contains only 3–5% of the amount present in air and fish in captive conditions are usually kept at higher densities than in the wild, so dissolved oxygen levels can become limiting, with potentially fatal consequences. Low oxygen levels may be a problem in, for example, heavily stocked outdoor ponds in summer with extensive planting or 'green water' caused by algae. Summer weather may lead to particularly low levels because warm water can contain less oxygen, increased fish activity increases their oxygen use, and respiration by plants and algae uses up oxygen. Therefore, increased aeration may be necessary for ponds in summer. Adequate oxygenation is achieved by exposing the water to oxygen from the atmosphere, allowing carbon dioxide to be driven off, and this can be enhanced by turbulence (e.g. using a 'spray bar' or 'airstones'). The oxygen requirements of fish vary, but levels should usually be maintained as close to saturation as possible (which can vary depending on water temperature).

Alongside maintaining good water quality, fish should also be given adequate environmental enrichment that is appropriate for the species concerned, such as rocks, plants, and substrates. This helps ensure adequate mental stimulation and allows fish to express the normal behavioural repertoire for their social interactions and life stage. For any species, owners should consider the fish's natural environment, appropriate company, and life history (e.g. breeding behaviour) and how this can be reproduced in the ornamental aquarium. For example, surgeonfish may use moving brushes that simulate the tactile movement of cleaner wrasse, potentially reducing stress (Soares et al. 2011). Any enrichment and substrates should be kept adequately clean.

However, owners should be careful when altering the aquarium environment and ensure disturbance is minimised. Regular cleaning should be carried out routinely and predictably so the animals may habituate to the disturbance or adapt by taking evasive action. Owners should avoid rearranging aquarium décor once a suitable environment has been created. Similarly, owners should avoid exposing their fish to sudden, loud noises such as banging on the aquarium glass. Fish are particularly sensitive to vibrations and so the use of cleaning tools (vacuums) or the banging of doors in the vicinity of their tank needs consideration. Recent research on rainbow trout in fish farms suggested that playing Mozart continuously improved growth and other indicators of welfare compared to fish held in standard conditions (Papoutsoglou et al. 2013). One possible explanation for these results is that the background noise of the music drowns out sudden noises that may act as fear causing stimuli, so fish exhibit better performance. Transportation and acclimatisation to new environments can also be stressful; for example, journey times of more than 24 hours are stressful for common clownfish (D. Wolfenden et al. personal communication).

22.2.3 Animal Interactions

Fish differ in their social behaviour from territoriality through to a variety of social structures. Aggressive or territorial species can, therefore, bully tank mates and present a chronic stressor resulting in mortality. Unless the tank is especially large, territorial species should be kept as individuals to prevent territory overlap and unnecessarily high rates of aggression. Other fish can form complex relationships, such as cooperative breeding where nonbreeding Lyretail cichlids help raise the offspring of related individuals. Sticklebacks may investigate predators as a group, reducing the risks of individuals being eaten. The selection of tank mates in the aquarium requires consideration of the natural social disposition of the species (e.g. territorial, solitary, or shoaling) and of group composition of group-living species (e.g. providing suitable numbers of males and females and sufficient numbers for shoaling to occur).

Some fish may prefer particular tank mates. For example, adult guppy males can continuously harass females for mating opportunities, and females prefer the company of other females when given a choice (Smith and Sargeant 2006). Female Siamese fighting fish (*Betta*) and angelfish prefer to be with similarly coloured females, although in the angelfish this depended on rearing conditions (Blakeslee et al. 2009; Gomez-Laplaza 2009). Preference for similarly coloured fish may be an anti-predator strategy because similarly coloured individuals may appear as one large fish from a distance or an individual may be less conspicuous in a group if they are same colour or pattern. Some fish also appear able to identify related fish compared with non-relatives, which demonstrates that they form social relationships with others within their species and have the cognitive ability to recognise them (Griffiths and Ward 2011). Conversely, new tank mates may also present a fear stimulus, although gradual stocking can be important to maintain water quality.

In some fish, increasing group size may positively affect natural shoaling behaviour (e.g. neon tetras and white cloud mountain minnows, Sloman et al. 2011). However, aquaria confine fish within a limited space and reduce their ability to avoid one another, which could represent an inescapable stressor. There is debate about how to calculate acceptable numbers of fish. Surface area influences oxygen uptake, and one method is based on total fish length in relation to the surface area of the aquarium. Water volume can influence quality parameters, and another method is based on total fish length (excluding tail) relative to aquarium volume (e.g. $2.5\,cm\,9\,l^{-1}$ for marine fish systems). These calculations are based on adult fish length, so the capacity of the fish to grow needs to be ultimately taken into account. These stocking densities are only guidelines because of factors such as the species and filtration efficiency significantly influence the system's capacity to support life. Such stocking guidelines are also unsuitable for large-bodied fish, which may generate relatively large amounts of waste. Routine testing of the water should be carried out for ammonia, nitrite, nitrate, and pH because these parameters give an absolute indication of the overall health of the system.

Many fish species breed easily in the home tank environment, and breeding fish in captivity can have a positive effect on reducing the capture of wild fish and producing a sustainable supply of fish for the ornamental industry. However, care of the offspring needs in-depth knowledge on the mating and spawning requirements of the adults as well as the nutritional needs of the offspring. Some species such as discus fish form breeding pairs that generally need to be kept in isolation during reproduction and the subsequent guarding of the eggs and fry (the fry feed off the parents' skin mucus). Many 'non-guarder' species provide no parental care and fertilised eggs must be removed immediately as adults can be known to cannibalise young. Other 'guarder' species may care for the eggs and young; and 'bearers' may carry eggs and live young in the mouth, pouch, gills, or are fertilised internally (Moyle and Cech Jr 2004). Breeders should ensure they have in-depth knowledge of the species' specific courtship behaviour, provision of nesting materials, and brooding behaviour.

Keeping fish in a 'community' of mixed species can have various effects. For example, the presence of freshwater angelfish in a tank containing neon tetras, white cloud mountain minnows and tiger barbs can reduce aggression between and within species (Sloman et al. 2011). However, compatibility varies tremendously between fish species. Extremely shy fish are best maintained in a single-species tank and large aggressive predators may be suited only to specialised systems. Larger species may be perceived as predatory by smaller fish and predators should never be held with their prey in small home ornamental aquaria where there is no escape. Knowledge of their social or aggressive behaviour before buying any fish is essential. 'Compatibility charts' can provide a useful guide, although species-specific behaviours should be researched in detail. The choice of marine fish can also depend on whether the system is set up as fish-only, fish only with live rock, or as a true reef aquarium. Similarly, the choice of freshwater fish may depend on whether they are in a 'biotope' aquarium. In general, nonterritorial fish should be allowed to establish themselves before adding a territorial species to reduce the stressful impact of territorial aggression.

One interspecific relationship is the client-cleaner relationship between blue-streak cleaner wrasse which eat the parasites and dead skin off their client fish (Alfieri and Dugatkin 2011). Many fish in the marine environment visit cleaner wrasse at cleaning stations on the reef. These client fish benefit from the smaller cleaner wrasses eating parasites and dead skin from them. Cleaning may also act as tactile stimulation or massage. Surgeonfish were much less stressed when allowed access to a moving brush to allow them to simulate the tactile movement of cleaner wrasse and spent a significantly greater amount of time with the moving brush than an immobile brush (Soares et al. 2011) suggesting a pleasurable or rewarding component.

Fish (particularly marines) are often kept with invertebrate species in community tanks. Some fish form close associations with invertebrates (e.g. goby and shrimp; clownfish and anemone). For example, the common clownfish lives in close contact with anemones, so it is vital when keeping this popular marine fish that anemones are available to allow the fish to perform natural symbiotic behaviours. However, if hungry, some fish species may eat their invertebrate tank mates. Terrestrial pets may also pose a threat to fish. Owners should ensure there is a secure, ventilated lid on tanks to prevent these attacks. Preventing predation can be harder in outdoor ponds where other predators, such as birds, can also be a threat.

22.2.4 Human Interactions

There is no evidence that human companionship benefits fish in aquaria, other than that fish in captivity totally rely on humans for the provision of food and correct environmental conditions. Fish can be stressed or disturbed by humans. Chasing with a net can elicit escape attempts. Emersion in air is acutely stressful with gill collapse, skin desiccation, sudden thermal and light intensity changes, the full effect of gravity on the fish's internal organs and potential suffocation. Fish are sensitive to touch, and damage to the fish's skin can result in loss of mucus and increase the risk of infection.

Fish should be disturbed as little as possible, and human interactions such as netting, capture, and handling need to be kept to a minimum. Capture should be as quick as possible to minimise chase-related stress to the fish and disturbance to other fish. One method to avoid emersion is to use a net to usher the fish into a small glass vessel or beaker containing tank water, which is then used to transport the fish. Fish training is not recommended because of the fragility of these creatures but if carried out should only be by using positive rewards.

22.2.5 Health

A wide variety of diseases can affect pet fish, including viruses (e.g. lymphocystis virus and koi herpes virus); bacteria (e.g. mycobacterial diseases and *Aeromonas* bacteria that cause skin ulcers; Figure 22.5); fungi (e.g. water mould infections such as *Saprolegnia* spp.); protozoa (e.g. whitespot [*Ichthyophthirius*] in freshwater fish and [*Cryptocaryon*] in marine fish); helminths (e.g. skin and gill flukes, tapeworms, and nematode worms), and parasitic crustaceans (e.g. fish lice; anchor worm). Some parasites (e.g. whitespot parasites) have a broad host range and can overwhelm an entire mixed-species community of fish. In the wild, pathogens (bacterial, viral, and parasitic disease causing agents) are normally kept in check by the fish's immune system, so that they rarely cause serious disease or death. However, in captivity, fish are often held at higher stocking densities, exposed to 'exotic' pathogens to which they have no natural immunity, and stressed by transportation, handling, and captive environments, which can reduce their immunity. If untreated, pathogens can rapidly proliferate.

Fish present a limited risk of spreading zoonotic diseases to humans because of the wide taxonomic differences (i.e. teleost to mammal) and environmental barriers (i.e. water to air). The majority of zoonotic diseases from fish are bacterial, most notably mycobacterioses (*Mycobacterium* spp.; Decostere et al. 2004). In humans, fish-borne mycobacterioses are generally restricted to lesions of the hand and generally respond to a prolonged course of antibiotics. Other fish-borne zoonotic bacteria include species of

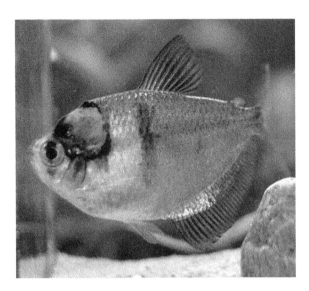

Figure 22.5 Severe ulceration on a black-widow tetra (*Source:* courtesy Peter Burgess).

Salmonella, Aeromonas, and *Staphylococcus.* Care should be taken when handling fish and cleaning tanks, wearing rubber gloves to protect any skin breaches to the hand or arm which represent a possible infection route. Owners should also avoid mouth siphoning.

A key aspect of disease prevention is to keep fish under optimal environmental conditions to maintain good immunity. Routine vaccination of pet fish is not undertaken, and the few suitable vaccines that exist were primarily developed for food fish, notably salmonids. Nets and equipment should be disinfected, for example, with alcohol, proprietary disinfectants or bleach, and then rinsed to remove traces of disinfectant (no chlorine smell) before reuse. Prophylactic treatment may be implemented where appropriate, for example, low doses of copper during the quarantine of marine fish to eradicate certain parasites, and the use of ultraviolet irradiation and ozone.

All new fish should be quarantined before mixing with established stock. Quarantine enables newly acquired fish to be closely monitored for outward signs of disease. If an infectious disease does arise, the fish can then be medicated in isolation. Quarantine may additionally serve as a period of acclimation, for example where new fish need to be slowly adapted to a different set of water parameters, or where wild-caught specimens need to be acclimated to conditions of captivity and perhaps become accustomed to artificial diets. The quarantine unit should be physically isolated from other fish-housing systems to avoid the accidental spread of disease by water droplets or aerosols. The quarantine unit must be of sufficient size to comfortably accommodate the fish and must provide optimal water conditions and filtration. A simple sponge filter may be sufficient for small fish; otherwise quarantine tanks may require a bio-filter prematured in another disease-free aquarium or chemical-filtration media. The quarantine unit also requires basic lighting, aeration, a heater, and thermostat (for tropical species) and enrichment that can be easily sterilised. Water quality needs to be tested regularly and maintained at optimal levels throughout. The length of quarantine should be determined on a case-by-case basis, although 30 days is a sensible minimum.

When disease outbreaks do occur, prompt treatment is vital because some diseases can quickly overwhelm fish. Accurate disease diagnosis usually requires the services of a specialist fish health scientist or veterinary surgeon. Water quality tests should also always form part of any disease investigation because underlying water problems are often a direct or contributory cause of ill health. Currently there are no effective chemical treatments for viral diseases of pet fish, but there are commercial treatments for other pathogen and parasite groups, and most are added to the water notably antibacterials (e.g. oxolinic acid, antibiotics); anti-fungals (e.g. salt, formalin); anti-parasitics (e.g. formalin, salt, copper sulphate); and anthelmintics (e.g. praziquantel). Other forms of treatment include ultraviolet irradiation, ozone, and altering the water temperature (e.g. 30 °C can kill the freshwater whitespot parasite). Several medications (e.g. formalin and copper) have a low safety margin for fish or aquatic invertebrates, so must be used at the correct dose to avoid toxicity. Some fish may not tolerate high temperatures, which may rule out thermal treatments.

Unfortunately, certain diagnostic procedures may themselves stress fish. For example, fish can be damaged during capture and through net abrasion. Gill and skin scrapes (to check for ecto-parasites) will cause localised damage and be painful. Such invasive techniques should therefore be used only where appropriate. Fish can be anaesthetised and given painkilling (i.e. analgesic) drugs to reduce the pain of tissue-damaging diagnostic procedures. However, this requires expert knowledge, and analgesic drugs are mostly not available without veterinary prescription. Some anaesthetics can be bought over the counter, but owners need to adhere to the instructions to avoid overdose and subsequent mortality (Sneddon 2012). Only a few analgesics have been tested in fish, and again only in a handful of species; for example, morphine and lidocaine can reduce pain related responses without side effects in tested species (Sneddon 2012). Many of these drugs are injected into the fish, which would need to be conducted by a veterinarian.

Certain health issues of ornamental fish relate to methods used in their capture and transportation. For example, 80–90% of ornamental marine fish exported from the Philippines were reported as being captured with sodium cyanide (Lecchini et al. 2006), which is a potent toxin to fish and coral communities. Accidental overdoses of chemicals used to stun fish to aid capture and the incidental poisoning of nontarget species are common (Morrissey and Sumich 2012). Fortunately, the practice of cyanide fishing appears to have reduced in recent years. As a result of capture methods and the stress of transportation, mortality rates can be high amongst wild-caught fish (Townsend 2011). Studies on individual shipments of ornamental fish report mortality from less than 1% up to around 30% (Ploeg 2007). For example, around 30% of marine fish caught off the waters of Sri Lanka died during capture, shipping and transfer to stockists in the United Kingdom with up to 75% mortality reported (Morrissey and Sumich 2012). Ideally wild-caught freshwater and marine species should be harvested in a sustainable fashion, using nondestructive techniques that cause minimal harm to both target and nontarget species as well as their environment.

Some ornamental fish are artificially dyed to increase their appeal and market value. Dye colouring is usually an invasive procedure, involving the delivery of dye(s) by injection or tattooing (Fossa 2004). There are anecdotal accounts of high mortalities following dye injection, and injected dyes may cause histological changes within the skin (e.g. glassfish [*Pseudambassis ranga*] Gomez 2012) and may perhaps transmit viruses via the needles (e.g. lymphocystis; Figure 22.6). Such dyeing procedures therefore, could be considered as unacceptable, as are fin cutting and mouth surgery for aesthetic, commercial, or identification purposes.

22.2.6 Euthanasia

The euthanasia of fish can be challenging especially the decision as to whether to humanely kill a fish or not. As discussed, there are many medications to treat fish disease, so the decision to euthanise should be carefully considered. However, where the chances of the fish recovering are poor, euthanasia is necessary to prevent unnecessary suffering. Euthanasia should be performed in two stages. The first is to cause unconsciousness. Hitting the top of the skull, which is composed of soft bone or cartilage in many species, can render the fish immediately unconscious and may also cause brain death. However, this technique should only be conducted by trained, experienced personnel and is impractical for large fish with strong bony plates on their skull (e.g. some catfishes). Anaesthetic overdoses by immersion can take up to 1 hour to be effective, and some anaesthetics may be aversive or irritant if not buffered. For example, zebrafish perceive MS222 and benzocaine as aversive, while 2,2,2 tribromoethanol (TBE) and etomidate are less aversive (Readman et al. 2013). Placing fish in Alka-Seltzer can cause significant pain because of carbon dioxide levels (Mettam et al. 2012), and methods such as flushing fish down the sewer, air suffocation, chilling, or freezing are unacceptable. Fish brains are tolerant of low oxygen and low blood flow, so any method should ensure death. Once all gill movements have ceased for a prolonged period, the second stage of euthanasia is to destroy the brain by pithing or exsanguination (see Table 22.2).

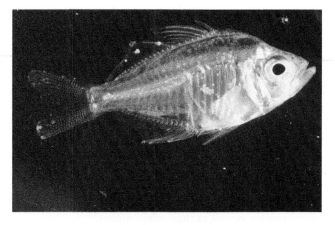

Figure 22.6 Glassfish (*Pseudambassis ranga*) injected with a coloured dye and infected with lymphocystis (the whitish lumps on body and fins) (*Source:* courtesy Peter Burgess).

Table 22.2 Methods of euthanasia of ornamental fish. The method, approach, and welfare issues are identified and whether these are approved by the UK Home Office (fish used in research) and by the American Veterinary Medical Association as being the most humane.

Method		Issues	Approved by UK home office	Approved by AVMA 2013
Immersion in a chemical agent (overdose) that kills the animal	Buffered MS222 or Benzocaine (>250–$500\,\mathrm{mg}\,\mathrm{L}^{-1}$) CO_2 saturated water (use of sodium bicarbonate preparations) Ethanol (95% at 10–30 mL/L) Eugenol, isoeugenol, clove oil (17 mg/L) Isofluorane, sevofluorane (5–20 mg/L) Quinaldine sulfate (>100 mg/L) 2-phenoxyethanol (Aquased, 0.5–0.6 mL/L or 0.3–0.4 mg/L) Metomidate, etomidate (>10 mg/L)	Fish central nervous system is resistant to hypoxia so overdose may not ensure brain death unless animals are left for a long time ~1h CO_2 excites nociceptors and may give rise to pain Effects of ethanol unknown and may be aversive	No; this must be followed by a secondary method such as brain destruction (pithing) or exsanguination (blood loss)	Yes, if fish are left for 10 min with cessation of gill and eye movement Metomidate and etomidate not approved for euthanasia
Overdose followed by secondary method	As above but on cessation of gill and eye movements, a physical method is employed to ensure brain destruction or blood loss	Operator must be trained in secondary techniques as ineffective brain destruction or blood loss may mean fish regain consciousness and experience pain	Yes	Yes

(*Continued*)

Table 22.2 (Continued)

Method		Issues	Approved by UK home office	Approved by AVMA 2013
Physical methods	Decapitation followed by pithing	Operator must be trained in physical techniques as ineffective brain destruction or blood loss may mean fish regain consciousness and experience pain, stress or fear	Yes for methods followed by pithing	Yes
	Cervical transection (severing spinal cord) followed by pithing			
	Cranial concussion followed by pithing			
	Maceration	Maceration involves the use of quickly moving blades to fragment and instantly kill the animal but is only suitable for embryos and larval fish	Maceration only of embryos and small larval fish	
	Rapid chilling at 2–4 °C in small tropical species only (adults left for 10 min; fry >4 d post fertilisation left for 20 min; fry <3 d post fertilisation followed by treatment in sodium or calcium hypochlorite 500 mg/L)	Rapid chilling is not considered humane because ice crystals may form in the tissues and be painful. Studies have shown if fish do not come into actual contact with ice in the anaesthetic bath ice crystal formation is avoided.	Rapid chilling not considered humane	
Unacceptable methods	Flushing into sewer Slow chilling in fridge or freezer Freezing Suffocation in air Caustic chemicals	Potential stress, fear and pain using these methods	No	No

Source: AVMA (2013).

22.3 Signs of Welfare Problems

22.3.1 Pathophysiological Signs

Various pathophysiological signs of various body systems can indicate a variety of health and welfare problems, such as reddening or colour loss of the gills, flared opercula, enhanced opercular beat, or puffing out of the scales (Table 22.3). Any alterations in shape, colour, fin posture, behaviour, and obvious signs of disease are symptoms of welfare problems. However, given the wide diversity of fish, the normal appearance of one species may be abnormal for another.

Table 22.3   Key pathophysiological signs of welfare compromises in ornamental fish.

Body area	Specific symptoms	Potential welfare issues
Surface	Ulcers	Bacterial or viral infection (pre-existing physical or chemical damage may be contributory)
	Haemorrhaging ('bruising')	Bacterial or viral pathogens
		Adverse water conditions
	Scale loss	Handling damage
		Damage by sharp or abrasive object (e.g. rock) within tank or pond
		Damage by other fish, or by fighting
	Distended (scales normal)	'Dropsy'
		Tapeworms
		Female fish with eggs
		Polycystic kidney (goldfish)
		Tumour
	Distended (scales stick out)	'Dropsy'
		Spring Viraemia of Carp virus (in koi)
	Covered in small grey-white spots	Protozoal disease (e.g. *Ichthyophthirius in* freshwater fish; *Cryptocaryon* in marine fish)
	White patches	Bacterial or protozoal disease
	White or light lumps	Virus infection such as lymphocystis or fish pox
	Skin-coloured lumps	Tumour (pigment cell tumour)
		Fluke larvae (under skin)
	Black spots or lumps	Melanoma
		Larval flukes
	Large lump under mouth	Goitre (common in captive sharks)
	Increased mucus production	Pain; stress; disease; water quality
	Altered colour	Stress; disease; water quality

(Continued)

Table 22.3 (Continued)

Body area	Specific symptoms	Potential welfare issues
Fins	Ragged, frayed	Bacterial infection
		Adverse water conditions
	Haemorrhaging	Adverse water conditions
		Viral or bacterial infection
	Milky colour	Bacterial or protozoal infection
Operculum and gills	Mucus trails	Adverse water conditions; gill parasites
	Reddening or loss of colour	Pain; fear; stress; disease; water quality; dietary deficiency; anaemia.
	Increased opercular beat rate	Pain; fear; stress; disease; water quality
	Reduced opercular beat rate	Disease; water quality
	Flared opercula	Stress; disease; water quality
Eyes	Bulge out (= exophthalmia)	Water quality problem
		Bacterial infection
		Vitamin deficiency
	Cloudy (opacity of eye surface or eye lens).	Water quality problem (e.g. chlorine toxicity)
		Bacterial infection
		Vitamin A deficiency.
		Eye fluke (causing cataracts)
		Physical damage (e.g. handling abrasion)
		Ultraviolet light damage (causing cataracts)
	Missing	Fighting
		Physical injury.
Vent	Stringy faeces	Nutritional problem
		Gut infection

Challenges to the fish's physiological balance can result in a stress response that is strikingly similar to that of mammals, whether environmental (e.g. adverse water conditions; extremes of temperature; aggression by tank-mates), biological (e.g. disease), or perceived (e.g. disturbances by the owner). Activation of the sympathetic nervous system results in the release of various hormones, including adrenaline and noradrenaline from the chromaffin tissue around the kidney and corticosteroids from the hypothalamus-pituitary-interrenal axis (HPI; Figure 22.7). Adrenaline and noradrenaline increase heart rate and blood pressure alongside an increase in blood glucose concentration and metabolism as a result of increased cortisol that prepares the animal for action and is commonly known as the 'fight-or-flight' response. These hormones can also trigger a second phase of the stress response (Pottinger 2008). This involves rapid physiological

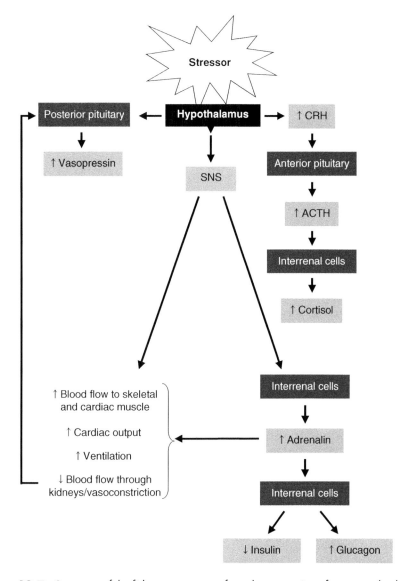

Figure 22.7 Summary of the fish stress response from the perception of a stressor by the brain to cortisol production by interrenal cells. ACTH = adrenocorticotropic hormone; CRH = corticotropin-releasing hormone; SNS = sympathetic nervous system.

changes, including an increased respiratory rate, increased vasodilation to maximise blood flow to the gills, and increased stroke volume of the heart. These effects, coupled with mobilisation of fat and carbohydrate stores and increased alertness, prime the fish for immediate action (Wendelaar-Bonga 1997).

If stressors are experienced for an extended period of time, or severely stressful experiences are encountered frequently, a tertiary stress response can be initiated

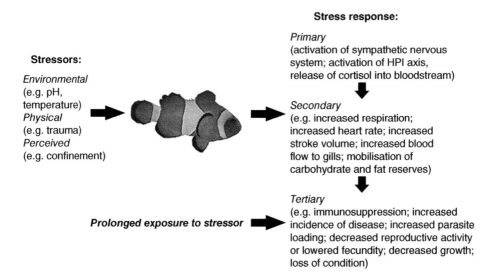

Stressors:

Environmental
(e.g. pH,
temperature)
Physical
(e.g. trauma)
Perceived
(e.g. confinement)

Stress response:

Primary
(activation of sympathetic nervous
system; activation of HPI axis,
release of cortisol into bloodstream)

Secondary
(e.g. increased respiration;
increased heart rate; increased
stroke volume; increased blood
flow to gills; mobilisation of
carbohydrate and fat reserves)

Tertiary
(e.g. immunosuppression; increased
incidence of disease; increased parasite
loading; decreased reproductive activity
or lowered fecundity; decreased growth;
loss of condition)

Prolonged exposure to stressor

Figure 22.8 Summary of the teleost primary, secondary, and tertiary stress responses.
HPI = hypothalamus-pituitary interrenal.

(Figure 22.8). Prolonged rises in cortisol and catecholamines can suppress growth, reproduction, and the immune system, which can lead to further diseases. Chronically stressed fish may therefore show a general lack of condition, reduced growth and reproduction, and increased risk of parasitic and other diseases (Conte 2004). The tertiary response may also cause pronounced changes in the ability of the fish to osmoregulate because of the influence of stress hormones on gill, and possibly skin, permeability (Wendelaar-Bonga 1997; Barton 2002; Pottinger 2008).

22.3.2 Behavioural Signs

A variety of behavioural signs can indicate problems (Table 22.4). Common behavioural responses to disease or stress include a change in activity including increased swimming activity, restlessness, or hyperactivity. However, poor welfare can also be indicated by reduced activity, for example, fish resting on the substrate or hovering for long periods (Sneddon 2009, 2011). This may often be accompanied by a reduced feeding response or anorexia where fish show no interest in food or altered behaviour during feeding, and this is frequently one of the first behavioural signs of stress. In shoaling species, diseased or injured individuals may be ostracised from the group or swim away from the others and are often behaviourally unresponsive to external stimuli such as disturbance to the tank.

   In the short term, acute pain may be indicated by fish tending to avoid feeding, cease engaging in normal behaviour, or exhibiting anomalous behaviours and enhanced physiological responses. For example, zebrafish substantially reduce activity when subject to injection of acetic acid or tail fin clipping and have an enhanced opercular (gill cover) beat rate (Reilly et al. 2008; Maximino 2011). In acetic acid tests where mild acid in injected subcutaneously, fish may perform pain-related behaviours for 3 to 6 hours

Table 22.4 Key behavioural signs of welfare compromises in ornamental fish.

Aspect of behaviour	Specific responses	Potential welfare issues
Swimming	Abnormal sinking or floating	Water quality; disease
	Flashing where fish rub their sides against solid object	Disease; water quality
	Flashing at surface where fish show the flanks in an erratic manner	Fear; stress
	Erratic bursts followed by periods of inactivity	Pain; fear; stress; disease; water quality
	Hovering	Pain; fear; stress; disease; water quality
	Darting	Fear; stress; water quality
Activity (excluding feeding)	Reduced (periods of inactivity and freezing)	Pain; fear; stress; disease
	Increased	Pain; fear; stress; disease; water quality
Feeding	Reduced or absent	Pain; fear; stress; disease; water quality
Abnormal behaviour	Repeated body rubbing against substrate or solid objects; repeated fin twitching	Pain; fear; stress; disease; water quality; skin parasites
	Rocking on substrate	Pain
	Tail wafting	Pain
	Head shaking	Pain
	Surface piping, gasping; fast opercular beats	Stress; disease; water quality; low dissolved oxygen level (environmental hypoxia); gill disease or damage; nitrite poisoning
Posture and position	Altered fin posture	Stress; disease; water quality
	Buoyancy problems (e.g. float to surface; sink to substrate) or nonupright swimming	Swim-bladder hyperinflation or collapse
Altered habitat use	Use of crevices and overhangs more than normal	Fear; stress
	Reduced shoaling where individual(s) swim away from the group	Stress; disease; water quality
Unresponsive to external stimuli	Easy to net, no response to disturbance	Pain; stress; disease; water quality

(Sneddon 2009, 2011). Fin clipping (for identification purposes) in fish resulted in altered behaviour for up to 24 hours afterwards (Roques et al. 2010). Fish injected with vaccines in an adjuvant that causes internal tissue damage showed reduced interest in food and decreased activity for 3 days after vaccination (Bjorge et al. 2011). This indicates potential longer term pain in fish.

Fear or anxiety may be indicated by behaviours such as avoidance of new objects. Fish may swim at the tank's walls rather than the middle of the tank or sink to the bottom of the tank for prolonged periods. In some cases fish may start swimming fast and then dive to the bottom. Excessive darting and flashing of the flank (swimming where the side of the fish is shown) are general signs of stress or increased anxiety. Escape attempts, freezing, and other natural anti-predator behaviours may also indicate the fish perceives a threat (Sneddon 2013). Hiding in crevices or within tank furniture may also indicate fear, although it may also be normal in crepuscular species or may be related to spawning activity.

Abnormal behaviours include rocking on the substrate; tail wafting; rubbing of mouth, opercula or body; and head shaking. Fish may show abnormal swimming patterns, including stereotyped route-pacing or swimming in an unnatural posture (e.g. floating, head down, or lying on one side); difficulty maintaining an upright position (poor equilibrium). Fish may gasp (or 'pipe') at the surface to obtain additional oxygen. However, given the wide diversity of fish, the normal behaviour for one species may be abnormal for another. For example, marine shrimpfishes naturally swim in a vertical, head-down, posture, but for most other fish, this would a clear sign of ill health. Similarly, the behaviour and appearance of a fish may alter significantly with age and during breeding times. Owners should therefore identify what is normal for the individual. Given that many owners buy ornamental fish to watch them, they should be ideally placed to detect any changes in their normal behaviour.

22.4 Action Plan for Improving Animal Welfare in Fish Worldwide

Fish are relatively inexpensive pets (some species retail for around €1 per animal), and generally speaking any adult can purchase aquarium or pond fish. Prospective owners may know absolutely nothing about keeping fish save that they require water and food. The diversity of fish species means that their care requires comprehensive knowledge of the species-specific requirements and regular monitoring of water quality, equipment, and fish health. However, this is rarely the case, and such failure can result in serious welfare problems. Anyone contemplating buying an aquarium requires access to good sources of information of the fish that they plan to keep. There is a paucity of aquatics training courses for amateur fish keepers, and this is something that needs to be addressed.

Unfortunately, the low retail cost of some pet fish may make them seem dispensable in some people's minds. However, owners might be encouraged to provide better care in their own interests. In ornamental aquaria and ponds, healthy fish display bright colours, interesting behaviours, and provide many years (up to 43 years in goldfish) of pleasure to the owner. In comparison, sick fish in poor condition provide little satisfaction because their colouration becomes dull, fins droop, and they become unresponsive to external stimuli displaying lethargy or restlessness. Reputable pet and aquatics stores should take time to enquire about and advise new customers on tank size, water conditions and any other factors relevant to the fish species being sought.

Training in fish care and welfare is also needed for those involved in the fish industry, including Internet traders (in some cases shop staff are required to obtain fish husbandry and health qualifications). For example, many ornamental fish importers and aquatics retail shops routinely quarantine new stock, but unfortunately this is not universal. Ideally pet shops should also be inspected and licensed, with properly accredited aquatics training programmes for pet store inspectors. At a higher level, better policing of the global pet fish industry should be considered, with internationally agreed standards of husbandry and welfare that are based on good practice. These proposals will require the education of politicians and law enforcement agencies.

Despite fish probably being the most 'populous' pet in terms of numbers of individual pet fish (PFMA 2014), pet fish are rarely presented as patients at veterinary clinics. Consequently, disease diagnosis is often limited to the owner's 'best-guess' based on any outward symptoms (e.g. visible spots, ulcers) and occasionally techniques such as mucus or skin scrapes. In contrast to most other pets, post-mortems and other disease diagnostic services are rarely undertaken on pet fish, except in the case of high-value species such as koi carp. This may be partly because of the challenges associated with presenting a fish patient at a veterinary surgery. However, it may also be the result of the relative costs of veterinary services compared to the purchase cost of the fish (except koi and some aquarium species). The situation is exacerbated by lack of fish specialist veterinary surgeons and general lack of fish medicine knowledge within the profession. Better undergraduate and more widely available postgraduate fish medicine courses are needed.

There is also a need for more veterinary research. For example, further research into the most effective dosages and administration routes for pain killers, including dosing by dissolving drugs in the tank water. More generally, there is a need for more research in fish pain across a wider number of species, beyond those of aquaculture importance (e.g. Atlantic salmon, rainbow trout, and tilapia); goldfish, koi carp, and zebrafish are the few that have behavioural and physiological indicators identified. These examples suggest that behavioural responses are species-specific, so each species need to be individually assessed for its repertoire of pain-related behaviours. Studies are also needed to investigate chronically painful situations such as large skin lesions.

Legislation could be used to address three issues. The first to consider a ban on the trade in mutilated pet fish, such as those who have been dye- or dye-injected or undergone 'cosmetic' surgery. These are done for aesthetic and commercial reasons, particularly in parts of Asia. Occasionally, mutilated pet fish are exported to other countries, and there should be legislation against the trade in such animals. More controversial and difficult to achieve would be a ban on trade in certain 'man-made', artificially selected strains that are of welfare concern (e.g. celestial eyed goldfish; scoliotic parrot cichlid hybrids; balloon mollies that experience swimming problems due to unnatural body shape). Restrictions on the import of unsuitable species that grow too large for the home aquaria should be considered. Species to be avoided include pacu, giant gourami, large catfish species (e.g. *Pangassius*, red tailed catfish and shovel-nosed catfish), common pleco, arowana, high fin banded loach, bala shark, tin foil barb, and sturgeons. These fish grow too large and either die prematurely or end up being rehomed, where possible, at public aquaria. The international ornamental fish industry should be encouraged to regulate and restrict the trade in large 'problem' species.

International regulation and voluntary cooperation is also necessary if the aim is to improve the capture and trade of wild fish. By developing sustainable breeding programmes in the importer's country, it is possible to circumvent many of these problems and reduce length of transport and sustain natural populations thereby improving both native and captive-bred fish welfare. If fish are wild-caught, ideally they should be harvested in a sustainable fashion, using nondestructive techniques that cause minimal harm to the target, as well as nontarget, species and their environment. Additional political and public will for making such improvements may come from environmental concerns. Improvements in wild capture may reduce damage to the environment and maintain the biodiversity of tropical marine ecosystems. At the very least, there is a commercial reason to ensure sustainability of natural fish populations.

Bibliography

Alfieri, M.S. and Dugatkin, L.A. (2011). Cooperation and cognition in fishes. In: *Fish Cognition and Behavior*, 2e (ed. C. Brown, K. Laland and J. Krause), 258–276. Oxford: Wiley Blackwell.

Andrews, C., Exell, A., and Carrington, N. (2011). *The Manual of Fish Health*. Surrey: Interpet Ltd.

AVMA (American Veterinary Medical Association). (2013). AVMA Guidelines for the Euthanasia of Animals: 2013 Edition. Available at https://www.avma.org/KB/Policies/Pages/Euthanasia-Guidelines.aspx. Accessed 7 October 2015.

Barton, B. (2002). Stress in fishes: a diversity of responses with particular references to changes in circulating corticosteroids. *Integrative and Comparative Biology* 42: 517–525.

Bjorge, M.H., Nordgreen, J., Janczak, A.M. et al. (2011). Behavioural changes following intraperitoneal vaccination in Atlantic salmon (*Salmo salar*). *Applied Animal Behaviour Science* 133: 127–135.

Blakeslee, C., McRobert, S.P., Brown, A.C., and Clotfelter, E.D. (2009). The effect of body coloration and group size on social partner preferences in female fighting fish (*Betta splendens*). *Behavioural Processes* 80: 157–161.

Branson, E.J. (ed.) (2008). *Fish Welfare*. Oxford: Blackwell Publishing.

Brown, C., Laland, K., and Krause, J. (eds.) (2011). *Fish Cognition and Behavior*, 2e. Oxford: Wiley Blackwell.

Camargo, J.A., Alonso, A., and Salamanca, A. (2005). Nitrate toxicity to aquatic animals: a review with new data for freshwater invertebrates. *Chemosphere* 58: 1255–1267.

Conte, F.S. (2004). Stress and the welfare of cultured fish. *Applied Animal Behaviour Science* 86: 205–223.

Davenport, K.E. (1996). Characteristics of the current international trade in ornamental fish, with special reference to the European Union. *Revue Scientifiqueet Technique de l'Office International des Epizooties* 15: 435–443.

Decostere, A., Hermans, K., and Haesebrouk, F. (2004). Piscine mycobacteriosis: a literature review covering the agent and the disease it causes in fish and humans. *Veterinary Microbiology* 99: 159–166.

Fishbase (2014). Available on http://fishbase.org (retrieved 2 September 2014)

Fossa, S.A. (2004). Man-made fish: domesticated fishes and their place in the aquatic trade and hobby. *OFI Journal* 44: 1–19.

Gomez, S. (2012). Histological lesions induced by exogenous pigment in dyed Indian glass-fish, *Pseudambassis ranga* (Hamilton). *Journal of Fish Diseases* 35: 953–954.

Gomez-Laplaza, L.M. (2009). Recent social environment affects colour-assortative shoaling in juvenile angelfish (*Pterophyllum scalare*). *Behavioural Processes* 82: 39–44.

Griffiths, S.W. and Ward, A. (2011). Social recognition of conspecifics. In: *Fish Cognition and Behavior*, 2e (ed. C. Brown, K. Laland and J. Krause), 186–216. Oxford: Wiley Blackwell.

Lecchini, D., Polti, S., Nakamura, Y. et al. (2006). New perspectives on aquarium fish trade. *Fisheries Science* 72: 40–47.

Lewbart, G.A. (1998). Clinical nutrition of ornamental fish. *Seminars in Avian and Exotic Pet Medicine* 7: 154–158.

Maximino, C. (2011). Modulation of nociceptive-like behavior in zebrafish (*Danio rerio*) by environmental stressors. *Psychology and Neuroscience* 4: 149–155.

Mettam, J.J., McCrohan, C.R., and Sneddon, L.U. (2012). Characterisation of chemosensory trigeminal receptors in the rainbow trout, *Oncorhynchus mykiss*: responses to chemical irritants and carbon dioxide. *Journal of Experimental Biology* 215: 685–693.

Morrissey, J.F. and Sumich, J.L. (2012). *Introduction to the Biology of Marine Life*, 10e. London: Jones and Bartlett Learning International.

Moyle, P.B. and Cech, J.J. Jr. (2004). *Fishes: An Introduction to Ichthyology*, 5e. London: Pearson.

Papoutsoglou, S.E., Karakatsouli, N., Skouradakis, C. et al. (2013). Effect of musical stimuli and white noise on rainbow trout (*Oncorhynchus mykiss*) growth and physiology in recirculating water conditions. *Aquacultural Engineering* 55: 16–22.

Oliver, K. (2001) *The ornamental fish market*. FAO/GLOBEFISH Research Programme, Volume 67, FAO, Rome.

Oliver, K. (2003). World trade in ornamental species. In: *Collection, Culture and Conservation* (ed. J.C. Cato and C.L. Brown), 49–64. Iowa: Blackwell Publishing.

PFMA (2014). Available at https://www.pfma.org.uk/pet-population-2014. Accessed 24 August 2018.

Ploeg, A. (2007). Facts on in shipments of ornamental fish. In: *International Transport of Live Fish in the Ornamental Aquatic Industry* (ed. A. Ploeg, S.A. Fossa, G. Bassler, et al.), 115–122. Montfoort, The Netherlands: Ornamental Fish International.

Pottinger, T.G. (2008). The stress response in fish – mechanisms, effects and measurement. In: *Fish Welfare* (ed. E.J. Branson), 32–48. Oxford: Blackwell Publishing.

Readman, G.D., Owen, S.F., Murrell, J.C., and Knowles, T.G. (2013). Do fish perceive Anaesthetics as aversive? *PLOS One* doi: 10.1371/journal.pone.0073773.

Reilly, S.C., Quinn, J.P., Cossins, A.R., and Sneddon, L.U. (2008). Behavioural analysis of a nociceptive event in fish: comparisons between three species demonstrate specific responses. *Applied Animal Behaviour Science* 114: 248–259.

Roques, J.A.C., Abbink, W., Geurds, F. et al. (2010). Tailfin clipping, a painful procedure: studies on Nile tilapia and common carp. *Physiology & Behavior* 101: 533–540.

Sea Shepherd (2012). https://seashepherd.org/2012/11/24/wildlife-species-are-a-public-trust-not-disposable-trinkets.

Sloman, K.A., Baldwin, L., McMahon, S., and Snellgrove, D. (2011). The effects of mixed-species assemblage on the behaviour and welfare of fish held in home aquaria. *Applied Animal Behaviour Science* 135: 160–168.

Smith, C.C. and Sargent, R.C. (2006). Female fitness declines with increasing female density but not male harassment in the western mosquitofish, *Gambusia affinis*. *Animal Behaviour* 71: 401–407.

Sneddon, L.U. (2009). Pain perception in fish: indicators and endpoints. *Institute for Laboratory Animal Research Journal* 50: 338–342.

Sneddon, L.U. (2011). Pain perception in fish: evidence and implications for the use of fish. *Journal of Consciousness Studies* 18: 209–229.

Sneddon, L.U. (2012). Clinical anesthesia and analgesia in fish. *Journal of Exotic Pet Medicine* 21: 32–43.

Sneddon, L.U. (2013). Do painful sensations and fear exist in fish? In: *Animal Suffering: From Law to Science* (ed. T. Auffret Van Der Kemp and M. Lachance), 93–112. Toronto: Carswell.

Soares, M.C., Oliveira, R.F., Ros, A.F.H. et al. (2011). Tactile stimulation lowers stress in fish. *Nature Communications* doi: 10.1038/ncomms1547.

Tacon, A.G. (1992). *Nutritional Fish Pathology. Morphological Signs of Nutrient Deficiency and Toxicity in Farmed Fish*, FAO Fisheries Technical Paper, vol. 330, 75. Rome: Food and Agriculture Organization.

The Telegraph (2012). One in ten Britons now have pet fish. Available at https://www.telegraph.co.uk/lifestyle/pets/9217643/One-in-ten-Britons-now-have-pet-fish.html. Accessed 2 September 2014.

Townsend, D. (2011). Sustainability, equity and welfare: a review of the tropical marine ornamental fish trade. *SPC Live Reef Fish Information Bulletin* 20: 2–12.

UFAW (2013). Genetic welfare problems of companion animals an information resource for prospective pet owners. Available at https://www.ufaw.org.uk/fish/fish. Accessed 2 September 2014.

Walster, C. (2008). The Welfare of Ornamental Fish. In: *Fish Welfare* (ed. E.J. Branson), 271–290. Oxford, UK: Blackwell.

Wendelaar-Bonga, S.E. (1997). The stress response in fish. *Physiological Reviews* 77: 591–625.

Wheaton, F. (2002) Recirculating aquaculture systems: an overview of waste management. In: Proceedings of the Fourth International Conference on Recirculating Aquaculture, eds. MB Timmons JM Ebeling, FW Wheaton, ST Summerfelt, BH Vinci. Virginia Polytechnic and State University, Sea Grant Program. Blacksburg, Virginia, pp. 57–68.

Wood, E. and Dakin, N. (2003). *The Responsible Marine Aquarist*. Ross-on-Wye, Hereford: Marine Conservation Society.

Yanong, R.P.E. (2001). Nutritional disorders. In: *BSAVA Manual of Ornamental Fish*, 2e (ed. W.H. Wildgoose), 225–231. Gloucester: British Small Animal Veterinary Association.

Goldfish (*Carassius auratus*)

23

Culum Brown, David Wolfenden, and Lynne Sneddon

23.1 History and Context

23.1.1 Natural History

Goldfish (*Carassius auratus*) are members of the cyprinid family (carp and their relatives). They originated in Southeast Asia, although the cyprinid family covers a far wider global range. Because of accidental and deliberate introduction into the wild (Angeler et al. 2002), goldfish are now found worldwide, with a few exceptions such as Greenland and Antarctica. *C. auratus* are classified as least concern (IUCN 2015).

Goldfish are usually considered a temperate water fish; however, they may survive in temperatures below 10 °C and up to 30 °C. Collectively, their broad environmental tolerances mean that they can be found inhabiting a very wide range of habitats. Their natural diet is very varied, with wild goldfish eating anything from terrestrial insects to vegetation to detritus (Richardson et al. 1995; Pinto et al. 2005). Goldfish show a variety of social behaviours and are often found in the company of other goldfish (Pitcher and Magurran 1983). Breeding typically occurs in spring, and males chase and court gravid females. Mate attraction and species recognition involves pheromones (Sisler and Sorensen 2008). Females lay eggs in aquatic vegetation, and the eggs are

Companion Animal Care and Welfare: The UFAW Companion Animal Handbook,
First Edition. Edited by James Yeates.

adhesive and hatch in 2 to 3 days. Under optimal conditions, fry grow rapidly and can be sexually mature within a year. In captivity, goldfish typically live for 5–10 years, but in large ponds they can live for up to 30 years. The oldest goldfish on record died aged 43.

As shallow water fish, goldfish vision is most sensitive to red, green, blue, and ultraviolet wavelengths (Neumeyer 1992). Their vision often corresponds best to vertical orientated stimuli, e.g. aquatic vegetation (Mednick and Springer 1988; Warburton 1990). Goldfish can differentiate certain shapes, colours, and sounds (e.g. Wyzisk and Neumeyer 2007; Shinozuka et al. 2013) and can remember associations for as long as a year (Brown et al. 2006), which can help foraging in anti-predator behaviour (Brown et al. 2011). They can also sense vibration, and their hearing capabilities are sensitive across a broad range of frequencies (Fay and Popper 1974). Goldfish can also detect different odours in the water, which they can use to find food, avoid predators, or preferentially associate with one another (Sisler and Sorensen 2008). Their skin cells can release an alarm substance when the skin is damaged that prompts other goldfish to display anti-predator responses such as shoaling or reduced feeding (Zhao and Chivers 2005; Brown and Laland 2011).

23.1.2 Domestic History

Goldfish were originally kept in China at least 2000 years ago, where they were primarily raised as food fish. By around 800 CE, rearing the orange (gold) morph in ponds became commonplace and goldfish had an important role in Chinese culture. Goldfish were exported to Japan and then to Portugal and the rest of Europe (Brewster and Fletcher 2004). Goldfish are also used in laboratory research (e.g. to study memory, Rodríguez et al. 2006). Once goldfish were being reared indoors, a number of morphs were produced through selective breeding (Zhen 1988). Today, more than 120 varieties exist which vary in their shape, colours, fin structure, and the morphology of their eyes (Komiyama et al. 2009), including the 'comet' variety, which closely resembles the wild type. Various extreme morphologies have been developed, such as 'bubble eye' goldfish, selected for large sacs under each eye (UFAW 2013). Many, if not all, of these lines can revert to wild type in just a few generations after being released to the wild.

23.2 Principles of Fish Welfare

23.2.1 Diet

Goldfish are generalist omnivores and eat a range of food varieties, from insects to plants. A balanced diet can be provided with some standard commercial flake and pellet foods, with other food types added. As a rule of thumb, goldfish should be fed only as much as they can eat in a few minutes, so that the breakdown of additional food does not cause nitrates, nitrites, and ammonia to build up in the water, which can cause irreversible gill and other damage.

Goldfish are motivated to forage amongst substrates and aquatic vegetation. They appear to forage more in sandy substrates than gravel, pebbles, or cobbles, suggesting that these latter substrates are less suitable (Smith and Gray 2011). The addition of live food such as mosquito larvae or bloodworms can be a source of additional enrichment for the fish. Goldfish can rapidly learn the time and place of feeding (Gee et al. 1994) and may show signs of anticipation when it is meal time, for example looking at their owner and waiting in a designated feeding area. They therefore respond well to routine, so long as it is maintained. This learning can also allow owners to train goldfish to feed themselves, for example using 'demand feeders' that deliver food when a submerged lever is nudged by the fish.

23.2.2 Environment

All goldfish need adequate space for shoaling, keeping adequate distances between individuals, maintaining adequate water quality, and allowing all goldfish to reach their full size potential. This requires ponds and aquaria to be many times the expected adult sizes, depending on the number of fish kept together. Common goldfish can reach as much as 60 cm in length in suitable conditions (Orme 1991). Tanks and ponds should be secure and situated so as to ensure that the fish cannot escape into nearby waterbodies during floods.

Although goldfish may tolerate some variation in water parameters, poor water quality can be fatal, and some fancy varieties are at particular risk. It is better to perform small, frequent water changes than change all the water together to avoid causing chemical or thermal shock. The volume and frequency of water changes depend on the water quality, and owners should measure water parameters regularly and carefully using standard aquarium test kits (Table 23.1), particularly in small aquaria where the water quality can quickly deteriorate. Any new water should be dechlorinated before being added to the tank because excessive chlorine can be toxic. Goldfish are relatively resilient to changes in salinity, but acute exposure to high salt concentrations can result in high mortality.

Goldfish may be kept indoors or outdoors, although optimal temperature ranges depend on the strain. As examples, outdoor ponds may be suitable for comet variety goldfish even in cool climates, whereas some 'fancy' fish are less hardy. Similarly, although goldfish may survive in low dissolved oxygen levels, this is unsuitable. Goldfish may obtain additional oxygen by gulping air at the water surface. Full spectrum lighting designed for shallow, tropical species normally suit goldfish, although too much light, particularly direct sunlight, can encourage algal growth. Prolonged exposure to noise can result in hearing loss and high levels of stress (Smith et al. 2004). Indoor goldfish

Table 23.1 Ideal aquarium water quality conditions for goldfish.

Ammonia	<0.1 ppm
Nitrite	<0.1 ppm
Nitrate	<75 ppm
pH	6.5–7.5
KH	70–140 ppm
GH	150 ppm
Temp	18–24 °C

tanks should therefore be kept in places that are relatively free from loud noises, particularly repeated tapping on the glass by people or disturbance by pets.

Tank substrates should be provided to meet behavioural needs for manipulation and foraging, such as appropriate freshwater sand. The manipulation of sifting the sand with their mouths may be a behavioural need, which cannot be fulfilled with larger pebbles or cobbles (Smith and Gray 2011). Substrates and sediments should be kept clean, particularly to remove debris from gravel and to prevent anaerobic fauna development in sand. Sand is a compact substrate but is prone to becoming anaerobic, which can cause problems in aquarium hygiene if not kept clean. Sufficient live aquatic vegetation may be provided, but plant cover should not exceed 50% of the area of the aquarium. Goldfish often dig plants up while they are searching for food, so plants should be given time to become established before any fish are introduced. Care should be taken not to uproot plants during cleaning.

In consideration of the relatively complex cognitive abilities goldfish display, their environment should allow for expression of natural behaviour. However, some degree of familiarity may allow fish to adapt to their environment (Pitcher and Magurran 1983) and avoid fear of novelty.

When transporting goldfish, care should be taken to minimise thermal and physical disturbances. Goldfish are often sold and transported in small plastic bags (Figure 23.1). These risk being shaken, cooling, and being located next to sources of fear such as other pets such as dogs or cats. In addition, leaving goldfish too long in the transportation container can lead to changes in water quality such as deoxygenation and a build up of ammonia. Following transportation, goldfish need to be acclimatised to the water into which they will be put, to avoid any sudden thermal or other shocks.

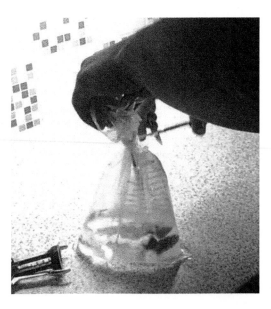

Figure 23.1   A fish in a small transportation bag (this fish was then swallowed whole, leading to a successful animal welfare prosecution) (*Source:* Courtesy RSPCA.)

23.2.3 Animal Company

Goldfish are motivated to shoal and may form schools in large ponds. The strength of this motivation is shown by the fact that, in one study, goldfish would pay a cost (receiving electric shocks) to access the social company of another goldfish (Dunlop et al. 2006). Moreover, isolation stress can interfere with memory formation (Laudien et al. 1986). Apart from being a natural defence against predators, shoaling has other benefits. Larger shoals are more likely to discover the location of new foraging patches because they are able to copy the behaviour of their shoal mates (Pitcher et al. 1982). The behaviour of one fish on finding food attracts others to the location.

However, although goldfish tend not to be aggressive to one another, owners should ensure that fish are compatible and avoid environmental challenges such as overcrowding that may lead to aggression. Maintaining stable groups of familiar tank mates may also reduce the potential for stress during introductions. Given their sensitivity to alarm substances, the presence of injured goldfish may induce stress and unusual behaviour in others, such as food avoidance, tight schooling, or hiding. Anecdotal evidence suggests that some fish may show signs of aggression to injured fish, and fish may need short-term isolation during treatment.

Goldfish may be kept with certain other species of fish, provided such fish do not out-compete or attack the goldfish. Goldfish may perceive other pets as predators, such as cats, dogs, and terrapins. In particular, outdoor ponds should be protected to prevent predation by birds.

23.2.4 Human Interactions

Direct handling and disturbances should be minimised to avoid injury. Anecdotal evidence from owners suggests that goldfish can distinguish between different members of the human family based on vision alone. However, it seems unlikely that goldfish form particular affiliative relationships with humans or enjoy the interactions with humans in general, beyond any response to feeding. Their learning ability also allows goldfish to be trained to perform particular actions (Mackintosh et al. 1971; Breuning et al. 1981). Any such training should be carried out in ways that minimise disturbances to the goldfish, use rewards rather than punishment, and that aim at providing enrichment for the animals' benefit, rather than teaching tricks for humans'. At the same time, their learning ability may also be expected to increase fear responses following previous unpleasant interactions, such as handling or environmental disturbance.

23.2.5 Health

Goldfish can be affected by a variety of health problems (Table 23.2), including bacterial infections (e.g. fin-rot and ulcers; Figure 23.2), fungus outbreaks (e.g. fungal growths on the skin), and parasitic infestations (e.g. whitespot disease [*Ichthyophthirius multifiliis*]). They may also suffer from noninfectious diseases such as skin tumours (e.g. benign fibromas; Figure 23.3). Many common health problems are linked to poor water conditions, such as skin or gill damage arising from high levels of ammonia in the water, which generally indicate a lack of water changes or inadequate filtration. New fish should be quarantined to reduce the risk of introducing infectious diseases. The feeding of wild-harvested live foods (e.g. pond collected water fleas and aquatic worms)

Table 23.2 Selected health problems in goldfish.

Condition			Welfare effects
Infectious or parasitic	Bacteria	*Aeromonas* species	Skin ulcers; osmoregulatory stress; secondary infections.
		Flavobacterium columnare	Fin rot
	Fungi (water moulds)	*Saprolegnia* spp.	Mild to severe skin damage.
	Internal Parasites	Gut nematodes and gut cestodes	Mild to moderate debilitation; emaciation; lethargy
		Ichthyophthirius (whitespot disease)	Skin, fin and gill damage; respiratory stress; secondary infections
	External Parasites	Various ecto-parasitic protozoa (e.g. *Chilodonella*; *Ichthyobodo*; *Trichodina*)	Skin and fin damage; gill damage and respiratory stress (caused by certain species of parasitic protozoa); secondary infections
		Argulus (fish-louse)	Skin damage; anaemia; secondary infections
Water quality problems		Low dissolved oxygen (e.g. as a result of overcrowding; inadequate aeration; water pollution)	Respiratory stress
		Chlorine poisoning (caused by failure to dechlorinate tapwater)	Gill damage; respiratory stress.
		Ammonia poisoning	Gill damage; respiratory stress
		Nitrite poisoning	Respiratory stress.
Tumours		Skin fibroma	Generally benign
Buoyancy problems		Positive buoyancy (fish floats at surface); negative (fish sinks)	Distress; difficulty in obtaining food; drying of air-exposed skin in cases of positive buoyancy
Traumatic		Physical handling by owner	Distress; skin damage; skin infection
		Aerial emersion	Distress; skin and gill damage; respiratory stress

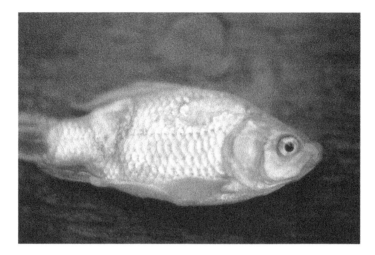

Figure 23.2   Goldfish with skin ulceration (probably as a result of *Aeromonas* bacteria) (*Source:* courtesy Peter Burgess).

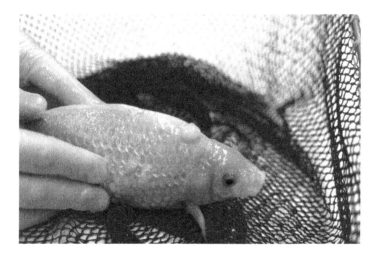

Figure 23.3   Goldfish with skin fibroma (*Source:* courtesy Peter Burgess and Stan McMahon).

is inadvisable because these wild prey organisms can transmit certain diseases (e.g. parasitic worms) to goldfish. Owners should also regularly check their goldfish closely for signs of diseases, such as the 1-mm small white spots on body and fins that suggest *Ichthyophthirius*.

Treatments depend on the disease. Some conditions require a water change or a salt bath (e.g. fungal diseases may respond to salt concentrations of about 2–3 g/L). Others may require commercial disease remedies added to the water, following the manufacturer's instructions. More serious diseases, such as internal bacterial infections, require antibiotics. Many treatments have a low safety margin and can be highly stressful to fish if the recommended dosage is exceeded (e.g. formalin and malachite green). Many treatments can also kill the beneficial waste-removing bacteria in the filter and gravel, with potentially catastrophic effects on water quality (e.g. some antibiotics and methylene blue). For some diseases it may be necessary to medicate the whole aquarium or pond, particularly for diseases caused by organisms that have free-living stages in the water (e.g. whitespot parasites). In other cases, the affected fish may be treated in isolation.

Some of the more extreme phenotypes, such as bubble eye or fancy fins, have implications for welfare and health (Table 23.3). The bubbles under the eye are prone to rupture if sharp objects are in the aquarium, with likely subsequent pain and risks of infection. Varieties with very fancy fins (e.g. butterfly tail) can have issues with sustained swimming. Certain fancy strains of goldfish are particularly prone to buoyancy problems due to swim bladder disorders and may float at the surface or sink to the bottom. Although the average life span is around 10–15 years, some fancy strains tend to live for shorter periods. Owners should obtain goldfish with less extreme body shapes which have been bred to be healthy pets.

23.2.6 Euthanasia

Acceptable methods of the euthanasia of goldfish are listed in Table 23.4. The most efficient method should involve two stages, the first to cause unconsciousness and the second to ensure death. Sedation may also be valuable for some methods. The first stage should involve either head trauma or an anaesthetic overdose by immersion or in larger goldfish, injection. Immersion can be slower and goldfish should be left in the anaesthetic for at least 10 minutes after cessation of opercular movement (Neiffer and Stamper 2009). Some immersion anaesthetics (e.g. MS-222) are highly acidic and will need to be buffered to a neutral pH. In any case, once all gill movements have ceased for a prolonged period, the second stage of euthanasia is to destroy the brain by pithing or exsanguination (blood loss). The owner needs to be competent and legally permitted

Table 23.3 Welfare issues associated with the breeding of some fancy goldfish strains.

Strain	Trait selected for	Impact on the fish
Bubble eye	Fluid-filled sacs under the eyes	Impaired vision and behaviour; injury; infection; pain
Celestial eye	Abnormal eye position where eyes point upwards to the 'stars'	Retinal degeneration and blindness; impaired behaviour
	Absence of dorsal fin	Movement affected; lack of stability and agility
Eggfish Pompom	Absence of dorsal fin	Movement impaired; lack of stability and agility
Lionhead Ranchu	Excessive facial tissue	Restricted vision and breathing; infection; pain
Lionchu	Absence of dorsal fin	Movement affected; lack of stability and agility

Source: UFAW (2013) www.ufaw.org.uk/fish.php.

Table 23.4 Methods of euthanasia for goldfish kept as companion animals (followed by a method to ensure death such as brain destruction or blood loss).

Method	Restraint required	Welfare risks
Anaesthetic overdose, immersion	Containment in limited water volume	Irritation of product (varies with type of anaesthetic drug used)
Anaesthetic overdose, injection into a vein	Handling for immobility Sedation advised	Must be done by a veterinarian to ensure efficiency of injection. Involves handling and emersion which will cause stress
Concussion	Handling for immobility in air Sedation advised	Emersion Possibility of recovery of consciousness if concussion not done properly or pithing or exsanguination does not take place immediately after concussion

to use the appropriate method. Flushing goldfish down the toilet may lead to a slow death or spread diseases into the natural waterways and is unacceptable.

23.3 Signs of Welfare Problems

23.3.1 Pathophysiological signs

Decreased survival or growth can generally indicate some sort of welfare issue, such as poor water conditions or insufficient space. Fast initial growth is normal but once fish reach maturity, growth should slow considerably. Signs of disease include an increased respiratory rate (i.e. faster gill beats per minute) and changes to the fins, skin, eyes, and overall body shape. A change in colour can be indicative of stress or disease; however, goldfish naturally alter in colour over time and may become very pale, even silver, as they reach old age. 'Dropsy', in which the body becomes distended with fluid and the scales stick out to give a pine-cone appearance to the body contour is normally a sign of poor osmotic balance which is commonly caused by bacterial infections.

23.3.2 Behavioural Signs

Reduced levels of activity, listlessness, a reduction of feeding behavior, or unusual levels of hiding are all signs that can indicate a problem such as poor water quality. A loss of buoyancy is indicative of swim bladder or diet-related issues or a variety of causes (Wildgoose 2007). Fish gulping at the surface may be normal feeding behaviour or a sign of poor water quality. Goldfish show anomalous rubbing behaviour when experimentally injected with acetic acid that is reduced by the analgesic drug morphine (Newby et al. 2009). This suggests that goldfish are capable of feeling discomfort and pain, which is alleviated through the administration of analgesics. Rubbing is also seen in the case of external pathogens which may be an attempt to remove them or may be a sign of itchiness of the infection. Another carp species, koi, exhibit reduced feeding, decreased activity and spend more time lower in the water column post-surgery (Harms et al. 2005; Baker et al. 2013).

23.4 Action Plan for Improving Goldfish Welfare Worldwide

It is important to raise public awareness that goldfish have feelings, perceive pain, and so on. – such that they should be treated with the same care and respect as any other pet. Owners should be made aware that goldfish are not unintelligent or inactive, so that they provide adequate environments to meet their genuine needs. This is a cycle: keeping goldfish in more suitable and enriched environments may mean owners see a wider range of their potential behaviour. Goldfish should not be seen as disposable ornaments but as individual pets. Goldfish should only be kept by owners who have the commitment and knowledge to look after them for their entire lifetime, which is potentially for several decades. This means goldfish should not be given as prizes (e.g. at fairs) or as mascots as in the Chinese tradition of giving goldfish to wish good fortune.

Governments should set out minimum care standards specifically for pet goldfish, particularly with reference to minimal size of tank and isolating goldfish. In the absence of such legislation, responsible pet shops should ensure they only sell aquaria that can properly accommodate the fish as adults and sell goldfish in pairs or possibly as established groups dependent upon the owner's tank size. Greater research is also needed into the requirements of pet goldfish, for example, in terms of precise space requirements, environmental enrichment, and social housing. Research is also needed to evaluate the welfare issues associated with fancy forms that have impairments such as eye deformities and distorted backbones. When particular strains are shown to have health problems, they should not be bred or sold. Education of purchasers and breeders about the welfare impact of these genetic conditions is important and there may even be a case for regulation, although dog breed-specific legislation has proven problematic. More generally, veterinary surgeons need to have a greater involvement in the care of goldfish. Owners may be reluctant to obtain veterinary advice because of the difficulty of moving goldfish, their low financial value, high veterinary care costs, and the ease of obtaining nonprescription medicines. Veterinary surgeons need appropriate training so that they can provide sound advice.

Bibliography

Angeler, D.G., Álvarez-Cobelas, M., Sánchez-Carrillo, S., and Rodrigo, M.A. (2002). Assessment of exotic fish impacts on water quality and zooplankton in a degraded semi-arid floodplain wetland. *Aquatic Sciences* 64: 76–86.

Baker, T.R., Baker, B.B., Johnson, S.M., and Sladky, K.K. (2013). Comparative analgesic efficacy of morphine sulfate and butorphanol tartrate in koi (*Cyprinus carpio*) undergoing unilateral gonadectomy. *Journal of the American Veterinary Medical Association* 243 (6): 882–890.

Brewster, B. and Fletcher, N. (2004). *Keeping Goldfish*. England: Interpet publishing.

Breuning, S.E., Ferguson, D.G., and Poling, A.D. (1981). Second-order schedule effects with goldfish: a comparison of brief-stimulus, chained, and tandem schedules. *Pyschological Record* 31: 437–445.

Brown, C. and Laland, K.N. (2011). Social learning in fishes. In: *Fish cognition and behavior* (ed. C. Brown and K.N. Laland), 186–202. UK, Blackwell: Chichester.

Brown, C., Laland, K., and Krause, J. (2006). *Fish Cognition and Behaviour*. Oxford: Blackwell Publishing.

Brown, C., Laland, K., and Krause, J. (2011). *Fish Cognition and Behaviour*, 2e. Oxford: Wiley-Blackwell Publishing.

Dunlop, R., Millsopp, S., and Laming, P. (2006). Avoidance learning in goldfish (Carassius auratus) and trout (Oncorhynchus mykiss) and implications for pain perception. *Applied Animal Behaviour Science* 97: 255–271.

Fay, R.R. and Popper, A.N. (1974). Acoustic stimulation of the goldfish (*Carassius auratus*). *The Journal of Experimental Biology* 61: 243–260.

Gee, P., Stephenson, D., and Wright, D.E. (1994). Temporal discrimination in operant feeding in goldfish (Carassuis auratus). *Journal of the Experimental Analysis of Behaviour* 62: 1–13.

Harms, C.A., Lewbart, G.A., Swanson, C.R. et al. (2005). Behavioral and clinical pathology changes in Koi carp (*Cyprinus carpio*) subjected to anesthesia and surgery with and without intra-operative analgesics. *Comparative Medicine* 55 (3): 221–226.

IUCN (2015). IUCN Red List of threatened species. Available at http://www.iucnredlist.org/photos/2015. Accessed 14 June 2018.

Komiyama, T., Kobayashi, H., Tateno, Y. et al. (2009). An evolutionary origin and selection process of goldfish. *Gene* 430: 5–11.

Laudien, H., Freyer, J., Erb, R., and Denxer, D. (1986). Influence of isolation stress and inhibited protein biosynthesis on learning and memory in goldfish. *Physiology and Behavior* 38 (5): 621–628.

Mackintosh, N.J., Lord, J., and Little, L. (1971). Visual and spatial probability learning in pigeons and goldfish. *Psychonomic Science* 24: 221–223.

Mednick, A.S. and Springer, A.D. (1988). Asymmetric distribution of retinal ganglion cells in goldfish. *Journal of Comparative Neurology* 268: 49–59.

Neumeyer, C. (1992). Tetrachromatic color vision in goldfish: evidence from color mixture experiments. *Journal of Comparative Physiology A* 171 (5): 639–649.

Newby, N.C., Wilkie, M.P., and Stevens, E.D. (2009). Morphine uptake, disposition and analgesic efficacy in the common goldfish (*Carassiusauratus*). *Canadian Journal of Zoology* 87: 388–399.

Neiffer, D.L. and Stamper, A. (2009). Fish sedation, anesthesia, analgesia, and euthanasia: considerations, methods, and types of drugs. *ILAR Journal* 50: 343–360.

Orme, F.W. (1991). *Fancy Goldfish Culture*, 2e. Concord, MA, USA: Paul & Co Pub Consortium.

Pinto, L., Chandrasena, N., Pera, J. et al. (2005). Managing invasive carp (*Cyprinus carpio* L.) for habitat enhancement in at Botany Bay, Australia. *Aquatic Conservation: Marine and Freshwater Ecosystems* 15: 447–462.

Pitcher, T.J. and Magurran, A.E. (1983). Shoal size, patch profitability and information exchange in foraging goldfish. *Animal Behaviour* 31: 546–555.

Pitcher, T.J., Magurran, A.E., and Winfield, I. (1982). Fish in larger shoals find food faster. *Behavioral Ecology and Sociobiology* 10: 149–151.

Richardson, M.J., Whoriskey, F.G., and Roy, L.H. (1995). Turbidity generation and biological impacts of an exotic fish *Carassius auratus*, introduced into shallow seasonally anoxic ponds. *Journal of Fish Biology* 47: 576–585.

Rodríguez, F., Broglio, C., Durán, E. et al. (2006). Neural Mechanisms of Learning in Teleost Fish. In: *Fish Cognition and Behavior* (ed. C. Brown, K. Laland and J. Krause), 243–277. Oxford, UK: Wiley.

Sisler, S.P. and Sorensen, P.W. (2008). Common carp and goldfish discern conspecific identity using chemical cues. *Behaviour* 145: 1409–1425.

Shinozuka, K., Ono, H., and Watanabe, S. (2013). Reinforcing and discriminative stimulus properties of music in goldfish. *Behavioural Processes* 99: 26–33.

Smith, A. and Gray, H. (2011). Goldfish in a tank: the effect of substrate on foraging behaviour in aquarium fish. *Animal Welfare* 20: 311–319.

Smith, M.E., Kane, A.S., and Popper, A.N. (2004). Noise-induced stress response and hearing loss in goldfish (*Carassius auratus*). *Journal of Experimental Biology* 207: 427–435.

UFAW. (2013). Genetic Welfare Problems of Companion Animals. Available at https://www.ufaw.org.uk/fish/fish. Accessed 8 November 2015

Warburton, K. (1990). The use of local landmarks by foragin goldfish. *Animal Behaviour* 40: 500–505.

Wildgoose, W.H. (2007). Buoyancy disorders of ornamental fish: a review of cases seen in veterinary practice. *Fish Veterinary Journal* 9: 22–37.

Wyzisk, K. and Neumeyer, C. (2007). Perception of illusory surfaces and contours in goldfish. *Visual Neuroscience* 24: 291–298.

Zhen, L.i. (1988). *Chinese Goldfish*, vol. 1988, 13–26. Beijing, China: Foreign Language Press.

Zhao, X. and Chivers, D.P. (2005). Response of juvenile goldfish (Carassius auratus) to chemical alarm cues: relationship between response intensity, response duration and the level of predation risk. In: *Chemical Signals in Vertebrates*, vol. 10 (ed. R.T. Mason, M.P. LeMaster and D. Müller-Schwartze), 334–341. Berlin Heidelberg New York: Springer.

Index

adjunctive pecking, 367
adrenal gland, 135, 173, 197, 210, 212
adrenaline, 458–9
Aeromonas, 451–2, 472–3
aestivation, 427
Agapornis fischeri see lovebird
Aleutian disease *see* parvovirus
Alligator mississippiensis see American
    alligator
Alopecia, 70, 133, 136, 138–9
alpaca, 250, 258
American alligator, 372
Amphiprion ocellaris see clownfish
amyloidosis, 211, 328
anaemia, 65, 93–4, 98, 133, 135, 276,
    305, 327, 363, 418, 444, 458, 472
Anodorhynchus hyacinthinus see
    macaw
Ara ararauna see macaw
Ara macao see macaw
Ara rubrogenys see macaw
Aratinga jandaya see conure
Aratinga solstitialis see conure
argon, 242
Argulus, 472

Artemisia, 218
Aspergillus, 21, 211, 301–2, 305, 327, 363
Astronotus ocellatus see oscar
Atoxoplasma, 326–7
Aviopoxvirus, 363

ball python, 372–4, 380, 382
barbering, 150, 156, 238–9, 244
Bassariscus astutus see ringtail cat
Bengalese finch, 294, 297, 303, 309
Betta splendens, 400–1, 449 *see* Siamese
    fighting fish
binkying, 177–8
blenny, 441
bobcat, 40
Bordetella bronchiseptica, 194–5
Brachylophus vitiensis see Fijian crested
    iguana
brumation, 372–3, 396, 399–400
budgerigar, 295, 338–40, 344–5, 347
Burkholderia mallei see glanders
burn, 376, 406–7, 414, 418, 430, 435

Cacatua alba see cockatoo
Cacatua galerita see cockatoo

Companion Animal Care and Welfare: The UFAW Companion Animal Handbook,
First Edition. Edited by James Yeates.
© 2019 Universities Federation for Animal Welfare. Published 2019 by John Wiley & Sons Ltd.

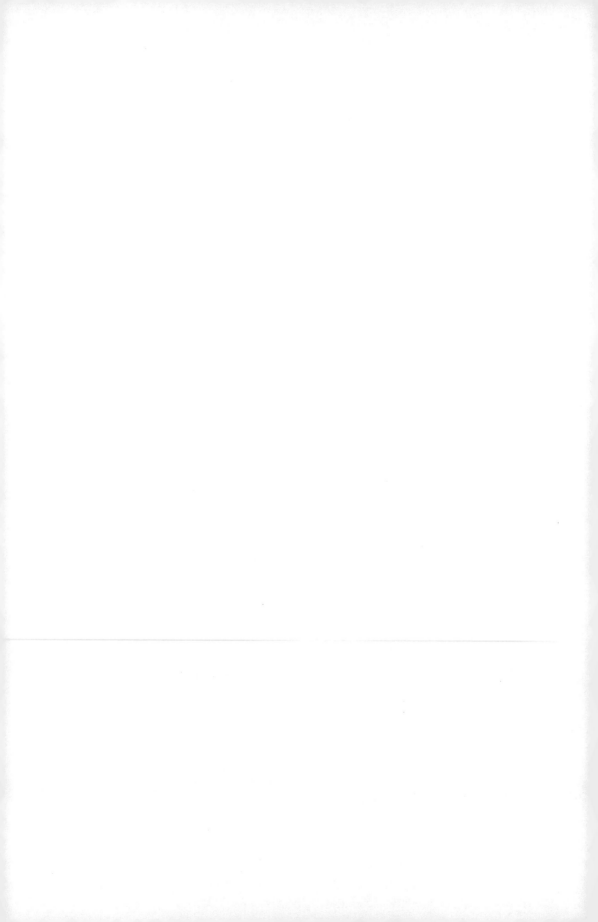

Printed and bound by CPI Group (UK) Ltd, Croydon, CR0 4YY

09/06/2025

14686003-0001